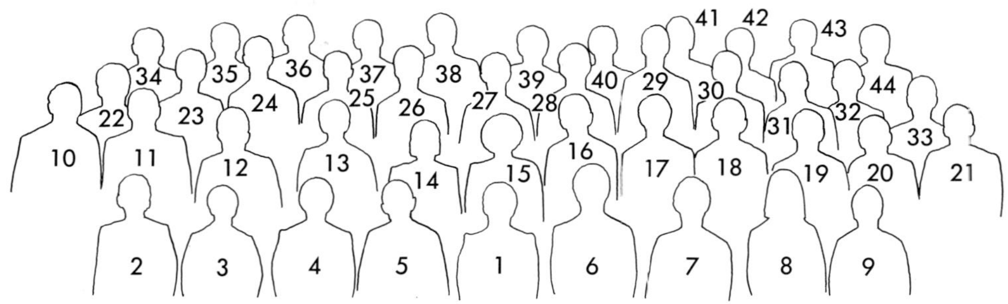


PARTICIPANTS

1. H.I.H. Princess Takamatsu
2. Mrs. Anders
3. Mrs. Talalay
4. Mrs. Ernster
5. Dr. Ernster
6. Dr. Gelboin
7. Mrs. Gelboin
8. Dr. Perera
9. Mrs. Tannenbaum
10. Dr. Adamson
11. Dr. Anders
12. Dr. Talalay
13. Dr. Board
14. Mrs. Board
15. Mrs. Monnervik
16. Dr. Monnervik
17. Dr. Weber
18. Dr. Estabrook
19. Dr. Tannenbaum
20. Dr. Kato
21. Dr. Burchell
22. Dr. Hashimoto
23. Dr. Muramatsu
24. Dr. Gonzalez
25. Dr. Guengerich
26. Dr. Simpson
27. Dr. Randerath
28. Dr. Gustafsson
29. Dr. Kadlubar
30. Dr. Marnett
31. Dr. Nishi
32. Dr. Fujii
33. Dr. Orrenius
34. Dr. Sugimura
35. Dr. Sugano
36. Dr. Toyoshima
37. Dr. Ito
38. Dr. Kawajiri
39. Dr. Wada
40. Dr. Tsuruo
41. Dr. Yamazoe
42. Dr. Takayama
43. Dr. Nishimura
44. Dr. Esumi

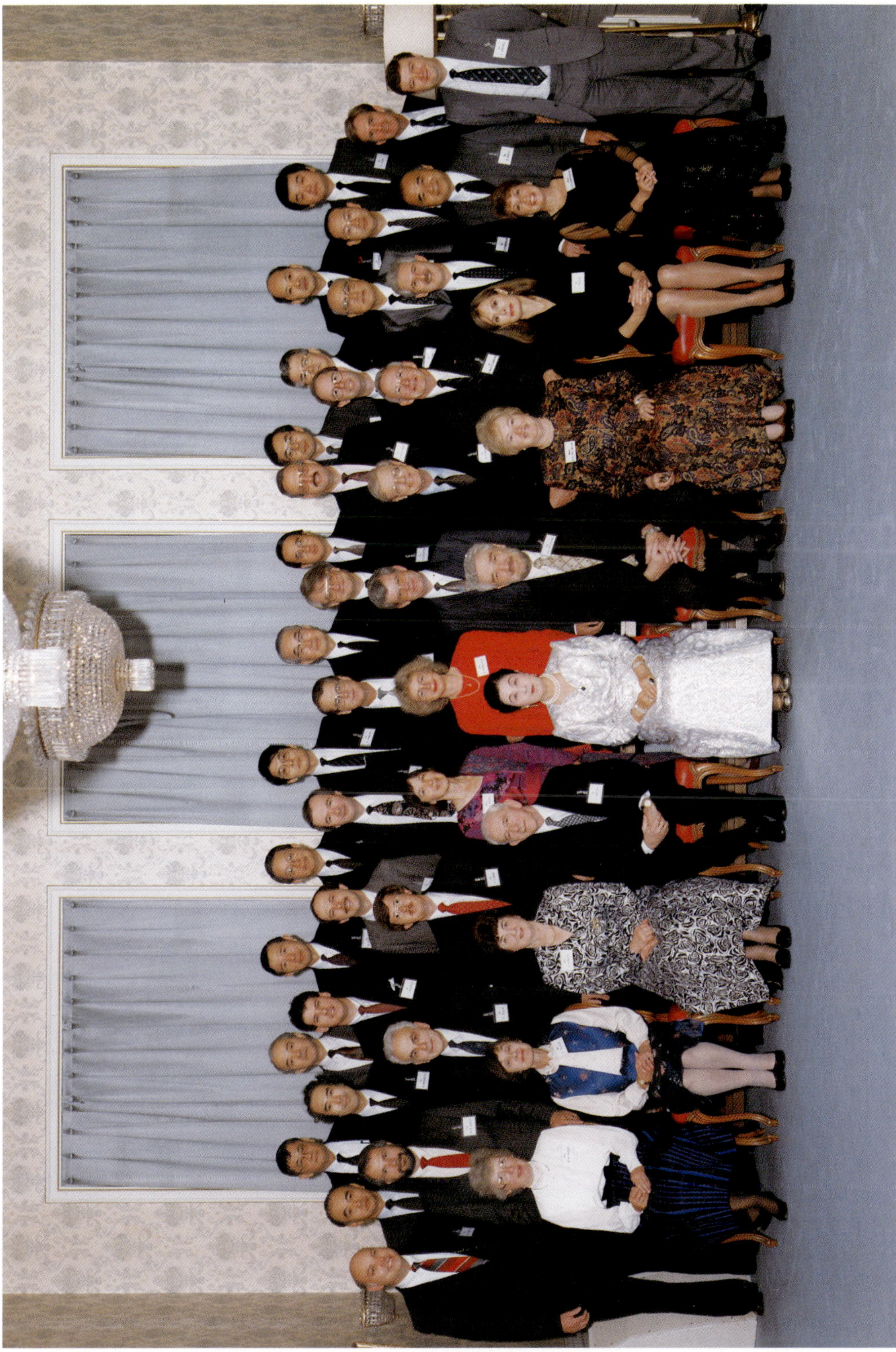

XENOBIOTICS AND CANCER

Proceedings of the 21st International Symposium of
The Princess Takamatsu Cancer Research Fund, Tokyo, 1990

# XENOBIOTICS AND CANCER

## Implications for Chemical Carcinogenesis and Cancer Chemotherapy

Edited by
LARS ERNSTER, HIROYASU ESUMI,
YOSHIAKI FUJII, HARRY V. GELBOIN,
RYUICHI KATO, and TAKASHI SUGIMURA

JAPAN SCIENTIFIC SOCIETIES PRESS, Tokyo
TAYLOR & FRANCIS LTD., London and Bristol

Published jointly by:
JAPAN SCIENTIFIC SOCIETIES PRESS
Hongo 6-2-10, Bunkyo-ku, Tokyo 113, Japan
ISBN 4-7622-4667-0
and
TAYLOR & FRANCIS LTD.
4 John Street, London WCIN 2 ET, UK
1900 Frost Road, Suite 101, Bristol, Pennsylvania 19007, U.S.A.
ISBN 0-74840-037-0

Distributed in all areas outside Japan and Asia between Pakistan and Korea by TAYLOR & FRANCIS LTD.

Printed in Japan

## Princess Takamatsu Cancer Research Fund

## Organizing Committee of the 21st International Symposium

Lars ERNSTER
Department of Biochemistry, Arrhenius Laboratories, University of Stockholm, S-106 91 Stockholm, Sweden

Hiroyasu ESUMI
Biochemistry Division, National Cancer Center Research Institute, Tokyo 104, Japan

Yoshiaki FUJII
Department of Chemistry, Faculty of Science, Tohoku University, Sendai 980, Japan

Harry V. GELBOIN
Laboratory of Molecular Carcinogenesis, National Cancer Institute, National Institutes of Health, Bethesda, Maryland 20892, U.S.A.

Ryuichi KATO
Department of Pharmacology, School of Medicine, Keio University, Tokyo 160, Japan

Takashi SUGIMURA
National Cancer Center, Tokyo 104, Japan

## Preface

Recent developments in cancer research have revealed that there are divergent causes of the multiple genetic alterations found in human cancers. The presence of many potential carcinogens in the everyday environment is represented by newly identified carcinogens in cooked food. Carcinogens are one class of xenobiotics to which human beings are continuously exposed; therefore, not only the amount of carcinogenic xenobiotics but also human response to those xenobiotics are important determinants of human carcinogenesis. Cancer chemotherapeutic agents are also xenobiotics, and the response of cancer cells to chemotherapeutic agents sometimes adversely results in a cancer which is drug resistant. Better primary cancer prevention and better cures for this disease thus depend strongly on a deeper understanding of biological responses to xenobiotics.

A meeting covering recent advances in chemical carcinogenesis and cancer chemotherapy was appropriate because molecular findings in those two areas have greatly progressed during the past decade. The 21st International Symposium of the Princess Takamatsu Cancer Research Fund, which was held November 13 to 15, 1990, was entitled "Xenobiotics and Cancer" and merged these two areas. Scientists who had followed separate paths shared their common interests and focused their attention on one subject, namely, better control of cancer. The outcome of the Symposium was quite fruitful and is presented in this Proceedings.

Lars ERNSTER
Hiroyasu ESUMI
Yoshiaki FUJII
Harry V. GELBOIN
Ryuichi KATO
Takashi SUGIMURA

Contents

## Xenobiotics and Gene Regulation



## Drug Resistance

## Xenobiotics as a Cause of Human Cancer



## Biomonitoring

## Contributors


| | |
|---|---|
| Richard H. ADAMSON | Division of Cancer Etiology, National Cancer Institute, National Institutes of Health, Bethesda, Maryland 20892, U.S.A. |
| Bruce N. AMES | Division of Biochemistry and Molecular Biology, University of California, Berkeley, California 94720, U.S.A. |
| M. W. ANDERS | Department of Pharmacology, School of Medicine and Dentistry, University of Rochester, Rochester, New York 14642, U.S.A. |
| Irwin M. ARIAS | Department of Physiology, Tufts University School of Medicine, Boston, Massachusetts 02111, U.S.A. |
| Philip BOARD | Division of Clinical Sciences, Human Genetics Group, John Curtin School of Medical Research, Australian National University, Canberra ACT 2601, Australia |
| Brian BURCHELL | Department of Biochemical Medicine, Ninewells Hospital and Medical School, University of Dundee, Dundee DD1 9SY, U.K. |
| Lars ERNSTER | Department of Biochemistry, Arrhenius Laboratories, University of Stockholm, S-106 91 Stockholm, Sweden |
| Ronald W. ESTABROOK | Department of Biochemistry, The University of Texas, Southwestern Medical Center, Dallas, Texas 75235, U.S.A. |
| Hiroyasu ESUMI | Biochemistry Division, National Cancer Center Research Institute, Chuo-ku, Tokyo 104, Japan |
| Yoshiaki FUJII | Department of Chemistry, Faculty of Science, Tohoku University, Aoba-ku, Sendai 980, Japan |
| Harry V. GELBOIN | Laboratory of Molecular Carcinogenesis, National Cancer Institute, National Institutes of Health, Bethesda, Maryland 20892, U.S.A. |
| Frank J. GONZALEZ | Laboratory of Molecular Carcinogenesis, National Can- |

| | |
|---|---|
| | cer Institute, National Institutes of Health, Bethesda, Maryland 20892, U.S.A. |
| F. Peter GUENGERICH | Department of Biochemistry and Center in Molecular Toxicology, Vanderbilt University School of Medicine, Nashville, Tennessee 37232–0146, U.S.A. |
| Jan-Åke GUSTAFSSON | Department of Medical Nutrition, Karolinska Institute, Huddinge University Hospital F60, Novum, S-141 86 Huddinge, Sweden |
| Yoshiyuki HASHIMOTO | Department of Hygienic Chemistry, Faculty of Pharmaceutical Sciences, Tohoku University, Aoba-ku, Sendai 980, Japan |
| Fred F. KADLUBAR | Public Health Service, Food and Drug Administration, The National Center for Toxicological Research, Jefferson, Arkansas 72079, U.S.A. |
| Ryuichi KATO | Department of Pharmacology, School of Medicine, Keio University, Shinjuku-ku, Tokyo 160, Japan |
| Kaname KAWAJIRI | Departments of Biochemistry and Epidemiology, Saitama Cancer Center Research Institute, Ina-machi, Kitaadachi-gun, Saitama 362, Japan |
| Bengt MANNERVIK | Department of Biochemistry, Biomedical Center, University of Uppsala, 751 23 Uppsala, Sweden |
| Lawrence J. MARNETT | A. B. Hancock Memorial Laboratory for Cancer Research, Departments of Biochemistry and Chemistry, Center in Molecular Toxicology, Vanderbilt University School of Medicine, Nashville, Tennessee 37232 U.S.A. |
| Masami MURAMATSU | Department of Biochemistry, University of Tokyo, Faculty of Medicine, Bunkyo-ku, Tokyo 113, Japan |
| Sten ORRENIUS | Department of Toxicology, Karolinska Institute, S-104 01 Stockholm, Sweden |
| Frederica P. PERERA | Division of Environmental Sciences, Columbia University, School of Public Health, New York, New York 10032, U.S.A. |
| Kurt RANDERATH | Division of Toxicology, Department of Pharmacology, Baylor College of Medicine, Houston, Texas 77030, U.S.A. |
| Evan R. SIMPSON | Cecil H. and Ida Green Center for Reproductive Biology Sciences, Departments of Obstetrics-Gynecology and Biochemistry, The University of Texas Southwestern Medical Center, Dallas, Texas 75235-9051, U.S.A. |
| Takashi SUGIMURA | National Cancer Center, Chuo-ku, Tokyo 104, Japan |
| Paul TALALAY | Department of Pharmacology and Molecular Sciences, The Johns Hopkins University School of Medicine, Baltimore, Maryland 21205, U.S.A. |
| Steven R. TANNENBAUM | Department of Chemistry, Division of Toxicology, Massachusetts Institute of Technology, Cambridge, Massachusetts 02139, U.S.A. |

| | |
|---|---|
| Takashi TSURUO | Institute of Applied Microbiology, University of Tokyo, Bunkyo-ku, Tokyo 113, Japan |
| Wendell W. WEBER | Department of Pharmacology, University of Michigan, Ann Arbor, Michigan 48109-0626, U.S.A. |
| Yasushi YAMAZOE | Department of Pharmacology, School of Medicine, Keio University, Shinjuku-ku, Tokyo 160, Japan |

# Opening Address

H.I.H. Princess Kikuko Takamatsu

It is my delightful duty to deliver the opening address at the 21st International Symposium of the Princess Takamatsu Cancer Research Fund. I extend my sincere welcome to all of you, especially to those of you from abroad who have traveled far to be with us here.

Our Foundation, the Princess Takamatsu Cancer Research Fund, initiated its activity about 20 years ago. During these two decades, many remarkable achievements were done in cancer research. A rapid progress in understanding fundamental mechanism of development of cancer also seems to promise us cancer prevention and better cure of cancer eventually. However, unfortunately, still many people are suffering from cancer and dying of cancer.

The title of this year's Symposium is, "Xenobiotics and Cancer: Implications for Chemical Carcinogenesis and Cancer Chemotherapy". I hope that the presentations and discussion at this symposium will contribute to a better understanding of those mechanisms and will be a big milestone in both the prevention of cancer and increasing cured numbers of cancer patients.

I would like to express my sincere thanks to Dr. Harry V. Gelboin of The National Cancer Institute in the United States, and to Dr. Lars Ernster of the University of Stockholm in Sweden for their valuable assistance as members of the Organizing Committee of this Symposium.

Now, I declare open the 21st International Symposium of the Princess Takamatsu Cancer Research Fund. I am confident that the Symposium will be successful.

Dr. Lars ERNSTER

Your Imperial Highness:

On behalf of Dr. Gelboin and myself, and of all participants of this Symposium, it is my great honor and privilege to express our warm thanks for your opening address and for the gracious hospitality extended to us on this occasion. We feel the deepest compassion with you on the loss of three members of your family, your mother, your husband Prince Takamatsu and, last year, His Majesty Emperor Showa, because of cancer.

We have come here from distant continents, America, Australia, and Europe, to discuss with our Japanese colleagues the latest developments in cancer research, in particular the role of xenobiotics—*i.e.*, foreign compounds—in chemical carcinogenesis and chemotherapy.

Cancer research has deep roots in Japan. It was here that the first observations were made, in the early 1910s, indicating that cancer can be transmitted by a cell-free tumor extract. Shortly thereafter, another group of Japanese scientists demonstrated that coal tar can cause skin cancer. These early observations were forerunners of the discovery of oncogenic viruses and of chemical carcinogens. The latter were subsequently identified as polycyclic hydrocarbons, which are the carcinogenic components of cigarette smoke. Another category of chemical carcinogens, consisting of azodyes, were discovered in Japan in the 1930s, and yet another group of compounds, nitroquinoline oxides, in the 1950s. The latter discovery opened the way, through research initiated in the 1970s at the National Cancer Center in Tokyo, to the identification of a number of heterocyclic amines as powerful carcinogens occurring in cooked food.

Today we know that many components of our natural environment, including our daily food, contain chemicals that are carcinogenic or can be converted to carcinogens by our own enzymes. Several of these enzymes—oxygenases, and in particular the family of enzymes called cytochrome P450—act by inserting molecular oxygen into these compounds; and, again, Japanese scientists have made fundamental contributions to identifying and characterizing these enzymes.

Much of the program of the present Symposium will deal with current knowledge about the metabolic activation of chemical carcinogens by way of these enzymes, as well as the available information concerning physiological and pharmacological defense mechanisms against their action. Recent advances in the fields of biochemistry and molecular biology have led to a most important development in our understanding of the chemical background of these processes and their implications for the genetic, immunological, pharmacological and clinical aspects of cancer research. It is thus highly appropriate to devote this 21st International Symposium of the Princess Takamatsu Cancer Research Fund to a discussion of these developments.

In closing, I would like to thank you again, Your Imperial Highness, for your generous support and encouragement, and to convey to you our warmest congratulations on the occasion of this 20th anniversary of these Symposia, with our best wishes for the continued successful activity of your Cancer Research Fund for the benefit of mankind.

# LECTURES

XENOBIOTICS AND CANCER, L. ERNSTER ET AL. (EDS.),
JAPAN SCI. SOC. PRESS, TOKYO/TAYLOR & FRANCIS LTD., LONDON, pp. 3–16, 1991

KEYNOTE LECTURE

# Mapping of Cytochrome P-450 Distribution and Function with Monoclonal Antibodies and cDNA Expression

H. V. GELBOIN,*[1] S. S. PARK,*[1] T. AOYAMA,*[1] T. FUJINO,*[1] C. L. CRESPI,*[2] and F. J. GONZALEZ*[1]

*Laboratory of Molecular Carcinogenesis, National Cancer Institute, Bethesda, Maryland 20892*[1] and Gentest Corporation, Woburn, Massachusetts 01801, U.S.A.*[2]*

*Abstract:* A large number of cytochrome P-450 forms are responsible for the metabolism and detoxification as well as the mutagenic and carcinogenic activation of numerous classes of xenobiotics. These include drugs and carcinogens and other environmental chemicals. The cytochrome P-450 enzymes are also responsible for the metabolism of endogenous substrates including fatty acids, prostaglandins and all classes of steroids. In order to fully understand the role of each P-450 in a specific metabolic reaction, it is necessary to know both the substrate and product specificity of each P-450 as well as the contribution of the individual P-450 to the total metabolism catalyzed in a tissue containing many P-450 forms. Our laboratory has cloned and expressed, with various vectors, a number of rodent and human P-450s. This technique has enabled us to determine the specificity of individual forms of P-450 for certain substrate utilization and product formation, as well as for the metabolic activation of promutagens to their mutagenic forms. The latter has been measured with the Ames mutagen detection system coupled to mutagen activation by vaccinia expressed single P-450s. Mutagenesis and DNA binding have also been measured with a human cell line stably expressing a single P-450. The former approach determines the specificity of single P-450s in cell lysates and the latter determines P-450 specificity in the living cell. In a complementary approach, we have prepared, characterized and utilized inhibitory monoclonal antibodies to six epitope specific classes of P-450. The inhibitory antibodies block the enzymatic activities of specific P-450s in tissue preparations and thus define the contribution of the single P-450 to the total reaction. This approach can be used to measure many P-450 functions, *e.g.*, substrate utilization, product formation, stereochemical metabolism, mutagen activation, drug toxicity, and DNA binding. The two complementary techniques of cDNA expression and immunoinhibition have been used to examine a number of different classes of compounds with respect to their metabolism and mutagen activation. These approaches may eventually yield an atlas of individual P-450 function and their contribution to the total metabolism of xenobiotics and endobiotics.

The cytochrome P-450s are the primary enzyme interface between xenobiotics and all higher organisms as well as many lower organisms. Thus, P-450s are the key enzymes responsible for the initial metabolism of a variety of xenobiotics including most drugs, carcinogens, and pesticides. The P-450s also metabolize numerous classes of endobiotics such as steroids, fatty acids, and prostaglandins. P-450 catalyzed metabolism may be either beneficial or harmful leading to detoxified products that are conjugated and safely excreted or to activated metabolites that may be toxic, mutagenic, or carcinogenic (*1*, *2*). There are thirteen known human P-450 families or subfamilies, each containing numerous subtypes and more than a hundred different P-450s from various species have been characterized (*3*, *4*). P-450 enzyme multiplicity, complex distribution, and overlapping positional, stereo-, and regio-selectivity for different substrates and products has limited to a large extent our ability to define the precise distribution and contribution of the different P-450s to the metabolism and activation of individual xenobiotics and endobiotics. Further, the complex P-450 multiplicity has made difficult the understanding of genetic and environmental factors in the interindividual variation in drug and carcinogen sensitivity that relate to cytochrome P-450.

### *Monoclonal Antibodies (MAbs) and cDNA Expression*

MAbs to different forms of P-450 (*5*) and cDNA expression of cloned cDNAs in different expression vectors enable the mapping and construction of an atlas of P-450 distribution and function. The MAbs are useful for the direct measurement of the distribution of epitope specific individual or classes of P-450 by radioimmunoassay (RIA), enzyme-linked immunosorbent assay (ELISA), or by Western blotting and can determine the content of a specific or class of P-450 in a tissue, organ, or species under different conditions of enzyme induction or different nutritional, developmental, or hormonal states (*5*). MAbs have also been successfully used in the immunohistochemical localization of specific P-450s. This localization of a specific P-450 has been successful in liver (*6*), lung (*7*), and brain (*8*) as well as subcellularly in the nuclear membrane of liver cells (*9*). Figure 1 shows how the use of inhibitory MAbs and cDNA expression can be used to define the specificity and contribution of individual P-450s to specific reactions.

MAbs inhibitory to enzyme activity can determine the contribution of the MAb specific P-450 to the total reaction of an individual substrate in a tissue preparation such as microsomes. The degree of inhibition by the MAb measures the contribution

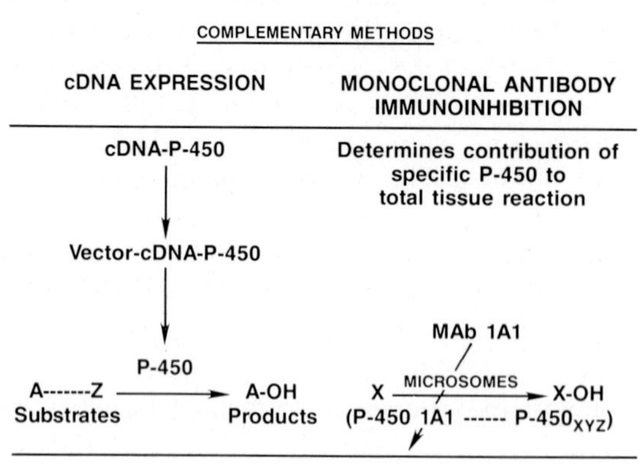


FIG. 1. Cytochrome P-450 specificity and metabolic role.

of the individual or class of P-450. This technique is applicable to a cytochrome P-450 dependent reaction or its consequences such as substrate disappearance, product formation, positional, regio- or stereo-specificity, mutagen activation, formation of DNA or protein adducts, or the formation of transforming or toxic products. We have termed this technique "reaction phenotyping" (*5*) since it describes the quantitative contribution of individual P-450s in tissue metabolism. The use of cDNA expression complements the use of MAbs. cDNA expression produces a single pure P-450 product from a cloned cDNA and thus is useful for the determination of the specificity of pure individual P-450s. With this technique (*10*, *11*), the cloned cDNA is incorporated into a vector such as vaccinia or transfected stably (*12*) with an Epstein-Barr vector into a cell which then expresses the single P-450. The single P-450 can be studied for the large variety of P-450 functions described above.

### *Library of MAbs to Cytochromes P-450*

The cytochromes P-450 are very suitable for investigation with MAbs since they are present in multiple forms with some at very low concentrations. Table 1 depicts our current library of MAbs to different forms of P-450 and to cytochrome $b_5$. In 1980, we reported the first preparation of MAbs to a P-450, and we have reviewed the usefulness of MAbs in P-450 research (*5*).

Table 1 also shows the use of synthetic peptides to elicit antibodies directed against a single P-450 enzyme. Two peptide sequences each with 17 amino acids from P-450 IA2 were synthesized, coupled to ovalbumin and used as antigens to generate anti-peptide monoclonal and polyclonal antibodies. Antisera to both peptides reacted with rat IA2 but not the structurally similar IA1 form as determined by ELISA. However, antisera to both peptides detected both rat IA2 and IA1 on immunoblots. Immunoblots of human liver microsomes, however, revealed that both antisera recognized human IA2 but not IA1. The utility of anti-peptide antisera as a practical approach for the generation of P-450 specific antibodies seems promising.

### *Immunohistochemical Studies*

*Liver* (*6*): MAbs specific for P-450 IA1/IA2 and 2B1/2 were used to investigate the intralobular distribution and induction sites of the hemoproteins within the livers of CD-1, C57BL/6, and DBA/2 mice. Cytochromes P-450 IA1 and IA2 were localized

TABLE 1. Library of Monoclonal Antibodies to Cytochromes P-450

| P-450 | Positive clones (RIA) | Inhibitory clones | % inhibition | Reference |
|---|---|---|---|---|
| IA1/IA2 | 10 | 3 | 90 | (*13*) |
| IA1 | 15 | 0 | 0 | (*13*) |
| IA2 (17 amino acid peptide) | 2 | 0 | 0 | (*14*) |
| IIB1/IIB2 | 10 | 4 | 90 | (*15*) |
| IIE1 | 31 | 1 | 90 | (*16*) |
| scup (IA1) | 8 | 4 | 87–94 | (*17*) |
| IIC11/IIC12 | 6 | 2 | 90 | (*18*) |
| IIIA1/IIIA2 | 11 | 0 | 0 | (*19*) |

predominantly in centrilobular hepatocytes of control mice from all strains and were present at higher levels in CD-1 and C57BL/6 mice than in DBA/2 mice. Treatment with either 3-methylcholanthrene (MC) or $\beta$-naphthoflavone (BNF) produced striking increases of P-450 IA1/IA2 in hepatocytes from all regions of the hepatic lobule in DC-1 and C57BL/6 mice, but not in DBA-2 mice. Cytochromes P-450 IIB1/IIB2 were localized in hepatocytes throughout all segments of the lobule in control mice with slightly greater hemoprotein content in centrilobular hepatocytes. Treatment with phenobarbital resulted in enhancement of P-450 that was visualized in hepatocytes in all regions of the lobule. Strain-related differences were not observed for phenobarbital-specific P-450. These results demonstrate that constitutive levels of P-450 IA1/IA2 and phenobarbital-specific cytochromes P-450II are localized predominantly in centrilobular hepatocytes of murine livers, and induction of the hemoproteins is manifested to the greatest extent in periportal hepatocytes, resulting in a more uniform distribution throughout the hepatic lubule (*5*).

*Lung* (*7*): The same techniques were used to study the distribution of P-450 IA1/IA2 and IIB1/2 in the lungs of "responsive" C57BL/6 and "nonresponsive" DBA/2 mice (*7*). P-450IA1 and P-450IA2 were found in the alveolar septa, including type II cells, as well as endothelial cells lining blood vessels. IA1 (MAbs 1-31-2, 1-36-1) is localized in type II cells of the alveolar septa but is not found in endothelial cells. Patterns of immunoreactivity indicate that alveolar septal cells possess IA1 and IA2, whereas endothelial cells of the vasculature contain IA2 and do not contain IA1. An MAb which recognizes IIB1/IIB2 is reactive with P-450s localized in type II alveolar and bronchiolar epithelial cells, including nonciliated Clara cells. The epitope for IIB1/2 is present in constitutive lung but does not appear to be responsive to induction by phenobarbital (PB). In contrast, epitopes for P-450 IA1/IA2 are not expressed constitutively but are only detected when induced by MC. The regional and cellular selectivities exhibited by lung tissues for the major IA1/2 and IIB1/2 forms of P-450 emphasize unique tissue specificities with regard to the expression of certain forms of P-450.

The presence of P-450 IA1/IA2 in rat brain (*8*) was studied by immunohistochemistry using polyclonal antibodies. Immunoreactive nerves were observed only in brain sections incubated with immunoglobulin-G to MC-induced P-450 (IA1/IA2). The most abundant concentration of nerve fibers with P-450 immunoreactivity was observed in the globus pallidus. Immunoreactive fibers were also observed in the caudate putamen, amygdala, septum, ventromedial nucleus of the hypothalamus, medial forebrain bundle, ansa lenticularis, and ventromedial portion of the internal capsule of crus cerebri. Cell bodies with P-450 immunoreactivity were observed in the caudate putamen and in the perifornical area of the hypothalamus. This P-450 isozyme was detected in brain areas which metabolize morphine and convert estradiol and estrone into catecholestrogens, which suggests a role for this enzyme in the metabolism of both exogenous and endogenous compounds in brain. Cytochrome P-450 IA1/IA2 was also detected in nuclear membranes of rat liver with immunohistochemistry with electron microscopy (*9*).

*1. Quantitative analyses of P-450 distribution*

A variety of immunodetection techniques can be used for the quantitative assay

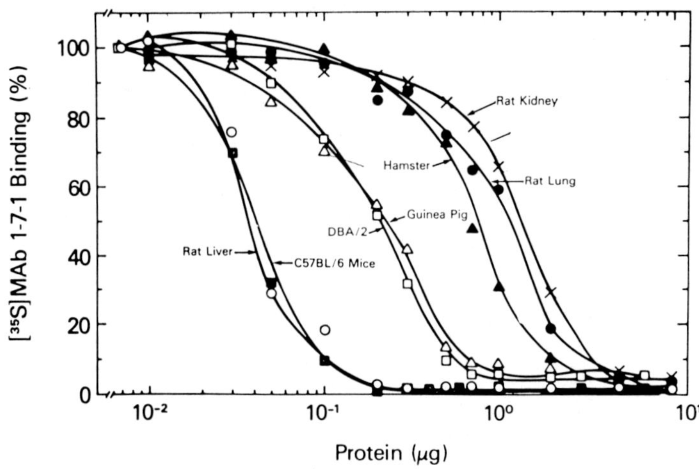


FIG. 2. MAb 1-7-1 competitive immunoquantitation of P-450 IA1/IA2 in MC-treated animal species and tissues.

of P-450 with MAbs. These include direct as well as competitive RIA as well as ELISA. Figure 2 shows the quantitative distribution of P-450 IA/IA2 in tissues of MC-treated animals with MAb 1-7-1 in a competitive RIA (*20, 21*). Microsomes from tissues of different species differentially competed with the well-coated liver microsomes of MC-treated rats for binding with MAb-1-7-1. The binding of [$^{35}$S]MAb 1-7-1 to the well was reduced in the presence of competing liver microsomal proteins from MC-treated rats, with a 50% reduction ($I_{50}$) of the binding occurring with 0.042 μg of microsomal proteins. Microsomes from C57BL/6 mice competed as effectively for the binding, whereas DBA/2 mice, which is relatively noninducible for aryl hydrocarbon hydroxylase activity, only moderately competed for the binding. Microsomes from guinea pigs and hamsters competed much less effectively than rats for binding to [$^{35}$S]MAb 1-7-1. The effectiveness of liver microsomes of MC-treated animals in competing for binding decreased in the following order: rats ($I_{50}=0.042$ μg); C57 BL/6 mice ($I_{50}=0.050$ μg); guinea pigs ($I_{50}=0.21$ μg); DBA/2 mice ($I_{50}=0.23$ μg); hamsters ($I_{50}=0.78$ μg); lung microsomes of rats ($I_{50}=1.02$ μg); and kidney microsomes of rats ($I_{50}=1.04$ μg). The presence of antigens of similar affinities for MAb 1-7-1 in different microsomal preparations was indicated by the horizontal displacement of the competitive binding curves. Thus, the differential competition reflects quantitative differences in levels of P-450 IA1/IA2 in the microsomal preparations examined.

2. *Monoclonal antibody-based "reaction phenotyping"*

The cytochromes P-450 collectively catalyze the oxidation of literally thousands of xenobiotic and endobiotic substrates including a large variety of different classes of chemicals. MAbs that inhibit the enzyme activity of the epitope containing P-450 are useful for "reaction phenotyping". The inhibitory MAb is added to the tissue preparation at saturating levels, and the amount of inhibition is a measure of the minimum contribution of the MAb-sensitive P-450 to the total reaction of the tissue.

Table 2 shows the use of MAbs for identifying the type of P-450 responsible for a specific drug or carcinogen reaction (*22, 23*) and the level of liver aryl hydrocarbon

TABLE 2. MAb Inhibition of Hepatic AHH and ECD of Different Species and Strains

| Species | Induction | AHH (pmole/min/mg) P-450 IA1 Control | 1-7-1 | Inhibition (%) | ECD (nmole/min/mg) (P-45 IA1/IA2) Control | 1-7-1 | Inhibition (%) |
|---|---|---|---|---|---|---|---|
| Rat | None | 367 | 384 | 0 | 0.82 | 0.95 | 0 |
| Sprague- | PB | 600 | 615 | 0 | 1.27 | 1.16 | 8 |
| Dawley | MC | 11,704 | 2,872 | 75 | 5.28 | 1.56 | 71 |
| Mouse | None | 88 | 87 | 1 | 6.4 | 5.6 | 12 |
| C57BL/6 | PB | 128 | 125 | 2 | 7.0 | 5.8 | 17 |
| | MC | 5,716 | 699 | 88 | 21.9 | 13.2 | 39 |
| Mouse | None | 70 | 70 | 0 | 4.0 | 3.5 | 11 |
| DBA/2 | PB | 51 | 94 | 0 | 4.7 | 3.6 | 25 |
| | MC | 501 | 486 | 3 | 16.9 | 18.9 | 0 |
| Guinea pig | None | 282 | 209 | 25 | 2.0 | 2.1 | 0 |
| | PB | 703 | 722 | 0 | 2.9 | 3.0 | 0 |
| | MC | 1,642 | 804 | 47 | 5.3 | 6.2 | 0 |
| Hamster | None | 100 | 136 | 0 | 8.7 | 9.1 | 0 |
| Golden | PB | 192 | 219 | 0 | 18.0 | 17.0 | 5 |
| Syrian | MC | 387 | 204 | 51 | 22.1 | 23.7 | 0 |

hydroxylase (AHH) and ethoxycoumarin deethylase (ECD) of four different species exposed to different inducers. The liver enzymes in rats are highly induced by MC for both AHH and ECD and are induced by PB to a lesser extent. MAb 1-7-1 inhibits AHH activity 75% in MC-induced rats. This is due to inhibition of IA1. We know this to be IA1 since cDNA expressed IA2 does not exhibit AHH activity and MAb 1-7-1 recognize only IA1 and IA2. Thus, the MAb-sensitive P-450 IA1 contributes 75% of the total activity of rat liver MC microsomes. IA1 contributes none of the AHH or ECD activity of either the rat liver control or PB microsomes since there is no inhibition by MAb 1-7-1. With the highly inducible C57 mouse strain, 87% of liver AHH activity but only 39% of ECD activity is a function of the P-450 IA1/IA2. Thus, 60% of ECD depends on a P-450 that is different than the MAb1-7-1-sensitive P-450. In both control and induced guinea pigs and hamsters, none of the ECD is sensitive to MAb 1-7-1 and is therefore catalyzed by a P-450 other than that sensitive to MAb 1-7-1. In control guinea pigs, 25% of AHH is due to MAb 1-7-1-sensitive P-450. Thus, the MC-induced form of AHH in guinea pigs and hamsters is inhibited by MAb 1-7-1 as it is in rats, but to a lesser extent.

Table 3 shows the contribution of P-450IA, P-450IIB, P-450IIC11, and P-450IIE1 to the oxidative metabolism of benzene, 7-ethoxyresorufin and 7-pentoxyresorufin in liver microsomes from fed, 1-day fasted, PB-, MC-, and ethanol treated rats (*24*). MAb 1-91-3 against P-450IIE1 did not influence ethoxyresorufin dealkylation but inhibited benzene aromatic hydroxylase (BAH) in relation to its increasing inducibility as follows: MC, PB ($\leq$48%) $<$ fed ($\leq$59%) $<$ fasted ($\leq$70%) $<$ ethanol ($\leq$91%). MAbs 2-66-3, 4-7-1, and 4-29-5, all against P450IIB, had no effect on 7-ethoxyresorufin O-deethylase (EROD) but inhibited the activities of high $K_m$ BAH ($\geq$58%) and 7-pentoxyresorufin O-depentylase (PROD) ($\geq$96%) in PB-treated

TABLE 3. Cytochromes P-450 Reaction Phenotyping of BAH, EROD, and PROD Metabolism by MAb Inhibition

| Treatment | Fold induction | MAbs[a)] (Nomenclature of P-450) | | | | | |
|---|---|---|---|---|---|---|---|
| | | 1-7-1 (P-450IA) | 2-66-3 (P-450IIB) | 4-7-1 (P-450IIB) | 4-29-5 (P-450IIB) | 1-68-11 (P-450IIC11) | 1-91-3 (P-45IIE1) |
| | | Degree of inhibition | | | | | |
| BAH low-$K_m$/high $K_m$ | | | | | | | |
| Fed | 1.0/1.0 | 0/0 | 0/0 | 0/0 | 0/0 | 0/+ | ++/+ |
| Fasted | 2.6/2.1 | 0/0 | 0/0 | 0/0 | 0/0 | 0/+ | ++/++ |
| PB | 1.3/3.5 | 0/0 | 0/++ | 0/++ | 0/++ | 0/0 | +/0 |
| MC | 0.9/1.7 | 0/+ | 0/0 | 0/0 | 0/0 | 0/+ | +/+ |
| Ethanol | 6.9/5.2 | 0/0 | 0/0 | 0/0 | 0/0 | 0/0 | +++/+++ |
| EROD | | | | | | | |
| Fed | 1.0 | 0 | 0 | 0 | 0 | ++ | 0 |
| Fasted | 1.5 | 0 | 0 | 0 | 0 | ++ | 0 |
| PB | 3.7 | 0 | 0 | 0 | 0 | +++ | 0 |
| MC | 222.0 | +++ | 0 | 0 | 0 | 0 | 0 |
| Ethanol | 2.3 | 0 | 0 | 0 | 0 | ++ | 0 |
| PROD | | | | | | | |
| Fed | 1.0 | 0 | 0 | 0 | 0 | +++ | 0 |
| Fasted | 1.3 | 0 | 0 | 0 | 0 | +++ | 0 |
| PB | 75.0 | 0 | +++ | +++[b)] | +++[b)] | 0 | 0 |
| MC | 6.7 | ++ | 0 | 0 | 0 | 0 | 0 |
| Ethanol | 1.3 | 0 | 0 | 0 | 0 | +++ | 0 |

a) Relative inhibitory effect of MAb: 0, ≤15%; +, 16–49%; ++, 50–74%; +++, 40.74%; ≥75%.
b) 200 μg MAb/200 μg microsomal protein.

microsomes. MAb 1-7-1 against P450IA inhibited EROD (79%), PROD (50%), and high $K_m$ BAH (42%) activities in MC-microsomes. MAb 1-68-11 against P450IIC11 inhibited EROD, PROD, and high $K_m$ BAH activities. Thus, P-450IIE1 contributed to benzene metabolism as a low $K_m$ BAH but not to ethoxyresorufin metabolism. P-450IIB was responsible besides for the major part of 7-pentoxyresorufin metabolism and benzene hydroxylation at high benzene concentration. P-450IA contributed primarily to 7-ethoxyresorufin metabolism and only slightly to PROD and high $K_m$ BAH activities. P-450IIC11 contributed slightly to high $K_m$ BAH and to ethoxyresorufin metabolism.

### 3. *cDNA expression of cytochrome P-450*

A number of expression systems including yeast, COS cells, vaccinia virus, and Herpes virus have been used to express enzymatically active P-450. The expression potential of vaccinia virus-expressed P-450 cDNA is considerably greater than that of the yeast or the COS cell system. In one study, expression vectors were constructed containing P-450 cDNAs for mouse P-450IA1 and P-450IA2 and for rat P-450IIA1 in a modified vaccinia virus vector. These cDNAs were expressed into their respective P-450 proteins, characterized immunochemically by immunoblots, by their enzymatic activities, and by their ability to activate a number of carcinogens of different classes to mutagenic forms (*25*).

TABLE 4. AHH, ECD, Testosterone 7α-hydroxylase, and AcOH Activities of Vaccinia-expressed cDNA P-450s

| Virus | pmol/min/mg Hep G2 cell lysate | | | |
|---|---|---|---|---|
| | AHH | ECD | Testosterone 7α-hydroxylase | AcOH |
| Control | 0.2 | ND | ND | 1 |
| vTF7-P-450IIA1 | 0.7 | 0.3 | 0.43 | 8 |
| vTF7-P-450IA1 | 193.0 | 10.5 | ND | 9 |
| vTF7-P-450IA2 | 4.5 | 22.2 | ND | 220 |

Analysis of enzyme activities revealed that all of the expressed enzymes were capable of oxidizing model substrates when expressed in Hep G2 cells. The level of AHH, ECD, testosterone 7α-hydroxylase, and acetanilide *p*-hydroxylase (AcOH) activities were assayed in lysates of the human cell line, Hep G2 infected by either control vvWT or vaccinia virus containing cDNAs for P-450a, P-450IA1, and P-450IA2 (Table 4). IA1 cDNA produced AHH at high levels in Hep G2 cells; the Hep G2 cells exhibited an 8-fold higher level of AHH activity than the $TK^-$ cells (data not shown). No AHH activity was detected in cells infected with the wild-type virus, and negligible or no AHH activity was observed in cells infected with virus expressing either IA2 or IIA1. Testosterone 7α-hydroxylase activity appeared only in the lysates of cells infected with vTF7-P-450IIA1 and was not detectable in the lysates of the cells infected by vvWT, IA1, or IA2. Thus, a high level of specificity was observed for each of the four enzyme activities, with each of the P-450s expressed from their respective cDNAs; AHH was specific for IA1, AcOH for IA2, and testosterone 7α-hydroxylase for IIA1. In the case of ECD enzyme activity, both IA1 and IA2 were active, and IA2 was twice as active as IA1. No ECD activity was detected in cells infected with wild-type virus or with vTF7-IIA1. AcOH was exhibited only by IA2 and not by the other P-450.

4. *Mutagen activation by expressed P-450s* (*Table 5*)

The expressed IA1 exhibited moderate mutagen activation for B[a]P and DMBA and to a much lesser extent for MC. The lysate containing either wild-type virus, IA2, or IIA1 showed essentially no mutagen activation for B[a]P and DMBA. The B[a]P-7, 8-diol is an intermediate of B[a]P metabolism and an immediate precursor of the highly mutagenic B[a]P-diol epoxides. With the B[a]P-7, 8-diol, both the expressed IA1 and IA2 showed very high mutagenic activation, which was much greater than shown by S-9. The IA2, which is not usually associated with polycyclic aromatic hydrocarbon metabolism, showed mutagen activation 50% that of IA1. B[a]P and DMBA were activated only by IA1 and to a relatively low level, compared with S-9, which suggests that additional P-450s may be involved in the activation of B[a]P and DMBA in the S-9 preparation.

The aromatic amine class of carcinogens were highly activated to mutagens by the expressed cytochrome IA2 and to a lesser degree in some cases by IA1. IA2 was very active in acetylaminofluorene (AAF) activation while IA1 and P-450a were inactive. The activity of IA2 towards AAF was greater than the S-9. The *N*-hydroxy metabolite of AAF was activated most strongly by IA2 and to a lesser extent by IA1 and IIA1.

TABLE 5. Mutagen Activation by cDNA-expressed P-450 (*25*)

| Promutagens | S-9 rat liver | IA1 | IA2 | IIA1 |
|---|---|---|---|---|
| B[a]P | 820 | 262 | 14 | 5 |
| B[a]P-7, 8 diol | 754 | 2,108 | 1,108 | 73 |
| DMBA | 459 | 317 | 47 | 49 |
| MC | 449 | 44 | 12 | 5 |
| 2-AAF | 73 | 35 | 878 | 18 |
| 4-Aminobiphenyl (4-ABP) | 70 | 13 | 89 | 8 |
| N-OH-4-ABP | 29 | 13 | 49 | 24 |
| 2-Naphthylamine | 180 | 17 | 87 | 11 |
| Aflatoxin $B_1$ | 954 | 21 | 37 | 21 |
| Trp-P1 | 1,580 | 680 | 2,015 | 5 |
| Trp-P2 | 2,527 | 2,227 | 5,179 | 2 |
| Glu-P1 | 12,435 | 385 | 2,700 | 9 |
| Glu-P2 | 224 | 12 | 71 | 7 |
| IQ | 15,217 | 718 | 6,353 | 9 |

A series of heterocyclic amine pyrolysis products of certain common foods have been found to require metabolic activation for their very high mutagenic activity. Five of these pyrolysis products, Trp-P1, Trp-P2, Glu-P1, Glu-P2, and IQ, were examined for their activation to mutagenic compound by the vaccinia-expressed P-450s. IIA1 was essentially inactive to each of the latter compounds. Trp-P1 was activated by both IA2 and IA1; IA2 was 3-fold more active. Trp-P2 was also activated by IA2 as well as by IA1, and the IA2 was twice as active. With Trp-P2, the IA1 showed activity twice that of the S-9. With Glu-P1, the IA2 was about one-fourth as active as the S-9 and the IA1 was one-sixth as active as the IA2. When the IQ was activated by IA2, it showed the highest mutagenic activity of any compound tested, and the IA2 was about 9-fold more effective in this activation than the IA1.

### *Mouse and Human cDNA Expressed P-450s*

The vaccinia virus cDNA expression system was also used to produce human P-450 IA2 in a hepatoma cell line that is devoid of significant basal levels of P-450 (*26*). The expressed enzyme yielded a reduced carbon monoxide-bound difference spectrum with a $\lambda_{max}$ of 449 nm. Catalytic activities and mutagen activation ability of the human enzyme were assessed and directly compared with the expressed orthologous mouse IA2. Both the human and mouse enzymes catalyzed the *p*-hydroxylation of aniline. Mouse IA2 also catalyzed ethoxyresorufin O-deethylation, and its activity was 7-fold greater than expressed human IA2. The mouse and human enzymes also activated several promutagens and procarcinogens. Mouse IA2 was 5- to 7-fold more active than the human enzyme for activation of the procarcinogens 2-acetylamino-fluorene and benzo[a]pyrene-*trans*-7, 8-dihydrodiol and the promutagens Glu-P-2 and Trp-P1. Comparable activities of the human and mouse P-450s were observed with 2-aminoanthracene, 2-aminofluorene, and Glu-P-1 (*26*).

### *cDNA Expression of Eight Human P-450s: Mutagen Activation* (*27*)

Eight forms of human liver microsomal P-450 were individually expressed in human hepatoma Hep G2 cells with a vaccinia virus cDNA. Each expressed P-450 was examined for its ability to mutagen activate 2-amino-3-methylimidazo[4,5-f]quinoline (IQ), 2-amino-3,4-dimethylimidazo[4,5-f]quinoline (methyl IQ), 2-amino-3,8-dimethylimidazo[4,5-f]quinoxaline (methyl IQx), and 2-amino-3,4,8-trimethylimidazo-[4, 5-f]quinoxaline (dimethyl IQx), respectively. Three forms of human P-450 significantly activated 2-amino-3-methylimidazo[4, 5-f]quinoline when the latter was at high substrate concentrations, but only a single form, P-450IA2, showed very high activation of all promutagens at lower substrate concentrations (Table 6). Human IA2 is likely the predominant P-450 enzyme responsible for their mutagenic activation in human liver.

### *Aflatoxin Mutagenic Activation with Twelve Human P-450s* (*28*)

Twelve forms of human hepatic P-450 were expressed in hepatoma cells from re-

TABLE 6. Activation of Promutagens by Human P-450s (*27*)

| P-450 activation system | Promutagens (revertant/mg lysate) | | | |
|---|---|---|---|---|
| | IQ | Methyl IQ | Methyl IQx | Dimethyl IQx |
| IA2 | 2,851±266 | 1,172±105 | 4,134±316 | 2,840±123 |
| IIB7 | 17±6 | 25±11 | 9±3 | 13±6 |
| IIC8 | 32±8 | 29±7 | 6±2 | 28±11 |
| IIC9 | 253±20 | 176±19 | 2±2 | 18±8 |
| IID6 | 8±6 | 35±11 | 5±4 | 7±2 |
| IIE1 | 7±2 | 10±6 | 5±2 | 6±2 |
| IIIA4 | 255±31 | 397±30 | 70±16 | 329±22 |
| IIIA5 | 69±9 | 89±15 | 22±5 | 38±11 |
| WT | 10±6 | 26±8 | 7±2 | 11±6 |
| Human liver S-9 | 6,053±501 | 1,802±105 | 7,917±517 | 4,873±469 |

TABLE 7. Aflatoxin $B_1$: Mutagenic Activation and DNA Binding Catalyzed by Vaccinia Expressed Human P-450s (*28*)

| P-450 | Mutagen activation (revertants/plate) | DNA binding (dpm/mg DNA $10^3$) |
|---|---|---|
| Virus control | 198 | 0.9 |
| IA2 | 381 | 52.6 |
| IIA3 | 320 | 39.4 |
| IIB1 | 643 | 20.1 |
| IIIA4 | 976 | 22.6 |
| IIIA5 | 774 | 21.0 |
| IIC8 | 113 | 1.0 |
| IIC9 | 130 | 0.9 |
| IID6 | 125 | 2.6 |
| IIE1 | 142 | 1.0 |
| IIF1 | 117 | 0.9 |
| IIIA6 | 168 | 4.3 |
| IVB1 | 243 | 1.5 |

TABLE 8. Aflatoxin $B_1$ in P-450 IA2 Transfected AHH TK−/+ Cells (*29*)

| | Toxicity | | Mutagenicity | |
|---|---|---|---|---|
| | Relative survival | | Mutant fraction ($\times 10_6$) | |
| AFB$_1$ ($\mu$g/ml) | AHH-1 control | AHH-1 P-450 IA2 | AHH-1 control | AHH-1 P-450 IA2 |
| None | 1.0 | 1.0 | 4.4 | 2.8 |
| 0.003 | — | 0.76 | — | 10.8 |
| 0.01 | — | 0.69 | — | 14.3 |
| 0.03 | 1.02 | 0.45 | — | 16.1 |
| 0.06 | 1.05 | 0.26 | — | 24.4 |
| 1.0 | — | — | 7.8 | — |
| 2.0 | — | — | 8.2 | — |

TABLE 9. Binding of [$^3$H]-Aflatoxin $B_1$ to Cellular DNA

| Cell line | Binding (dpm/$\mu$g DNA) (mean$\pm$SD) |
|---|---|
| AHH-1 TK+/− (untransfected) | Not detectable $<0.2$ |
| AHH-1 TK+/− with pMF6 | Not detectable $<0.2$ |
| AHH-1 TK+/− with pMF6/1A2 | $16.3\pm0.9$ |

combinant vaccinia virus and analyzed for activation of the potent hepatocarcinogen aflatoxin $B_1$ to metabolites having mutagenic or DNA-binding properties (Table 7). Five forms, P-450s, IA2, IIA3, IIB1, IIIA4, and IIIA5, activated aflatoxin $B_1$ to mutagenic metabolites. The same P-450s catalyzed the conversion of aflatoxin $B_1$ to DNA-bound derivatives. Seven other human P-450s, IIC8, IIC9, IID6, IIE1, IIF1, IIIA6, and IVB1, did not significantly activate aflatoxin $B_1$. Thus, metabolic activation of aflatoxin $B_1$ in human liver involves the contribution of multiple forms of P-450.

*Stable Expression of Human Cytochrome P-450IA2 cDNA in a Human Lymphoblastoid Cell Line: Metabolic Activation of Aflatoxin $B_1$*

A human lymphoblastoid cell line stably expressing human P-450IA2 was constructed and expressed P-450IA2 and estradiol 2-hydroxylase activity, neither of which was detected in the parental cell line. The recombinant cell line was also approximately 1,000-fold more sensitive to the cytotoxicity and mutagenicity of aflatoxin $B_1$ than the parent cell line (Table 8). The latter was paralleled by a corresponding increase in the level of aflatoxin $B_1$ binding to DNA (*12*) (Table 9). Stability of P-450IA2 expression in the transfected cell line was evaluated by examining the cytotoxicity of aflatoxin $B_1$ as a function of growth in culture. Sensitivity to the cytotoxicity of aflatoxin $B_1$ was maintained in cells that were propagated continuously for more than 60 days.

*Epilogue*

Our studies demonstrate the facility and utility of a combination of methods utilizing MAbs and cDNA expression of cytochrome P-450s for the mapping of the distribution and function of the complex multiform-enzyme family of cytochrome

P-450s. These systems seem highly applicable to the study of the large multiplicity of forms of cytochrome P-450 and their complex distribution. These techniques separately and in combination characterize P-450 function and distribution which exist in a variety of constellations in different species, strains, tissues, and organs and vary in different developmental, hormonal, and nutritional states. Since P-450 is the primary enzyme metabolizing drugs, carcinogens, and xenobiotics, knowledge of the dynamics of P-450 function and distribution should well serve drug design, optimizing drug efficacy and reducing adverse toxic side effects. Further knowledge of the specific P-450s engaged in carcinogen and mutagen activation would promote our understanding of the interindividual differences in cancer incidence and their relationship to polymorphism of P-450 in the human population (*29*). This knowledge would also serve the development of risk assessment systems utilizing DNA expressed human P-450s and appropriate human host cells (*11*). The utility of these systems would also be large when applied to endobiotic regulatory metabolism such as that concerned with prostaglandins, fatty acids, and steroids. The construction of an atlas of P-450 distribution and function that we propose would serve well the manifold goals of P-450 research.

## REFERENCES

1. Lu, A. Y. H. Multiplicity of mammalian microsomal cytochrome P-450. Pharmacol. Rev., *31*: 277–295, 1980.
2. Gelboin, H. V. Benzo[a]pyrene metabolism, activation, and carcinogenesis: role and regulation of mixed function oxidases and related enzymes. Physiol. Rev., *60*: 1107–1166, 1980.
3. Nebert, D. W., Adesnik, M., Coon, M. J., Estabrook, R. W., Gonzalez, F. J., Guengerich, F. P., Gunsalus, I. C., Johnson, E. F., Kemper, B., Levin, W., Phillips, I. R., Sato, R., and Waterman, M. R. The P450 gene superfamily: recommended nomenclature. DNA, *6*: 1–11, 1987.
4. Gonzalez, F. J. The molecular biology of cytochrome P450s. Pharmacol. Rev., *40*: 243–287, 1989.
5. Gelboin, H. V., and Friedman, F. K. Monoclonal antibodies for studies on xenobiotic and endobiotic metabolism: cytochromes P-450 as paradigm. Biochem. Pharmacol., *34*: 2225–2234, 1985.
6. Forkert, P. G., Mirehouse-Brown, P., Park, S. S., and Gelboin, H. V. Distribution and induction sites of phenobarbital- and 3-methylcholanthrene-inducible cytochromes P-450 in murine liver; immunohistochemical localization with monoclonal antibodies. Mol. Pharmacol., *34*: 736–743, 1988.
7. Forkert, P. G., Vessey, M. L., Park, S. S., Gelboin, H. V., and Cole, S. P. C. Cytochromes P-450 in murine lung: An immunohistochemical study with monoclonal antibodies. Drug Met. Disposition, *17*: 551–555, 1989.
8. Kapitulnik, J., Gelboin, H. V., Guengerich, F. P., and Jacobowitz, B. M. Immunohistochemical localization of cytochrome P-450 in rat brain. Neuroscience, *20*: 829–834, 1987.
9. Brands, R., Snider, M. D., Hino, Y., Park, S. S., Gelboin, H. V., and Rothman, J. E. Retention of membrane proteins by the endoplasmic reticulum. J. Cell Biol., *101*: 1724–1732, 1985.
10. Battula, N., Sagara, J., and Gelboin, H. V. Expression of $P_1$-450 and $P_3$-450 DNA

coding sequences as enzymatically active cytochromes P-450 in mammalian cells. Proc. Natl. Acad. Sci. U.S.A., *84*: 4073–4077, 1987.

11. Gonzalez, F. J., Crespi, C. L., and Gelboin, H. V. cDNA-expressed human cytochrome P450s: a new age of molecular toxicology and human risk assessment. Mutat. Res., in press.
12. Crespi, C. L., Steimel, D. T., Aoyama, T., Gelboin, H. V., and Gonzalez, F. J. Stable expression of human cytochrome P-450 IA2 cDNA in human lymphoblastoid cell line: Role of the enzyme in the metabolic activation of aflatoxin B-1. Molec. Carc., *3*: 5–8, 1990.
13. Park, S. S., Fujino, T., West, D., Guengerich, F. P., and Gelboin, H. V. Monoclonal antibodies that inhibit enzyme activity of 3-methylcholanthrene-induced cytochrome P-450. Cancer Res., *42*: 1798–1808, 1982.
14. Myers, M. J., Liu, G., Miller, H., Gelboin, H. V., Robinson, R. C., and Friedman, F. K. Synthetic peptide antigens elicit monoclonal and polyclonal antibodies to cytochrome P-450 IA2. Biochem. Biophys. Res. Commun., *169*: 171–176.
15. Park, S. S., Fujino, T., Miller, H., Guengerich, F. P., and Gelboin, H. V. Monoclonal antibodies to phenobarbital induced rat liver cytochrome P-450. Biochem. Pharmacol., *33*: 2071–2081, 1984.
16. Ko, I., Park, S. S., Song, B. J., Pattern, C., Tan, Y., Ha, Y. C., Yang, C. S., and Gelboin, H. V. Monoclonal antibodies to ethanol-induced rat liver cytochrome P-450 that metabolizes aniline and nitrosamines. Cancer Res., *47*: 3101–3109, 1987.
17. Park, S. S., Miller, H., Klotz, A. V., Kloepper-Sams, P. J., Stegeman, J. J., and Gelboin, H. V. Monoclonal antibodies to liver microsomal cytochrome P-450E of the marine fish *Stenotomus chrysops* (scup): cross reactivity with 3-methylcholanthrene induced rat cytochrome P-450. Arch. Biochem. Biophys., *249*: 339–350, 1986.
18. Park, S. S., Waxman, D. J., Lapenson, D. P., Schenkman, J. B., and Gelboin, H. V. Monoclonal antibodies to rat liver cytochrome P-450 2c/RLM5 that regiospecifically inhibit steroid metabolism. Biochem. Pharmacol., *38*: 3067–3074, 1989.
19. Park, S. S., Waxman, D. J., Miller, H., Robinson, R., Attisano, C., Guengerich, F. P., and Gelboin, H. V. Preparation and characterization of monoclonal antibodies to pregnenolone-16-$\alpha$-carbonitrile inducible rat liver cytochrome P-450. Biochem. Pharmacol., *35*: 2859–2867, 1986.
20. Song, B. J., Fujino, T., Park, S. S., Friedman, F. K., and Gelboin, H. V. Monoclonal antibody-directed radioimmunoassay of specific cytochrome P-450. J. Biol. Chem., *259*: 1394–1397, 1984.
21. Cheng, K., Gelboin, H. V., Song, B. J., Park, S. S., and Friedman, F. K. Detection and purification of cytochrome P-450 in animal tissues with monoclonal antibodies. J. Biol. Chem., *259*: 12279–12284, 1984.
22. Fujino, T., Park, S. S., West, D., and Gelboin, H. V. Phenotyping of cytochromes P-450 in human tissues with monoclonal antibodies. Proc. Natl. Acad. Sci. U.S.A., *79*: 3682–3686, 1982.
23. Fujino, T., West, D., Park, S. S., and Gelboin, H. V. Monoclonal antibody-directed phenotyping of cytochrome P-450 dependent aryl hydrocarbon hydroxylase and 7-ethoxycoumarin deethylase in mammalian tissues. J. Biol. Chem., *259*: 9044–9050, 1984.
24. Nakajima, T., Elovaara, E., Park, S. S., Gelboin, H. V., Hietanen, E., and Vainio, H. Monoclonal antibody-directed characterization of benzene, ethoxyresorufin and pentoxyresorufin metabolism in rat liver microsomes.
25. Aoyama, T., Gonzalez, F. J., and Gelboin, H. V. Mutagen activation by cDNA-expressed $P_1450$, $P_3450$, and P450a. Molec. Carc., *1*: 253–259, 1989.
26. Aoyama, T., Gonzalez, F. J., and Gelboin, H. V. Human cDNA-expressed cytochrome

P450 IA2: Mutagen activation and substrate specificity. Molec. Carc., *2*: 192–198, 1989.

27. Aoyama, T., Gelboin, H. V., and Gonzalez, F. J. Mutagenic activation of 2-amino-3-methylimidazo [4, 5-f] quinoline (IQ) by cDNA-expressed human liver P450. Cancer Res., *50*: 2060–2063, 1990.
28. Aoyama, T., Yamano, S., Guzelian, P. S., Gelboin, H. V., and Gonzalez, F. J. Five of 12 forms of vaccinia virus-expressed human hepatic cytochrome P450 metabolically activate aflatoxin $B_1$. Proc. Natl. Acad. Sci. U.S.A., *87*: 4790–4793, 1990.
29. Gelboin, H. V. Carcinogens, drugs, and cytochromes P-450. N. Engl. J. Med., *309*: 105, 1983.

XENOBIOTICS AND CANCER, L. ERNSTER ET AL. (EDS.),
JAPAN SCI. SOC. PRESS, TOKYO/TAYLOR & FRANCIS LTD., LONDON, pp. 17–29 1991

NAKAHARA MEMORIAL LECTURE

# Chemical Carcinogenesis and Its Prevention: Is There a Common Denominator?

Lars ERNSTER

*Department of Biochemistry, Arrhenius Laboratories, Stockholm University, S-106 91 Stockholm, Sweden*

*Abstract:* Chemical carcinogenesis is generally recognized as a multistep process consisting of initiation, promotion and progression. Today there is substantial evidence that the process involves reactive species of oxygen, which are generated through enzymic or nonenzymic transformation of xenobiotics and their metabolites, and which can alter nucleic acids, proteins, and lipids, thereby interfering with normal cell growth and differentiation. Most cells possess powerful defense mechanisms against these effects, both in the form of antioxidants acting as free-radical scavengers, and of various enzymes capable of preventing the formation of facilitating the removal of reactive species of oxygen. The present paper is a brief survey of current knowledge concerning these mechanisms. The available information is consistent with the concept that chemical carcinogenesis and its prevention share a common denominator, namely, the metabolic activation of a xenobiotic that can lead, on one hand, to the generation of reactive species of oxygen and thereby cancer initiation, promotion and progression, and, on the other hand, to an induction of antioxidant enzymes that can prevent these effects. The final outcome will depend on the relative impact of the two events. Elucidation of the underlying molecular mechanisms may provide a rationale for devising drugs that enhance resistance against chemical carcinogenesis without themselves being carcinogenic.

It is a great honor to be this year's Nakahara Memorial Lecturer, and I thank Dr. Sugimura and his colleagues in the Organizing Committee for this privilege.

Waro Nakahara has been one of the pioneers in the study of chemical carcinogenesis and a founding father of this field of research in Japan. As Director of the National Cancer Center Research Institute he organized in 1970 the First International Symposium of the Princess Takamatsu Cancer Research Fund, and it is thus highly appropriate to honor his memory at these Symposia.

When Nakahara began his scientific career, over 70 years ago, cancer research was in its infancy. Rous (*1*) had just discovered his sarcoma virus, a discovery which Nakahara followed with great interest (*cf.* ref. *2*). Biology was still strongly influenced by the vitalistic ideology, and it was difficult to imagine that a cancer cell could arise under the influence of a cell-free agent. However, at about the same time, Yamagiwa and Ishikawa (*3*) described the induction of skin cancer in rabbits by coal tar, *i.e.*, by chemicals. These were subsequently identified by Kennaway (*4*) as polycyclic hydrocarbons.

In 1932, Yoshida (*5*), and soon thereafter Kinoshita *et al.* (*6*), discovered another group of chemical carcinogens, the azodyes. A few years later, Nakahara and his coworkers (*7*) made the interesting observation that the carcinogenicity of 4-dimethylaminoazobenzene (DAB) was obliterated by dried yeast which contained a flavoprotein acting as an azoreductase—an enzyme that, in retrospect, may be related to DT-diaphorase. In any case, this was the first indication that an enzyme may act as an anticarcinogen (*cf.* ref. *8* for review).

In 1957, Nakahara *et al.* (*9*) discovered the carcinogenicity of 4-nitro-quinoline-1-oxide. In contrast to DAB, the carcinogenic effect of this compound was subsequently found to be enhanced by reduction *via* DT-diaphorase to the corresponding hydroxylamine (*10*). The introduction of these compounds in the study of chemical carcinogenesis opened the way to the investigation of heterocyclic amines as environmental carcinogens. This development culminated in the identification by Sugimura and his colleagues (*11*) of a number of carcinogenic compounds commonly occurring in cooked food.

Much of the progress in this field has been made possible by the application of the bacterial mutagenicity test developed by Ames and his associates (*12*), and the demonstration of a good correlation between mutagenicity as revealed by the Ames test and the carcinogenicity of various compounds in experimental animals and in humans (*13*). Today we know that many chemicals in our natural environment, including our daily food, are mutagens and carcinogens; and, moreover, that due to this circumstance, we have evolved a battery of protective devices against such agents (*14, 15*). The subject of this lecture is to highlight some aspects of this relationship between chemical carcinogenesis and its prevention, primarily in the context of the coordinate regulation of cellular pro- and antioxidant mechanisms.

### *The Multistep Model of Chemical Carcinogenesis and the Role of Reactive Species of Oxygen*

Beginning with the pioneering observations of Berenblum (*16*) and of Rous and Kidd (*17*) almost 50 years ago, chemical carcinogenesis is now widely recognized as a multistep process, consisting of initiation, promotion and progression. Today we know that this is a somewhat simplified model, behind which there is a highly complex pattern of disturbances in what has been referred to as the "regulatory circuit of cellular phenotype" (*18*), including activation of various oncogenes, receptor-mediated inter- and intracellular responses to histocompatibility antigens, growth factors and hormones, regulation of enzymes governing protein phosphorylation, phosphatidyl inositol metabolism, $Ca^{2+}$ homeostasis, pro- and antioxidant status, *etc.*—events that only in recent years have become accessible to study at the molecular level. According to current concepts (*cf.* refs. *19, 20*), initiation consists of a permanent modification of a gene (or genes), *i.e.*, a mutation, most often somatic, which remains dormant until a promoter activates its expression, leading to selective clonal expansion of the cells concerned, and finally resulting in progression through a breakdown of contact inhibition and an invasiveness towards neighboring cells and tissues.

In recent years substantial evidence has accumulated which indicates that chemical carcinogenesis involves reactive species of oxygen (*21–23*). These include the superoxide ($O_2\cdot^-$) and hydroxyl ($OH\cdot$) radicals, hydrogen peroxide ($H_2O_2$), organic peroxides, and singlet oxygen ($^1O_2$). Various sources and consequences of oxygen-radical production in animal cells are schematically illustrated in Fig. 1. Some details of this scheme have been discussed elsewhere (*24, 25*), and will not be further elabo-

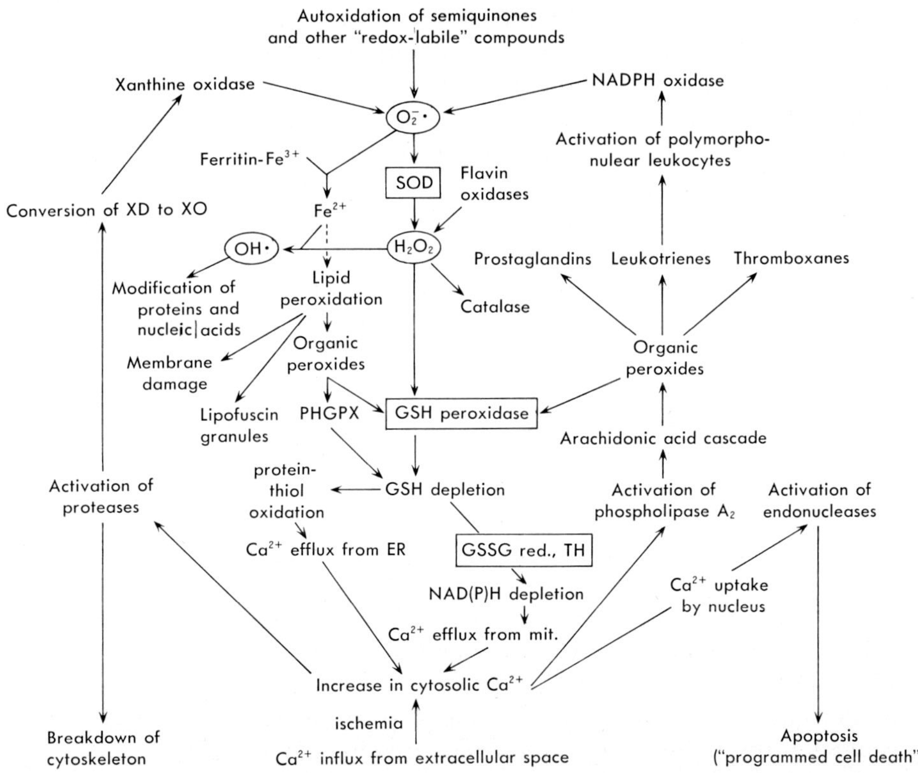


FIG. 1. Sources and consequences of oxygen-radical production in animal cells. Abbreviations: SOD, superoxide dismutase; GSH, glutathione; GSSG, glutathione disulfide; PHGPX, phospholipid hydroperoxide glutathione peroxidase; GSSG red., glutathione reductase; TH, nicotinamide nucleotide transhydrogenase; ER, endoplasmic reticulum; mit., mitochondria; XD, xanthine dehydrogenase; XO, xanthine oxidase. (Updated from ref. *25*. For further explanation, see text.)

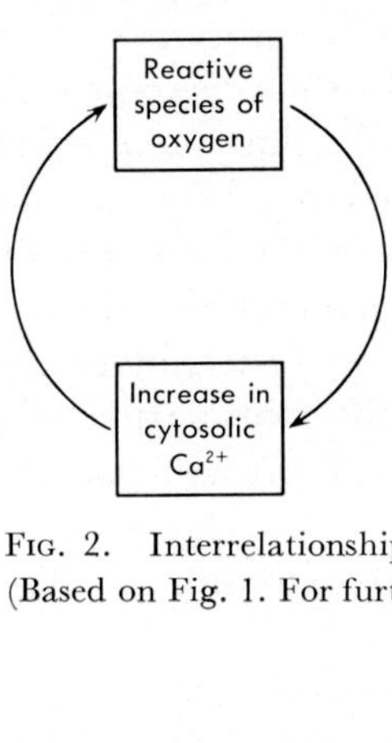


FIG. 2. Interrelationship between reactive species of oxygen and increase in cytosolic calcium. (Based on Fig. 1. For further explanation, see text.)

rated on here. Briefly, the effects of reactive oxygen species can be divided into two categories: primary and secondary. Primary effects are those caused by oxygen radicals directly on cell components and functions. They require Fe and lead to perferryl-radical initiated lipid peroxidation, with ensuing membrane damage and deposition of lipofuscin granules, and to hydroxyl-radical induced modification of proteins and nucleic acids, resulting in enzyme inactivation and DNA strand-breaks. Secondary effects consist of a perturbation of cellular $Ca^{2+}$ homeostasis, leading to an increase in cytosolic $Ca^{2+}$ and a consequent activation of $Ca^{2+}$-dependent cytosolic enzymes including proteases and phospholipases. The latter effects result, in turn, in a breakdown of the cytoskeleton and an activation of enzymes, such as xanthine oxidase and NADPH oxidase, that give rise to further oxygen-radical formation as depicted in a simplified way in Fig. 2. Thus, the two types of effect may amplify one-another in a synergistic fashion, *i.e.*, any agent that gives rise to oxygen-radical production is a potential inducer of an increase in cytosolic $Ca^{2+}$ and, *vice versa*, any agent that causes an increase in cytosolic $Ca^{2+}$ is a potential inducer of oxygen-radical generation. It should be noted (*cf.* Fig. 1) that $H_2O_2$ and organic peroxides have a central role in this interplay by being, on one hand, the products of oxygen-radical metabolism and, on the other hand, the sources—by way of GSH peroxidase—of the perturbation of $Ca^{2+}$ homeostasis.

The mechanisms outlined above may provide a rational framework for the possible roles of oxygen activation in the various phases of chemical carcinogenesis, which may be summarized as follows:

*Initiation*, resulting from a chemical alteration of DNA, may consist of the covalent addition of electrophiles produced through the cytochrome P-450-linked monooxygenation of polycyclic hydrocarbons, giving rise to arene epoxides (*26*). Polycyclic hydrocarbons can also be activated by organic peroxides (*27*) or free radicals (*28, 29*) to epoxides or quinones that act as mutagens (*30*). Furthermore, DNA may be modified by cross-linking *via* malondialdehyde derived from lipid peroxides (*31*), or by base oxidations by way of OH• (*32*), leading to strand-breaks. Finally, DNA may undergo degradation through endonucleases activated by an enhanced $Ca^{2+}$ uptake by the cell nuclei as a consequence of the increase in cytosolic $Ca^{2+}$ concentration (*33*; *cf.* Fig. 1).

*Promotion* has been studied extensively in recent years with respect to its relationship with oxygen toxicity (*cf.* ref. *22*). A role of oxygen radicals in tumor promotion has been considered mainly on three grounds: a) different classes of tumor promoters evoke the cellular generation of oxygen radicals; b) they modulate antioxidant enzyme activities *in vivo*; and c) their effect can be prevented by free-radical scavengers. Regarding the chemical nature of the commonly studied promoters and their cellular targets it appears, on the basis of the foregoing discussion, that their effects may be classified mostly as "secondary" in terms of oxygen toxicity, *i.e.*, that they act by perturbing cellular $Ca^{2+}$ homeostasis. Activation of protein kinase C by altered thiol disulfide status (*34*), enhanced induction of ornithine decarboxylase—the rate-limiting enzyme in polyamine biosynthesis—by the phorbol ester 12-O-tetradecanoylphorbol-13-acetate (TPA) and other tumor promoters (*35*), or the stimulation of poly-ADP ribosylation and other factors activating transcription of growth-related protooncogenes (*20*) are likely examples of this type of effect.

*Progression*, which is generally considered to be an extension of the effects of initiators and/or promoters, may involve membrane damage arising from lipid peroxidation or from the breakdown of cytoskeleton through a $Ca^{2+}$-activated protease, resulting in impaired cell-cell interaction and consequent loss of contact inhibition.

It should be pointed out in this connection that carcinogenesis is but one example of the manifestations of oxygen toxicity. Others are radiation damage, hyperoxygenation injury, toxic effects of various xenobiotics, inflammatory processes, autoimmune diseases, the "ischemia-reperfusion syndrome", the process of *apoptosis* ("programmed cell death") and, last but not least, the physiological aging of cells (*cf.* refs. *36–38*). The exponential increase of cancer incidence with age is on good grounds believed to be a reflection of diminished antioxidant capacity.

*Regulation of Pro- and Antioxidant Mechanisms of Its Implications for Chemical Carcinogenesis*

It is now well established that various xenobiotics can act as inducers of enzymes involved both in the formation and the removal of active metabolites that are responsible for carcinogenesis. Such compounds may, in principle, act both as carcinogens and anticarcinogens. For example, certain polycyclic hydrocarbons and azodyes are potent inducers, as first shown in 1956–57 by Conney *et al.* (*39, 40*), of "hydroxylases" —now known as isozymes of cytochrome P-450—which are the key enzymes in the metabolic activation of these carcinogens. However, as first demonstrated as early as 1951 by Richardson and Cunningham (*41*), and subsequently found in several laboratories (*cf.* ref. *42*), low doses of these compounds can make rats resistant to the toxic and carcinogenic effects of these chemicals. A striking example of this phenomenon is shown in Table 1. Moreover, as demonstrated by Huggins and associates in the early 1960s (*42–44*), the protective effect of these substances was accompanied by the induction of a "menadione reductase", which proved to be identical to an enzyme described in our laboratory in 1960 under the name DT-diaphorase (*45*).

Over the last 30 years, DT-diaphorase (EC 1.6.99.2) has been studied extensively in several laboratories (and under various names) with respect to its catalytic properties, structure and regulation (*cf.* ref. *46* for a historical review). It is an NAD(P)H-oxidizing flavoprotein occurring in the cytosol, microsomes and mitochondria of mammalian tissues and catalyzing the reduction of a variety of quinones. A prominent feature of DT-diaphorase, demonstrated in 1970 by Iyanagi and Yamazaki (*47*), is that it is a two-electron transfer enzyme. In this respect it differs from

TABLE 1. Azodye-induced Prevention of Leukemia in Rats Treated with a Carcinogenic Polycyclic Hydrocarbon

| Sudan III (mg) | Number of rats | Rats with leukemia | |
|---|---|---|---|
| | | Number | Percent |
| 0 | 13 | 12 | 92 |
| 1 | 16 | 1 | 6 |
| 10 | 14 | 0 | 0 |

Beginning at age 50 days, L-E male rats were given a series of four intravenous injections of the polycyclic hydrocarbon 7, 8, 12-trimethylbenzanthracene, 35 mg/kg, at biweekly intervals. The azodye Sudan III (1-(*p*-phenylazo-phenylazo)-2-naphthol), 1 mg or 10 mg, dissolved in 2 ml sesame oil was fed by gastric instillation at 40 hr and again at 24 hr before each injection. Controls were fed 2 ml sesame oil. (Quoted from ref. *42*) other known quinone reductases—*e.g.*, the mitochondrial NADH dehydrogenase and the microsomal NADH-cytochrome $b_5$ and NADPH-cytochrome P-450 reductases—which are one-electron quinone reductases, giving rise to semiquinones prone to autoxidation and $O_2 \cdot^-$ generation. DT-diaphorase was shown to prevent this "redox cycling" and thus to promote the detoxication of quinones by conjugation (*48*). DT-diaphorase is also active in reducing and detoxifying azodyes (*49*) and hexavalent chromium compounds (*50*). Furthermore, it can act as a nitroreductase, but in this case the reduction may result in the activation of a carcinogen (*10, 51*). Likewise, reduction *via* DT-diaphorase has been implicated in the cytotoxicity of certain quinonoid drugs in human tumor cells (*52, 53*).

Another mechanism of quinone detoxication in which DT-diaphorase may be involved relates to the antioxidant function of superoxide dismutase (SOD). It was found that certain hydroquinones as formed by way of DT-diaphorase were still readily autoxized but could be stabilized by Cu, Zn-SOD as revealed by an inhibition of NAD(P)H oxidation, $O_2$ consumption and $H_2O_2$ accumulation (*54*). This was in contrast to the effect of SOD in the case of one-electron quinone reductases, *e.g.*, NADPH-cytochrome P-450 reductase, where SOD stimulated NADPH and $O_2$

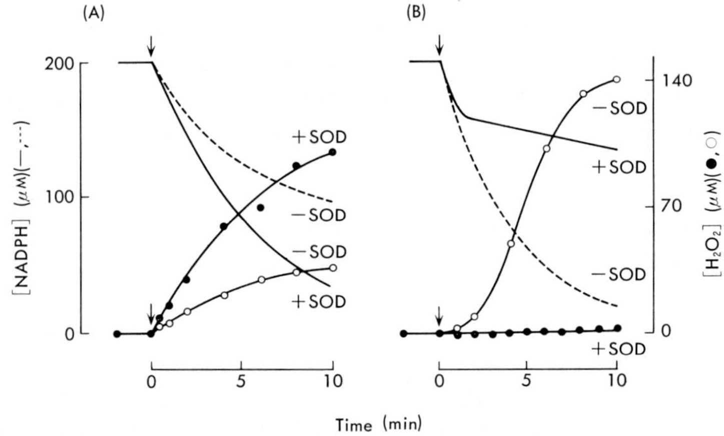


FIG. 3. Effect of SOD on NADPH oxidation and $H_2O_2$ formation lowing the reduction of 2, 3-dimethoxy-1,4-naphthoquinone by NADPH-cytochrome P-450 reductase or DT-diaphorase. The reaction was started by the addition of NADPH-cytochrome P-450 reductase (A) or DT-diaphorase (B) as indicated by the arrow. (From ref. *55*)

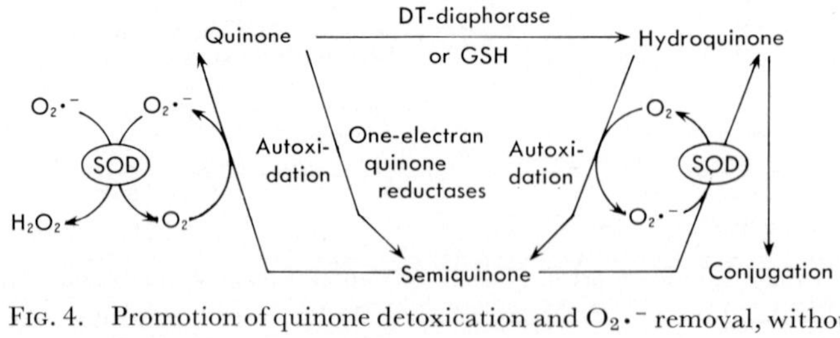


FIG. 4. Promotion of quinone detoxication and $O_2 \cdot^-$ removal, without the concomitant accumulation of $H_2O_2$, through the concerted action of SOD and either DT-diaphorase or the reductive addition of GSH.

consumption and $H_2O_2$ formation (*55*). The experiment shown in Fig. 3 illustrates this contrast, using 2,3-dimethoxy-1,4-naphthoquinone (a quinone that has recently been shown (*34*) to cause an activation of protein kinase C in isolated hepatocytes, due to an altered thiol/disulfide status of the enzyme). The SOD effect in preventing hydroquinone autoxidation was dependent on the structure of the quinone; for example, it did not occur with 5-hydroxy-1,4-naphthoquinones (*56*). Autoxidation of hydroquinones that were produced by the reductive addition of glutathione was likewise inhibited by SOD (*56, 57*), and Cu,Zn- and Mn-SOD were equally active (*57*).

On the basis of the above findings it has been suggested (*54*) that SOD in addition to its well-recognized function, may act as "superoxide-semiquinone oxidoreductase", as schematically illustrated in Fig. 4. Alternatively, it has been proposed (*58*) that SOD may prevent hydroquinone autoxidation by suppressing a $O_2\cdot^-$-dependent free radical propagation. Arguments for and against either mechanism have been considered (*55, 59, 60*), and the final answer will have to await further investigation. Regardless of the underlying mechanism, however, the ability of SOD to prevent the autoxidation of hydroquinones produced by DT-diaphorase or by the reductive addition of GSH represents an important new aspect of the antioxidant function of SOD, which enables the enzyme to remove $O_2\cdot^-$ *without* the concomitant accumulation of $H_2O_2$. As pointed out above, there is growing evidence for a central role of $H_2O_2$ in oxygen toxicity, both as a precursor of OH•—the radical species directly responsible for DNA and protein damage—and as an oxidant of GSH through GSH peroxidase, thus perturbing protein thiol/disulfide status and $Ca^{2+}$ homeostasis. In addition, $H_2O_2$ is an inhibitor of SOD (*cf.* ref. *61* and refs. therein), a circumstance that may be especially critical in the context of quinone redox metabolism, which probably constitutes a major potential source of cellular oxygen-radical production from xenobiotics.

In this context, it seems appropriate to discuss some aspects of the regulation of chemoprotective enzymes in general and DT-diaphorase in particular. This topic has been the subject of numerous reviews over the years (*cf.*, *e.g.*, refs. *62–65*) and will only briefly be considered here. Chemoprotective enzymes may be defined as those involved in the removal of reactive metabolites that are derived from toxic xenobiotics. They are often referred to as "Phase II enzymes", as opposed to the "Phase I enzymes" responsible for the formation of the reactive metabolites; the latter are as a rule members of the cytochrome P-450 "superfamily" of enzymes. This classification seemed to be useful as a basis for studying the genetic regulation of the enzymes involved—the "*Ah* gene battery"—under various experimental, physiological and pathological conditions, an approach extensively pursued especially in Nebert's laboratory (*65*). At the same time, however, it has its shortcomings, both from the point of view of definition and in its functional implications. For example, DT-diaphorase may be defined as a "Phase II enzyme" as a quinone reductase, and a "Phase I enzyme" as a nitroreductase. In addition, it is now clear that there is no compulsory functional link between the two classes of enzymes. For example, DT-diaphorase can be induced in a cell line that lacks functional aryl hydrocarbon monooxygenase, as elegantly demonstrated by Prochaska and Talalay (*66*). At the same time, highly interesting recent results by Favreau and Pickett (*67*) reveal the occurrence of two separate regulatory elements associated with the 5′-flanking region of the DT-diaphorase gene,

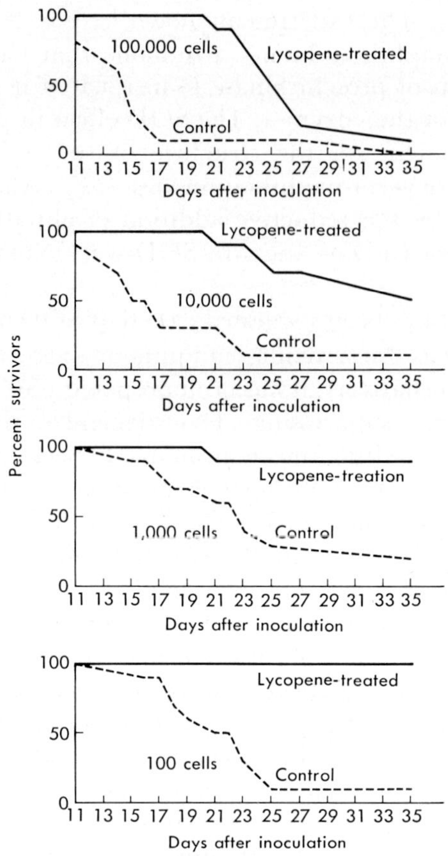


FIG. 5. Effect of lycopene on the lethality of Ehrlich ascites tumor growth in mice. When indicated, the mice were treated with 1 mg lycopene injected intraperitoneally 24 hr before inoculation of the amount of Ehrlich ascites tumor cells as indicated. (From ref. *75*)

one responsive to planar aromatic xenobiotics (XRE) and identical with the XRE found in the cytochrome P-450 IA1 gene; and one to antioxidants that act as inducers of the enzyme (ARE). Similar and structurally closely related elements are found in the gene of the *Ya* subunit of glutathione-S-transferases (*68*), another "Phase II enzyme". Clearly, XRE responds to polycyclic hydrocarbons regardless of whether or not these can be metabolized, *i.e.*, probably to the *Ah* receptor rather than to the active cytochrome P-450. The ARE may respond to antioxidants or their metabolites or, as indicated by recent work from Talalay's laboratory (*69*), to electrophiles that are Michael reaction acceptors and substrates to glutathione-S-transferase. In the last analysis, it may respond simply to $H_2O_2$, similar to Ames and associates' bacterial *oxy*R gene regulator (*70*), possibly through a peroxide- and GSH-modulated thiol group of a regulatory protein (*71*).

A final question relates to the role of dietary antioxidants in chemoprotection. There is growing evidence that especially carotenoids and vitamin E may exert a protective effect against chemical carcinogenesis (*cf.* ref. *72*). Among the carotenoids, particular interest has recently been focused on lycopene, by demonstrating that it quenches $^1O_2$ with higher efficiency than does β-carotene (*73*). In this connection, it is interesting to recall that a little over 30 years ago, lycopene has been reported to induce a remarkable resistance in mice against radiation damage (*74*), bacterial toxicity, and Ehrlich ascites tumor growth (Fig. 5) (*75*). Of further interest is the fact that cancer cells have been shown to exhibit a strikingly poor ability to undergo lipid peroxidation and that this feature seems to be related to an enhanced capacity of these cells to store dietary antioxidants, mainly vitamin E (*76*).

*Concluding Remarks*

Viewed from the perspective of chemical carcinogenesis, it seems that there is today a great deal of information that has been derived from studies of cytochrome P-450 and DT-diaphorase, their metabolic function and genetic regulation, and their relationship to other pro- and antioxidant enzymes including various types of quinone reductase, carbonyl reductase, glutathione transferase and peroxidase, SOD, catalase, epoxide hydrolase, *etc*. The picture that emerges suggests that chemical carcinogenesis and its prevention share a common denominator, namely, the metabolic activation of a xenobiotic that can lead, on one hand, to the initiation, promotion and progression of the carcinogenic process through reactive species of $O_2$, and, on the other hand, to an induction of antioxidant mechanisms that prevent these effects. The final outcome will depend on the relative impact of the two events.

To assess this, we need better insight into the mechanisms that are responsible for the coordinate regulation of the enzymes and other factors involved. The demonstration of a coordinate regulation of DT-diaphorase and glutathione-S-transferase at the gene level is an important step in this direction and will hopefully open the way to an understanding of the factors that govern the expression of the two genes. For example, growing Zajdela ascites tumor in the rat induces liver DT-diaphorase but not glutathione-S-transferase (*77*). Another important problem is to understand the regulation of SOD *versus* DT-diaphorase. Many tumors contain high DT-diaphorase levels (*78*) but low SOD (*79*); there is also an example of the converse situation, in diethylstilbestol-induced kidney tumor in golden hamsters (*80*). As discussed earlier in this paper, DT-diaphorase, in order to act efficiently as an antioxidant enzyme requires SOD; and *vice versa*, SOD may require DT-diaphorase as a "partner" to detoxify $O_2{\cdot}^-$ produced by hydroquinone autoxidation. What, if any, are the mechanisms for the coordination of DT-diaphorase and SOD biosynthesis?

In conclusion, an elucidation of the molecular mechanisms by which cells can acquire resistance against chemical carcinogens may provide a rationale for devising drugs that protect against these chemicals without themselves being carcinogenic.

*Acknowledgments*

I wish to express my thanks to Drs. Enrique Cadenas (Los Angeles), Joseph W. DePierre (Stockholm), and Cecil B. Pickett (Montreal) for stimulating discussions, and to Ms. Ann Nielsen and Ms. Kerstin Nordenbrand for excellent editorial help during the preparation of this paper. Work quoted from the author's laboratory has been supported by the Swedish Cancer Foundation, the Swedish Medical and Natural Science Research Councils, and the National Cancer Institute, National Institutes of Health, U.S.A.

## REFERENCES

1. Rous, P. Transmission of malignant new growth by means of a cell-free filtrate. J. Am. Med. Assoc., *56*: 198, 1911.
2. Toyoshima, K. Nakahara Memorial Lecture at the 17th International Symposium of the Princess Takamatsu Cancer Research Fund, Tokyo, 1986.
3. Yamagiwa, K. and Ishikawa, K. Experimentelle Studie über die Pathogenese der Epithegeschwülste. Mitt. Fak. K. Jpn. Univ. Tokyo, *15*: 295–344, 1916.
4. Kennaway, E. L. The formation of cancer-producing substance from isoprene (2-methyl-butadiene). J. Pathol. Bacteriol., *27*: 233–238, 1924.
5. Yoshida, T. Proc. Imp. Acad. Tokyo, *8*: 464–467, 1932 (quoted from ref. *8*).
6. Kinoshita, R. Osaka Igakukai Zasshi, *35*: 403–406, 1936 (in Japanese).
7. Nakahara, W., Fujiwara, T., and Mori, K. Inhibiting effect of yeast feeding on experimental production of liver cancer. Gann, *33*: 57–65, 1939.
8. Sugimura, T. Studies on environmental chemical carcinogenesis in Japan. Science, *233*: 312–318, 1988.
9. Nakahara, W., Fukuoka, F., and Sugimura, T. Carcinogenic action of 4-nitroquinoline-N-oxide. Gann, *48*: 129–137, 1957.
10. Sugimura, T., Okabe, K., and Nagao, M. The metabolism of 4-nitroquinoline-N-oxide. Cancer Res., *26*: 1717–1721, 1966.
11. Sugimura, T. Carcinogenicity of mutagenic heterocyclic amines formed during the cooking process. Mutat. Res., *150*: 33–41, 1985.
12. Ames, B. N., Durston, W. E., Yamasaki, E., and Lee, F. D. Carcinogens are mutagens. A simple test system combining liver homogenates for activation and bacteria for defection. Proc. Natl. Acad. Sci. U.S.A., *70*: 2281–2285, 1973.
13. Ames, B. N., Lee, F. D., and Durston, W. E. An improval test system and classification of mutagens and carcinogens. Proc. Natl. Acad. Sci. U.S.A., *70*: 782–786, 1973.
14. Ames, B. N., Profet, M., and Gold, L. S. Dietary pesticides (99.99% all natural). Proc. Natl. Acad. Sci. U.S.A., *87*: 7777–7781, 1990.
15. Ames, B. N. and Gold, L. S. Natural chemicals, synthetic chemicals, risk assessment and cancer. This volume, pp. 303–314.
16. Berenblum, I. The carcinogenic action of croton resin. Cancer Res., *1*: 44–48, 1941.
17. Rous, P. and Kidd, J. G. Conditional neoplasms and subthreshold neoplastic states. A study of tar tumors in rabbits. J. Exp. Med., *73*: 365–390, 1941.
18. Bishop, J. M. Retroviruses and oncogenes II. Les Prix Nobel 1989, Almqvist & Wiksell, Stockholm, 1990, pp. 214–238.
19. Maskens, A. P., Ebbesen, P., and Burny, A. (eds.). Concepts and Theories in Carcinogenesis, Excerpta Medica, Vol. 732, Elsevier, Amsterdam, 1987.
20. Cerutti, P. Response modification creates promotability in multistage carcinogenesis. Carcinogenesis, *9*: 519–526, 1988.
21. Ames, B. N. Dietary carcinogens and anticarcinogens. Science, *221*: 1256–1264, 1983.
22. Kensler, T. W. and Trush, M. A. Role of oxygen radicals in tumor promotion. Environ. Mutagen., *6*: 593–616, 1984.
23. Cerutti, P. Prooxidant states and tumor promotion. Science, *227*: 375–380, 1985.
24. Ernster, L. Oxygen as an environmental poison. Chem. Scr., *26*: 525–534, 1986.
25. Ernster, L. Biochemistry of reoxygenation injury. Crit. Care Med., *16*: 947–953, 1988.
26. Miller, E. C. and Miller, J. A., Searches for ultimate chemical carcinogens and their reactions with cellular macromolecules. Cancer, *47*: 2327–2345, 1981.
27. Marnett, L. J. and Reed, G. A. Peroxidatic oxidation of benzo(a)pyrene and prosta-

glandin biosynthesis. Biochemistry, *18*: 2923-2929, 1979.
28. Cavalieri, E. and Rogan, E. Role of radical cations in aromatic hydrocarbon carcinogenesis. Environ. Health Persp., *64*: 69–84, 1985.
29. Marnett, L. J., Reddy, A., Pruess-Schwartz, D., and Ji, C. Oxidation of polycyclic hydrocarbons by oxygen radicals. This volume, pp. 63–73.
30. Chesis, P. L., Levin, D. E., Smith, M. T. S., Ernster, L., and Ames, B. N. Mutagenicity of quinones: Pathways of metabolic activation and detoxification. Proc. Natl. Acad. Sci. U.S.A., *81*: 1696–1700, 1984.
31. Vaca, C. E., Wilhelm, J., and Harms-Ringdahl, M. Interaction of lipid peroxidation products with DNA: A review. Mutat. Res., *195*: 137–149, 1988.
32. Anderson, D. (ed.). Effect of active oxygen species on the genetic apparatus. Mutat. Res. (special issue), 1988.
33. Jones, D. P., McConkey, D. J., Nicotera, P., and Orrenius, S. Calcium-activated DNA fragmentation in rat liver nuclei. J. Biol. Chem., *264*: 6398–6403, 1989.
34. Kass, G. E. N., Duddy, S. K., and Orrenius, S. Activation of hepatocyte protein kinase C by redox-cycling quinones. Biochem. J., *260*: 499–507, 1989.
35. Fujiki, H. and Sugimura, T. New potent tumour promotors: teleocidin, lyngbyatoxin A and aplysiatoxin. Cancer Survey, *2*: 539–556, 1983.
36. Bulkley, G. B. The role of oxygen free radicals in human disease processes. Surgery, *94*: 407–411, 1983.
37. Saul, R. L., Gee, P., and Ames, B. N. Free radicals, DNA damage, and aging. *In*; H. R. Warner *et al.* (eds.), Modern Biological Theories of Aging, pp. 113–129, Raven Press, New York, 1987.
38. Kass, G. E. N., Nicotera, P., and Orrenius, S. Effects of xenobiotics on signal transduction and $Ca^{2+}$ mediated processes in mammalian cells. This volume, pp. 213–226.
39. Conney, A. H., Miller, E. C., and Miller, J. A. The metabolism of methylated aminoazo dyes. V. Evidence for induction of enzyme synthesis in the rat by 3-methylcholanthrene. Cancer Res., *16*: 450–459, 1956.
40. Conney, A. H., Miller, E. C., and Miller, J. A. Substrate-induced synthesis and other properties of benzpyrene hydroxylase in rat liver. J. Biol. Chem., *228*: 753–756, 1957.
41. Richardson, H. L. and Cunningham, L. The inhibitory action of methylcholanthrene on rats fed the azo dye 3′-methyl-4-dimethylaminoazobenzene. Cancer Res., *11*: 274, 1951.
42. Huggins, C. B. Experimental Leukemia and Mammary Cancer. Inducton, Prevention, Cure, University of Chicago Press, Chicago, 1979.
43. Williams-Ashman, H. G. and Huggins, C. Oxidation of reduced pyridine nucleotides in mammary gland and adipose tissue following treatment with polynuclear hydrocarbons. Med. Exp., *4*: 223–226, 1961.
44. Huggins, C. and Fuknnishi, R. Induced protection of adrenal cortext against 7,12-dimethylbenz[a]anthracene. Influence of ethionine. Induction of menadione reductase. Incorporation of thymidine-$^3$H. J. Exp. Med., *119*: 923–942, 1964.
45. Ernster, L., Ljunggren, M., and Danielson, L. Purification and some properties of a highly dicoumarol sensitive liver diaphorase. Biochem. Biophys. Res. Commun., *2*: 88–92, 1960.
46. Ernster, L. DT-Diaphorase: A historial review. Chem. Scr., *27A*: 1–13, 1987.
47. Iyanagi, T. and Yamazaki, I. One-electron transfer reactions in biochemical systems. V. Difference in the mechanism of quinone reduction by the NADH dehydrogenase and NAD(P)H dehydrogenase (DT-diaphorase). Biochim. Biophys. Acta, *216*: 282–294, 1970.
48. Lind, C., Hochstein, P., and Ernster, L. DT-diaphorase as a quinone reductase: a

cellular control device against semiquinone and superoxide radical formation. Arch. Biochem. Biophys., *216*: 178–185, 1982.

49. Huang, M.-T., Miwa, G. T., and Lu, A. Y. H. Rat liver cytosolic azoreductase. Purification and characterization. J. Biol. Chem., *254*: 3930–3934, 1979.
50. De Flora, S., Morelli, A., Basso, C., Romano, M., Serra, D., and De Flora, A. Prominent role of DT-diaphorase as a cellular mechanism reducing chromium (VI) and reverting its mutagenicity. Cancer Res., *45*: 3188–3196, 1985.
51. Knox, R. J., Boland, M. P., Friedlos, P., Coles, B., Southan, C., and Roberts, J. J. The nitroreductase enzyme in Walker cells that activates 5-(aziridin-1-yl)-2, 4-dinitrobenzamide (CB 1954) to 5-(aziridin-1-yl)-4-hydroxylamino-2-nitrobenzamide is a form of NAD(P)H dehydrogenase (quinone) (EC 1.6.99.2). Biochem. Pharmacol., *37*: 4671–4677, 1988.
52. Siegel, D., Gibson, N. W., Preusch, P. C., and Ross, D. Metabolism of diaziquinone (AZQ) by NAD(P)H: (quinone acceptor) oxidoreductase (DT-diaphorase): role in AZQ-induced DNA damage and cytotoxicity in human colon carcinoma cells. Cancer Res., *50*: 7239–7300, 1990.
53. Siegel, D., Gibson, N. W., Preusch, P. C., and Ross, D. Metabolism of mitomycin C by DT-diaphorase: role in mitomycin C-induced DNA damage and cytotoxicity in human colon carcinoma cells. Cancer Res., *50*: 7483–7489, 1990.
54. Cadenas, E., Mira, D., Brunmark, A., Lind, C., Segura Aguilar, J., and Ernster, L. Effect of superoxide dismutase on the autoxidation of various hydroquinones. A possible role of superoxide dismutase as superoxide: semiquinone oxidoreductase. Free Rad. Biol. Med., *5*: 71–79, 1988.
55. Öllinger, K., Buffinton, G. D., Ernster, L., and Cadenas, E. Effect of superoxide dismutase on the autoxidation of substituted hydro- and semi-naphthoquinones. Chem. Biol. Interact., *73*: 53–76, 1990.
56. Buffinton, G. D., Öllinger, K., Brunmark, A., and Cadenas, E. DT-diaphorase-catalyzed reduction of 1,4-naphthoquinone derivatives and glutathione-quinone conjugates. Effect of substitution on autoxidation rates. Biochem. J., *257*: 561–571, 1989.
57. Llopis, J., Ernster, L., and Cadenas, E. Effects of glutathione on the redox transistions of naphthoquinone derivatives formed during DT-diaphorase catalysis. Free Rad. Res. Commun., *8*: 271–285, 1990.
58. Winterbourn, C. C., Cowden, W. B., and Sutton, H. C. Auto-oxidation of dialuric acid, divicine, and isouramil. Superoxide dependent and independent mechanisms. Biochem. Pharmacol., *38*: 611–618, 1989.
59. Ishii, T. and Fridovich, I. Dual effects of superoxide dismutase on the autoxidation of 1,4-naphthohydroquinone. Free Rad. Biol. Med., *8*: 21–24.
60. Bandy, B., Moon, J., and Davison, A. J. Multiple actions of superoxide dismutase: why can it both inhibit and stimulate reduction of oxygen by hydroquinones? Free Rad. Biol. Med., *9*: 143–148, 1990.
61. Salo, D. C., Pacifici, R. E., Lin, S. W., Giulivi, C., and Davies, K. J. A. Superoxide dismutase undergoes proteolysis and fragmentation following oxidative modification and inactivation. J. Biol. Chem., *265*: 11919–11927, 1990.
62. DePierre, J. W. and Ernster, L. The metabolism of polycyclic hydrocarbons and its relationship to cancer. Biochim. Biophys. Acta, *473*: 49–106, 1978.
63. Ernster, L., Estabrook, R. W., Hochstein, P., and Orrenius, S. (eds.). DT-diaphorase: A Quinone reductase with special functions in cell metabolism and detoxication. Chem. Scr., *27A*: 1987.
64. Pickett, C. B. and Lu, A. Y. H. Glutathione-S-transferases: Gene structure, regulation, and biological function. Annu. Rev. Biochem., *58*: 743–764, 1989.

65. Nebert, D. W., Petersen, D. D., and Fornace, A. J. Cellular responses to oxidative stress: the [*Ah*] gene battery as a paradigm. Environ. Health Persp., *88*: 13–25, 1990.
66. Prochaska, H. J. and Talalay, P. Regulatory mechanisms of monofunctional and bifunctional anticarcinogenic enzyme inducers in mouse liver. Cancer Res., *48*: 4776–4782, 1988.
67. Favreau, L. V. and Pickett, C. B. Transcriptional regulation of the rat liver NAD(P)H: quinone reductase gene. J. Biol. Chem., *266*: 4556–4561, 1991.
68. Rushmore, T. H., King, R. G., Paulson, K. E., and Pickett, C. B. Regulation of glutathione-S-transferase *Ya* subunit gene expression: Identification of a unique xenobiotic-responsive element controlling inducible expression by planar aromatic compounds. Proc. Natl. Acad. Sci. U.S.A., *87*: 3826–3830, 1990.
69. Talalay, P., De Long, M. J., and Prochaska, H. J. Identification of common chemical signal regulating the induction of enzymes that protect against chemical carcinogenesis. Proc. Natl. Acad. Sci. U.S.A., *85*: 8261–8265, 1988.
70. Storz, G., Tartaglia, L. A., and Ames, B. N. Transcriptional regulator of oxidative stress-inducible genes: Direct activation by oxidation. Science, *248*: 189–194, 1990.
71. Talalay, P., Prochaska, H. J., and Spencer, S.R. Regulation of enzymes that detoxify the electrophilic forms of chemical carcinogens. This volume, pp. 177–187.
72. Di Mascio, P., Murphy, M. E., and Sies, H. Antioxidant defense systems: The role of carotenoids, tocopherols, and thiol. Am. J. Clin. Nutr., *53*: 194S–200S, 1991.
73. Di Mascio, P., Kaiser, S., and Sies, H. Lycopene as the most efficient biological carotenoid singlet oxygen quencher. Arch. Biochem. Biophys., *274*: 532–538, 1989.
74. Forssberg, A., Lingen, C., Ernster, L., and Lindberg, O. Modification of the X-irradiation syndrome by lycopene. Exp. Cell Res., *16*: 7–14, 1959.
75. Lingen, C., Ernster, L., and Lindberg, O. The promoting effect of lycopene on the non-specific resistance of animals. Exp. Cell Res., *16*: 384–393, 1959.
76. Cheesman, K. H., Collins, M., Proudfoot, K., Slater, T. F., Burton, D. W., Webb, A. C., and Ingold, K. U. Studies on lipid peroxidation in normal and tumour tissues. The Novikoff rat liver tumour. Biochem. J., *235*: 507–514, 1986.
77. Beyer, R. E., Segura-Aguilar, J., and Ernster, L. The anticancer enzyme DT-diaphorase is induced selectively in liver during ascites hepatoma growth. Anticancer Res., *8*: 233–238, 1988.
78. Schor, N. A. DT-Diaphorase and the cancer cell. Chem. Scr., *27A*: 135–139, 1987.
79. Oberley, L. W. Superoxide dismutase and cancer. *In;* Oberley, L. W., (ed.), Superoxide Dismutase, Vol. II, pp. 127–165, CRC Press, Boca Raton, 1982.
80. Segura-Aguilar, J., Cortés-Vizcaino, V., Llombart-Bosch, A., Ernster, L., Monsalve, E., and Romero, F. J. The levels of quinone reductases, superoxide dismutase, and glutathione-related enzymatic activities in diethylstilbestrol-induced carcinogenesis in the kidney of male Syrian golden hamsters. Carcinogenesis, *11*: 1727–1732, 1990.

# BIOACTIVATION OF XENOBIOTICS

XENOBIOTICS AND CANCER, L. ERNSTER ET AL. (EDS.),
JAPAN SCI. SOC. PRESS, TOKYO/TAYLOR & FRANCIS LTD., LONDON, pp. 33–44, 1991

# Cytochrome P-450s as Toxicogenic Catalysts: The Influence of Dehydroepiandrosterone

Ronald W. ESTABROOK,*[1] Leon MILEWICH,*[1] and Russell A. PROUGH*[2]

*Department of Biochemistry and Obstetrics and Gynecology and the Cecil H. and Ida M. Green Center for Reproductive Biology Sciences, University of Texas Southwestern Medical Center, Dallas, Texas 75235, U.S.A.*[1] and the Department of Biochemistry, University of Louisville Medical Center, Louisville, Kentucky 40292, U.S.A.*[2]*

*Abstract:* The cytochrome P-450s catalyze the oxidative transformation of a large number of endogenous and exogenous chemicals in plants, insects, and mammals. One consequence of this type of reaction is the generation of highly reactive electrophilic metabolites that can react with intracellular macromolecules. It has been postulated that the initiation reaction for chemical carcinogenesis and/or cellular toxicity involves the metabolism of xenobiotics by P-450s.

The naturally occurring steroid dehydroepiandrosterone (DHEA), when administered as a supplement to the diet of rodents, has been reported to have anti-carcinogenic and other chemoprotective activities. A change in the inventory of liver P-450s occurs during treatment of rodents with DHEA, the most pronounced being that involved in the omega-hydroxylation of medium-chain length fatty acids. In addition, changes in the activities of other liver P-450s, *viz.*, P-450IIB1, P-450IIC11, and P-450IIIA, occur as shown by *in vitro* experiments to assess the P-450-dependent formation of hydroxylated metabolites of testosterone and androstenedione. The effect of feeding rodents a diet supplemented with DHEA mimics some of the changes seen when animals are treated with hypolipidemic drugs (such as ciprofibrate, and other chemicals which are known to be peroxisome proliferators).

Studies comparing the enzymatic functions of the heterologous expressed recombinant forms of $P\text{-}450_{17\alpha}$, responsible for the two step conversions of progesterone and pregnenolone to the $C_{19}$-steroids, androstenedione, and DHEA, respectively, illustrated the marked differences in enzymatic properties between the human and the rat orthologues. The findings serve to demonstrate that DHEA is an obligatory intermediate for the synthesis of androgens in the human, but not in the rodent.

The biochemical changes responsible for the anti-carcinogenic properties of DHEA remain to be identified. The studies presented here suggest that DHEA, when administered as a dietary supplement, functions like a xenobiotic, and that its effects may result from alterations in the inventory of cellular P-450s, thereby influencing the balance of metabolic activities associated with the initiation phase of chemical carcinogenesis and/or toxicity.

Understanding the event(s) that trigger the transformation of a normal cell to a cancer cell is a major challenge for modern biology. In many instances exposure of an animal to a variety of different chemicals results in the formation of either preneoplastic nodules and/or tumors or in a change in cellular homeostasis associated with tissue necrosis. Is there a common pathway that leads to both uncontrolled cell proliferation, *i.e.*, loss of regulation of cell growth and division associated with cancer, and the onset of cell death, *i.e.*, as the result of toxic reactions? Once understood, will it be possible to modify the cell environment and thereby attenuate the subsequent sequence of reactions that lead to tumor formation? Similar questions can be asked about the reactions associated with cellular toxicity.

Cytochrome P-450s are members of a gene superfamily of hemoproteins that catalyze the oxidative metabolism of a great variety of chemicals, both endogenous and exogenous. It is recognized that one or more of these P-450s play a key role in the activation of inert precarcinogenic chemicals (xenobiotics), a process that leads to the formation of highly reactive electrophilic products that can chemically alter critical intracellular macromolecules. A number of different P-450s have been shown to catalyze reactions leading to the formation of reactive metabolites, *e.g.*, P-450IA1 (polycyclic aromatic hydrocarbons), P-450IA2 (acetylaminofluorene, biphenyl or aromatic amines), P-450IIB (bromobenzene or carbon tetrachloride), P-450IIC and P-450IIIA (aflatoxins), to name but a few. In addition to activating inert xenobiotics, P-450s frequently act as detoxifying enzymes by catalyzing the conversion of many pharmacologically active drugs and other foreign chemicals to inactive metabolites. Thus P-450s should be considered as having a duality of function, *viz.*, the detoxification of some chemicals to less active hydrophobic metabolites or the activation of inert chemicals to reactive toxic compounds. It is in this latter role that we propose a toxicogenic function—that is, capable of producing atoxic substance—for P-450s as the common thread for both chemical carcinogenesis and cell toxicity (Fig. 1).

In addition to the role of P-450s in the oxidative metabolism of xenobiotics, these hemoproteins are believed to be responsible, in part, for the generation of reactive

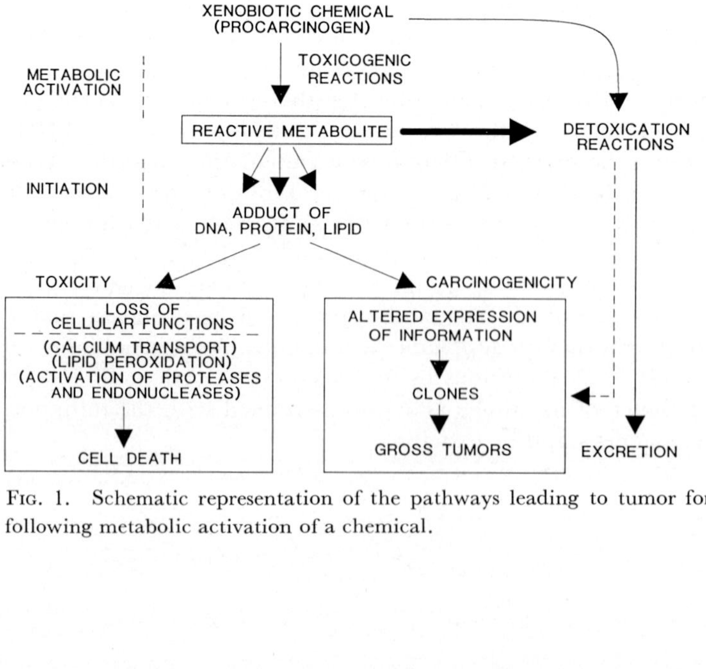


FIG. 1. Schematic representation of the pathways leading to tumor formation or cell toxicity following metabolic activation of a chemical.

species of oxygen, such as superoxide or hydrogen peroxide (*1*). These reactive oxygen species can be formed either directly by decomposition of the key intermediate oxyP450—the ternary complex of reduced P-450, molecular oxygen, and substrate—or by the further oxidation of primary metabolites to secondary metabolites, such as quinones—which can then undergo redox cycling.

Thus, a better understanding of changes in the activity or types of P-450s in tissue sites of action may provide important information concerning the initial events critical to the onset of carcinogenesis or cellular toxicity.

### *The Cytochrome P-450s*

The P-450s are intracellular, membrane-bound hemoproteins found associated with either the mitochondria or the endoplasmic reticulum of many cells. The P-450s are lipophilic proteins that occur as monomers with molecular weights between 45,000–60,000 Daltons. These hemoproteins are widely distributed in Nature where they play an important role in the synthesis of such varied compounds as flavors and pigments of plants, moulting hormones of insects, physiologically important steroid hormones such as androgens and estrogens and metabolites of polyunsaturated fatty acids such as thromboxane and prostacyclin, among others. The P-450s can be major contributors to the inventory of proteins in cells, *e.g.*, in rodent liver the P-450s may contribute up to 4% of the total cellular protein, representing as much as 20% of the protein of the endoplasmic reticulum.

Our knowledge of the number and variety of the P-450s continues to expand at a rapid pace. Recently (*2*) it has been reported that 146 different P-450s have been cloned and sequenced. The genes encoding these hemoproteins have been described in 24 eukaryotes (including 10 mammalian and 1 plant species) and 4 prokaryotes. For each P-450 gene that has been studied in detail, one can estimate that there are at least three or more additional genes being evaluated or awaiting identification. The P-450s that have been characterized can be classified into 26 gene families (Fig. 2)

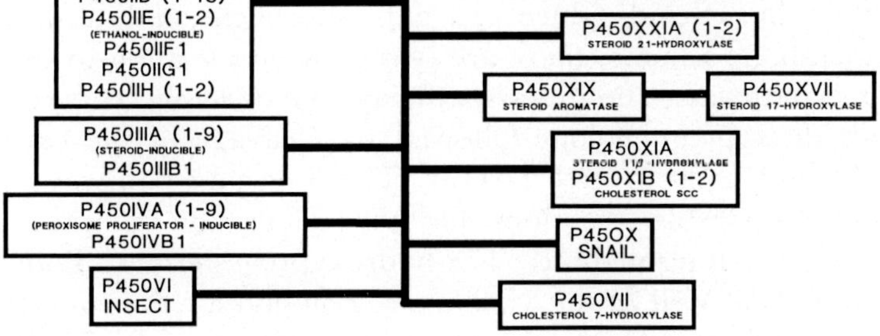


FIG. 2. The superfamily of cytochrome P-450s. A P-450 whose protein sequence is more than 40% similar to those of other P-450s is assigned to a specific gene family. The numbers in brackets indicate the number of P-450s in a family or subfamily.

based on protein sequence similarity: in most cases, the members of a P-450 family will have greater than 40% amino acid sequence similarity. Clearly, the P-450s represent a large superfamily of hemoproteins that are present across the breadth of phylogeny.

The P-450s have a number of unique properties, among which the following are most notable:

1. P-450s have divergent mechanisms of regulation of synthesis because they are expressed in specific tissues during various stages of development and frequently are under transcriptional or translational control, *i.e.*, they are rapidly induced on exposure of an animal to many xenobiotics;

2. P-450s have a special chemistry for oxygen activation that involves a thiolate-ligand for the heme prosthetic group. Many P-450s have been shown to function as oxygenases, peroxygenases as well as oxidases. The P-450s are believed to function by facilitating hydrogen abstraction from the chemical to be metabolized. This generates a highly reactive free radical intermediate capable of reacting with activated oxygen (a caged hydroxyl radical) to form an oxidized (hydroxylated) product. In addition, the P-450s can catalyze a cooxygenation reaction with many organic peroxides or they can catalyze the rearrangement of endo- and exoperoxides of polyunsaturated fatty acid metabolites, *e.g.*, the prostaglandins or hydroperoxyeicosatrienoic acids;

3. In many instances P-450s have a high specificity for the substrate metabolized suggesting a unique active site geometry for the enzyme. In many other instances, P-450s are known to be very promiscuous with a broad substrate specificity. The latter property is most common for those P-450s involved in the metabolism of xenobiotics;

4. It is believed that many P-450s have a defined membrane topology that permits them to act in concert with other membrane-bound P-450s, as well as enzymes that catalyze the Phase II metabolism of products formed following the oxidation of xenobiotics.

These are but a few examples of some of the properties of the P-450s. Clearly, these hemoproteins represent a remarkable and important group of enzymes.

### *Chemopreventive Effects of Dehydroepiandrosterone (DHEA)*

One of the most important physiological roles for P-450s is the catalysis of reactions for the synthesis and metabolism of steroid hormones. At least *five* well characterized P-450s are involved in the metabolic sequence of reactions that lead to the conversion of cholesterol to mineralocorticoids, glucocorticoids, androgens, and estrogens (Fig. 3). As shown in this metabolic scheme, there are two pathways leading to the formation of $C_{19}$ steroids. One pathway—the delta$^5$-pathway—involves the conversion of pregnenolone to 17$\alpha$-hydroxypregnenolone followed by cleavage of the carbon-carbon bond between C-17 and C-20 to give DHEA. The alternate pathway—the delta$^4$-pathway—involves comparable reactions for the conversion of progesterone to androstenedione *via* the intermediate, 17$\alpha$-hydroxyprogesterone. Both the 17$\alpha$-hydroxylation of steroids as well as the 17,20-lyase reaction for the conversion of the $C_{21}$-steroids to $C_{19}$-steroids are catalyzed by a single cytochrome P-450 (P-450$_{17\alpha}$).

In recent years great interest has focussed on the $C_{19}$-steroid DHEA (3$\beta$-hydroxy-5-androsten-17-one) (*3, 4*). As shown in Fig. 3 (highlighted) this steroid is a key inter-

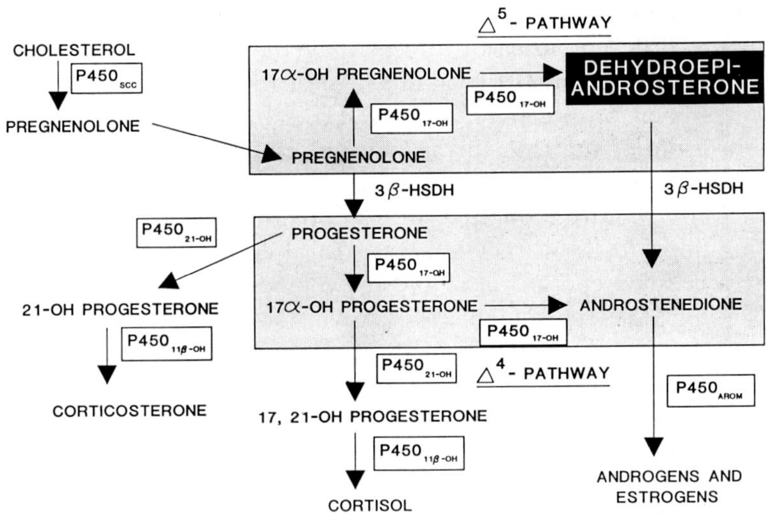


FIG. 3. Schematic representation of the pathway of cholesterol metabolism leading to the formation of mineralocorticoids, glucocorticoids, androgens, and estrogens. The various P-450s involved in the pathways of metabolism are indicated. The position of DHEA in the metabolic pathway has been highlighted.

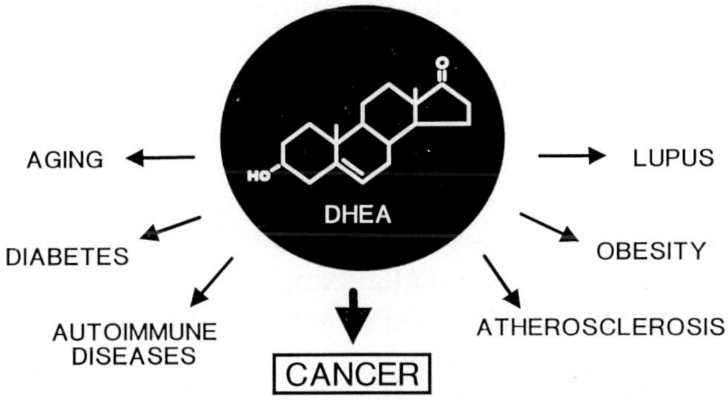


FIG. 4. The chemopreventive role of DHEA in designated disease states.

mediate in the delta$^5$-pathway, which leads to the formation of androgens and estrogens.

DHEA, administered as a supplement to the diet, has been reported to have remarkable chemopreventive effects on a variety of disease processes. For example, when rodents are provided DHEA as a dietary supplement (0.2–0.8% of the diet) beneficial effects have been observed in the normal progression of tumor formation (*5*), lupus erythematosus (*6*), obesity (*7*), diabetes (*8*), atherosclerosis (*9*), and the process of aging and loss of memory (*10*), to name but a few (Fig. 4). Of greatest interst is the reported action of this steroid as an anti-neoplastic agent and its demonstrated protective effect against the spontaneous formation of mammary cancer in female CH3 mice (*11*) and the onset of tumor formation after exposure of animals to chemical carcinogens (such as 7,12-dimethylbenz(a)anthracene or 1,2-dimethylhydrazine) and promoters, such as 12-O-tetradecanoylphorbol-13-acetate (*12, 13*).

Is there a biochemical rational for explaining the multiple beneficial effects of DHEA on so many different disease processes? What types of biochemical changes occur during the feeding of DHEA to rodents? And can one extrapolate these findings to humans? It has been proposed (*14*) that DHEA inhibits the enzyme, glucose-6-phosphate dehydrogenase, and that this inhibition results in a reduced rate of generation of NADPH with a consequent reduction in the rate of synthesis of pentose phosphates, which are required for the synthesis of ribonucleosides and deoxyribonucleosides, the building blocks of nucleic acids. An alternate hypothesis proposes that DHEA influences cellular energy metabolism by modifying ATP synthesis in mitochondria (*15*) or by participating in an energy utilizing futile cycle of fatty acid acylationdeacylation (*16*). Of interest to the present study is the proposal (*11*) that feeding large amounts of DHEA to rodents may influence cytochrome P-450-dependent mixed-function oxidation reactions, thereby reducing the amount (or rate) of formation of reactive metabolites generated from xenobiotics. Support for this last hypothesis is the recent study by Prasanna *et al.* (*17*) who showed that DHEA-feeding caused a 3-fold reduction in the covalent binding of 7,12-dimethylbenz(a)anthracene or aflatoxin metabolites to the DNA of liver.

### *DHEA as an Inducer of Liver Enzymes*

In the 1960s Selye (*18*) studied the ability of various steroids to protect animals from toxic agents. One of the most powerful of these "catatoxic" steroids was pregnenolone 16α-carbonitrile (PCN). Subsequent studies by Lu *et al.* (*19*) showed that administration of this steroid to rats in pharmacological doses—greater than 10 mg per kg body weight—resulted in the pronounced induction of what we know today as Family III P-450s (see Fig. 2). This P-450 family is recognized as the dominant type of P-450 in human livers where they catalyze the metabolism of a large number of drugs and other xenobiotics, *e.g.*, cyclosporin, aflatoxin, erythromycin.

Based on the earlier studies with PCN, experiments were initiated (*20*) to determine whether there was a comparable change in the content and type of P-450s in the livers of rats fed DHEA. For these studies, the rates of P-450-directed metabolism

TABLE 1. Effect of DHEA-feeding on Liver Enzymes

| | Control (nmole/min/mg protein) | DHEA-fed |
|---|---|---|
| Microsomal P-450 activities | | |
| Ethylmorphine | 7.5 | 3.6 |
| Benzphetamine | 5.8 | 5.5 |
| Aniline | 1.39 | 1.21 |
| Ethoxyresorufrin | 0.033 | 0.032 |
| Laurate 12- | 0.35 | 5.90 |
| 11- | 0.32 | 0.74 |
| Testosterone | 2.16 | 2.10 |
| Androstenedione | 1.96 | 2.10 |
| Peroxisome enzymes | | |
| Palmitoyl-CoA oxidase | 4.4 | 40.7 |
| Catalase | 45 | 86 |

of a number of different compounds were determined (Table 1) using liver microsomes prepared from untreated or DHEA-treated rats. In general the changes seen were minimal, although the observed greater than 50% decrease in the rate of ethylmorphine demethylation is considered significant. A greater than 80% increase in the activity of the flavoprotein, NADPH-cytochrome *c* (P-450) reductase, was noted also in the microsomes from rats fed DHEA. This increase in the activity of liver microsomal NADPH-cytochrome *c* reductase is similar to that seen following treatment of animals with phenobarbital. Most significant is the greater than 15-fold increase in the rate of omega-hydroxylation of the medium-chain length fatty acid, lauric acid. The induction of P-450IVA1, the P-450 that catalyzes the omega-hydroxylation of fatty acids, has been shown (*21*) to occur when animals are treated with drugs that act as peroxisome proliferators, such as the hypolipidemic drug ciprofibrate, or the plasticizer, di(2-ethylhexyl)phthalate (*22*).

Studies were conducted to determine whether other enzymes, known to increase in activity during treatment of rodents with agents that cause peroxisome proliferation, were affected by DHEA (*20, 23*). Indeed, as presented in Table 1, large increases in the activities of palmitoyl-CoA oxidase and catalase were seen during treatment of rats with DHEA. A similar conclusion was made by Leighton *et al.* (*24*) following treatment of animals with DHEA-acetate.

Tamburini *et al.* (*21*) had shown that purified P-450IVA1 was a poor metabolizer of steroids such as testosterone. The data presented in Table 1 shows no change in the overall rate of metabolism of testosterone or androstenedione following incubation with microsomes prepared from untreated or DHEA-treated rats. However, when the individual metabolites formed during the metabolism of testosterone or androstenedione were compared by use of HPLC (Fig. 5), it was apparent that major changes in the types of P-450 in the liver of DHEA-treated rats had occurred. As different P-450s catalyze unique site-specific hydroxylations of steroids, the rate of formation of individual metabolites generated from testosterone or androstenedione can serve as a "fingerprint" of the different P-450s present in liver tissue. The data presented

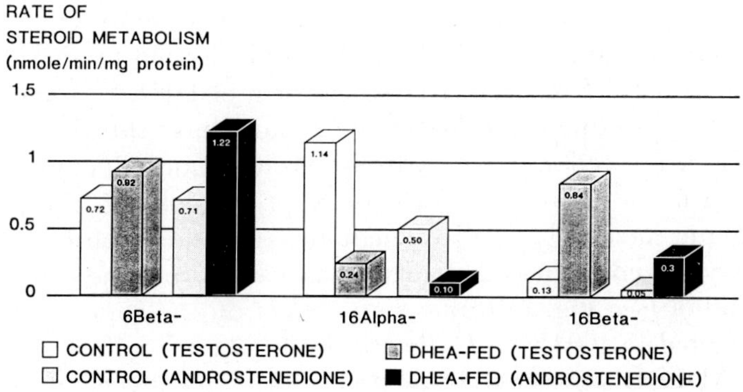


FIG. 5. Rates of site-specific hydroxylation of testosterone and androstenedione. Microsomes were prepared from livers of rats fed either a control diet (AIN-76A) or the same diet supplemented with DHEA (0.45%). The experiments were carried out by incubating microsomes (1 mg protein/ml) with steroid (100 $\mu$M), NADPH (0.2 mM) plus a generating system consisting of isocitrate and isocitrate dehydrogenase. Aliquots of the reaction mixtures were sampled, extracted with methylene chloride, and the metabolites were separated by HPLC and quantified as described (*20*).

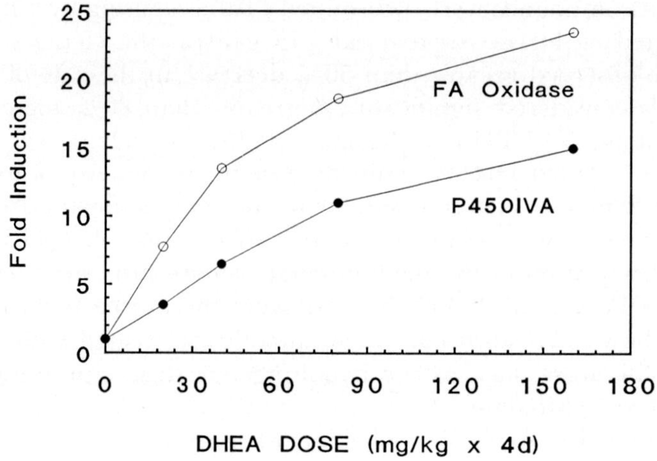


FIG. 6. Induction of liver P-450IVA and palmitoyl-CoA oxidase following treatment of male rats with varying concentrations of DHEA by intraperitoneal injection for 4 consecutive days (*20*).

in Fig. 5 indicates increases in the activities associated with P-450IIB1 (the major phenobarbital-inducible P-450), P-450IIIA (the PCN-inducible P-450), P-450IVA1 (the P-450 induced by peroxisome proliferators) and a decrease in the activity of P-450IIC11 (the male-specific P-450 of rat liver). From these results it is apparent that the activities of many different P-450s and those of other liver enzymes undergo changes following DHEA-treatment of rodents.

An extension of these studies showed (*20*) that DHEA, administered by intraperitoneal injection, was just as effective for inducing specific liver enzymes as was dietary DHEA. As shown in Fig. 6, daily injections of DHEA for 4 days at concentrations of about 100 mg per kg body weight caused large increases in the activities of the P-450 responsible for the omega-hydroxylation of lauric acid (P-450IVA) and the peroxisomal enzyme, palmitoyl-CoA oxidase. The convenience of the intraperitoneal technique for DHEA administration permitted the testing of many other steroids to evaluate their effectiveness as mimics of DHEA. The only steroid to give results comparable to those seen with DHEA was the reduced form of DHEA, 5-androstene-3$\beta$, 17$\beta$-diol (ADIOL). *In vitro* studies using liver homogenates have shown that the major metabolite of DHEA, produced by 17$\beta$-hydroxysteroid oxidoreductase catalysis, is ADIOL. Of interest was the failure of 17$\alpha$-hydroxypregnenolone—the precursor of DHEA in steroidogenic tissues—, androstenedione—the metabolite formed from DHEA on the pathway to androgen and estrogen synthesis—, and the active hormones testosterone and estradiol (see Fig. 3) to have any effect on the content or activity of the liver enzymes affected by DHEA (*4*). These results argue against the hypothesis that DHEA and/or ADIOL serve merely as precursors for conversion to active sex steroids that then can manifest the multiple biological effects seen at target tissues.

Using the technique of Western blot analysis, it was shown that DHEA or ADIOL-treatment of animals resulted also in the induction of P-450IVA in the kidney and lung of rodents. ADIOL and DHEA are equally effective for the induction of P-450IVA in liver. Of interest is the observation that ADIOL is far more effective than DHEA in inducing the protein in lung, while DHEA is more effective in inducing P-450IVA in kidney. The basis for these differences are currently under investigation.

*Heterologous Expression of Human and Rat P-$450_{17\alpha}$(s)*

Can the results of experiments carried out with rodents be extrapolated to humans? Is the role of DHEA in the pathway of steroid metabolism in rats the same as in humans? One approach to answer these questions is to examine the enzymatic properties of the key enzyme for the synthesis of DHEA—P-$450_{17\alpha}$—from rat and human. In recent years P-$450_{17\alpha}$(s) from a number of different species have been cloned and sequenced. Moreover, the cloned cDNAs for P-$450_{17\alpha}$ have been expressed as functional enzymes in COS cells (*25, 26*). It was of interest to compare the activities associated with recombinant P-$450_{17\alpha}$(s) of human and rat. For these experiments, the full length cDNAs were inserted in suitable viral vectors (pCMV—a plasmid derived from the cytomegalovirus) and transfected into COS cells (SV-40 transformed cells derived from the kidney of the African green monkey). Active enzyme is transiently expressed in the transfected COS cells that permits the determination of metabolism of different steroids (see ref *27* for summary). Studies with P-$450_{17\alpha}$(s) of rat and human showed comparable activities for the conversion of pregnenolone to 17α-hydroxypregnenolone and then to DHEA (*cf.* Fig. 3). However, when progesterone was used as the substrate, using similar transformed COS cells, it was noted that only the rat P-$450_{17\alpha}$ was competent for catalyzing the conversion of progesterone to androstenedione *via* 17α-hydroxyprogesterone (*28, 29*). The results of one series of

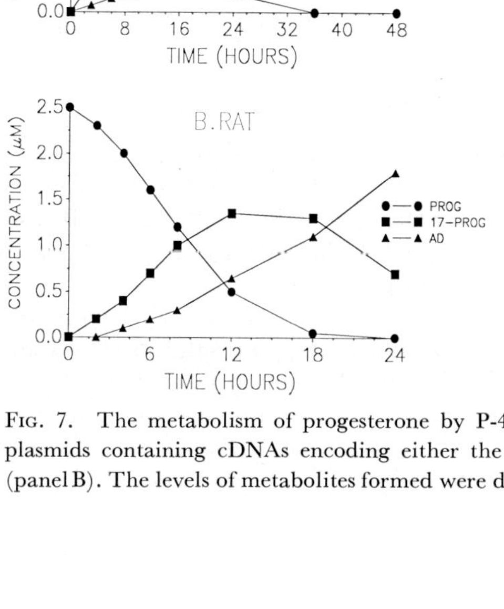


FIG. 7. The metabolism of progesterone by P-$450_{17\alpha}$ expressed in COS cells transfected with plasmids containing cDNAs encoding either the human enzyme (panel A) or the rat enzyme (panel B). The levels of metabolites formed were determined by HPLC analysis, as described (*27*).

experiments illustrating this difference in the ability of human P-450$_{17\alpha}$ and rat P-450$_{17\alpha}$ to metabolize progesterone is shown in Fig. 7. These results provide a direct demonstration that the delta$^5$-pathway of steroid metabolism *via* DHEA is the *only* pathway to androgens and estrogens in humans, while the delta$^4$-pathway is operative in rodents, such as the rat.

*Discussion*

It is well recognized that DHEA has remarkable effects on diverse biological systems: greatest interest are those associated with the prevention of various types of cancer. The present report summarizes some of the effects resulting from DHEA treatment of rats. The activities of a number of liver enzymes are affected, in particular the activities of some of the cytochrome P-450s that metabolize xenobiotics. The changes in activities observed are similar to those noted when rats are treated with peroxisome proliferators such as hypolipidemic drugs and phthalate derivatives. It is proposed that a contributor to the beneficial effects of DHEA action is exerted *via* an alteration of the inventory of the P-450 enzymes that participate in the metabolic activation of chemicals. This hypothesis would provide one explanation for the modification of the course of tumor formation following exposure to xenobiotics. In support of this hypothesis is the observation (Fig. 6) that high concentrations of DHEA are required to observe an effect on the liver enzymes.

The present studies also indicate that the reduced metabolite of DHEA, ADIOL, is equally or more effective than DHEA for inducing liver microsomal and peroxisomal enzymes. Whether peroxisome proliferation is directly linked to the many beneficial effects of DHEA or whether it is a secondary consequence of other alterations in cellular metabolism remains to be determined.

Interest in chemopreventive, anti-neoplastic agents is a worthwhile activity (*30*). The vast literature that has developed during the last decade documenting the chemotherapeutic effects of DHEA, warrants the further study of this remarkable chemical.

*Acknowledgments*

This work was supported in part by grants from the U.S. Public Health Service: NIGMS 16488, NIEHS 04244, NCI 43839 and 43311, and the Robert A. Welch Fundation: I0959.

REFERENCES

1. Estabrook, R. W., Weiss, R. H., Werringloer, J., and Peterson, J. A. The cytochromes P450 and oxygen stress. *In;* K. J. A. Davies (ed.), Oxidative Damage and Repair: Chemical, Biological and Medical Aspects, Proceedings of the 5th Biennial General Meeting of the International Society for Free Radical Research, Pasadena, CA, November 14–20, 1990, Pergamon Press, 1991, in press.
2. Nebert, D. W., Nelson, D. R., Coon, M. J., Estabrook, R. W., Feyereisen, R., Fujii-Kuriyama, Y., Gonzalez, F. J., Guengerich, F. P., Gunsalus, I. C., Johnson, E. F., Loper, J. C., Sato, R., Waterman, M. R., and Waxman, D. J. The P450 superfamily: Update on new sequences, gene mapping, and recommended nomenclature. DNA Cell. Biol., *10*: 1–14, 1991.
3. Abstracts of the Symposium Pharmaco-Clinique Roussel UCLAF No. 9, Dehydro-

epiandrosterone Revisited, Paris, France, January 19–20, 1989.

4. Various papers. *In;* M. Kalimi and W. Regelson (eds.), The Biologic Role of Dehydroepiandrosterone (DHEA), Walter de Gruyter, New York, 1990.
5. Schwartz, A. G., Pashko, L., and Whitcomb, J. B. Inhibition of tumor development by dehydroepiandrosterone and related steroids. Toxicol. Pathol., *14*: 357–362, 1986.
6. Lucas, J. A., Ahmed, S. A., Casey, M. L., and MacDonald, P. C. Prevention of autoantibody formation and prolonged survival in NZB/NZW $F_1$ mice fed dehydroepiandrosterone. J. Clin. Invest., *75*: 2091–2093, 1985.
7. Various papers. *In;* Hormones, Thermogenesis, and Obesity, H. Lardy and F. Stratman (eds.), Proceedings of the Eighteenth Steenbock Symposium, June 12–16, 1988, Madison, WI, Elsevier, New York, 1989.
8. Coleman, D. L., Leiter, E. H., and Schizer, R. W. Therapeutic effects of dehydroepiandrosterone (DHEA) in diabetic mice. Diabetes, *31*: 830–833, 1984.
9. Gordon, G. B., Bush, D. E., and Weissman, H. F. Reduction of atherosclerosis by administration of dehydroepiandrosterone. A study in the hypercholesterolemic New Zealand white rabbit with aortic intimal injury. J. Clin. Invest., *82*: 712–720, 1988.
10. Flood, J. F. and Roberts, E. Dehydroepiandrosterone sulfate improves memory in aging mice. Brain Res., *448*: 178–181, 1988.
11. Schwartz, A. G., Whitcomb, J. M., and Nyce, J. W. Oral feeding prevents spontaneous formation of breast tumors in mice and chemically induced tumors in lung and colon. Adv. Cancer Res., *51*: 391–424, 1988.
12. Nyce, J. W., Magee, P. N., Hard, G. C., and Schwartz, A. G. Inhibition of 1,2-dimethylhydrazine-induced colon tumorigenesis in Balb/c mice by dehydroepiandrosterone. Carcinogenesis, *5*: 57–62, 1984.
13. Prasanna, R., Hart, R. W., and Magee, P. N. Effect of short-term exposure of rats to dehydroepiandrosterone on the hepatic metabolism of dimethylnitrosamine. Biochem. J. *262*: 985–988, 1989.
14. Shantz, L. M., Talalay, P., and Gordon, G. B. Mechanism of inhibition of growth of 3T3-L1 fibroblasts and their differentiation to adipocytes by dehydroepiandrosterone and related steroids: Role of glucose-6-phosphate dehydrogenase. Proc. Natl. Acad. Sci. U.S.A., *86*: 3852–3856, 1989.
15. Mohan, P. F. and Clary, M. P. Dehydroepiandrosterone and related steroids inhibit mitochondrial respiration *in vitro*. Int. J. Biochem., *21*: 1103–1107, 1989.
16. Mohan, P. F. and Cleary, M. P. Effect of short term DHEA administration on liver metabolism of lean and obese rats. Am. J. Physiol., *255*: E1–E8, 1988.
17. Prasanna, H. R., Hart, R. W., and Magee, P. N. Effect of dehydroepiandrosterone (DHEA) on the mechanism of 7,12-dimethylbenz(a)anthracene (DMBA) in rats. Carcinogenesis, *10*: 953–955, 1989.
18. Selye, H. Hormones and resistance. J. Pharm. Sci., *60*: 1–28, 1971.
19. Lu, A. Y., Somogyi, A., West, S., Kuntzman, R., and Conney, A. H. Pregnenolone-16-alpha-carbonitrile: A new type of inducer of drug-metabolizing enzymes. Arch. Biochem. Biophys., *152*: 457–462, 1972.
20. Wu, H-Q., Masset-Brown, J., Tweedie, D. J., Milewich, L., Frenkel, R. A., Martin-Wixtrom, C., Estabrook, R. W., and Prough, R. A. Induction of microsomal NADPH-cytochrome P-450 reductase and cytochrome P1450IVA1 (P-$450_{LAw}$) by dehydroepiandrosterone in rats: A possible peroxisome proliferator. Cancer Res., *49*: 2337–2343, 1989.
21. Tamburini, P. P., Masson, H. A., Bains, S. K., Makowski, R. J., Morris, B., and Gibson, G. G. Multiple forms of hepatic cytochrome P-450. Purification, characterization and comparison of a novel clofibrate-induced isozyme with other major forms of cytochrome

P-450. Eur. J. Biochem., *139*: 235–246, 1984.

22. Okita, R. T. and Chance, C. Induction of laurate $\omega$-hydroxylase by di(2-ethylhexyl)-phthalate in rat liver microsomes. Biochem. Biophys. Res. Commun., *121*: 304–309, 1984.
23. Frenkel, R. A., Slaughter, C. A., Orth, K., Moomaw, C. R., Hicks, S. H., Snyder, J. M., Bennett, M., Prough, R. A., Putnam, R. S., and Milewich, L. Peroxisome proliferation and induction of peroxisomal enzymes in mouse and rat liver by dehydroepiandrosterone feeding. J. Steroid Biochem., *35*: 333–342, 1990.
24. Leighton, B., Tagliaferro, A. R., and Newsholme, E. A. The effect of dehydroepiandrosterone acetate on liver peroxisomal enzyme activities of male and female rats. J. Nutr., *117*: 1287–1290, 1987.
25. Zuber, M. X., Simpson, E. R., and Waterman, M. R. Expression of bovine 17$\alpha$-hydroxylase cytochrome P-450 cDNA in nonsteroidogenic (COS 1) cells. Science, *234*: 1258–1261, 1986.
26. Zuber, M. X., Mason, J. I., Simpson, E. R., and Waterman, M. R. Simultaneous transfection of COS-1 cells with mitochondrial and microsomal steroid hydroxylases: incorporation of a steroidogenic pathway into nonsteroidogenic cells. Proc. Natl. Acad. Sci. U.S.A., *85*: 699–703, 1988.
27. Estabrook, R. W., Mason, J. I., Simpson, E. R., Peterson, J. A., and Waterman, M. R. The heterologous expression of cytochromes P450: A new approach for the study of enzyme activities and synthesis. *In;* G. Weber (ed.), Regulation of Enzyme Activity and Synthesis in Normal and Neoplastic Tissues, pp. 365–383, Pergamon Press, London, 1991.
28. Namiki, M., Kitamura, M., Buczko, E., and Dufau, M. L. Rat testis P-450(17)$\alpha$ cDNA: the deduced amino acid sequence, expression and secondary structural configuration. Biochem. Biophys. Res. Commun., *15*: 157, 1988.
29. Fevold, H. R., Lorence, M. C., McCarthy, J. L., Trant, J. M., Kagimoto, M., Waterman, M. R., and Mason, J. I. Rat P450 (17$\alpha$) from testis: characterization of a full-length cDNA encoding a unique steroid hydroxylase capable of catalyzing both delta 4- and delta 5-steroid-17, 20-lyase reaction. Mol. Endocrinol., *3*: 968–975, 1989.
30. Wattenberg, L. W. Inhibition of carcinogenesis by naturally-occurring and synthetic compounds. Basic Life Sci., *52*: 155–166, 1990.

XENOBIOTICS AND CANCER, L. ERNSTER ET AL. (EDS.),
JAPAN SCI. SOC. PRESS, TOKYO/TAYLOR & FRANCIS LTD., LONDON, pp. 45–53, 1991

# Pharmacogenetics and Polymorphism of Human P-450 Which Activates and Detoxicates Xenobiotics and Carcinogens

Ryuichi KATO, Yasushi YAMAZOE, and Toshio YASUMORI

*Department of Pharmacology, School of Medicine, Keio University, Tokyo 160, Japan*

*Abstract:* Stereoselective hydroxylation of mephenytoin is expressed polymorphically in the Japanese population: the occurrence of the poor metabolizer was approximately 20% in Japanese, which was 5 to 8 times higher than that in Caucasians. Microsomal 4′-hydroxylation of S-mephenytoin, but not of R-mephenytoin, was correlated to the content of cytochrome P-450 human-2. P-450 human-2 cDNA was cloned and expressed in yeast cells. The expressed P-450 showed stereoselectivities similar to those in human livers for hydroxylations of mephenytoin and hexobarbital enantiomers. The P-450 catalyzed benzo[a]pyrene and tolbutamide hydroxylations and cyclophosphamide oxidation, but showed low activity for the mutagenic activation of IQ (2-amino-3-methylimidazo[4, 5-*f*]quinoline). Two cDNAs (MP-8 and λhPA6), which are two amino acids mutated and deleted, respectively, from P-450 human-2 cDNA were expressed in yeasts. These two expressed P-450s revealed complete loss of the stereoselectivity in the hydroxylation of mephenytoin and hexobarbital. These results indicate that many xenobiotics and carcinogens are detoxicated and activated by the human liver in quite different manners among individuals by reason of genetic differences.

In recent years, several genetically determined polymorphisms of cytochrome P-450-mediated drug oxidations in humans have been discovered. Genetic polymorphisms of drug oxidations cause impaired biotransformation of certain drugs in the so-called "poor metabolizer" (*1*). Because of their frequent occurrence, genetic polymorphisms of drug oxidations are major determinants of individual differences in therapeutic and toxic responses to numerous clinically important drugs (*1*, *2*). There is only a limited amount of evidence available on the influence of polymorphic oxidation of mutagenic and carcinogenic compounds on the occurrence of human cancer. However, it is important to note that clear ethnic differences exist in polymorphic metabolism of a variety of drugs as shown in Table 1 (*1*, *3*).

We earlier purified a cytochrome P-450, termed P-450 human-2, which showed activity for benzo[a]pyrene and mephenytoin hydroxylation (*4*).

An anticonvulsant agent, mephenytoin, has been reported to undergo hydroxylation with high stereoselectivity and to exhibit a polymorphism in human populations

TABLE 1. Ethnic Differences in Polymorphic Drug Metabolism in Human

| | |
|---|---|
| 1) | Debrisoquine type (P-450IID) |
| | PM: 5% in Caucasian, <1% in Japanese |
| 2) | Nifedipine type (P-450IIIA) |
| | PM: 15% in Caucasian, ?% in Japanese |
| 3) | Mephenytoin type (P-450IIC) |
| | PM: 3% in Caucasian, 20% in Japanese |
| 4) | N-acetylation of arylamine |
| | PM: 50% in Caucasian, 15% in Japanese |

PM, poor metabolizer.

(*5–8*). Poor metabolizers were detected at low frequency in white subjects (3%) but at considerably higher frequency (more than 20%) in Japanese subjects by analysis of the urinary excretion of unmetabolized R- and S-mephenytoins after administration of the racemates (*6–8*). Several cytochrome P-450 isozymes with identical amino-terminal sequences of amino acids have been reported to participate in polymorphic S-(+)-mephenytoin 4′-hydroxylation (*9–13*). In addition, several cDNAs assumed to encode human S-mephenytoin 4′-hydroxylase have been isolated, but none of these cDNAs were demonstrated to encode a functionally active S-mephenytoin 4′-hydroxylase (*10–14*).

We have recently isolated a cDNA clone, termed P-450 human 2-cDNA, from a λgtll cDNA library using anti-P-450 human-2 sera (*10*). Moreover, we ascertained that the cDNA encodes a functionally active S-mephenytoin 4′-hydroxylase by the expression of the cDNA in yeast cells using an expression vector containing a galactose-inducible gene (*GAL7*) promotor and terminator (*15, 16*). These P-450s expressed in the yeast cells show stereoselectivities similar to those observed in human liver samples.

In the present study, we have sought to assess whether the percentage of poor metabolizers for S-mephenytoin 4′-hydroxylase in Japanese liver samples is as high as suggested by the study on urinary analysis of excreted metabolites after administration of racemic mephenytoin, and to find out whether the activity of stereoselective S-mephenytoin hydroxylase is correlated to the content of P-450 human-2. Moreover, we have expressed three P-450 IIC9/10 cDNAs, termed P-450 human-2 cDNA, MP-8 (*13*) and λhPA6 (*14*) in yeast cells to clarify which one really encodes stereoselective mephenytoin 4′-hydroxylase.

### *Determination of the Phenotype of Human Liver Microsomes for Mephenytoin Hydroxylation —Correlation to P-450 Human-2 Content*

Stereoselective metabolisms of R-(−)-mephenytoin and S-(+)-mephenytoin to each 4′-hydroxy-metabolite were determined with 19 liver microsomal samples of Japanese subjects (Fig. 1). The R/S ratios of 4-hydroxy metabolites in 14 samples were less than 0.3, and the values in the remaining 5 samples ranged from 0.71 to 2.47 (Fig. 2) (*17*). Thus we defined those subjects who showed ratios of more than 0.5 as poor metabolizers. The frequency of poor metabolizers in Japanese subjects was found to be more than 20%. This value is in close agreement with previous studies in which

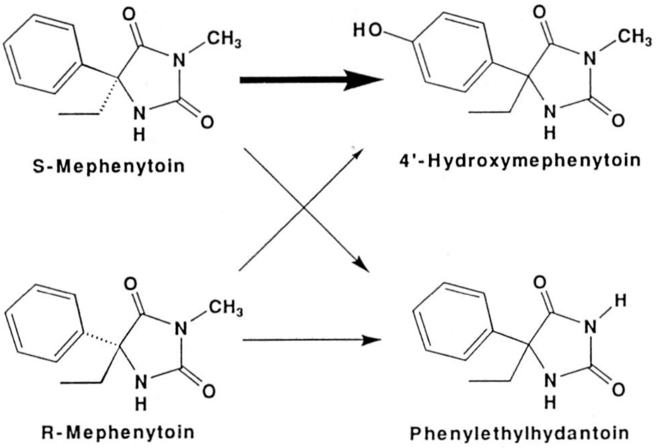


FIG. 1. Metabolic fate of S- and R-mephenytoin in human livers.

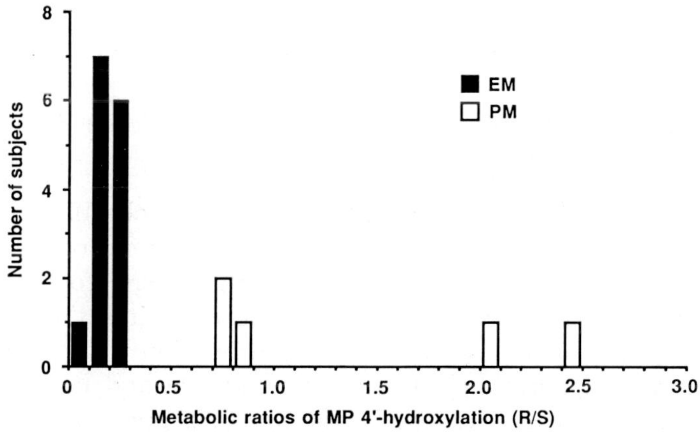


FIG. 2. Distribution of extensive metabolizers (EM) and poor metabolizers (PM) for mephenytoin (MP) hydroxylation determined by the metabolic ratios of hydroxylation of the R- and S-isomers. (Yasumori *et al.*, 1990)

the frequency of the poor metabolizer was shown to be much higher in Japanese subjects than in Caucasians, as determined by the urinary excretion ratio of unmetabolized R- and S-mephenytoin after ingestion of racemic mephenytoin (*7*). S-mephenytoin 4′-hydroxylations in livers of extensive metabolizer (EM) and poor metabolizer (PM) were $0.55 \pm 0.15$ and $0.09 \pm 0.04$ nmol/hr/mg protein, respectively, whereas the activity for R-mephenytoin was $0.11 \pm 0.04$ and $0.11 \pm 0.08$ nmol/hr/mg protein, respectively, for EM and PM. Thus, R/S ratio was $0.21 \pm 0.07$ for EM and $1.36 \pm 0.82$ for PM.

As shown in Fig. 3, a good correlation was observed between the rate of S-mephenytoin 4′-hydroxylation and the content of immunochemically determined P-450 human-2 in human livers (*17*). However, no significant correlation was observed between the rate of R-mephenytoin 4′-hydroxylation and P-450 human-2 content. Moreover, no significant correlation was observed between P-450 human-2 content and the rates of R- or S-mephenytoin N-demethylations.

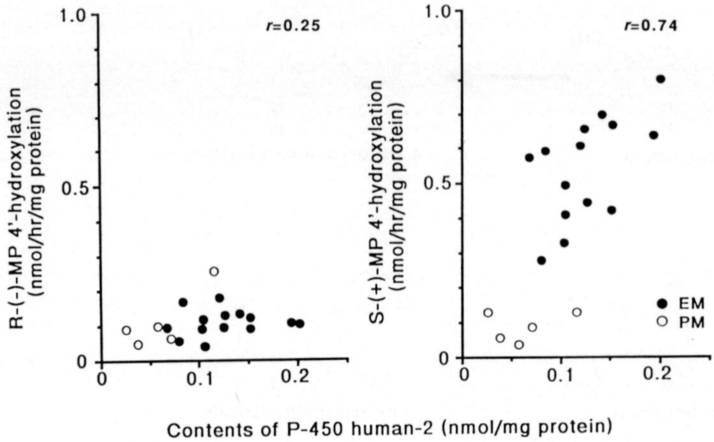


FIG. 3. Correlation between rate of mephenytoin (MP) 4′-hydroxylation and immunochemically determined P-450 human-2 content in human liver microsomes (Yasumori *et al.*, 1990). Symbols represent different individual livers of Japanese EM and PM.

*Stereoselective and Stereospecific Hydroxylations of Hexobarbital in Human Liver Microsomes from Extensive and Poor Metabolizers*

The stereoselective and stereospecific hydroxylations of hexobarbital were studied using R-(−)-hexobarbital and S-(+)-hexobarbital (*17*). The rates of S-hexobarbital 3′β-hydroxylation and R-hexobarbital 3′α-hydroxylation were correlated to the content of P-450 human-2. However, the rates of S-hexobarbital 3′α-hydroxylation and R-hexobarbital 3′β-hydroxylation showed poor correlation with P-450 human-2 content. The R/S ratio for 3′α-hydroxylation in livers of EM and PM was 4.61 and 0.87, respectively, and that for 3′β-hydroxylation was 0.32 and 1.25 (Fig. 4) (*17*). On the other hand, α/β ratio for R-hexobarbital in livers of EM and PM was 1.94 and 0.72, respectively, and that for S-hexobarbital was 0.14 and 0.99. It is of interest to note that the extensive metabolizers are capable of stereoselectively hydroxylating R-hexobarbital to 3′α-hydroxy-metabolites, contrary to the hydroxylation of S-mephenytoin in which the extensive metabolizers hydroxylate S-enantiomer stereoselectively.

*Correlation between P-450 Human-2 Content and Benzo[a]pyrene Hydroxylation in Human Liver Microsomes*

The extensive metabolizer for S-mephenytoin hydroxylation extensively hydroxylated benzo[a]pyrene (14.4±12.0 pmol/min/mg protein). Although there was a 23-fold difference in the activity of benzo[a]pyrene hydroxylase between extensive and poor metabolizers, there was no clear correlation between the content of P-450 human-2 and benzo[a]pyrene hydroxylation in human liver samples (Fig. 5).

These results indicate that P-450 human-2 may be one of the major enzymes responsible for the hydroxylation of benzo[a]pyrene in human liver microsomes, but that other cytochromes may also be involved in the hydroxylation.

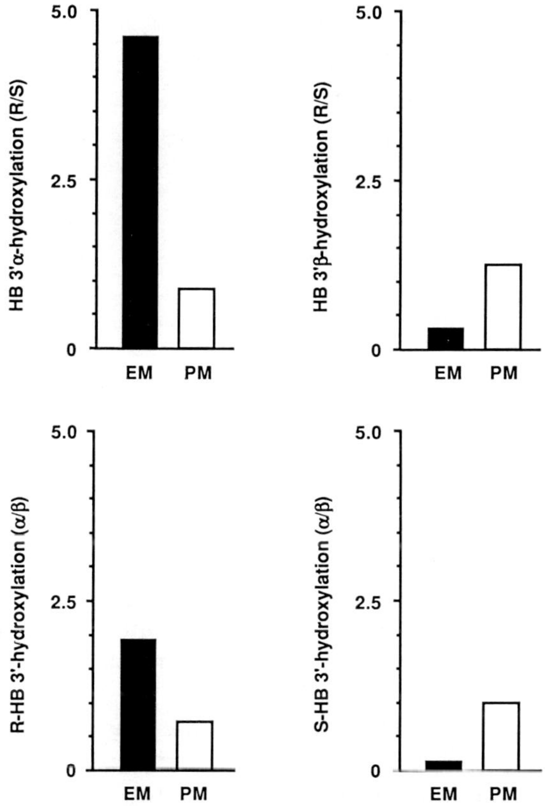


FIG. 4. Metabolic ratios of hexobarbital (HB) 3′-hydroxylation from liver microsomes of EM and PM.

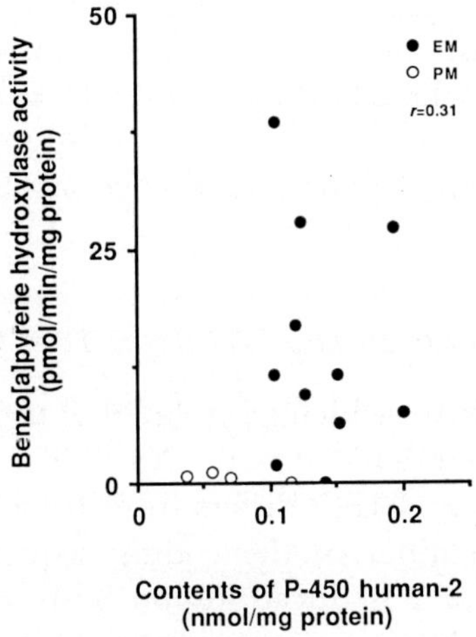


FIG. 5. Relationship between P-450 human-2 content and benzo[a]pyrene hydroxylase activity in human liver samples.

TABLE 2. Stereoselective Mephenytoin 4′-Hydroxylation and Hexobarbital 3′-Hydroxylation in Microsomes of Yeasts and Human Livers from Extensive Metabolizers

| | Yeast microsomes | Human microsomes |
|---|---|---|
| R-MP 4′-Hydroxylation[a] | 10.5±2.0 | 110±40 |
| S-MP 4′-Hydroxylation[a] | 46.5±6.0 | 550±150 |
| R/S ratio | 0.23 | 0.21±0.07 |
| R-HB 3′α-Hydroxylation[b] | 23.5±2.0 | 460±230 |
| S-HB 3′α-Hydroxylation[b] | 5.5±1.0 | 130±120 |
| R/S ratio | 4.27 | 4.61±2.20 |
| R-HB 3′β-Hydroxylation[b] | 6.5±1.5 | 280±160 |
| S-HB 3′β-Hydroxylation[b] | 51.5±4.0 | 960±570 |
| R/S ratio | 0.13 | 0.32±0.14 |

Data are shown as mean±standard deviation of at least 3 different determinations for yeast samples and of 14 different EM subjects. The content of cytochrome P-450 in yeast and human microsomes was 50 and 270±70 pmol/mg protein, respectively.

[a] The activity is expressed as pmol/hr/mg protein.

[b] The activity is expressed as pmol/min/mg protein.

### *Comparison of the Metabolic Activity of Yeast-expressed P-450 Human-2 with That of Human Liver*

The hydroxylations of S- and R-mephenytoin by P-450 human-2 expressed in microsomes of yeasts and human livers of extensive metabolizers are given in Table 2. The stereoselectivity in mephenytoin hydroxylation of the yeast microsomes was similar to that of human liver microsomes. The activities in the yeast microsomes were lower than those in the human liver microsomes, but the addition of cytochrome $b_5$ and dilauroyl phosphatidylcholine stimulated the activities about 10-fold without any change of the stereoselectivity (*18*, *19*).

Moreover, the S- and R-hexobarbital 3′α-hydroxylation and S- and R-hexobarbital 3′β-hydroxylation by yeast microsomes of expressed P-450 human-2 showed stereoselectivities similar to those obtained with human liver microsomes. R/S ratio of hexobarbital 3′α-hydroxylation in the yeast and human liver microsomes was 4.27 and 4.61, respectively, and R/S ratio of hexobarbital 3′β-hydroxylation was 0.13 and 0.32.

Moreover, the $K_m$ for S-mephenytoin hydroxylation in the yeast and human liver microsomes were almost identical.

### *Expresions of P-450 Human-2 cDNA and Two Closely Related cDNAs in Yeast Cells*

Recently, two cDNA clones, MP-8 and λhPA6, which are related to mephenytoin 4-hydroxylase, have been reported by Guengerich's group (Nashville, TN) and Kamataki's group (Sapporo, Japan), respectively. MP-8 differs from P-450 human-2 cDNA in two silent and two non-silent nucleotides in the coding sequences (*13*). A truncated clone, λhPA6, has 6 bp-deletion for 2 deduced amino acids in human-2 cDNA sequence (Table 3) (*14*). Therefore, we have constructed plasmids containing MP-8 and λhPA6, termed pGY450 and pKY450, respectively, by modification of P-450 human-2 cDNA through site-directed mutagenesis. The original plasmid, pTF450,

TABLE 3. Microheterogeneity between P-450 Human-2 cDNA and Two Closely Related cDNAs

| cDNA | Differences in the deduced amino acid sequences | | | |
|---|---|---|---|---|
| | 273 274 | 358 | 417 | |
| P-450 human-2 cDNA | .........Lys-Glu | ..........Tyr | ........Gly | ........ |
| MP-8 | .........Lys-Glu | ..........Cys | ........Asp | ........ |
| λhPA6 | .......... | ..........Tyr | ........Gly | ........ |

P-450 human-2 cDNA encodes 490 amino acids in the sequence. No obvious similarity was observed between P-450 human-2 cDNA and MP-8 in their 3′noncoding sequences, except for the first 75 bases, or in the length of the complete sequences.

and two other related plasmids were each introduced into yeast MT8-1. MT8-1-[pTF450] (P-450 human-2) microsomes hydroxylated mephenytoin at a 5-fold higher rate toward S-enantiomer than R-enantiomer. However, the activities of MT8-1 [pGY450] and MT8-1[pKY450] microsomes were almost non-stereoselective. MT8-1 [pTF450] microsomes hydroxylated S-mephenytoin at the rate of 0.93 nmol/hr/nmol P-450, which was respectively 4.4-fold and 2.4-fold higher than those of MT8-1 [pGY450] and MT8-1[pKY450] microsomes.

In addition, MT8-1[pTF450] microsomes stereospecifically ($\alpha/\beta$) hydroxylated both R- and S-enantiomers of hexobarbital, and also stereoselectively (R/S) at both $3'\alpha$- and $3'\beta$-positions, while the two other cDNA-derived proteins hydroxylated in less stereospecific ($\alpha/\beta$) and stereoselective (R/S) manners.

These results clearly showed that the change of Tyr-358 and Gly-417 of P-450 human-2 to Cys-358 and Asp-417, respectively, and the deletion of Lys-273 and Glu-274 completely abolished stereoselectivity in the hydroxylations of mephenytoin and hexobarbital.

On the other hand, these three P-450 showed a relatively high activity for hydroxylation of tolbutamide, but the activity of P-450 human-2 was higher than MP-8 and λhPA6 derived cytochrome P-450s.

### *The Metabolic Activation of Mutagens and Carcinogens by P-450 Human-2 and Two Related Cytochrome P-450s Expressed in the Yeast and Human Liver Microsomes*

The activities of benzo[a]pyrene hydroxylase of the P-450 expressed in the yeast cells are stipulated in Table 4. The microsomes from MT8-1[pKY450] showed an activity similar to those from MT8-1[pTF450]. However, the activity of MT8-1

TABLE 4. Benzo[a]pyrene Hydroxylation and Cyclophosphamide Oxidation by Yeast Microsomes and Human Liver Microsomes

| Measurement | Yeast microsomes | | | | Human microsomes |
|---|---|---|---|---|---|
| | MT8-1[pTF450] | MT8-1[pKY450] | MT8-1[pGY450] | MT8-1[pAA7][c] | |
| Benzo[a]pyrene Hydroxylation[a] | 0.34±0.06[d] | 0.25±0.05 | 0.11±0.03 | <0.005 | 2.51±2.83[e] |
| Cyclophosphamide Oxidation[b] | 0.36±0.02 | 0.03±0.01 | <0.01 | <0.01 | 0.75±0.63[e] |

[a] The activity is expressed as nmol/hr/nmol P-450. [b] The activity is expressed as nmol/min/nmol P-450. [c] Expression vector pAA7 contained only *GAL7* promoter and terminator. [d] Data represent the mean values of at least three different determinations. [e] Data represent the mean±standard deviation of 14–15 subjects.

[pGY450] microsomes was lower than that of MT8-1[pTF450] microsomes. The cyclophosphamide oxidase activity of MT8-1[pTF450] microsomes was about 10 times higher than that of MT8-1[pGY450] and MT8-1[pTF450] microsomes, while that of P-450 human-2 expressed in the yeast was quite comparable to that of human liver microsomes. There was no clear correlation, however, between cyclophosphamide oxidase activity and P-450 human-2 content in human liver samples. These results indicate that the oxidation of cyclophosphamide in human liver microsomes is not mediated by P-450 human-2 alone.

The N-hydroxylation of IQ (2-amino-3-methylimidazo[4,5-*f*]quinoline) (*20*) was low in three yeast cells in which human cytochrome P-450s were expressed (unpublished data).

Further studies will thus be needed to elucidate the possible role of P-450 human-2 in the detoxification and activation of carcinogens relative to the susceptibility in chemical carcinogenesis.

## REFERENCES

1. Kalow, W. Genetic variation in the human hepatic cytochrome P-450 system. Eur. J. Clin. Pharmacol., *31*: 633–641, 1987.
2. Guengerich, F. P. Polymorphism of cytochrome P-450 in humans. TIPS., *10*: 107–109, 1989.
3. Meyer, U. A., Skoda, R. C., and Zanger, U. M. The genetic polymorphism of debrisoquine/sparteine metabolism—molecular mechanisms. Pharmacol. Ther., *46*: 297–308, 1990.
4. Kawano, S., Kamataki, T., Yasumori, T., Yamazoe, Y., and Kato, R. Purification of human liver cytochrome P-450 catalyzing testosterone 6$\beta$-hydroxylation. J. Biochem., *102*: 493–501, 1987.
5. Küpfer, A., Roberts, R. K., Schenker, S., and Branch, R. A. Stereoselective metabolism of mephenytoin in man. J. Pharmacol. Exp. Ther., *218*: 193–199, 1981.
6. Küpfer, A. and Preisig, R. Pharmacogenetics of mephenytoin: a new drug hydroxylation polymorphism in man. Eur. J. Clin. Pharmacol., *26*: 753–759, 1984.
7. Nakamura, K., Goto, F., Ray, W. A., McAllister, C. B., Jacqz, E., Wilkinson, G. R., and Branch, R. A. Interethnic differences in genetic polymorphism of debrisoquin and mephenytoin hydroxylation between Japanese and Caucasian populations. Clin. Pharmacol. Ther., *38*: 402–408, 1985.
8. Jurima, M., Inaba, T., Kadar, D., and Kalow, W. Genetic polymorphism of mephenytoin *p*(4′)-hydroxylation: difference between Orientals and Caucasians. Br. J. Clin. Pharmacol., *19*: 483–487, 1985.
9. Shimada, T., Misono, K. S., and Guengerich, F. P. Human liver microsomal cytochrome P-450 mephenytoin 4-hydroxylase, a prototype of genetic polymorphism in oxidative drug metabolism: purification and characterization of two similar forms involved in the reaction. J. Biol. Chem., *261*: 909–921, 1986.
10. Yasumori, T., Kawano, S., Nagata, K., Shimada, M., Yamazoe, Y., and Kato, R. Nucleotide sequence of a human liver cytochrome P-450 related to the rat male specific form. J. Biochem., *102*: 1075–1082, 1987.
11. Ged, C., Umbenhauer, D. R., Bellew, T. M., Bork, R. W., Srivastava, P. K., Shinriki, N., Lloyd., R. S., and Guengerich, F. P. Characterization of cDNAs, mRNAs, and proteins related to human liver microsomal cytochrome P-450 (S)-mephenytoin 4′-hydroxylase. Biochemistry, *27*: 6929–6940, 1988.

12. Kimura, S., Pastewka, J., Gelvoin H. V., and Gonzalez, F. J. cDNA and amino acid sequences of two members of the human P-450IIC gene subfamily. Nucl. Acids Res., *15*: 10053–10054, 1987.
13. Umbenhauer, D. R., Martin, M. V., Lloyd, R. S., and Guengerich, F. P. Cloning and sequence determination of a complementary DNA related to human liver microsomal cytochrome P-450 S-mephenytoin 4-hydroxylase. Biochemistry, *26*: 1094–1099, 1987.
14. Ohgiya, S., Komori, M., Fujitani, T., Miura, T., Shinriki, N., and Kamataki, T. Cloning of human cytochrome P-450 cDNA and its expression in *Saccharomyces cerevisiae.* Biochem. Int., *18*: 429–438, 1989.
15. Yasumori, T., Murayama, N., Yamazoe, Y., Abe, A., Nogi, Y., Fukasawa, T., and Kato, R. Expression of a human P-450IIC gene in yeast cells using galactose-inducible expression system. Mol. Pharmacol., *35*: 443–449, 1989.
16. Kato, R., Yasumori, T., and Yamazoe, Y. Characterization of human P-450IIC isozyme by using a yeast expression system. Methods Enzymol., in press.
17. Yasumori, T., Murayama, N., Yamazoe, Y., and Kato, R. Polymorphism in hydroxylation of mephenytoin and hexobarbital stereoisomers in relation to hepatic P-450 human-2. Clin. Pharmacol. Ther., *47*: 313–322, 1990.
18. Yasumori, T., Yamazoe, Y., and Kato, R. Cytochrome P-450 human-2 (P-450IIC9) in mephenytoin hydroxylation polymorphism in human livers: differences in substrate and stereoselectivities among microheterogeneous P-450IIC species expressed in yeasts. J. Biochem., *109*: 711–717, 1991.
19. Aoyama, T., Nagata, K., Yamazoe, Y., Kato, R., Matsunaga, E., Gelboin, H. V., and Gonzalez, F. J. Cytochrome $b_5$ potentiation of cytochrome P-450 catalytic activity demonstrated by a vaccinia virus-mediated *in situ* reconstitution system. Proc. Natl. Acad. Sci. U.S.A., *87*: 5425–5429, 1990.
20. Yamazoe, Y., Shimada, M., Kamataki, T., and Kato, R. Microsomal activation of 2-amino-3-methylimidazo[4, 5-*f*]quinoline, a pyrolysate of sardine and beef extracts, to a mutagenic intermediate. Cancer Res., *43*: 5768–5774, 1983.

XENOBIOTICS AND CANCER, L. ERNSTER ET AL. (EDS.),
JAPAN SCI. SOC. PRESS, TOKYO/TAYLOR & FRANCIS LTD., LONDON, pp. 55–61, 1991

# Individual Differences in Lung Cancer Susceptibility in Relation to Polymorphisms of P-450IA1 Gene and Cigarette Dose

Kaname KAWAJIRI,*[1] Kei NAKACHI,*[2] Kazue IMAI,*[2] Shin-ichi HAYASHI,*[1] and Junko WATANABE*[1]

*Departments of Biochemistry*[1] *and Epidemiology,*[2] *Saitama Cancer Center Research Institute, Ina-machi, Saitama 362, Japan*

*Abstract:* Individual differences in susceptibility to chemical carcinogens are one of the most important host factors in the development of human cancer. We studied the etiological association of lung cancer with the DNA polymorphisms of P-450 IA1 gene, because cytochrome P-450IA1 is responsible for the metabolic activation of benzo(a)pyrene and other procarcinogens in cigarette smoking to the ultimate forms in the initiation process of lung cancer. Three polymorphisms of the gene were identified by restriction fragment length polymorphisms (RFLPs) with Msp I: the predominant homozygous allele (A type), the heterozygote (B type), and the homozygous rare allele (C type). A comparison of genotype frequencies between patients with lung cancer and a healthy population revealed that the individuals with genotype C were at higher risk than other types, and that this genetic risk elevation was specific to the Kreyberg I type of the cancer with relative risk of 3.21 but not to the Kreyberg II.

We further studied this genetic susceptibility to the squamous cell carcinoma of lung cancer in relation to cumulated cigarette smoking dose, and found that the genetically susceptible patients with genotype C contracted the cancer with less cigarette dose than other types. Our case-control study showed that the relative risk of genotype C was remarkably high at 7.31 with a low dose of cigarette consumption compared to genotypes A and B, and that risk elevation with increasing dose saturated at 13.17 at high dose levels where the risk of genotypes A and B was at 8.89.

It is now accepted that a great portion of human cancer is caused by man-made or natural chemical compounds in our environment. Many chemical carcinogens are metabolically activated to a form which may have a harmful effect on an organism(s) (*1*). This metabolic activation is an obligatory initiation step in chemical carcinogenesis (*1*), and the microsomal electron transport system, including cytochrome P-450s, plays the most important role in oxidation of chemical compounds (*2*, *3*).

Genetic variation among individuals in the metabolism of chemicals has been reported, and variations in the oxidative activation of chemical carcinogens might well explain differences in susceptibility of individuals to chemical carcinogenesis (*4–7*).

The metabolism of chemical carcinogens involves a variety of isozymes of P-450 (*3*), and differences in their genotypes (*8*) or phenotypes (*4–7*) may be one of the main factors responsible for differences among individuals in susceptibility to carcinogens.

Accumulated evidence (*6, 7*) suggests that increased risk of smoking-induced bronchogenic carcinoma is associated with high activity of aryl hydrocarbon hydroxylase (AHH), an inducibility phenotype of P-450IA1, which is responsible for the metabolism of polycyclic hydrocarbon procarcinogens including benzo(a)pyrene. In this presentation, we report that Msp I polymorphisms are associated with genetically determined differences among individuals in their susceptibility to lung cancer, and that the genetically susceptible individuals contracted lung cancer with less dose of cigarette smoking than other people.

*Detection of Msp I Polymorphisms*

Blood samples were obtained from both patients and controls, and DNAs were isolated from peripheral lymphocytes. The identification of the genotypes of P-450IA1 gene ascribed to Msp I site in the 3′-flanking region was carried out by two methods (Fig. 1): 1) RFLPs of P-450IA1 gene were determined by genomic Southern blotting, digesting the sample DNAs with Msp I and hybridizing with a probe 1 (Xba I-EcoR I fragment) (*8, 9*) (Fig. 1a); 2) DNAs were amplified using a polymerase chain reaction (*10*), and the amplified fragments including the polymorphic site were digested with Msp I and subjected to electrophoresis in 1.8% agarose gel (Fig. 1b). These two methods completely accorded with each other in the identification of the genotypes. Genotype A is the predominant homozygote, where the site of Msp I does not exist at the 3′ end, genotype C is a homozygous rare allele with this Msp I site, and genotype B is a heterozygous allele (*8*).

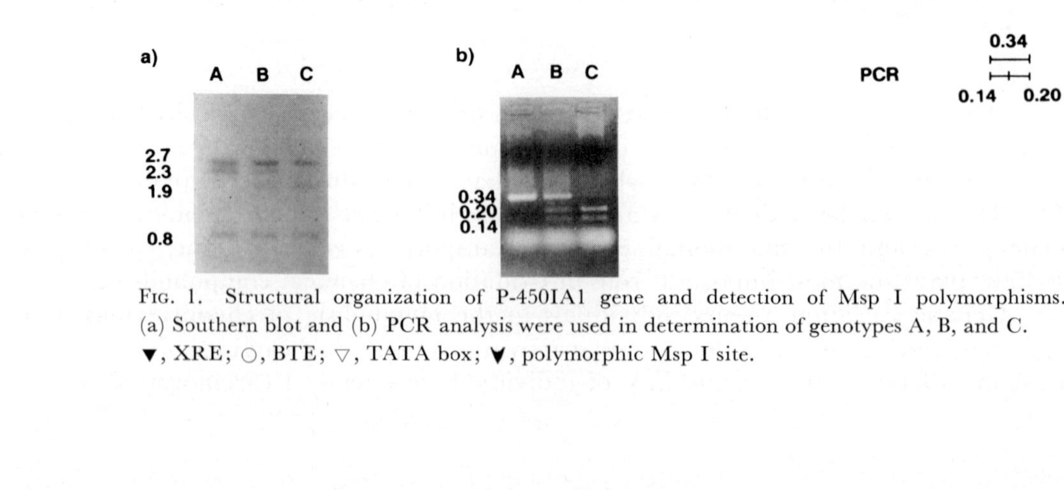


FIG. 1. Structural organization of P-450IA1 gene and detection of Msp I polymorphisms. (a) Southern blot and (b) PCR analysis were used in determination of genotypes A, B, and C. ▼, XRE; ○, BTE; ▽, TATA box; ▼, polymorphic Msp I site.

*Msp I Polymorphisms and Lung Cancer Incidence*

We determined the frequency of each type of Msp I polymorphisms in a general population. We isolated lymphocyte DNAs from a cohort of 2,500 persons over 40 years old and analyzed the DNA polymorphisms of 375 randomly selected subjects as healthy controls (Table 1). Types A (m1/m1), B (m1/m2), and C (m2/m2) were found, respectively, in 166, 169, and 40 of these healthy controls. This result gave a good fit to the Hardy-Weinberg equilibrium with a gene frequency of 0.67 for m1 and 0.33 for m2. The frequency of genotypes among lung cancer patients was different from those among healthy controls with statistical significance of $p<0.01$ ($\chi^2=10.191$, $df=2$). However, the frequency distribution among other cancer patients was the same as healthy controls (Table 1).

Histological classification of patients is very important, especially in studies of lung cancer because the carcinogenic mechanism and etiology are different. Among four main histological types of lung cancer, three types (squamous, small, and large cell carcinomas) are categorized as Kreyberg I and known to be closely associated with cigarette smoking. The frequency distribution of genotypes among Kreyberg I showed a remarkable difference from that of healthy controls with statistical significance of $p<0.001$ ($\chi^2=15.462$, $df=2$) (Table 2). The odds ratio estimate revealed that the individuals with C type had about 3-fold higher risk to the cancer than A type ($p<0.001$, $\chi^2=13.757$). On the other hand, the frequency among the adenocarcinoma

TABLE 1. Distribution of the 3 Types of P-450IA1 Gene among Healthy Controls and Cancer Patients

| Population | P-450IA1 genotype | | | Total | Gene frequency of m1 |
|---|---|---|---|---|---|
| | A (m1/m1) | B (m1/m2) | C (m2/m2) | | |
| Lung cancer | 61 (40.4) | 58 (38.4) | 32 (21.2) | 151 (100.0) | 0.596 |
| Stomach cancer | 45 (43.3) | 50 (48.0) | 9 ( 8.7) | 104 (100.0) | 0.673 |
| Colon cancer | 37 (47.5) | 32 (41.0) | 9 (11.5) | 78 (100.0) | 0.679 |
| Breast cancer | 15 (48.4) | 13 (41.9) | 3 ( 9.7) | 31 (100.0) | 0.693 |
| Healthy controls | 166 (44.3) | 169 (45.1) | 40 (10.6) | 375 (100.0) | 0.668 |

TABLE 2. Distribution of the 3 Types of P-450IA1 Gene among Histological Types of Lung Cancer Patients

| Histological type | P-450IA1 genotype | | | Total | Association with smoking |
|---|---|---|---|---|---|
| | A (m1/m1) | B (m1/m2) | C (m2/m2) | | |
| A) Kreyberg I type | (m1=0.538, m2=0.462) | | | | |
| Squamous cell carcinoma | 19 (33.3) | 23 (40.4) | 15 (26.3) | 57 (100.0) | Very high |
| Small cell carcinoma | 10 (41.8) | 7 (29.1) | 7 (29.1) | 24 (100.0) | High |
| Large cell carcinoma | 2 (20.0) | 6 (60.0) | 2 (20.0) | 10 (100.0) | Medium |
| | 31 (34.0) | 36 (39.6) | 24 (26.4) | 91 (100.0) | |
| | Odds ratio | | | | |
| | 1.000 | 1.141 | 3.213* | | |
| B) Kreyberg II type | (m1=0.683, m2=0.317) | | | | |
| Adenocarcinoma | 30 (50.3) | 22 (36.7) | 8 (13.3) | 60 (100.0) | Low |

* $\chi^2=13.757$, $p<0.001$.

(Kreyberg II) which shows little or no association with smoking, was almost identical to that among healthy controls.

*Difference of Susceptibility to Squamous Cell Carcinoma of the Lung in Relation to Smoking Dose*

The results we obtained indicate that the individuals with genotype C were more susceptible to smoking-induced cancers than other types. Accordingly, it is reasonable to examine the hypothesis that those highly susceptible patients contracted the carcinoma with less cigarette dose than other patients, because their metabolic activation of the carcinogens in cigarette smoking by P-450IA1 is expected to be high. We studied this focusing on the squamous cell carcinoma, which is most closely associated with smoking among Kreyberg I. Figure 2 compares the total cigarette amounts consumed over a lifetime among the patients with genotypes A, B, and C. We found that the distribution of the amounts of genotype C showed a lesser dose than the other two types. Since there was no difference in the distribution between genotypes A and B, we combined them as A+B and compared the mean cigarette consumption with that of genotype C. The mean value of 312,988 cigarettes ($n=12$, SD$=$128,059) was lower than the mean of 424,749 ($n=33$, SD$=$181,559) of genotypes A+B with statistical significance of $p<0.05$ ($t_0=2.12$ for $df=43$), noting that the two sample variances estimated the same parametric variance: $F=s^2_{A+B}/s^2_C=2.01<F_{0.1[32,11]}=2.08$.

We then designed a case-control study to estimate the susceptibility of the geno-

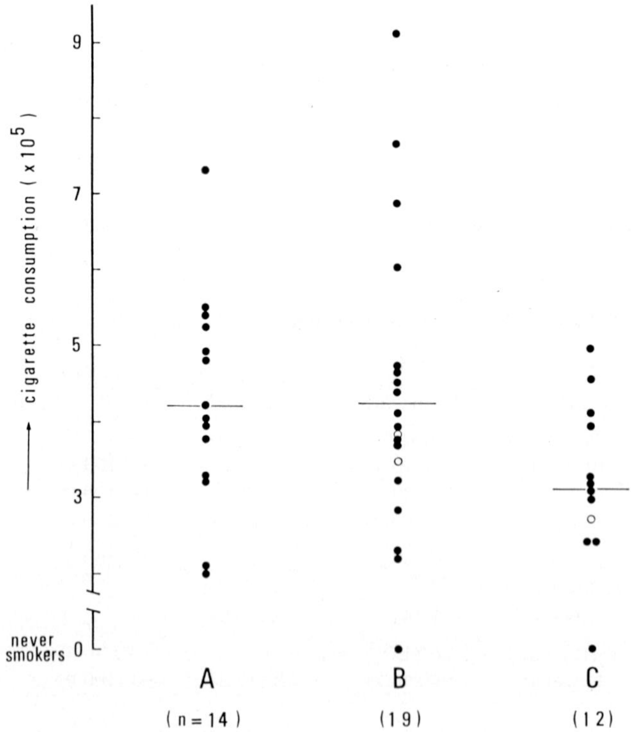


FIG. 2. Cigarette consumption of patients with squamous cell carcinoma of the lung in genotypes. ●, male; ○, female.

TABLE 3. Distribution of Patients and Controls by Genotype and Cigarette Dose and Relative Risk Estimate

<table>
<tr><th rowspan="2"></th><th rowspan="2">Genotype</th><th colspan="3">Cigarette consumption ($\times 10^5$)</th></tr>
<tr><th>3</th><th>3–4</th><th>4</th></tr>
<tr><td rowspan="2">Patients</td><td>C</td><td>5 (0.455)</td><td>4 (0.267)</td><td>3 (0.158)</td></tr>
<tr><td>A+B</td><td>6</td><td>11</td><td>16</td></tr>
<tr><td rowspan="2">Controls</td><td>C</td><td>9 (0.102)</td><td>4 (0.153)</td><td>3 (0.143)</td></tr>
<tr><td>A+B</td><td>79</td><td>22</td><td>18</td></tr>
<tr><td rowspan="4">Odds ratio</td><td rowspan="2">C</td><td rowspan="2">7.31*</td><td>13.17**</td><td>13.17**</td></tr>
<tr><td colspan="2">13.17**</td></tr>
<tr><td rowspan="2">A+B</td><td rowspan="2">1.0</td><td>6.58**</td><td>11.70**</td></tr>
<tr><td colspan="2">8.89**</td></tr>
<tr><td rowspan="2">Susceptibility of genotype C</td><td rowspan="2"></td><td rowspan="2">7.31*</td><td>2.00</td><td>1.13</td></tr>
<tr><td colspan="2">1.48</td></tr>
</table>

Frequency of genotype C is shown in parentheses.
* $p<0.01$. ** $p<0.001$.

types in relation to cigarette dose. Controls were randomly selected from our cohort population with DNA samples and individually matched to the patients with respect to sex and age. Three controls were selected for each patient. Among controls, mean cigarette consumption of the genotypes were identical to each other, in contrast with those among patients.

The distribution of patients and controls by genotype and cigarette dose level are shown in Table 3. The frequency of genotype C among controls was almost constant at all cigarette dose levels, while that among patients clearly depended on dose level: *i.e.*, the frequency reduced with increasing dose level. This indicated that the susceptibility of genotype C to the carcinoma varied as a function of cigarette dose, and we therefore estimated the odds ratios at different dose levels. These ratios are calculated in the same table, taking the risk of the controls with genotypes A+B at the lowest dose level of less than $3\times10^5$ cigarettes over a lifetime to be at a baseline of 1.0. We could not take the baseline of exposure as never-smokers, since there were only two never-smokers among the patients (Fig. 2). It was found that the odds ratio of genotypes C increased with cigarette dose and saturated at the dose of 3 to $4\times10^5$ cigarettes, while that of genotypes A+B increased linearly with dose. This was obvious even when we combined the two dose levels into one level of more than $3\times10^5$ cigarettes: *i.e.*, the large difference between the odds ratio of 7.31 of genotype C and 1.0 of A+B in the low dose level dropped drastically to a smaller difference of 13.17 and 8.89 at the high dose. This was clearly demonstrated by the susceptibility estimate in Table 3, where the susceptibility was odds ratio of genotype C to A+B at the same dose level and was equal to the ratio of odds ratios shown in Table 3. The relative risks by the genotypes in relation to cigarette dose are summarized in Fig. 3.

## *Concluding Remarks*

We have shown the results of two different approaches to investigate inter-individual differences in susceptibility to lung cancer: *i.e.*, a comparison of the genotype

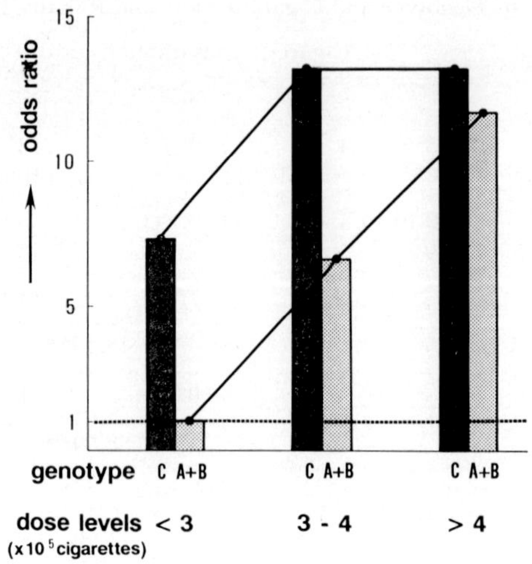


FIG. 3. Relative risk of the genotypes in relation to cigarette consumption.

frequencies between patients and a healthy population, and a relative risk estimate of susceptible individuals in relation to cigarette smoking dose. Our results of these approaches can be summarized: (1) a significant difference in frequencies of the genotypes was observed between patients with lung cancer and healthy controls, and the observed risk elevation of genotype C was specific to Kreyberg I type, not to Kreyberg II (adenocarcinoma). (2) An intrapatient study on cumulative cigarette dose for squamous cell carcinoma revealed that those with genotype C contracted the cancer with less cigarette consumption than other genotypes; the relative risk estimate based on a case-control study showed that the risk of people with genotype C to the carcinoma was remarkably high at a low dose of cigarette smoking, and that their risk elevation with increasing dose saturated at high dose levels, being closer to the risk of other genotypes.

Our study identified genetically susceptible individuals to lung cancer at the DNA level. We are now investigating the linkage of the polymorphic MspI site with a "real susceptibility site(s)" in the coding or regulatory regions of P-450IA1 gene by polymerase chain reaction (PCR) direct sequencing.

## REFERENCES

1. Heidelberger, C. Chemical carcinogenesis. Annu. Rev. Biochem., *44*: 79–121, 1975.
2. Nebert, D. W. and Gonzalez, F. J. P-450 genes: Structure, evolution, and regulation. Annu. Rev. Biochem., *56*: 945–993, 1987.
3. Guengerich, F. P. Roles of cytochrome P-450 enzymes in chemical carcinogenesis and cancer chemotherapy. Cancer Res., *48*: 2946–2954, 1988.
4. Ayesh, R., Idle, J. R., Ritchie, J. C., Crothers, M. J., and Hetzel, M. R. Metabolic oxidation phenotypes as markers for susceptibility to lung cancer. Nature, *312*: 169–170, 1984.
5. Kaisary, A., Smith, P., Jaczq, E., McAllister, C. B., Wilkinson, G. R., Ray, W. A., and Branch, R. A. Genetic predisposition to bladder cancer: ability to hydroxylate debrisoquine and mephenytoin as risk factors. Cancer Res., *47*: 5488–5493, 1987.

6. Kellermann, G., Shaw, C. R., and Luyten-Kellermann, M. Aryl hydrocarbon hydroxylase inducibility and bronchogenic carcinoma. N. Engl. J. Med., *298*: 934–937, 1973.
7. Kouri, R. E., McKinney, C. R., Slomiany, D. J., Snodgrass, D. R., Wray, N. P., and McLemore, T. L. Positive correlation between high aryl hydrocarbon hydroxylase activity and primary lung cancer as analyzed in cryopreserved lymphocytes. Cancer Res., *42*: 5030–5037, 1982.
8. Kawajiri, K., Nakachi, K., Imai, K., Yoshii, A., Shinoda, N., and Watanabe, J. Identification of genetically high risk individuals to lung cancer by DNA polymorphisms of the cytochrome P450IA1 gene. FEBS Lett., *263*: 131–133, 1990.
9. Kawajiri, K., Watanabe, J., Gotoh, O., Tagashira, Y., Sogawa, K., and Fujii-Kuriyama, Y. Structure and drug inducibility of the human cytochrome P-450c gene. Eur. J. Biochem., *159*: 219–225, 1986.
10. Mullis, K. B. and Faloona, F. A. Specific synthesis of DNA *in vitro via* a polymerase-catalyzed chain reaction. Methods Enzymol., *155*: 335–350, 1987.

XENOBIOTICS AND CANCER, L. ERNSTER ET AL. (EDS.),
JAPAN SCI. SOC. PRESS, TOKYO/TAYLOR & FRANCIS LTD., LONDON, pp. 63–73, 1991

# Oxidation of Polycyclic Hydrocarbons by Oxygen Radicals

Lawrence J. MARNETT, Ashok REDDY, Donna PRUESS-SCHWARTZ, and Chuan JI

*A. B. Hancock, Jr. Memorial Laboratory for Cancer Research, Departments of Biochemistry and Chemistry, Center in Molecular Toxicology, Vanderbilt University School of Medicine, Nashville, Tennessee 37232, U.S.A.*

*Abstract:* Dihydrodiolepoxides (BPDE) are reactive derivatives that appear to mediate the genotoxic effects of benzo[a]pyrene (BP) and several other polycyclic hydrocarbons. Their formation requires sequential epoxidation, hydration, and epoxidation steps. The first epoxidation step is catalyzed by cytochrome P-450 isoenzymes whereas the second is catalyzed by cytochromes P-450 and assorted species of oxygen radicals (in particular peroxyl radicals). The stereochemistry of epoxidation of the procarcinogen 7,8-dihydroxy-7,8-dihydrobenzo[a]pyrene (BP-7,8-diol) is a useful tool with which to dissect the contributions of cytochrome P-450-dependent and independent pathways. [$^{32}$P]-Postlabeling techniques were developed to analyze the diastereomeric composition of BPDE-deoxynucleoside-*bis*-phosphate adducts recovered from DNA of target tissues for BP tumorigenesis. Application of these techniques revealed that cytochrome P-450 is the major contributor to BPDE production in mouse skin *in vivo*. Following administration of BP or (+)-BP-7,8-diol to female CD-1 mice, only minor amounts of adducts derived from peroxyl radical epoxidation were detected. In contrast, pretreatment of the animals with the tumor promoter tetradecanoyl phorbol acetate (TPA) led to the formation of sizeable amounts of non-cytochrome P-450-dependent adducts following coincident administration of (+)-BP-7,8-diol with a second dose of TPA. The results demonstrate that although oxygen radicals appear to play a minor role in tumor initiation by BP, they may play a major role in tumor promotion by phorbol esters.

Polycyclic hydrocarbons represent an important class of xenobiotics (*1*, *2*). From the early reports of Potts that scrotal cancer in humans has an environmental etiology, advances in our understanding of polycyclic hydrocarbon disposition have provided insights into the mechanisms of chemical carcinogenesis. A rather complete picture now exists of the metabolic activation of a few polycyclic hydrocarbons and the structures of their conjugates to DNA (*3*). In most cases, conversion to dihydrodiolepoxides (BPDE) is critical to DNA binding, mutagenesis, and tumor initiation (*4–10*). Figure 1 illustrates the metabolic transformations that convert benzo[a]pyrene (BP) to BPDE. Epoxidation of the 7,8-double bond produces an arene oxide that

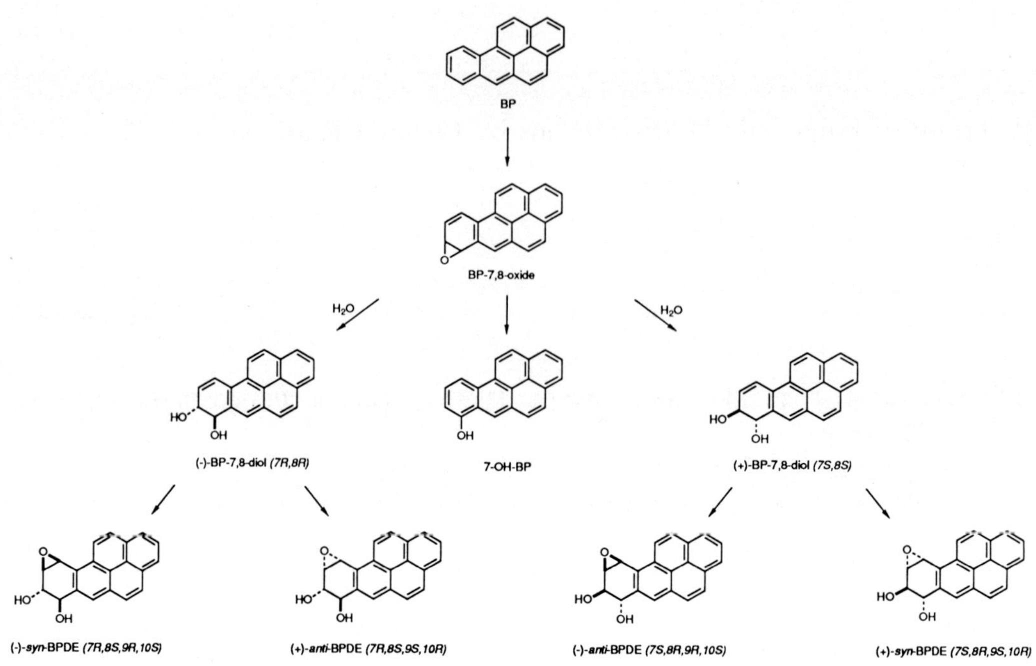


FIG. 1. Pathways of oxidation of BP to BPDE's.

isomerizes non-enzymatically to 7-hydroxy-BP or is hydrated enzymatically to 7,8-dihydroxy-7,8-dihydrobenzo[a]pyrene (BP-7,8-diol). Epoxidation of the 9,10-double bond of BP-7,8-diol produces highly reactive, mutagenic, and tumorigenic BPDE. Four diastereomers of BPDE exist but are not produced in equal amounts in all tissues (*11*). In fact, they are not produced in equal amounts in any tissues because of stereospecificity at each of the enzymatic steps illustrated in Fig. 1. Certain BPDE's exhibit potent mutagenicity and tumor-initiating activity in the mouse skin multiple stage carcinogenesis model (*12*). On this basis, they appear to be the major activated metabolites of BP. An alternate activation pathway for BP is one-electron oxidation which leads to DNA adducts derived from radical cations (*13, 14*). One-electron oxidation occurs *in vivo* but appears to be a relatively minor pathway of oxidative activation of BP in mouse skin (*15*).

Oxygenation of BP to BP-7,8-oxide is catalyzed by cytochromes P-450 *in vitro*. P-450IA1 (P-$450_c$) is the most active of the orthologs at the oxygenation of BP and the oxygenation of BP-7,8-diol (*16*). However, P-450IA1 is not a quantitatively important form in human liver so in this tissue the two oxygenation steps are catalyzed by different orthologs. BP oxidation to BP-7,8-oxide is catalyzed primarily by P-450IA2 in human liver microsomes whereas BP-7,8-diol oxidation to BPDE is catalyzed by P-450IIIA2 (*17*).

BP-7,8-diol oxygenation to BPDE is also effected by a variety of non-cytochrome P-450 catalysts. Enzyme reactions that generate peroxyl free radicals are particularly efficient in this regard (*18*). Peroxyl radicals insert oxygen atoms into the 9,10-double bond *via* the stepwise process depicted in Scheme 1. Peroxyl radical generation is associated with prostaglandin H (PGH) synthase and lipoxygenase catalyzed oxygenation of polyunsaturated fatty acids, NADPH- and ascorbate-dependent lipid peroxidation, peroxidase-dependent oxidation of β-dicarbonyl compounds, bisulfite, and hydroperoxides, and neutrophil-dependent superoxide generation (*19–26*).

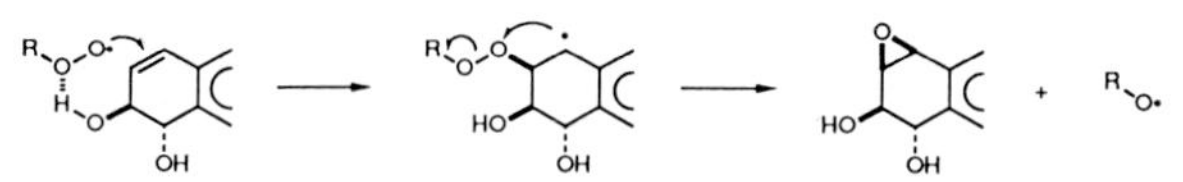

SCHEME 1.

The extent to which cytochrome P-450 and non-cytochrome P-450 processes contribute to BP-7,8-diol epoxidation *in vivo* is a matter of considerable interest. The principal diagnostic tool with which to answer this question is the differential stereochemistry of epoxidation of the (+)-enantiomer (*27, 28*). The major product of epoxidation of (+)-PB-7,8-diol by cytochromes P-450IA1 and IIIA2 is (+)-*syn*-BPDE (*17, 29, 30*). This outcome is determined by the orientation of the hydrocarbon at the active site of the protein (*31*). In contrast, non-cytochrome P-450 oxidations of (+)-BP-7,8-diol produce primarily (but not exclusively) (−)-*anti*-BPDE (*27, 28*). Hydrogen bonding of the 8-hydroxyl group with the approaching peroxyl radical apparently accounts for this result. By quantitating the extent of conversion of (+)-BP-7,8-diol to BPDE-derived products, it is possible to estimate the relative contribution of cytochrome P-450 and non-cytochrome P-450 processes to epoxidation. This approach has been used to demonstrate non-cytochrome P-450-dependent epoxidation of (+)-BP-7,8-diol in cultured C3H10T1/2 cells, cultured hamster trachea, freshly isolated mouse epidermal cells and epidermal homogenates, and mouse skin *in vivo* (*32–35*).

BPDE's are unstable and hydrolyze to *cis* and *trans*-tetrahydrotetraols (Scheme 2) (*36–38*). The tetraols can be separated by reversed phase HPLC to provide an indirect estimate of the stereochemistry of the BPDE's produced. This strategy was employed in all of the studies cited above. Radioactively-labeled (+)-BP-7,8-diol is commercially available which provides a high sensitivity method for detecting product formation. Tetrahydrotetraols are also commercially available so quantitating their formation is the straightforward method of choice for determining the contribution of non-cytochrome P-450 oxidations to BPDE formation. However, in certain situations this is not practical. For example, when BP-7,8-diol is administered to intact animals, both the diol and its oxidation products disappear rapidly from the tissues to which they are applied. This greatly complicates accurate quantitation of the pathways of BP-7,8-diol oxidation.

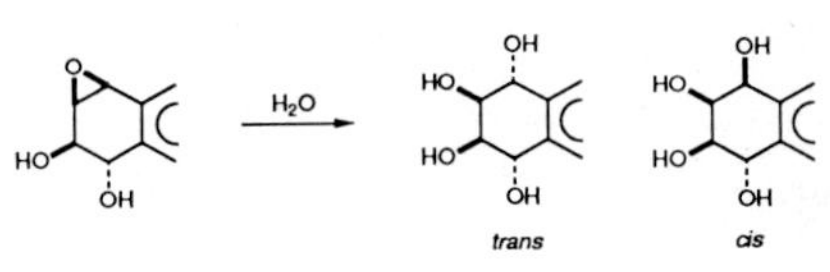


SCHEME 2.

## *DNA Adduction by BP in Mouse Skin In Vivo*

BPDE's also react with DNA and the levels of individual deoxynucleoside adducts can be used to evaluate the stereochemistry of (+)-BP-7,8-diol epoxidation

(*39–41*). Several practical problems limit the utility of this approach but it offers the potential advantage of integrating BPDE formation with time (in the absence of rapid DNA repair). Our laboratory utilized HPLC separation of BPDE-deoxynucleoside adducts to estimate the contribution of non-cytochrome P-450 pathways to BP-7,8-diol oxidation in mouse skin (*35*). Commercially available [$^3$H]-BP-7,8-diol was used for these experiments, but the low level of DNA adduction necessitated the use of large amounts of radiolabel (25 $\mu$Ci per animal) and 10–15 animals per datum point. This limited the variety of experiments that could be performed and precluded extensive studies of the effects of inhibitors, inducers, *etc*. Therefore, we have explored the possibility of using [$^{32}$P]-postlabeling techniques to analyze the diastereomeric BPDE-DNA adducts. The high sensitivity of postlabeling technology and the use of unlabeled BP-7,8-diol greatly enhances the flexibility of experimental design (*42*).

Standards of deoxynucleoside-*bis*-phosphates were prepared by reacting calf thymus DNA with (+)-*anti*-BPDE, (—)-*anti*-BPDE, (±)-*syn*-BPDE, and (+)-*syn*-BPDE. Standard Randerath postlabeling techniques were employed with a few modifications to maximize separation of the diastereomeric adducts (*42–44*). The most important modification was inclusion of 0.5 M boric acid and 0.5 M $MgCl_2$ in D4. The chromatographic system developed provides excellent separation of (+)-*syn*-BPDE and (—)-*anti*-BPDE adducts and acceptable separation of (+)-*anti*-BPDE adducts from them. The sensitivity of detection is sufficiently high that DNA from a single animal treated with BP or BP-7,8-diol can be analyzed for adduct content.

Figure 2 displays a chromatographic fingerprint of the adducts detected in the epidermal DNA from a female CD-1 mouse 4 hr after topical administration of BP. An intense spot is detected that cochromatographs with a standard of the *trans*-N$^2$-deoxyguanosine-(+)-*anti*-BPDE adduct. This result is consistent with previous literature reports on the identity of epidermal DNA adducts produced from BP (*39*, *40*, *44*, *45*). A minor adduct spot is detected that cochromatographs with the major DNA adduct produced by reaction with (+)-*syn*-BPDE. These observations are consistent with cytochrome P-450-catalyzed oxygenation of BP to (+)- and (—)-BP-7,8-diol

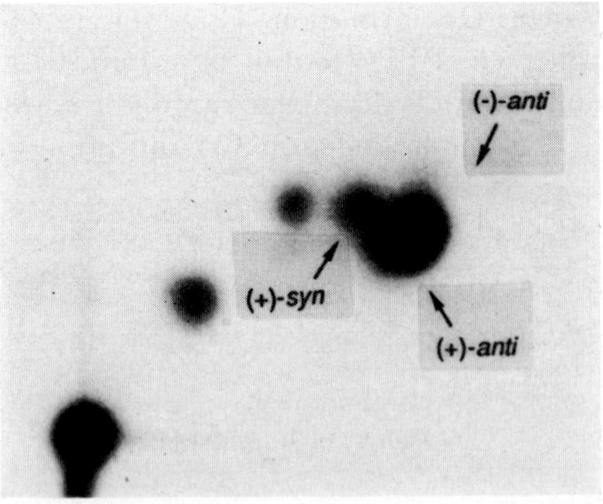


FIG. 2. Chromatographic fingerprint of deoxynucleoside-*bis*-phosphate adducts detected in mouse skin following administration of BP. BP=100 nmol/100 $\mu$l acetone. The major adduct cochromatographs with a standard of the N$^2$-deoxyguanosine-(+)-*anti*-BPDE adduct. No spots are observed in the region where adducts from (—)-*anti*-BPDE chromatograph.

followed by epoxidation of the BP-7,8-diol enantiomers to BPDE. It is noteworthy that a spot is not detected in the region of adducts formed by reaction of DNA with (—)-*anti*-BPDE. This implies that peroxyl radicals do not play a major role in the epoxidation of (+)-BP-7,8-diol produced from BP by cytochrome P-450. It is also unlikely that peroxyl radicals play a significant role in the epoxidation of the (—)-BP-7,8-diol produced from BP. Although peroxyl radicals and cytochrome P-450 oxidize (—)-BP-7,8-diol to the same product, (+)-*anti*-BPDE, the extent of epoxidation of the (+)- and (—)-BP-7,8-diol enantiomers by peroxyl radicals is the same. Thus, if they did not epoxidize the (+)-BP-7,8-diol enantiomer they would not be expected to epoxidize the (—)-enantiomer.

### *DNA Adduction by (+)-BP-7,8-diol in Mouse Skin In Vitro*

The conclusion of the experiment is that peroxyl radicals do not play a major role in metabolism of BP to DNA-binding derivatives in mouse skin *in vivo*. Conversely, cytochrome P-450 (ortholog unknown) appears to be the predominant catalyst for both epoxidations. The preeminence of cytochrome P-450 may be due to the ability of BP to induce synthesis of P-450IA1 in epidermal cells. Therefore, similar experiments were undertaken with (+)-BP-7,8-diol, which does not induce synthesis of cytochromes P-450 in mouse skin (*35*). Figure 3 displays a chromatogram from a typical experiment. Although a faint spot does appear at a position that cochromatographs with a (—)-*anti*-BPDE-DNA adduct, the major adduct is derived from (+)-*syn*-BPDE, the product of cytochrome P-450 epoxidation of (+)-BP-7,8-diol. Similar results were obtained over a wide range of doses of (+)-BP-7,8-diol and from times from 1–24 hr following administration of the diol. Taken with the results of the experiments with BP, these results provide strong evidence for the primacy of cytochrome P-450 in both epoxidation steps in the metabolic activation of BP to BPDE in mouse skin *in vivo*.

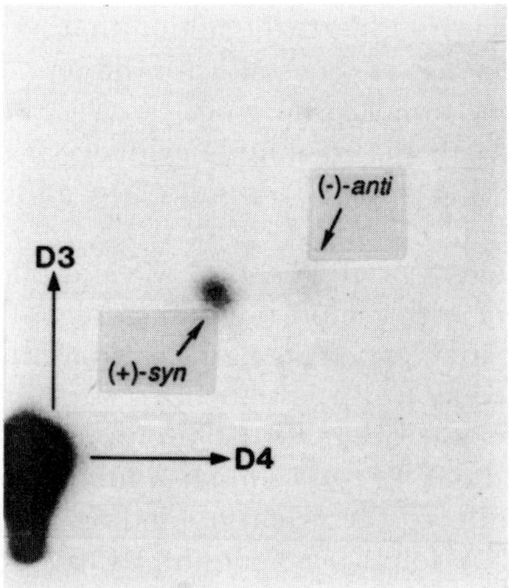


FIG. 3. Chromatographic fingerprint of deoxynucleoside-*bis*-phosphate adducts detected in mouse skin following administration of (+)-BP-7, 8-diol. BP-7, 8-diol=200 nmol/100 $\mu$l acetone. Diol left on skin 6 hr before sacrifice.

These results contrast with the results of previous investigations of the epoxidation of (+)-BP-7,8-diol by freshly isolated mouse epidermal cells, mouse epidermal homogenates, and intact mouse skin (*34*, *35*). All of the earlier studies monitored tetrahydrotetraol hydrolysis products rather than DNA adducts as indicators of BP-7,8-diol oxidation. It is conceivable that some degree of stereospecificity is observed in the reaction of (−)-*anti*-BPDE with DNA which limits its extent of adduction. Such stereospecificity is well-precedented for the reaction of (+)-*anti*-BPDE with DNA (*41*). If (−)-*anti*-BPDE reacts poorly with DNA, the use of DNA to trap it *in vivo* would significantly underestimate the extent of its formation in epidermal cells. Quantitative studies of the extent of DNA binding by each of the diastereomers of BPDE to mouse skin DNA *in vivo* are, therefore, in progress. Another potential explanation for the discrepancy between the present results and earlier reports on BP-7,8-diol oxidation is an altered metabolic capability of the various *ex vivo* epidermal preparations. Recent experiments in our laboratory reveal that BP-7,8-diol is extremely sensitive to peroxyl radical-dependent epoxidation during lipid peroxidation induced by tissue stress. This suggests that the procedures used to prepare "intact" keratinocytes and mouse skin homogenates may have led to a significant increase in lipid peroxidation which would have skewed the metabolic capabilities of the cells or homogenates in favor of peroxyl radical-dependent epoxidation.

### *Oxidant Generation in Mouse Skin by Phorbol Ester Tumor Promoters*

The experiments described above indicate that the levels of DNA adducts in mouse skin derived from peroxyl radical epoxidation products of (+)-BP-7,8-diol are quite low. This suggests (+)-BP-7,8-diol may be an ideal tool with which to probe for increases in non-cytochrome P-450 oxidant formation following pharmacological manipulation of the epidermis because there is a low background level of radical adduct formation. A particularly important application of this technology is to test for the production of oxidants following topical administration of tumor promoters. A considerable body of circumstantial evidence supports the notion that phorbol ester and non-phorbol ester tumor promoters increase oxygen radical production in mouse skin and that this is an important event in tumor promotion (*46–49*). However, a critical evaluation of the available data reveals that definitive evidence is lacking for the production of oxygen radicals in mouse skin *in vivo* as a result of the administration of tumor promoters.

Experiments were conducted in which (+)-BP-7,8-diol was applied to the shaven backs of female CD-1 mice coincident with tumor promoting doses (1–10 nmol) of tetradecanoyl phorbol acetate (TPA). After varying lengths of time, the animals were sacrificed and epidermal DNA analyzed by [$^{32}$P]-postlabeling as described above. At times up to 24 hr post-application, no alteration in the profile of adducts was observed relative to controls performed without TPA. A similar finding was reported several years ago by Kensler *et al.* who monitored the extent of binding of metabolites of [$^{3}$H]-(±)-BP-7,8-diol to epidermal DNA following coadministration of BP-7,8-diol and TPA (*26*). These workers also reported that pretreatment of the mice with TPA 16 hr prior to treatment with BP-7,8-diol and TPA increased the level of total binding by 30–60%. The identities of the adducts generated in these experiments were not established.

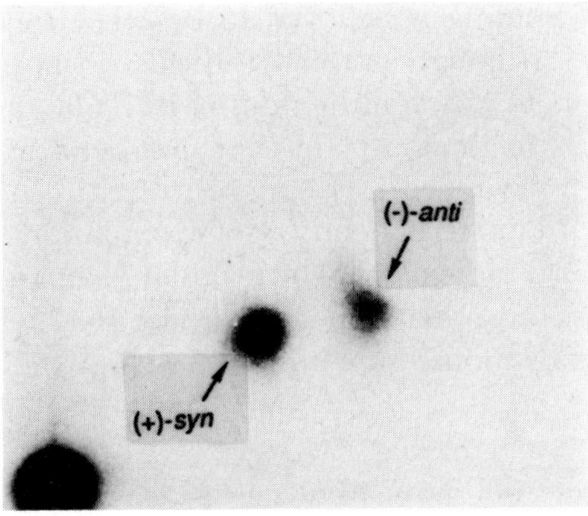


FIG. 4. Chromatographic fingerprint of deoxynucleoside-*bis*-phosphate adducts detected in mouse skin following administration of (+)-BP-7,8-diol and TPA, 24 hr after pretreatment with TPA. BP-7,8-diol=200 nmol/100 μl acetone. TPA=10 nmol/100 μl acetone. Diol left on skin 6 hr before sacrifice.

We, therefore, conducted experiments to evaluate the nature of the oxidants produced during multiple TPA treatments. Figure 4 compared the pattern of adducts detected by [$^{32}P$]-postlabeling following single or dual application of TPA. Similar results were obtained whether the animals were sacrificed 6 or 24 hr after administration of (+)-BP-7,8-diol. A significant alteration of the adduct profile is clear in the dual treatment experiments. The adducts that increase in abundance cochromatograph with the adducts produced by reaction of epidermal DNA with (−)-*anti*-BPDE, the non-cytochrome P-450 oxidation product of (+)-BP-7,8-diol. This suggests that sequential treatment of mouse skin with the phorbol ester tumor promoter TPA enhances generation of non-cytochrome P-450 oxidants. Similar experiments performed with the non-promoting phorbol ester 4-O-methyl-TPA, reveal no increase in the yield of the non-cytochrome P-450 adducts. This establishes that oxidant production is correlated with tumor promoting activity.

The identity of the oxidants produced in response to TPA administration is unknown. Kensler *et al.* demonstrated that pretreatment of mouse skin with TPA caused an infiltration of inflammatory cells and an attendant increase in myeloperoxidase activity (*26*). Activated neutrophils generate copious amounts of superoxide and therein hydrogen peroxide which is a substrate for myeloperoxidase. Thus, neutrophil recruitment may be an important component of the alteration of epidermal metabolism by the first TPA treatment. Activation of the recruited neutrophils may account for the requirement for a second TPA treatment. Experiments performed with a single TPA administration 24 hr before application of (+)-BP-7,8-diol (without the second TPA treatment) revealed no alteration of adducts relative to (+)-BP-7,8-diol alone. Thus, both TPA treatments are required; this may parallel the multiple treatments of phorbol ester tumor promotion.

*Conclusions*

The stereochemical approach outlined above established that cytochrome P-450 plays a predominant role in the oxidation of BP and BP-7,8-diol to DNA binding derivatives in mouse skin *in vivo*. This binding is believed to be a key step in tumor initiation by polycyclic hydrocarbons. Although peroxyl radicals do not appear to be quantitatively important contributors to DNA adduction by BP, adaptation of our basic experimental protocol enabled us to demonstrate that non-cytochrome P-450 oxidants (perhaps oxygen radicals) are produced in response to treatment of mouse skin with tumor promoters. The differential stereochemistry of epoxidation of (+)-BP-7,8-diol by cytochrome P-450 and peroxyl radicals may be a valuable diagnostic probe to evaluate the role of oxygen radicals and other non-cytochrome P-450 oxidants in the promotion and progression phases of mouse skin tumorigenesis.

*Acknowledgment*

This research was supported by a research grant from the National Cancer Institute (CA47479).

REFERENCES

1. Sims, P. and Grover, P. L. Epoxides in polycyclic aromatic hydrocarbon metabolism and carcinogenesis. Adv. Cancer Res., *20*: 165–774, 1974.
2. Harvey, R. G. Polycyclic hydrocarbons and cancer. Am. Sci., *70*: 386–393, 1982.
3. Dipple, A., Moschel, R. C., and Bigger, C.A.H. Polycyclic aromatic carcinogens. *In;* C. E. Searle (ed.), Chemical Carcinogens, Second edition, pp. 41–163, American Chemical Society, Washington, D. C., 1984.
4. Sims, P., Grover, P. L., Swaisland, A., Pal, K., and Hewer, A. Metabolic activation of benzo[a]pyrene proceeds by a diol-epoxide. Nature, *252*: 326–328, 1974.
5. Wood, A. W., Levin, W., Lu, A. Y. H., Yagi, H., Hernandez, O., Jerina, D. M., and Conney, A. H. Metabolism of benzo[a]pyrene and benzo[a]pyrene derivatives to mutagenic products by highly purified hepatic microsomal enzymes. J. Biol. Chem., *251*: 4882–4890, 1976.
6. Huberman, E., Sachs, L., Yang, S. K., and Gelboin, H. V. Identification of mutagenic metabolites of benzo[a]pyrene in mammalian cells. Proc. Natl. Acad. Sci. U.S.A., *73*: 607–611, 1976.
7. Wood, A. W., Wislocki, P. G., Chang, R. L., Levin, W., Lu, A. Y. H., Yagi, H., Hernandez, O., Jerina, D. M., and Conney, A. H. Mutagenicity and cytotoxicity of benzo(a)pyrene benzo-ring epoxides. Cancer Res., *36*: 3358–3366, 1976.
8. Levin, W., Wood, A. W., Chang, R. L., Slaga, T. J., Yagi, H., Jerina, D. M., and Conney, A. H. Marked differences in the tumor-initiating activity of optically pure (+)- and (−)-*trans*-7,8-dihydroxy-7,8-dihydrobenzo(a)pyrene on mouse skin. Cancer Res., *37*: 2721–2725, 1977.
9. Levin, W., Buening, M. K., Wood, A. W., Chang, R. L., Kedzierski, B., Thakker, D. R., Boyd, D. R., Gadaginamath, G. S., Armstrong, R. N., Yagi, H., Karle, J. M., Slaga, T. J., Jerina, D. M., and Conney, A. H. An enantiomeric interaction in the metabolism and tumorigenicity of (+)-and (−)-benzo[a]pyrene 7,8-oxide. J. Biol. Chem., *255*: 9067–9074, 1980.
10. Slaga, T. J., Gleason, G. L., Mills, G., Ewald, L., Fu, P. O., Lee, H. M., and Harvey, R. G. Comparison of skin tumor-initiating activities of dihydrodiols and diol epoxides of various polycyclic aromatic hydrocarbons. Cancer Res., *40*: 1981–1984, 1980.
11. Jerina, D. M., Lehr, R., Schaefer-Ridder, M., Yagi, H., Karle, J. M., Thakker, D. R., Wood, A. W., Lu, A. Y. H., Ryan, D., West, S., Levin, W., and Conney, A. H. Bay-region epoxides of dihydrodiols: A concept explaining the mutagenic and carcinogenic

activity of benzo[a]pyrene and benzo[a]anthracene. *In;* H. H. Hiatt, J. D. Watson, and J. A. Winsten (eds.), Origins of Human Cancer, pp. 639–658, Cold Spring Harbor Laboratory, Cold Spring Harbor, 1977.

12. Slaga, T. J., Bracken, W. J., Gleason, G., Levin, W., Yagi, H., Jerina, D. M., and Conney, A. H. Marked differences in the skin tumor-initiating activities of the optical enantiomers of the diastereomeric benzo[a]pyrene 7,8-diol-9,10-epoxides. Cancer Res., *39*: 67–71, 1979.
13. Rogan, E. G., Cavalieri, E. L., Tibbels, S. R., Cremonesi, P., Warnder, C. D., Nagal, D. L., Tomer, K. B., Cerny, R. L., and Gross, M. L. Synthesis and identification of benzo[a]pyrene-guanine nucleoside adducts formed by electrochemical oxidation and by horseradish peroxidase-catalyzed reaction of benzo[a]pyrene with DNA. J. Am. Chem. Soc., *110*: 4023–4029, 1988.
14. Kapitulnik, J., Wislocki, P. G., Levin, W., Yagi, H., Jerina, D. M., and Conney, A. H. Tumorigenicity studies with diol-epoxides of benzo[a]pyrene which indicate that (±)-*trans*-7β,8α-dihdryoxy-9α,10α-epoxy-7,8,9,10-tetrahydrobenzo[a]pyrene is an ultimate carcinogen in newborn mice. Cancer Res., *38*: 354, 1978.
15. Bodell, W. J., Devanesan P. D., Rogan, E. G., and Cavalieri, E. L. $^{32}$P-Postlabeling analysis of benzo[a]pyrene-DNA adducts formed *in vitro* and *in vivo*. Chem. Res. Toxicol., *2*: 312–315, 1989.
16. Thakker, D. R., Yagi, H., Lu, A. Y. H., Levin, W., Conney, A. H., and Jerina, D. M. Metabolism of benzo[a]pyrene: Conversion of (±)-*trans*-7,8-dihydroxy-7,8-dihydrobenzo[a]pyrene to highly mutagenic 7,8-diol-9,10-epoxides. Proc. Natl. Acad. Sci. U.S.A., *73*: 3381–3385, 1976.
17. Shimada, T., Martin, M. V., Pruess-Schwartz, D., Marnett, L. J., and Guengerich, F. P. Roles of individual human cytochrome P-450 enzymes in the bioactivation of benzo[a]pyrene, 7,8-dihydroxy-7,8-dihydrobenzo[a]pyrene, and other dihydrodiol derivatives of polycyclic aromatic hydrocarbons. Cancer Res., *49*: 6304–6312, 1989.
18. Marnett, L. J. Peroxyl free radicals: potential mediators of tumor initiation and promotion. Carcinogenesis, *8*: 1365–1373, 1987.
19. Marnett, L. J., Johnson, J. T., and Bienkowski, M. J. Arachidonic acid-dependent metabolism of 7,8-dihydroxy-7,8-dihydrobenzo[a]pyrene by ram seminal vesicles. FEBS Lett., *106*: 13–16, 1979.
20. Sivarajah, K., Mukhtar, H., and Eling, T. E. Arachidonic acid-dependent metabolism of (±)-*trans*-7,8-dihydroxy-7,8-dihydrobenzo[a]pyrene (BP-7,8-diol) to 7,10/8,9-tetrols. FEBS Letts., *106*: 17–20, 1979.
21. Dix, T. A. Fontana, R., Panthani, A., and Marnett, L. J. Hematin-catalyzed epoxidation of 7,8-dihydroxy-7,8-dihydrobenzo[a]pyrene (BP-7,8-diol) by polyunsaturated fatty acid hydroperoxides. J. Biol. Chem., *260*: 5358–5365, 1985.
22. Dix, T. A. and Marnett, L. J. Metabolism of polycyclic aromatic hydrocarbon derivatives to ultimate carcinogens during lipid-peroxidation. Science, *221*: 77–79, 1983.
23. Battista, J. R., Dix, T. A., and Marnett, L. J. The mechanism of hydroperoxide-dependent epoxidation of 7,8-dihydroxy-7,8-dihydrobenzo[a]pyrene by rat liver microsomes. Proc. Am. Assoc. Cancer Res., *25*: 114, 1984. (Abstract)
24. Reed, G. A., Brooks, E. A., and Eling, T. E. Phenylbutazone-dependent epoxidation of 7,8-dihydroxy-7,8-dihydrobenzo(a)pyrene: a new mechanism for prostaglandin H synthase-catalyzed oxidations. J. Biol. Chem., *259*: 5591–5595, 1984.
25. Reed, G. A., Curtis, J. F., Mottley, C., Eling, T. E., and Mason, R. P. Epoxidation of (±)-7,8-dihydroxy-7,8-dihydrobenzo[a]pyrene during (bi)sulfite autoxidation: Activation of a procarcinogen by a cocarcinogen. Proc. Natl. Acad. Sci. U.S.A., *83*: 7499–7502, 1986.

26. Kensler, T. W., Egner, T. A., Moore, K. G., Taffe, B. G., Twerdok, L. E., and Trush, M. A. Role of inflammatory cells in the metabolic activation of polycyclic aromatic hydrocarbons in mouse skin. Toxicol. Appl. Pharmacol., *90*: 337–346, 1987.
27. Panthananickal, A. and Marnett, L. J. Arachidonic acid-dependent metabolism of (±)-7,8-dihydroxy-7,8-dihydrobenzol[a]pyrene to polyguanylic acid-binding derivatives. Chem. Biol. Interactions, *33*: 239–252, 1981.
28. Dix, T. A. and Marnett, L. J. Detection of the metabolism of polycyclic aromatic hydrocarbon derivatives to ultimate carcinogens during lipid peroxidation. Methods Enzymol., *105*: 347–352, 1984.
29. Thakker, D. R., Yagi, H., Akagi, H., Koreeda, M., Lu, A. Y. H., Levin, W., Wood, A. W., Conney, A. H., and Jerina, D. M. Stereoselective metabolism of benzo[a]pyrene and benzo[a]pyrene-7,8-dihydrodiol to diol-epoxides. Chem. Biol. Interactions, *16*: 281–300, 1977.
30. Deutsch, J., Leutz, J. C., Yang, S. K., Gelboin, H. V., Chang, R. L., Vatsis, K. P., and Coon, M. J. Regio- and stereoselectivity of various forms of cytochrome P-450 in the metabolism of benzo[a]pyrene and (±)-7,8-dihydroxy-7,8-dihydrobenzo[a]-pyrene as shown by product formation and binding to DNA. Proc. Natl. Acad. Sci. U.S.A., *75*: 3123–3127, 1978.
31. Jerina, D. M., Michaud, D. P., Feldman, R. J., Armstrong, R. N., Vyas, K. P., Thakker, D. R., Yagi, H., Thomas, P. E., Ryan, D. E., and Levin, W. Stereochemical modeling of the catalytic site of cytochrome P-450c. *In;* R. Sato and R. Kato (eds.), Microsomes, Drug Oxidations, and Drug Toxicity, pp. 195–201, Wiley-Interscience, New York, 1982.
32. Boyd, J. A., Barrett, J. C., and Eling, T. E. Prostaglandin endoperoxide synthetase dependent cooxidation of (±)-*trans*-7,8-dihydroxy-7,8-dihydrobenzo[a]pyrene in C3H10T1/2 clone 8 cells. Cancer Res., *42*: 2828–2832, 1982.
33. Reed, G. A., Grafstrom, R. C., Krauss, R. S., Autrup, H., and Eling, T. E. Prostaglandin H synthase-dependent co-oxygenation of (±)-7,8-dihydroxy-7,8-dihydrobenzo[a]pyrene in hamster trachea and human bronchus explants. Carcinogenesis, *5*: 955–960, 1984.
34. Eling, T., Curtis, J., Battista, J., and Marnett, L. J. Oxidation of (+)-7,8-dihydroxy-7,8-dihydrobenzo[a]pyrene by mouse keratinocytes: evidence for peroxyl radical- and monoxygenase-dependent metabolism. Carcinogenesis, *7*: 1957–1963, 1986.
35. Pruess-Schwartz, D., Nimesheim, A., and Marnett, L. J. Peroxyl radical- and cytochrome P-450-dependent metabolic activation of (+)-7,8-dihydroxy-7,8-dihydrobenzo[a]pyrene in mouse skin *in vitro* and *in vivo*. Cancer Res., *49*: 1732–1737, 1989.
36. Keller, J. W., Heidelberger, C., Beland, F. A., and Harvey, R. G. Hydrolysis of syn- and anti-benzo[a]pyrene diol epoxides: stereochemistry, kinetics, and the effect of an intramolecular hydrogen bond on the rate of syn-diol epoxide solvolysis. J. Am. Chem. Soc., *98*: 8276–8277, 1976.
37. Yang, S. K., McCourt, D. W., Gelboin, H. V., Miller, J. R., and Roller, P. P. Stereochemistry of the hydrolysis products and their acetonides of two stereoisomeric benzo[a]-pyrene 7,8-diol 9,10-epoxides. J. Am. Chem. Soc., *99*: 5124–5130, 1977.
38. Whalen, D. L., Ross, A. M., Yagi, H., Karle, J. M., and Jerina, D. M. Stereoelectronic factors in the solvolysis of bay region diol epoxides of polycyclic aromatic hydrocarbons. J. Am. Chem. Soc., *100*: 5218–5221, 1978.
39. Weinstein, I. B., Jeffrey, A. M., Jennette, K. W., Blobstein, S. A., Harvey, R. G., Harris, C., Autrup, H., Kasai, H., and Nakanishi, K. Benzo[a]pyrene diol epoxides as intermediates in nucleic acid binding *in vitro* and *in vivo*. Science, *193*: 592–595, 1976.
40. Koreeda, M., Moore, P. D., Wislocki, P. G., Levin, W., Conney, A. H., Yagi, H., and

Jerina, D. M. Binding of benzo[a]pyrene 7,8-diol-9,10-epoxide to DNA, RNA, and protein of mouse skin occurs with high stereoselectivity. Science, *199*: 778–781, 1978.

41. Meehan, T. and Straub, K. Double-stranded DNA stereoselectively binds benzo[a]-pyrene diol-epoxides. Nature, *277*: 410–412, 1979.
42. Gupta, R. C., Reddy, M. V., and Randerath, K. $^{32}P$-Postlabeling analysis of non-radioactive aromatic carcinogen-DNA adducts. Carcinogenesis, *3*: 1081–1092, 1982.
43. Gupta, R. C. Enhanced sensitivity of $^{32}P$-postlabeling analysis of aromatic carcinogen-DNA adducts. Cancer Res., *45*: 5656–5662, 1985.
44. Randerath, K., Randerath, E., Agrawal, H. P., Gupta, R. C., Schurdak, M. E., and Reddy, M. V. Postlabeling methods for carcinogen-DNA adduct analysis. Environ. Health Perspect., *62*: 57–65, 1985.
45. Ashurst, S. W., Cohen, G. M., DiGiovanni, J., and Slaga, T. J. Formation of benzo[a]-pyrene-DNA adducts and their relationship to tumor initiation in mouse epidermis. Cancer Res., *43*: 1024–1029, 1983.
46. Troll, W. and Weisner, R. The role of oxygen radicals as a possible mechanism of tumor promotion. Annu. Rev. Pharmacol. Toxicol., *25*: 509–528, 1985.
47. Cerutti, P. Prooxidant states and tumor promotion. Science, *227*: 375–381, 1985.
48. Kensler, T. W. and Taffe, B. G. Free radicals in tumor-promotion. Adv. Free Rad. Biol., *2*: 347–387, 1986.
49. Perchellet, J.-P. and Perchellet, E. M. Phorbol ester tumor promoters and multistage skin carcinogenesis. ISI Atlas of Science: Pharmacology, 325–333, 1988.

XENOBIOTICS AND CANCER, L. ERNSTER ET AL. (EDS.),
JAPAN SCI. SOC. PRESS, TOKYO/TAYLOR & FRANCIS LTD., LONDON, pp. 75–87, 1991

# The Aromatase Enzyme: From Cloning to Cancer

Evan R. SIMPSON, Thomas PRICE, Jane AITKEN, Mala MAHENDROO, Gary MEANS, and Michael KILGORE

*Cecil H. and Ida Green Center for Reproductive Biology Sciences, and the Departments of Obstetrics-Gynecology and Biochemistry, The University of Texas Southwestern Medical Center at Dallas, Dallas, Texas 75235, U.S.A.*

*Abstract:* Estrogen production by adipose tissue has been implicated in the etiology of such human cancers as endometrial and breast cancer. Estrogen production by adipose cells is subject to complex multifactorial regulation by a number of growth factors and cytokines, including those produced by breast cancer cells. In order to understand the mechanisms responsible for aromatase regulation, the structural gene encoding aromatase cytochrome P-450 (P-$450_{AROM}$) was isolated from human genomic DNA. The gene spans at least 70 kb and is comprised of 10 exons, the first of which is untranslated. DNA sequence analysis indicates that the gene has a putative TATA (ATAAAA) sequence at −23 bp and putative CAAT binding sequences beginning at −41, −67, and −83 bp, that constitute a promoter region responsible for expression in placenta. However, this promoter does not appear to be responsible for expression in adipose, which may therefore be under the control of another, tissue-specific, promoter. Use of Polymerase Chain Reaction (PCR) technology has allowed for determination of expression of P-450AROM in samples of breast adipose. Preliminary results indicate that expression is highest in the upper lateral region, similar to the site of most frequent localization of tumors.

The biosynthesis of estrogens is catalyzed by an enzyme complex termed aromatase which is localized in the endoplasmic reticulum of cells in which it is expressed. The aromatase enzyme complex consists of two components (*1*): the first is a form of cytochrome P-450 known as aromatase cytochrome P-450 ($P450_{AROM}$; the product of the CYP19 gene). This heme protein is responsible for binding the $C_{19}$ steroid substrate and catalyzing the concerted series of reactions leading to the formation of the phenolic A ring. The second is a flavoprotein, NADPH-cytochrome P-450 reductase, which is an essentially ubiquitous protein in the endoplasmic reticulum of most cell types and is responsible for transferring reducing equivalents from NADPH to cytochrome P-450. Since there is only one gene encoding the reductase, this enzyme must be capable of transferring reducing equivalents to any form of microsomal cytochrome P-450 that it encounters (*2*). The aromatase reaction apparently utilizes 3 moles oxygen and 3 moles NADPH for every mole of $C_{19}$ steroid metabolized (*3*). The first 2 oxygen molecules are utilized in the oxidation of the $C_{19}$ angular methyl group. Considerable speculation continues as to the site and the mechanism of insertion of the third oxygen molecule. It has been suggested that this third site of oxygen attack is at the 2$\beta$-position (*4*) however, more recent work suggests that peroxidative attack, again involving the $C_{19}$ methyl group, may be involved instead (*5*).

The aromatization reaction occurs in a number of cells and tissues including ovarian granulosa cells (*6*), testicular Sertoli (*7*) and Leydig cells (*8, 9*), placenta, adipose tissue of both males and females (*10*), various sites of the brain including hypothalamus (*11*), amygdala, and hippocampus (*12*), as well as the preimplantation blastocyst (*13*). The principal sites of estrogen biosynthesis in the human female are the ovarian granulosa cells in the premenopausal woman, the placenta in the pregnant woman, and adipose tissue in the postmenopausal woman.

Recognition of the importance of adipose tissue as a source of estrogens in the postmenopausal woman came from the pioneering studies of MacDonald, Siiteri, and their colleagues in the 1970s, who determined the fractional conversion of plasma androstenedione to estrone in humans as a function of obesity and aging (*10, 14–17*). This parameter was shown to be correlated positively with excess body weight in both pre- and postmenopausal women, and may be increased as much as 10-fold in morbidly obese postmenopausal women. Furthermore, the fractional conversion of androstenedione to estrone is also increased with aging. This increase with both obesity and aging bears a striking relationship to the incidence of endometrial cancer, which is a disease primarily of elderly obese women. It is now generally accepted that the continuous production of estrogen by the adipose tissue in such women is a major causative factor in the etiology of this condition. Evidence also is accumulating suggestive of a role of estrogens produced by adipose tissue in the pathogenesis of certain forms of breast cancer. For example, in a recent report by Miller and colleagues (*18*) it was shown that aromatase activity of breast adipose tissue obtained from sites proximal to a tumor was higher than aromatase activity of breast adipose tissue removed from sites distal to the tumor. Thus, a relationship between the local production of estrogen by the adipose tissue of the breast and the presence of tumor cells within that region of the breast is strongly indicated.

### *Regulation of Expression of Cytochrome P-450$_{AROM}$ in Human Adipose Stromal Cells in Culture by Growth Factors*

With the isolation and characterization of P-450$_{AROM}$ cDNA inserts, it became possible to determine whether changes in the activity of aromatase were the consequence of changes in the absolute levels of this mRNA species. In order to do this we utilized the cDNA inserts as hybridization probes in Northern analysis of RNA extracted from adipose stromal cells incubated in the presence or absence of $(Bu)_2$-cAMP plus phorbol ester (Fig. 1). Hybridizable RNA was low in control cells but was detectable in RNA from cells treated with $(Bu)_2$cAMP. There was a marked increase in the levels of hybridizable RNA in cells treated with $(Bu)_2$cAMP plus phorbol ester. However, in cells treated with $(Bu)_2$cAMP plus phorbol ester plus a number of growth factors and cytokines, cytochrome P-450$_{AROM}$ mRNA was once again reduced to undetectable levels (*19*). These include epidermal growth factor (EGF), transforming growth factor-$\beta$, tumor necrosis factor, and interleukin-1$\beta$. Transforming growth

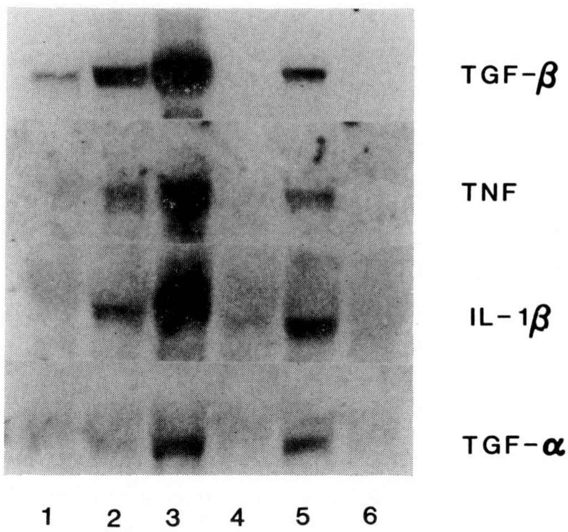


FIG. 1. Effects of various growth factors on the levels of mRNA encoding cytochrome P-$450_{AROM}$ as determined by Northern analysis. Lane 1: no additions; lane 2: $(Bu)_2cAMP$; lane 3: $(Bu)_2cAMP$ +PDA; lane 4: $(Bu)_2cAMP$+growth factor; lane 5: $(Bu)_2cAMP$+PDA+growth factor; lane 6: growth factor alone.

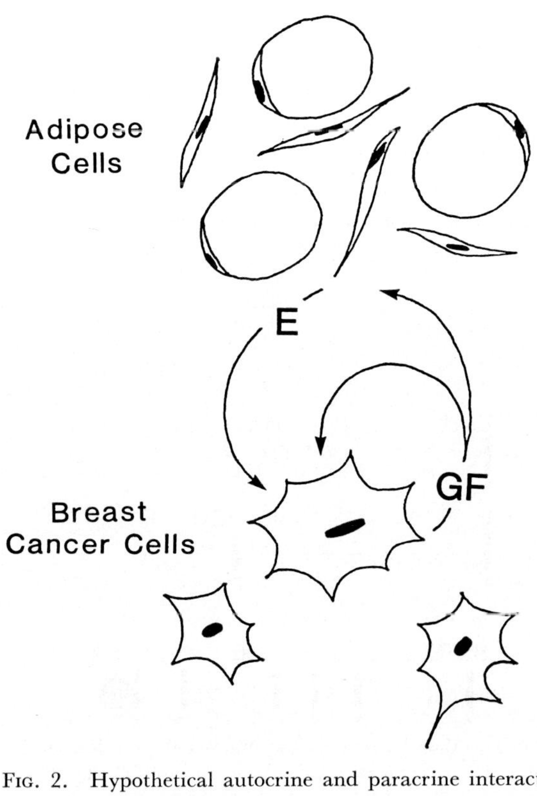


FIG. 2. Hypothetical autocrine and paracrine interaction between breast cancer cells and the the adipose cells in the breast surrounding the tumor. E, estrogen; GF, growth factors.

factor-α had a similar effect. Thus, all of these growth factors were markedly inhibitory of the expression of cytochrome P-450$_{AROM}$. In terms of mechanism, these results present a confusing picture at this time. For example, it is not unreasonable to imagine that at least some of the inhibitory growth factors act *via* protein kinase C activation, yet phorbol esters markedly potentiate the stimulatory action of cAMP analogs.

As mentioned previously, the results of Miller and colleagues (*18*) imply an interaction between breast tumors and proximal adipose cells in terms of the induction of aromatase activity. Since breast cancer cells, at least *in vitro*, produce a variety of growth factors in response to estrogens (*20*) it is tempting to attempt to rationalize the results of Miller and colleagues (*18*) in terms of a model such as that shown in Fig. 2. In this scheme, a local feedback loop operates within the breast, such that estrogens produced in breast fat surrounding the tumor regulate the production of growth factors by the tumor. These influence tumor growth and also act to regulate, in turn, the production of estrogen in the surrounding fat. However, until more is known about growth factors produced by breast tumors *in situ*, no conclusions can be drawn as to the likely factors that serve as autocrine and paracrine regulators of aromatase activity.

## *Structure of the Human Aromatase Cytochrome P-450 Gene*

As discussed above, aromatase activity of human adipose is subject, at least *in vitro*, to complex and multifactorial regulation which is correlated with changes in the levels of mRNA encoding this protein. In order to examine in greater detail the regulation of aromatase expression in the human, we have isolated and characterized the gene encoding P-450$_{AROM}$. Utilizing the full-length cDNA (*21*) and a primer extended cDNA insert as hybridization probes, four genomic clones encoding the entire P-450$_{AROM}$ structural gene have been isolated from two different human genomic libraries (*22*).

The gene is similar to that of other cytochrome P-450 species in that the structural

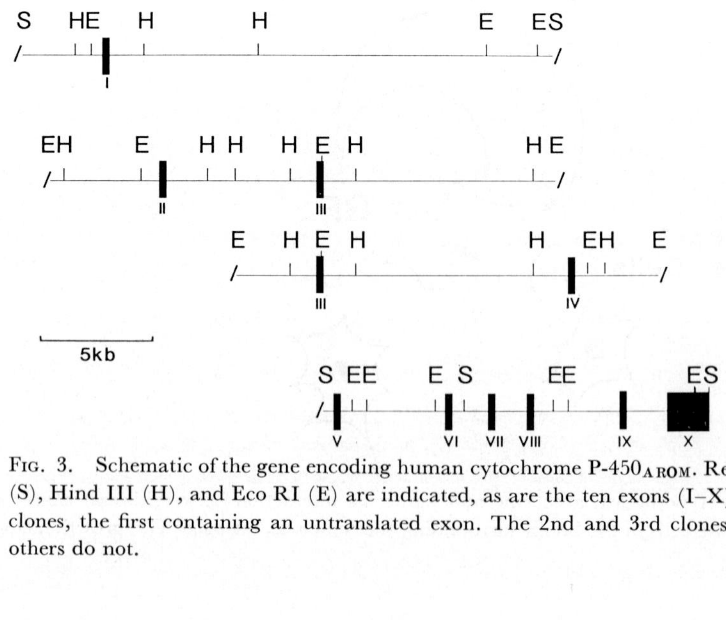


FIG. 3. Schematic of the gene encoding human cytochrome P-450$_{AROM}$. Restriction sites for Sal I (S), Hind III (H), and Eco RI (E) are indicated, as are the ten exons (I–X). The gene spans four clones, the first containing an untranslated exon. The 2nd and 3rd clones overlap, whereas the others do not.

gene comprises 10 exons (most cytochrome P-450 genes contain between 8 and 10 exons); the heme binding region and the entire 3′-untranslated region are encoded by the last exon (Fig. 3) (*23*). However, the gene is much larger than those of other steroidogenic cytochromes P-450 and may in fact be the largest cytochrome P-450 gene analyzed at this time. The entire gene spans at least 70 kb, and since there are two regions where the clones do not overlap, the actual size is unknown. By comparison, the genes for the other two microsomal steroidogenic cytochromes P-450, namely P-450$_{C21}$ (*24*) and P-450$_{17\alpha}$ (*25*) are 3.7 and 6.5 kb, respectively. Of the mitochondrial steroidogenic cytochrome P-450 species, the gene for bovine 11$\beta$-hydroxylase P-450 (P-450$_{11\beta}$) is 8 kb (*10*) long, whereas that for human cholesterol side chain cleavage cytochrome P-450 (P-450$_{SCC}$) is at least 20 kb long (*26*) and this also has an intron in which the clones do not overlap.

Analysis of the intron/exon boundaries reveals rather poor correlation with other steroidogenic cytochromes P-450. As shown in Fig. 4, the exon/intron boundaries of human P-450$_{17\alpha}$, and P-450$_{C21}$ agree rather well at least in the 3′ portion of the molecule, although there are several differences toward the 5′-end. On the other hand, the human P-450$_{AROM}$ gene shows no boundary identities when compared to those of P-450$_{17\alpha}$ and P-450$_{C21}$, although there are several boundaries in the 3′ portion of the molecule which are close to those of the other two microsomal P-450s. Toward the 5′-end of the molecule, however, attempts to align the boundaries with those of the other two microsomal P-450s become impossible. Poor exon/intron boundary alignment between the various genes is a characteristic feature of the cytochrome P-450 superfamily, leading to speculation that the ancestral gene had many more exons than the modern counterparts (*23*).

### *Number of Aromatase Cytochrome P-450 Genes Present in the Human Genome*

The issue of whether there is more than one aromatase enzyme in the human is an important one for several reasons. In the first place, it has been suggested (*27*) that different aromatase enzymes exist in placenta, ovary, and adipose tissue since the major estrogen produced in each of these tissues is different, namely estriol in the placenta, estradiol in the ovary, and estrone in the adipose. Equally, however, this could be due to the presentation to the same enzyme of different substrates, namely 16$\alpha$-hydroxylated androgens in the case of placenta, testosterone in the ovary, and androstenedione in the adipose tissue. The issue is also of importance clinically. At present there is much interest in the development of more effective inhibitors of aromatase for use clinically in the management of patients with breast cancer (*28*). However, the only source of aromatase available for the testing of such inhibitors is that derived from human placenta. Moreover, as discussed above, there is evidence to suggest that the estrogen which may be of consequence in the development of breast tumors is that produced in the breast adipose tissue surrounding the developing tumor. If the enzyme responsible for such estrogen in the adipose tissue were different from that in the placenta, then clearly inhibitors developed against the placental enzyme might be less efficacious toward the enzyme present in adipose.

Studies on the expression of the cDNA encoding P-450$_{AROM}$ (*21*) together with previous work on the purified enzyme (*29, 30*) suggest that a single enzyme is capable

```
          1                                                                                   80
P-450AROM MVLEMLNPIH YNITSIVPEA MPAATMSVLL LTGLFLLLWN YEGTSSIPGP GYCMGIGPLI SHGRFL..WM GSRSACNYYN
P-45017α  M......... .......... ...WELVALL LLTLAYLFWP KRRC.PGAKY PKSLLSLPLV GSLPFL..PR HGHMHNNFFK
P-450C21  MLL....... .......... ..LGLLLL.P LLAGARLLWN WWK....... LRSLHLPPLA PG..FLHLLQ PDLPIYLLG.

          81                                                                                 160
P-450AROM ..RVYGEFMR VWISGEE.TL II.SKSSSMF HIM..KHNHY SSRFGSKLGL QCIGMHEKGI IFNNNPELWK TTRP.FFMKA
P-45017α  LQKKYGPIYS VRMGTK..TT VIVGHHQLAK EVLI.KKGKD FSGRPQMATL DIASNNRKGI AFADSGAHWQ LHRRLAMATF
P-450C21  LTQKFGPIYR LHLGLQD.VV VLNSKRTIEE AMV..KKWAD FAGRPEPLTY KLVSKNYPDL SLGDYSLLWK AHKKLTRSAL

          161                                                                                240
P-450AROM LSG.PGLVRM VTVCAESLKT HLDRLEEVTN ESGY.VDVLT LLRRVMLDT. ...SNTLFLR IPLDESAIVV KIQGYFDAWQ
P-45017α  ALFKDGDQKL EKIICQEIST LCDML...AT HNGQSIDISF ...PVFVAVT NVISLICFNT SYKNGDPELN VIQNYNEGII
P-450C21  LLGIRDS..M EPVVEQLTQE FCERMRA... QPGTPVAIEE ...EFSLLTC SIICYLTFG. DKIKDDNLMP AYYKCIQEVL

          241                                                                                320
P-450AROM AL......L IKPDIFFKIS WLYKKY.... ......EKSV KDLKDAI... ......EVLI AEKRCRISTE EKLEECMDFA
P-45017α  DNL.SKDS.L VDLVPWLKIF PNKTLEKLK. SHVKIRNDLL NKILENYKEK FRSDSITNML DTLMQAKMNS DNGNAGPD..
P-450C21  KTWSHWSIQI VDVIPFLRFF PNPGLRRLKQ A.IEKRDHIV EMQLRQHKES LVAGQWRDMM DYMLQGVAQ. PSMEEGS...

          321                                                                                400
P-450AROM TELILAEKRG DLTRENVNQC ILEMLIAAPD TMSVSLFFML FLIAKHPNVE EAIIKEIQTV IG....ERDI KIDDIQKLKV
P-45017α  ......QDSE LLSDNHILTT IGDIFGAGVE TTTSVVKWTL AFLLHNPQVK KKLYEEIDQN VGFS...RTP TISDRNRLLL
P-450C21  ........GQ LL.EGHVHMA AVDLLIGGTE TTANTLSWAV VFLLHHPEIQ QRLQEELDHE LGPGASSSRV PYKDRARLPL

          401                                                                                480
P-450AROM MENFIYESMR YQPVVDLVM. RKALEDDVID GYPVKKGTNI ILNIGRMHRL E.FFPKPNEF TLENF..... .AKNVPYRYF
P-45017α  LEATIREVLR LRPVAPMLIP HKANVDSSIG EFAVDKGTEV IINLWALHHN EKEWHQPDQF MPERFLNPAG TQLISPSVSY
P-450C21  LNATIAEVLR LRPVVPLALP HRTTRPSSIS GYDIPEGTVI IPNLQGAHLD ETVWERPHEF WPDRFLEPGK NS......RA

          481                                                                                561
P-450AROM QPFGFGPRGC AGKYIAMVMM KAILVTLLRR FHVKTLQGQC VESIQKIHDL SLHPDETKNM LEMIFTPRNS DRCLEH
P-45017α  LPFGAGPRSC IGEILARQEL FLIMAWLLQR FDLEVPDDGQ LPSLEGIP.. KVVFLIDSFK VKIKVRQAWR EAQAEGST
P-450C21  LAFGCGAPVC LGEPLARLEL FVVLTRLLQA FTLLPSGD.A LPSLQPLPHC SVILKMQPFQ VRLQPRGM.. GAHSPGQNQ
```

FIG. 4. Comparison of the positions of introns in the coding regions of human P-$450_{AROM}$, P-$450_{17\alpha}$, and P-$450_{C21}$. Amino acids are denoted by their single letter designation. Solid arrowheads between amino acids indicate introns lying between codons; hatched arrowheads pointing to an amino acid indicate that the intron lies between the first and second bases of the corresponding codon; open arrowheads pointing to an amino acid indicate that the intron lies between the second and third bases of the corresponding codon. The data for human P-$450_{17\alpha}$ and P-$450_{C21}$ were derived from ref. *25*.

of metabolizing all three categories of $C_{19}$ substrate and that it is not necessary to postulate the presence of different enzymes in the different tissues which synthesize estrogens. Our present work on the characterization of the gene encoding P-$450_{AROM}$ is consistent with this view. In all of our restriction mapping and Southern analysis, we have obtained no evidence to suggest that there is more than one cytochrome P-$450_{AROM}$ gene within the human genome.

### *Characterization of the 5′-Untranslated Exon*

DNA sequence upstream from the bases encoding the start of translation contained putative CAAT and TATA boxes (Fig. 5), however, primer extension using

```
EXON II

cccaagaaat gtgttcttac tgtagaaact tactattttg atcaaaaaag tcattttggt caaaaagggg agttgggaga ttgccttttt   90
gttttgaaat tgatttggct tcaagggaag aagattgcct aaacaaaacc tgctgatgaa gtcacaaaat gactccacct ctggaatgag  180
ctttattttc ttataatttg gcaagaaatt tggctttcaa ttgggaatgc acgtcactct acccactcaa gggcaagatg ataaggttct  270
atcagaccaa gcgtctaaag gaacctgaga ctctaccaag gtcagaaatg ctgcaattca agccaaaaga tctttcttgg gcttccttgt  360
tttgacttgt aaccataaat tagtcttgcc taaatgtctg atcacattat aaaacagtaa gtgaatctgt actgtacagc accctctgaa  450

gcaacaggag ctatagatga accttttagg ggattctgta atttttctgt ccctttgatt tccacagGAC TCTAAATTGC CCCCTCTGAG  540
                1
GTCAAGGAAC ACAAGATGGT TTTGGAAATG CTGAACCCGA TACATTATAA CATCACCAGC ATCGTGCCTG AAGCCATGCC TGCTGCCACC  630
                MetVa lLeuGluMet LeuAsnProI leHisTyrAs nIleThrSer IleValProG luAlaMetPr oAlaAlaThr

ATGCCAGTCC TGCTCCTCAC TGGCCTTTTT CTCTTGGTGT GGAATTATGA GGGCACATCC TCAATACCAG gtaagtcagt catttatttc  720
MetProValL euLeuLeuTh rGlyLeuPhe LeuLeuValT rpAsnTyrGl uGlyThrSer SerIleProG

tgtatctaag gagattattt acttgggatt ttggtccatc atggtaaaga aaaattttgc aaaaaggaca aaaagcaaac ctggaaagat  810
ctctgaagac tatgtctgtg ttagcaaatg aggacttgga gaaatttcag accaattatc tg........ -6 kb......

EXON III

ttcaaatcac tttattcgtg attcacagat atacatcaca tgtacagaac acttagctat aaaagaacaa aaacaggagt aacacagaac   90
                                                            48
agttgcaatt tttggtgtaa ctaagatgtt gcttatgctc tgacacctgt cctagGTCCT GGCTACTGCA TGGGAATTGG ACCCCTCATC  180
                                                            lyPro GlyTyrCysM etGlyIleGl yProLeuIle

TCCCACGGCA GATTCCTGTG GATGGGGATC GGCAGTGCCT GCAACTACTA CAACCGGGTG TATGGAGAAT TCATGCGAGT CTGGATCTCT  270
SerHisGlyA rgPheLeuTr pMetGlyThr GlySerAlaC ysAsnTyrTy rAsnArgVal TyrGlyGluP heMetArgVa lTrpIleSer

GGAGAGGAAA CACTCATTAT CAGCAAgtga gtctgttcat aatcgaagac atacttttta aatcgaggct ggagtttttt ggagttaaga  360
GlyGluGluT hrLeuIleIl eSerLy

caactttatt ttgaatcttg atgtctttgt ttctaacgct atatttttac cactgaaatg aagtgagcaa tccccagaaa tctaacattg  450

caaacagaat aattgggttt tgcttgaatt gaagccagca gtacataaat aactaactct ggaaagttgg gaaattattt acaatctctg  540
tgagcagtga atgtggaaac ttagaagcca gataatttga ttttgacaaa .....-10 kb......
```

5-a

```
EXON IV

aaactgaact tagtaatcca caacttgatc ttggctcact cttatgtggc actttgatag ctggatgata cctggaggct gagttcttct   90
ggctctgtgt atggagggtt cagcttctta gcagcctgca gctctgactc catgtagtgg gtagtatttt ggtgaggtta gagaagaaag  180
agaagtaagg aatggtatat ggtgtgtgtg tgtgttttct atctttgtgg atagttgaaa cagggagtca gtaggtagaa atgattcaac  270
tggagaagga tgtcctcatg ctaacagaag tgcttattca acccgaatac tagaaatcat gcacattgca tttggagcaa catgcatttg  360
                                                                                                99
ctaagagagc tgcctcctag tcaaaatgta ccaccaggag ttctcctgac ccttaaaaat tgacaccaaa gtttcctgtc ttttcagGTC  450
                                                                                               sSe

CTCAAGTATG TTCCACATAA TGAAGCACAA TCATTACAGC TCTCGATTCG GCAGCAAACT TGGGCTGCAG TGCATCGGTA TGCATGAGAA  540
rSerSerMet PheHisIleM etLysHisAs nHisTyrSer SerArgPheG lySerLysLe uGlyLeuGln CysIleGlyM etHisGluLy

AGGCATCATA TTTAACAACA ATCCAGAGCT CTGGAAAACA ACTCGACCCT TCTTTATGAA AGgtaagcag gtacttagtt agctacaatc  630
sGlyIleIle PheAsnAsnA snProGluLe uTrpLysThr ThrArgProP hePheMetLy sA

ttcttttttg tctatgaatg tgcctttttt gaaatcatat ttttaaaata ttttatttat ttatttattt atttatttat ttattgagac  720
aggctctgac tctatcaccc aggcaggagt gaccttggct cacgaccttg gctcactgta acctccgcct cccaggactc aggcgattct  810
cccacctcag cctcgcgagt agctgggact acagaatgtg caccaccaat gcctggacaa atttttgtat tttttgtagc gatggggttt  900
cgccatattt gagaccaggc tgggctcaaa cacacggagt caaacgattg acctgcctcg gcctcccaaa gtgttgggat tacagggatg  990
agctatca..> 2.5 kb....


EXON V
                                                                         150
aaagcaaatg catgattgtg tgtgtgcctg gattctgtag gctgattctc tgtagtgtac tctgcagCTC TGTCAGGCCC CGGCCTTGTT   90
                                                                         laL euSerGlyPr oGlyLeuVal

CGTATGGTCA CAGTCTGTGC TGAATCCCTC AAAACACATC TGGACAGGTT GGAGGAGGTG ACCAATGAAT CGGGCTATGT GGACGTGTTG  180
ArgMetValT hrValCysAl aGluSerLeu LysThrHisL euAspArgLe uGluGluVal ThrAsnGluS erGlyTyrVa lAspValLeu

ACCCTTCTGC GTCGTGTCAT GCTGGACACC TCTAACACGC TCTTCTTGAG GATCCCTTTG GACGgtactg aaattttcac tctcacatct  270
ThrLeuLeuA rgArgValMe tLeuAspThr SerAsnThrL euPheLeuAr gIleProLeu AspG

tgaccatctg tcctttact....-3.5 kb....
```

5-b

```
EXON VI
       209
cctacagAAA GTGCTATCGT GGTTAAAATC CAAGGTTATT TTGATGCATG GCAAGCTCTC CTCATCAAAC CAGACATCTT CTTTAAGATT   90
       luS erAlaIleVa lValLysIle GlnGlyTyrP heAspAlaTr pGlnAlaLeu LeuIleLysP roAspIlePh ePheLysIle

TCTTGGCTAT ACAAAAAGTA TGAGAAGTCT GTgtaagtaa ttacaacttt ggaagattta tgagatcaat tggattggtt tttttccctt  180
SerTrpLeuT yrLysLysTy rGluLysSer Va

gtgtctttgc tgttttcttg gcctctcagg taacttttct gctctctaga gcccacaagg gagctgttga ttaagttgct gatgaaacac  270
tttttttacag caatttggct gcatttggcc agaccagaga gtaaatgaag cctttgctgg cagctctcgc agggct.... ˜3.0kb.....
```

```
EXON VII

atcttagcta actctggcac cttaacatga agtgtagggt ctatgtaatt taagggtatt tatgaagaaa taaaatagta attcacttac   90

tcataagcac caatgttttc aattaaagca gtcattttac ctaaatacat ggcaaataaa tctgtttcgc tagatgtcta aactgagtaa  180
                                248
aaatagacaa tattttgact tttttccag CAAGGATTTG AAAGATGCCA TAGAAGTTCT GATAGCAGAA AAAAGATGCA GGATTTCCAC  270
                               lLysAspLeu LysAspAlaI leGluValLe uIleAlaGlu LysArgCysA rgIleSerTh

AGAAGAGAAA CTGGAAGAAT GTATGGACTT TGCCACTGAG TTGATTTTAG CAGAGgtact gacctgaact aactgtaatt cccatgccac  360
rGluGluLys LeuGluGluC ysMetAspPh eAlaThrGlu LeuIleLeuA laGlu

atatgttatg actgtgtaga ggtgtgtaaa gatccccttt tgtaactgtt gcatatttct gcttttaaat acgggctcta gcagttctgt  450
aatcccaatc caaatagccc acacattaga tatttcagta aggcttttaa gattccaaca ttctagtaag actgactgct aagattgtga  540
ctctctgtgt aacagtataa atatgaaaca gt........ ˜2.5 kb...
```

5-c

```
EXON VIII

tacatataca tagacagtcg gcctatacgt tcatctttca gctaaagatt gtcatgtaaa atgtccacag tcaatcacag agacatgtgg   90
tttctatgat ttcattttgt tgaggttgtt gatccttgag tgtcacctcc cctcattttt tgaaactttg attcactttt ccaaattttt  180
                                                    286
cccatcttcc aatttgattc acttttccaa atttttccca tcttccaatt gttcagAAAC GTGGTGACCT GACAAGAGAG AATGTGAACC  270
                                                         LysA rgGlyAspLe uThrArgGlu AsnValAsnG

AGTGCATATT GGAAATGCTG ATCGCAGCTC CTGACACCAT GTCTGTCTCT TTGTTCTTCA TGCTATTTCT CATTGCAAAG CACCCTAATG  360
lnCysIleLe uGluMetLeu IleAlaAlaP roAspThrMe tSerValSer LeuPhePheM etLeuPheLe uIleAlaLys HisProAsnV

TTGAAGAGGC AATAATAAAG GAAATCCAGA CTGTTATTGg taagaattta tcaaataaat aatacatctt taaaaaccaa tttcttctga  450
alGluGluAl aIleIleLys GluIleGlnT hrValIleG

atatccattt cttatgtcct aagaatctga tatcaaacat gaaattttat aattgctcca accataagca agacattctg tcacatttga  540
ttacaccaga tagacggaaa gatagctctt tctgtgttc....... ˜2.5 kb........
```

```
EXON IX

tagatagagc acattttttt caccagagaa cgtctgtgaa aaaaatagaa gctttaatac caatcacaga tggaaactaa cattaccttc   90
                            340
tttgttcctt ttatctgttt ccacagGTGA GAGAGACATA AAGATTGATG ATATACAAAA ATTAAAAGTG ATGGAAAACT TCATTTATGA  180
                           lyGl uArgAspIle LysIleAspA spIleGlnLy sLeuLysVal MetGluAsnP heIleTyrGl

GAGCATGCGG TACCAGCCTG TCGTGGACTT GGTCATGCGC AAAGCCTTAG AAGATGATGT AATCGATGGC TACCCAGTGA AAAAGGGGAC  270
uSerMetArg TyrGlnProV alValAspLe uValMetArg LysAlaLeuG luAspAspVa lIleAspGly TyrProValL ysLysGlyTh

AAACATTATC CTGAATATTG GAAGGATGCA CAGACTCGAG TTTTTCCCCA AACCCAATGA ATTTACTCTT GAAAATTTTG CAAAGAATgt  360
rAsnIleIle LeuAsnIleG lyArgMetHi sArgLeuGlu PhePheProL ysProAsnGl uPheThrLeu GluAsnPheA laLysAsn

aaggagccca ttcctta... ~1.25 kb...
```

5-d

human placental poly A$^+$ RNA failed to reveal any start of transcription associated with these. Moreover, an oligonucleotide prepared against a region commencing 39 bp downstream from this putative TATA box failed to hybridize in Northern analysis of poly A$^+$ RNA from human placenta. We conclude, therefore, that an intron is present in the DNA 5′ of the exon encoding the start site of translation and that the intron/exon boundary occurs at the point where the genomic sequence and that of the cDNAs all become identical. A sequence similar to the splice junction consensus sequence is also present at this site (*31*). By contrast, the region of the gene which we have called exon I, therefore, fulfills the criteria of a 5′-untranslated exon (Fig. 6), although the clone that contains it does not overlap with the clones containing the exons en-

EXON X

```
                                                                                         421
ccagtttcag aatgaatcaa acagagactg agtgactcta gccttaatat tctggcaact gtctgatcat tttcatagGT TCCTTATAGG   90
                                                                                       Va lProTyrArg

TACTTTCAGC CATTTGGCTT TGGGCCCCGT GGCTGTGCAG GAAAGTACAT CGCCATGGTG ATGATGAAAG CCATCCTCGT TACACTTCTG  180
TyrPheGlnP roPheGlyPh eGlyProArg GlyCysAlaG lyLysTyrIl eAlaMetVal MetMetLysA laIleLeuVa lThrLeuLeu

AGACGATTCC ACGTGAAGAC ATTGCAAGGA CAGTGTGTTG AGAGCATACA GAAGATACAC GACTTGTCCT TGCACCCAGA TGAGACTAAA  270
ArgArgPheH isValLysTh rLeuGlnGly GlnCysValG luSerIleGl nLysIleHis AspLeuSerL euHisProAs pGluThrLys

AACATGCTGG AAATGATCTT TACCCCAAGA AACTCAGACA GGTGTCTGGA ACACTAGAGA AGGCTGGTCA GTACCCACTC TGGAGCATTT  360
AsnMetLeuG luMetIlePh eThrProArg AsnSerAspA rgCysLeuGl uHisEnd

CTCATCAGTA GTTCACATAC AAATCATCCA TCCTTGCCAA TAGTGTCATC CTCACAGTGA ACACTCAGTG GCCCATGGCA TTTTATAGGC  450

ATACCTCCTA TGGGTTGTCA CCAAGCTAGG TGCTATTGGT CATCTGCTCC TGTTCACACC AGAGAACCAG GCTACAAGAG AAAAAGCAGA  540

GGCCAAGAGT TTGAGGGGAG AAATAGTCGG TGAAGAAACC GTATCCATAA AGACCCGATT CCACCAAATG TGCTTTGAGA AGGATAGGCC  630

TTCATTAACA AAATGTATGT CTGGTTCCCC AGTAGAGCTC TACTGCCTCA ACCAAGGGGA TTTTTATGTC TGGGGCAGAA ACACTCAAGT  720

TGATTAGAAA GACCAGGCCA ATGTCAGGTA CCTGGGGCCA AACCCACCTG CTAGTGTGAA TTAAAGTACT TTAATTTTGT TTTCTGTGGA  810

GGTGGAAAAG CAACATTCAT AGTCTTTGGA GAAATGCTTA GAAATTCAGC ATTTGACCCT TGCTGTGAAT TAAGCCCAAT TAATTCCTGT  900

TTGTCTACAT ATGATCTGTC TGTGGCAAAA GTTTAATCAG AGGAAATTCT TTCCCAGTCT GTCGATTTAT GCCTCAGCCA CTTGCCTGTG  990

CTACAATTCA TTGTGTTACC TGTAGATTCA GGTAATACAA ACTATATATA ATCATCAAGT AATACAAACT AATTTAGTAA TAGCCTGGGT 1080

TAAGTATTAT TAGGGCCCTG TGTCTGCTGT AGAAAAAAAA ATTCACATGA TGCACTTCAA ATTCAAATAA AAATCCTTTT GGCATGTTCC 1170

CATTTTTGCT TAGCTCAATT AGTGTGGCTA ACCAAGAGAT AACTGTAAAT GTGACATTGA TTTGCTCTTA CTACAGCTTC AGTGATTGGG 1260

GGAGGAAAAG TCCCAACCCA ATGGGCTCAA ACTTCTAAGG GGTACTCCTC TCATCCCCTT ATCCTTCTCC CTCGACATTT TCTCCCTCTT 1350

TCTTCCCATG ACCCCAAAGC CAAGGGCAAC AGATCAGTAA AGAACGTGGT CAGAGTAGAA CCCCTGAAGT ATTTTTTAAT CCTACCTCAA 1440

AATTTAACAG TTACCTGAGA GATTTAACAT TATCTAGTTC ATTGAATCAT TGTATGTGGT CATGGATAAA TTGCACACCT TGGAATTCGC 1530

TTTCTAAAGG AAATCAAATG AATGGAGGAA CTTTCCAAAC ACCACTTTAC TTGTGTTATA TAGCCAATAT AACTATCTCT ACTGAATGTC 1620

ATTGAAAAAC TAAAAAATTA AACTTATTTA CAAATAGGTa aatatttgtc attgaatcca ttgccatccc atttgactgt tcttttcatc 1710

ctactgtcta gtaataagct gagtctaaga tgacagtgta actccctgaa agcaggagct acttctttct ttttgtaatc tatttccatc 1800
ccatttcctg tctgtctcct gtatcactcc agctcagtct gatagacatc tgctcagaga t
```

FIG. 5. Sequence of the exons and exon-intron boundaries of the translated portion of the P-450$_{AROM}$ gene (exons II–X). Exonic sequence is indicated by bold caps, intronic sequence by lower case letters. Exon-intron boundaries are underlined. The numbers in parentheses correspond to the positions with respect to the primary sequence of P-450$_{AROM}$ of the encoded amino acids. The putative membrane-spanning region is indicated by the boxed region of exon II, whereas the heme-binding region is indicated by the boxed region of exon X, with the cysteine believed to contribute the 5th coordinating ligand to the heme iron indicated by underlining. Internal EcoRI restriction sites in exon III and exon X are indicated by underlining, as are sequences established as not being CAAT and TATA boxes used as promoters in placenta, upstream from the translation start site. The polyadenylation signals which are used are also indicated by underlining in exon X and the start of each polyadenylate tail is indicated by a downstream arrow. The location of the second polyadenylate tail is taken from the work of Harada (*32*).

coding the translated gene product. This is based on the following criteria. In the first place, the clone contains sequence identical to that of the 5′-end of a cDNA (*32*) isolated from a primer extended human placental library which diverges at the exact same site identified as a splice junction. Secondly, an oligonucleotide prepared complementary to this region hybridizes to poly A$^{+}$ RNA from human placenta to give bands identical to those observed using the full-length cDNA as a hybridization probe. Thirdly, DNA hybridizing to this region can be amplified from human placental poly A$^{+}$ RNA by primer extension using an oligonucleotide complementary to a region of the first translated exon, now called exon II, indicating that it is present on the same mRNA species as is the first translated exon.

```
EXON I

aagctttgtc catttcctcc caactcaaac gttctgtgac ctacttgaag aactgtcatg tatccttatc tcttttcatc caggtatcag  -832
gtttagggcc aatggggagg agccactgag aagggagggt tgacactcag catcattcag atcttcattt aattcagtaa acacttaact  -742
gagcacttcc tgtgcctggt atgataatgg gcattggaga tacggaagta aaaaagacaa gcagattacc ctgtgagcag ctggaacacc  -652
gtggagcctt ctgggcttct ctttatccta acattcattg cagttactgt tgactgatca tctctcagca atacccacca ttaaccatgg  -562
aatagaagcc tcctgaggct agggccatgt cacccccaac acatagcaca gttcctgatt tggaattcac tattacccgt tgaataaatg  -472
agtgaatgaa cgaatgaata aatgaaaagc tgtatagtga aggcacttct atgtagaaca atgtggtgtg tggtgggggg tgtgatctta  -382
                                  GRE
tgattacatg tatatagatt tttgtccatg gttcttgtcc ataactccca tgacacttgc tgaggtcttt tgctataatg tagaggtgct  -292
                                                                                            CRE
ttaggcctca ggaaacagaa tatttctctg gccttctttg ccctcctttc atccacccaa ggcggactct ataatctgat tgtggtcata  -202
agaccctcat tccagaggag gtcatgcccc ataccctgga ggaaggaatg ctgcacaaag agaggaagaa gaatctggac agacagacct  -112
                                                                AP1
tgctgagatt agatcatacc cttttgtcc aatcacattt tgttcaatca catgcttcag tcatggacaa caaatgaaat ctccataaaa   -22
                      +1
ggcccaaagg acagggttca gGGAGTTTCT GGAGGGCTGA ACACGTGGAG GCAAACAGGA AGGTGAAGAA GAACTTAATC CTATCAGGAC    69
GGAAGGTCCT GTGCTCGGGA TCTTCCAGAC GTCGCgtatg tatctcttaa tctgactgag ccctcaacct gtgggatcag acactctttc   159
caggtagata gtgttggaac tgagttggag gacacccagc tggtgcccgc tgcttggtgt gtggggaaa atcccctaca tttggtcgca    249
gaagtcttct gtgttgatga ctgttgtcgt ggtgtgagag cagagggaaa acactgcttg agtgttttc tgaaatagga gggcctaaga    339
actatactgt tctatgccac agaactggcc ccctac.....>19 kb......
          GRE
```

FIG. 6. Sequence of exon I of the gene encoding cytochrome P-450$_{AROM}$. Exonic sequence is indicated by bold caps, upstream sequence and intronic sequence by lower case letters. The exon/intron boundary between exon I and intron I is indicated by underlining. The putative transcriptional start site is indicated by +1, and upstream from this, enclosed by boxes, are a putative TAT box and three putative CAAT boxes. Other sequences of potential regulatory significance are indicated in bold with underlining, and their possible roles so designated. GRE, glucocorticoid regulatory element; CRE, cAMP regulatory element.

### *Putative Regulatory Sequences within the Human Aromatase Cytochrome P-450 Gene*

5′-Flanking sequence comprising 918 bp upstream of exon I has been sequenced. Analysis of the 5′-Flanking region of exon I indicates the presence of a putative TATA box (ATAAA). Downstream from this (23 bp) is the site of transcription initiation as revealed by primer extension. Putative CAAT binding sequences are present at −54, −63, and −82 bp.

### *Are There Alternative Promoter Sequences?*

Sequencing of inserts from the primer-extended placental cDNA library revealed the presence of yet another divergent 5′-region upstream from the splice junction, suggestive of a second untranslated exon within the human cytochrome P-450$_{AROM}$ gene which may be subject to differential splicing. This, of course, raises the exciting possibility that these exons may be differentially spliced in different tissues which express aromatase, and that such differential splicing might account for some of the complexities of the regulation of expression of this gene which have been observed in these tissues.

More recently, we have found that this second promoter is responsible for the expression of a minor fraction of the P-450$_{AROM}$ mRNA species in human placenta, whereas the promoter present in exon I is the major promoter driving expression in placenta. However, neither of these exons is present in RNA derived from human ovary or adipose, indicative that neither of these placental promoters is responsible for P-$450_{AROM}$ expression in ovary or adipose. Conceivably therefore, the putative promoter upstream from exon II could be responsible for driving expression in either or both of these tissues, although further studies will be required to resolve this issue.

### *Determination of P-$450_{AROM}$ mRNA Levels in Samples of Breast Adipose Tissue*

Because of the evidence mentioned above, which is suggestive that estrogen production by breast adipose tissue might play a role in the development of breast tumors, it seemed important to measure the expression of aromatase in samples of breast fat and to relate this to the quadrant of the breast from which the sample was removed. However, in general, the expression of P-$450_{AROM}$ mRNA in samples of RNA from adipose tissue is too low to be detectable by northern analysis. Consequently, a more sensitive method was developed using Polymerase Chain Reaction (PCR) technology. To improve the quantification of this technique, an internal standard was utilized consisting of a rat P-$450_{AROM}$ cRNA. Equal amounts of this were added to each sample of breast fat RNA and then PCR amplification was achieved following first strand synthesis by means of priming oligonucleotides chosen because they were complementary to sequences identical in both the human and rat RNA. As probes, oligonucleotides were chosen to sequences which differed markedly in the rat and human RNAs. Thus, these oligonucleotides could be used to differentiate between the product of amplification of the human RNA and that from the rat RNA. This technique is being utilized to determine the expression of P-$450_{AROM}$ mRNA in samples of adipose taken from different quadrants of breast removed as a consequence of reduction mammoplasty as well as in samples of adipose from various body sites of individuals of different ages.

Preliminary results would indicate that the expression is highest in adipose removed from the lateral and superior areas rather than the medial and lower quadrants. Since these are the regions in which breast tumors are most frequently found, these preliminary observations raise the possibility that tumors most frequently develop in regions of the breast where aromatase expression is highest. The reason for this distribution of aromatase expression within the breast is, at present, not understood. It could conceivably be due to the distribution of breast tissue and, for example, if there are more stromal cells within this section of the breast, this would correlate well with our earlier findings that the highest levels of P-$450_{AROM}$ mRNA are in the stromal cell fraction of the breast tissue rather than the adipocytes.

Additionally, however, it is conceivable that the distribution of aromatase expression could be a consequence of gradients of growth factors produced locally within different regions of the breast which might influence the estrogen-producing cells in a paracrine fashion. Thus, it would appear that a study of the regional expression of several of these growth factors within the breast could yield interesting results.

### *Conclusions*

Understanding of the regulation of the biosynthesis of estrogens in the human is of great importance for a number of reasons, but in particular because a number of common human cancers, such as endometrial and breast cancer, are estrogen-dependent. For these reasons, therefore, understanding the differential regulation of aromatase in the various tissues in which it is expressed in the human, as well as understanding the developmental and tissue-specific expression of the enzyme are of great importance and interest. Characterization of the gene encoding human cytochrome P-$450_{AROM}$ should pave the way for studies addressing the issue of the different modes of regulation of this gene.

*Acknowledgments*

This work was supported, in part, by USPHS Grants AG08174 and AM31206. The expert editorial assistance of Sandra Finley is gratefully acknowledged.

## REFERENCES

1. Thompson, E. A., Jr. and Siiteri, P. K. Utilization of oxygen and reduced nicotinamide adenine dinucleotide phosphate by human placental microsomes during aromatization of androstenedione. J. Biol. Chem., *249*: 5364–5372, 1974.
2. Simmons, D. L., Lalley, P. A., and Kasper, C. B. Chromosomal assignments of genes coding for components of the mixed-function oxidase system in mice. J. Biol. Chem., *260*: 515–520, 1985.
3. Thompson, E. A. Jr. and Siiteri, P. K. The involvement of human placental microsomal cytochrome P450 in aromatization. J. Biol. Chem., *249*: 5373–5380, 1974.
4. Goto, J. and Fishman, J. Participation of a non-enzymatic transformation in the biosynthesis of estrogens from androgens. Science, *195*: 80–81, 1977.
5. Cole, P. A. and Robinson, C. H. A peroxide model reaction for placental aromatase. J. Am. Chem. Soc., *110*: 1284–1285, 1988.
6. McNatty, K. P., Baird, D. T., Bolton, A., Chambers, P., Corker, C. S., and McLean, H. Concentrations of oestrogens and androgens in human ovarian venous plasma and follicular fluid throughout the menstrual cycle. J. Endocrinol., *71*: 77–82, 1976.
7. Fritz, I. B., Griswold, M. D., Louis, B. F., and Dorrington, J. H. Similarity of responses of cultured Sertoli cells to cholera toxin and FSH. Mol. Cell. Endocrinol., *5*: 289–295, 1976.
8. Valladares, L. E. and Payne, A. H. Induction of testicular aromatization by luteinizing hormone in mature rats. Endocrinology, *105*: 431–436, 1979.
9. Tsai-Morris, C. H., Aquilano, D. R., and Dufau, M. L. Gonadotropic regulation of aromatase activity in the adult rat testis. Ann. NY Acad. Sci., *438*: 666–672, 1984.
10. Grodin, J. M., Siiteri, P. K., and MacDonald, P. C. Source of estrogen production in the postmenopausal women. J. Clin. Endocrinol. Metab., *36*: 207–213, 1973.
11. Naftolin, F., Ryan, K. J., Davis, I. J., Reddy, V. V., Flores, F., Petro, Z., and Kuhn, M. The formation of estrogen by central neuroendocrine tissues. Recent Prog. Horm. Res., *31*: 295–315, 1975.
12. Roselli, C. E., Horton, L. E., and Resko, J. A. Distribution and regulation of aromatase activity in the rat hypothalamus and limbic systems. Endocrinology, *117*: 2471–2476, 1985.
13. Sengupta, J., Roy, S. K., and Manchada, S. K. Effect of an oestrogen inhibitor, 1,4,6-androstatriene-3,17-dione, on mouse embryo development *in vitro*. J. Reprod. Fertil., *66*: 63–68, 1982.
14. Hemsell, D. L., Grodin, J., Breuner, P. F., Siiteri, P. K., and MacDonald, P. C. Plasma precursors of estrogen II correlation of the extent of conversion of plasma androstenedione to estrone with age. J. Clin. Endocrinol. Metab., *38*: 476–481, 1974.

15. Edman, C. D., MacDonald, P. C., and Combes, B. Extraglandular production of estrogens in subjects with liver disease. Gastroenterology, *69*: 819–824, 1975.
16. Edman, C. D. and MacDonald, P. C. Effect of obesity on conversion of plasma androstenedione to estrone in ovulatory and anovulatory young women. Am. J. Obstet. Gynecol., *130*: 456–461, 1978.
17. Gordon, G. G., Olivo, J., Rafii, F., and Southern, A. L. Conversion of androgens to estrogens in cirrhosis of the liver. J. Clin. Endocrinol. Metab., *40*: 1018–1083, 1975.
18. O'Neill, J. S., Elton, R. A., and Miller, W. R. Aromatase activity in adipose tissue from breast quadrants: a link with tumor site. Br. Med. J., *296*: 741–744, 1988.
19. Evans, C. T., Merrill, J. C., Corbin, C. J., Saunders, C., Simpson, E. R., and Mendelson, C. R. Regulation of estrogen biosynthesis in human adipose stromal cells. J. Biol. Chem., *262*: 6914–6919, 1987.
20. Dickson, R. B. and Lippman, M. E. Estrogenic regulation of growth and polypeptide growth factor secretion in human breast carcinoma. Endocr. Res., *8*: 29–40, 1987.
21. Corbin, C. J., Graham-Lorence, S., McPhaul, M., Mason, J. I., Mendelson, C. R., and Simpson, E. R. Isolation of a full-length cDNA encoding human aromatase cyotchrome P-450 and its expression in non-steroidogenic cells. Proc. Natl. Acad. Sci. U.S.A., *85*: 8948–8953, 1988.
22. Means, G. D., Mahendroo, M. S., Corbin, C. J., Mathis, J. M., Power, F. E., Mendelson, C. R., and Simpson, E. R. Structured analysis of the gene encoding aromatase cytochrome P450, the enzyme responsible for estrogen biosynthesis. J. Biol. Chem., *264*: 19385–19389, 1989.
23. Nebert, D. W. and Gonzalez, F. J. P-450 genes: structure, evolution and regulation. Annu. Rev. Biochem., *56*: 945–993, 1987.
24. White, P. C., New, M. I., and DuPont, B. Structure of human steroid 21-hydroxylase genes. Proc. Natl. Acad. Sci. U.S.A., *83*: 511–515, 1986.
25. Picado-Leonard, J. and Miller, W. L. Cloning and sequence of the human gene for $P450_{C17}$ (Steroid 17$\alpha$-hydroxylase/17,20 lyase): similarity with the gene for $P450_{C21}$. DNA, *6*: 439–448, 1987.
26. Morohashi, K., Sogawa, K., Omura, T., and Fujii-Kuriyama, Y. Gene structure of human cytochrome P450 (SCC), cholesterol desmolase. J. Biochem., *101*: 879–887, 1987.
27. Osawa, Y. and Igashiyama, T. M. J. *In;* Coon, A. H. Conney, R. W. Estabrook, H. V. Gelboin, J. R. Gillette, and P. J. O'Brian (eds.), Drug Oxidations and Chemical Carcinogenesis, pp. 225–232, Academic Press, New York, 1984.
28. Brodie, A. M., Coombes, R. C., and Dowsett, M. Aromatase inhibitor: basic and clinical studies. J. Steroid Biochem., *27*: 899–903, 1987.
29. Kellis, J. T. and Vickery, L. E. Purification and characterization of human placental aromatase cytochrome P-450. J. Biol. Chem., *262*: 4413–4420, 1987.
30. Osawa, Y., Yoshida, N., Franckowiak, M., and Kitawaki, J. Immunoaffinity purification of aromatase cytochrome P-450 from human placental microsomes, metabolic switching from aromatization to 1$\beta$ and 2$\beta$-monohydroxylation, and recognition of aromatase isozymes, Steroids, *50*: 11–28, 1987.
31. Mount, S. M. A catalogue of splice junction sequences. Nucl. Acids Res., *10*: 459–472, 1982.
32. Harada, N. Cloning a complete cDNA encoding human aromatase: immunochemical identification and sequence analysis. Biochem. Biophys. Res. Commun., *156*: 725–732, 1988.

XENOBIOTICS AND CANCER, L. ERNSTER ET AL. (EDS.),
JAPAN SCI. SOC. PRESS, TOKYO/TAYLOR & FRANCIS LTD., LONDON, pp. 89–99, 1991

# Glutathione-dependent Bioactivation of Xenobiotics: Implications for Mutagenicity and Carcinogenicity

M. W. ANDERS

*Department of Pharmacology, University of Rochester, Rochester, New York 14642, U.S.A.*

*Abstract:* Glutathione conjugate formation is now recognized as an important bioactivation mechanism for several classes of mutagenic and carcinogenic compounds. For example, dihalomethanes, 1,2-dihaloethanes, and 1,2,3-trihalopropanes are metabolized to glutathione conjugates that are direct-acting, *i.e.*, that require no further enzymatic processing, and that are cytotoxic or mutagenic, or both. Nephrotoxic and nephrocarcinogenic haloalkenes are metabolized by a multistep pathway that involves hepatic glutathione *S*-conjugate formation, conversion of the glutathione *S*-conjugates to cysteine *S*-conjugates, translocation of the cysteine *S*-conjugates to the kidney, and bioactivation by renal cysteine conjugate $\beta$-lyase. Fluoroalkene-derived conjugates are cytotoxic, whereas chloroalkene-derived conjugates are both cytotoxic and mutagenic. $\beta$-Lyase-dependent bioactivation may account for the observed nephrocarcinogenicity of hexachlorobutadiene, tetrachloroethylene, and trichloroethylene. Finally, glutathione conjugate formation has been implicated in the mutagenicity of Trp-P-2 and N-OH-Trp-P-2 and in the DNA damage produced by 1-methyl-4-phenyl-5-nitroimidazole. Glutathione may also play a role in the toxicity or action of several cancer chemotherapeutic agents, including *N*-methyl-*N*′-nitro-*N*-nitrosoguanidine (MNNG), *N*-methylformamide, cyclophosphamide, neocarzinostatin, and bleomycin.

Glutathione conjugate biosynthesis, followed by mercapturic acid formation and excretion, is an important detoxication mechanism for a range of compounds (*1*). Recently it has been recognized that glutathione conjugation is the key, initial step in the bioactivation of several classes of xenobiotics. Moreover, the observed mutagenicity or carcinogenicity, or both, of several groups of compounds is dependent on glutathione conjugate formation. Finally, glutathione-dependent reactions may be involved in the action of some chemotherapeutic agents.

This review will summarize briefly mechanisms of the glutathione-dependent bioactivation of xenobiotics with emphasis on the role of glutathione conjugate formation in the mutagenicity and carcinogenicity of xenobiotics. Reviews about glutathione-dependent xenobiotic toxicity have appeared (*2–4*).

*Direct-acting Glutathione Conjugates*

Direct-acting glutathione conjugates are toxic without the necessity of further enzymatic intervention, although nonenzymatic reactions are usually involved. This mechanism is important for the bioactivation of dihalomethanes, vicinal dihaloethanes, and 1,2,3-trihalopropanes.

*Dihalomethanes:* Dihalomethanes are metabolized to carbon monoxide *via* a cytochromes P-450-dependent pathway (*5*) and to formaldehyde *via* a glutathione *S*-transferase-dependent pathway (Fig. 1) (*6*). Chlorofluoromethane, dibromomethane, dichloromethane, and diiodomethane are directly mutagenic toward *Salmonella typhimurium* TA100 (*7–9*). Their mutagenicity is enhanced by the addition of S-9 fractions from Arochlor-treated rats and by the addition of hepatic cytosol and glutathione, indicating that both cytochromes P-450 and glutathione *S*-transferases may catalyze the formation of mutagenic metabolites(*7*). The observation of glutathione-dependent mutagenicity of dichloromethane is significant, because pharmacokinetic studies implicate glutathione *S*-transferase-catalyzed metabolism of dichloromethane in the development of lung and liver tumors seen after giving dichloromethane (*10*). Although the *S*-(chloromethyl)glutathione intermediate formed by the glutathione *S*-transferase-catalyzed reaction of glutathione with dichloromethane is highly reactive (Fig. 1) (*6*), dichloromethane-derived DNA adducts have not been detected (*10*).

*Vicinal dihaloethanes:* 1,2-Dibromoethane and 1,2-dichloroethane are cytotoxic and mutagenic (*11, 12*). Both cytochromes P-450 and glutathione *S*-transferases catalyze the metabolism of 1,2-dihaloethanes. For example, cytochromes P-450 convert 1,2-dibromoethane to bromoacetaldehyde, which gives rise to protein-bound

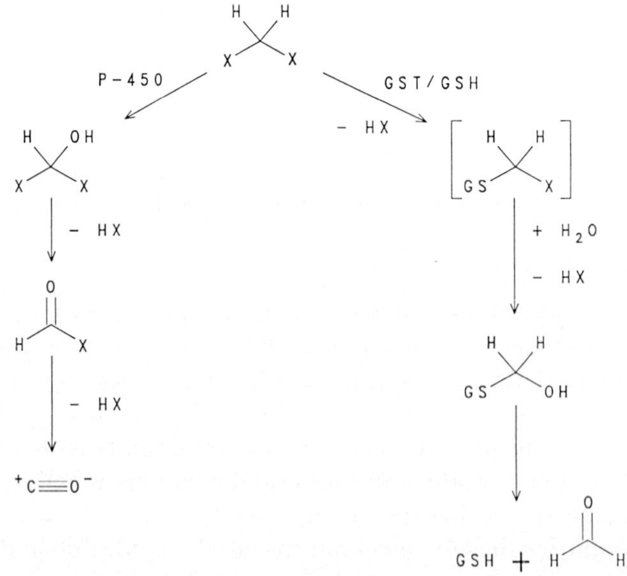


FIG. 1. Glutathione *S*-transferase- and cytochromes P-450-dependent metabolism of dihalomethanes. The *S*-(halomethyl)glutathione intermediate is shown in brackets. P-450, cytochromes P-450; GSH, glutathione; GST, glutathione *S*-transferases.

adducts, whereas glutathione *S*-transferases catalyze the formation of half-sulfur mustard metabolites that bind to DNA (Fig. 2) (*13*).

Although oxidative metabolism of 1,2-dibromoethane predominates *in vivo* (*14*), the genotoxicity of 1,2-dibromoethane is associated with glutathione conjugate formation. The mutagenicity of 1,2-dibromoethane toward *S. typhimurium* TA100 is increased by addition of cytosol and glutathione (*15*) and is lower in glutathione-deficient *S. typhimurium* strains (*16*). Moreover, [$^2H_4$]1,2-dibromoethane produces more DNA damage than 1,2-dibromoethane (*17*), which indicates a role for glutathione conjugate formation. Finally, the glutathione *S*-transferase-dependent metabolism of both 1,2-dibromoethane and 1,2-dichloroethane affords *S*-[2-($N^7$-guanyl)-ethyl]glutathione as a metabolite (Fig. 3) (*18, 19*). This adduct is formed by reaction of the episulfonium ion of *S*-(2-haloethyl)glutathione with DNA (*20*).

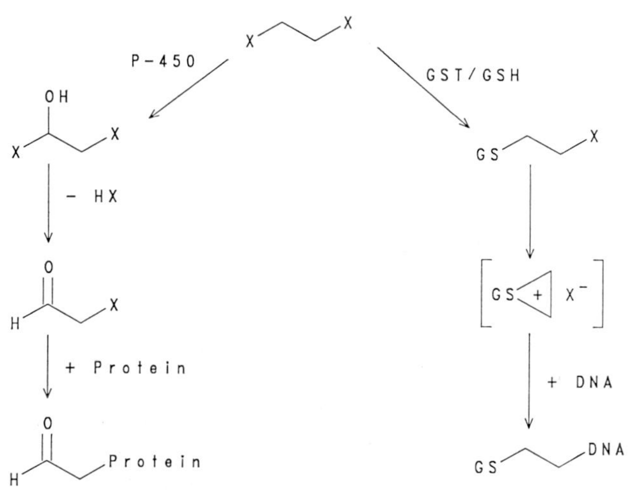


FIG. 2. Glutathione *S*-transferase- and cytochromes P-450-dependent metabolism of 1,2-dihaloethanes. The episulfonium-ion intermediate is shown in brackets.

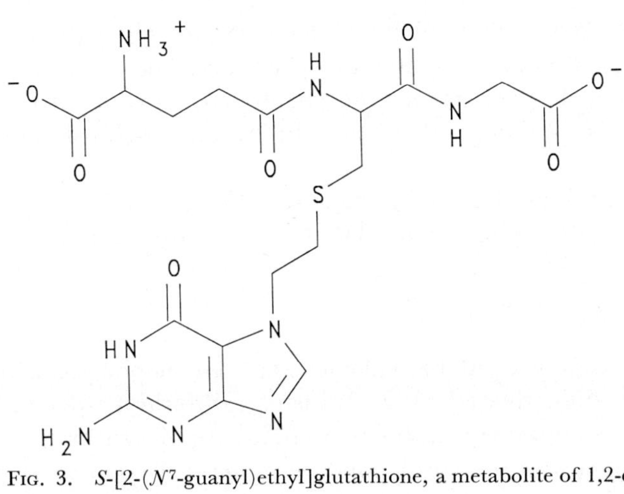


FIG. 3. *S*-[2-($N^7$-guanyl)ethyl]glutathione, a metabolite of 1,2-dibromoethane and 1,2-dichloroethane.

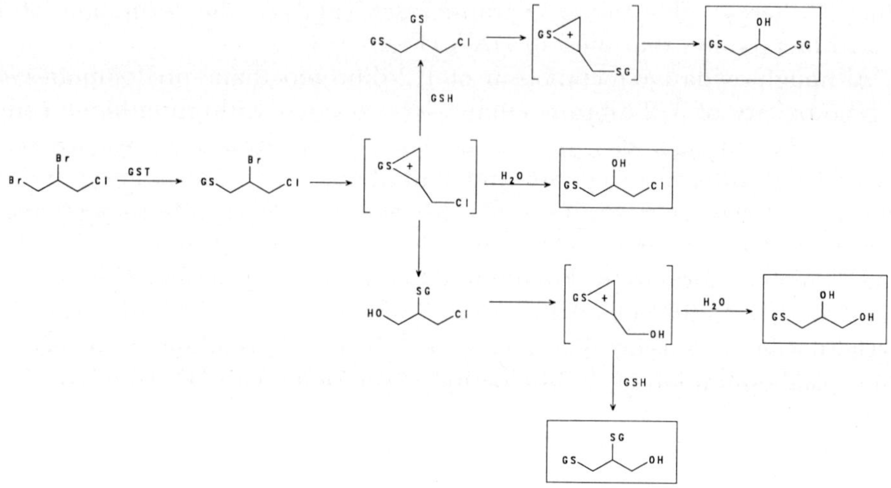


FIG. 4. Glutathione-dependent bioactivation of 1,2-dibromo-3-chloropropane. Episulfonium-ion intermediates are enclosed in brackets. Stable, terminal metabolites are enclosed in boxes. Modified from pearson *et al.* (*27*).

*1,2,3-Trihalopropanes:* 1,2-Dibromo-3-chloropropane is genotoxic in several bacterial and mammalian test systems, is carcinogenic in experimental animals, and is hepato- and nephrotoxic (*21*). In addition, exposure of humans to 1,2-dibromo-3-chloropropane leads to testicular damage, decreased spermatogenesis, and infertility.

The geno- and cytotoxicity of 1,2-dibromo-3-chloropropane appears to involve metabolism by both cytochromes P-450 and glutathione *S*-transferases. The mutagenicity of 1,2-dibromo-3-chloropropane in *S. typhimurium* strain TA100 is associated with its metabolism to 2-bromoacrolein by the cytochromes P-450 (*22*). Similarly, 1,2-dibromo-3-chloropropane-induced DNA damage in hepatocytes is associated with its metabolism by cytochromes P-450 (*23*). In contrast, studies with selectively methylated and deuterated analogs of 1,2-dibromo-3-chloropropane indicate that the *in vivo* testicular and renal bioactivation of 1,2-dibromo-3-chloropropane is glutathione-dependent (*24–26*), and chemical evidence for the glutathione-dependent metabolism of 1,2-dibromo-3-chloropropane to episulfonium-ion intermediates has recently been presented (Fig. 4) (*27*). Hence the extrahepatic toxicity of 1,2-dibromo-3-chloropropane appears to be dependent on glutathione *S*-transferase-catalyzed conjugate formation.

Evidence for the glutathione-dependent bioactivation of 1,2,3-trichloropropane to metabolites that bind covalently to hepatic DNA has recently been presented (*28*).

### *Cysteine Conjugate β-Lyase-dependent Bioactivation*

Recent studies show that several haloalkenes that are nephrotoxic or nephrocarcinogenic, or both, are bioactivated by a multistep, glutathione-dependent pathway. This pathway involves hepatic glutathione *S*-conjugate biosynthesis, metabolism of the glutathione *S*-conjugates to the corresponding cysteine *S*-conjugates, translocation of the cysteine *S*-conjugates to the kidney, and, finally, bioactivation by renal cysteine conjugate β-lyase. This pathway accounts for the kidney-selective toxicity of, for example, dichloroacetylene, hexachlorobutadiene, tetrachloroethylene, trichloroethylene, tetrachloroethylene, and chlorotrifluoroethylene. Several reviews of the β-lyase-dependent bioactivation of haloalkenes have appeared (*29–32*).

The first step in the glutathione-dependent bioactivation of haloalkenes is hepatic glutathione *S*-conjugate formation. Chloroalkenes are metabolized by an addition-elimination mechanism to *S*-(chlorovinyl)glutathione conjugates; for example, hexachlorobutadiene and trichloroethylene are metabolized to *S*-(pentachlorobutadienyl)glutathione and *S*-(1,2-dichlorovinyl)glutathione, respectively (Fig. 5) (*29–32*). Fluoroalkenes and dihaloacetylenes undergo a glutathione *S*-transferase catalyzed addition reaction; chlorotrifluoroethylene and dichloroacetylene are metabolized to *S*-(2-chloro-1,1,2-trifluoroethyl)glutathione and *S*-(1,2-dichlorovinyl)glutathione, respectively (Fig. 5). *In vitro* studies indicate that for all haloalkenes studied thus far, the microsomal glutathione *S*-transferase is a much better catalyst of conjugate formation than are the cytosolic glutathione *S*-transferases (*33*). Intracellular glutathione conjugate formation with chlorotrifluoroethylene is catalyzed selectively by the microsomal glutathione *S*-transferase (*34*).

Studies with the isolated, perfused rat liver show that glutathione *S*-conjugates of hexachlorobutadiene are eliminated from the liver in the bile, although some efflux *via* the blood is seen at high haloalkene concentrations (*35*). After infusion of *S*-(pentachlorobutadienyl)glutathione into the intestine *via* the bile duct, both *S*-

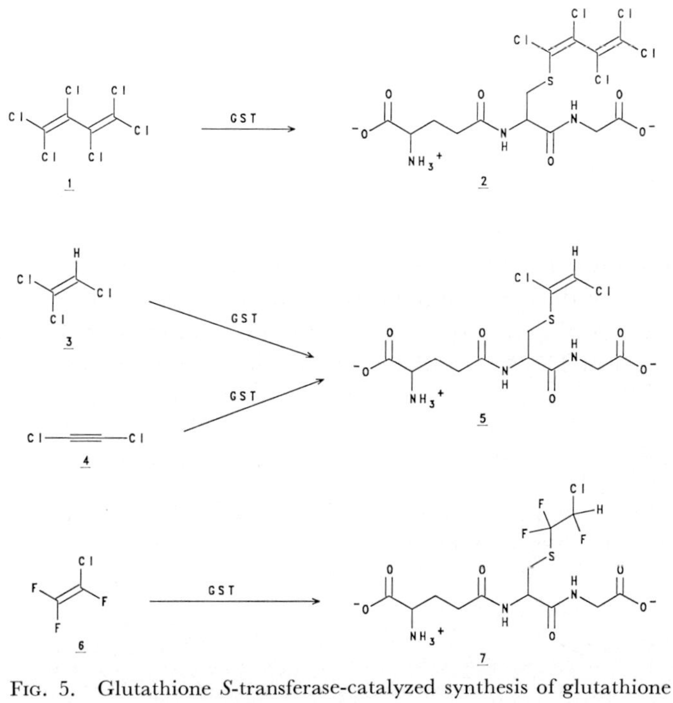

FIG. 5. Glutathione *S*-transferase-catalyzed synthesis of glutathione *S*-conjugates of haloalkenes and haloalkynes. 1, Hexachlorobutadiene; 2, *S*-(pentachlorobutadienyl)glutathione; 3, trichloroethylene; 4, dichloroacetylene; 5, *S*-(1,2-dichlorovinyl)glutathione; 6, chlorotrifluoroethylene; 7, *S*-(2-chloro-1,1,2-trifluoroethyl)glutathione.

(pentachlorobutadienyl)glutathione and *S*-(pentachlorobutadienyl)-L-cysteine were detected in portal blood, indicating uptake and partial hydrolysis of the glutathione conjugates in the intestine (*36*). Cysteine *S*-conjugates in the portal blood may be converted to the corresponding mercapturic acids by the liver. Hence glutathione *S*-conjugates, cysteine *S*-conjugates, and mercapturic acids may all be delivered to the kidney after exposure to chloro- or fluoroalkenes. In the kidney, glutathione *S*-conjugates are metabolized to L-cysteinylglycine *S*-conjugates by $\gamma$-glutamyltransferase, and the L-cysteinylglycine *S*-conjugates are metabolized to cysteine conjugates by the dipeptidases aminopeptidase M and cysteinylglycine dipeptidase. Moreover, mercapturic acids are metabolized to cysteine *S*-conjugates by acylase. Active transport systems exist in the kidney for the uptake of cysteine *S*-conjugates (*37*). These renal conjugate uptake and processing systems explain the observed kidney-selective toxicity of glutathione (*38, 39*), cysteinylglycine (*38*), and cysteine conjugates (*38, 39*) as well as of mercapturic acids (*40*).

The nephrotoxicity *in vivo* and cytotoxicity *in vitro* of cysteine *S*-conjugates is dependent on bioactivation by renal cysteine conjugate $\beta$-lyase. The pyridoxal phosphate-dependent $\beta$-lyase is identical with glutamine transaminase K and catalyzes transamination and elimination reactions of cysteine *S*-conjugates (*41*). The observations that aminooxyacetic acid, an inhibitor of pyridoxal phosphate-dependent enzymes, blocks the toxicity of cysteine *S*-conjugates and that $\alpha$-methyl analogs of cysteine *S*-conjugates are not toxic support the role of $\beta$-lyase in cysteine conjugate-induced cytotoxicity (*38, 39*). $\beta$-Lyase is present in both renal cytosol and mitochondria, which is consistent with the observation that cysteine *S*-conjugates are potent mitochondrial toxins (*42*).

The $\beta$-lyase-dependent metabolism of cysteine *S*-conjutaged yields pyruvate, ammonia, and fluoroalkylthiols (from fluoroalkene-derived conjugates) or chlorovinylthiols (from chloroalkene-derived conjugates) as metabolites (Fig. 6) (*30–32*). The fluoroalkylthiols lose hydrogen fluoride (HF) to afford thionoacyl fluorides that acylate cellular nucleophiles (*31*). Recent studies indicate that chlorovinylthiols give rise to thioketenes, which are potent acylating agents and dienophiles (*43*).

Although both chloroalkene- and fluoroalkene-derived cysteine *S*-conjugates are cytotoxic, only chloroalkene-derived conjugates are mutagenic in the Ames test (*31*). Metabolites of cysteine *S*-conjugates become covalently bound to kidney DNA and also induce the formation of DNA strand breaks in kidney cells *in vivo* and *in vitro*.

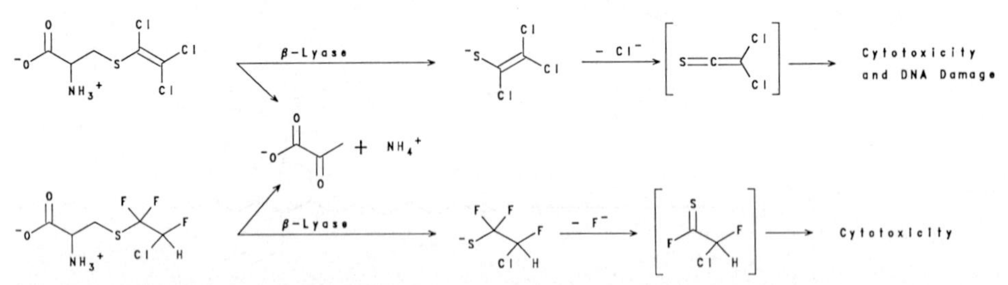


FIG. 6. Cysteine conjugate $\beta$-lyase-dependent bioactivation of *S*-(trichlorovinyl)-L-cysteine and *S*-(2-chloro-1,1,2-trifluoroethyl)-L-cysteine, the cysteine conjugates of tetrachloroethylene and chlorotrifluoroethylene. The thioketene and thionoacyl fluoride intermediates are shown in brackets.

Recent studies show that the pattern and temporal features of mitochondrial $Ca^{2+}$ depletion produced by cysteine *S*-conjugates resembles that caused by tumour promoters (*44*). The *β*-lyase-dependent DNA damage and perturbations of cellular calcium homeostasis caused by cysteine *S*-conjugates may contribute to the observed nephrocarcinogenicity of hexachlorobutadiene, trichloroethylene, and tetrachloroethylene (*31*, *32*).

### *Other Examples of Glutathione-dependent Bioactivation*

In addition to the glutathione-dependent bioactivation of xenobiotics by formation of direct-acting glutathione conjugates and by the cysteine conjugate *β*-lyase pathway, several other examples of glutathione-dependent bioactivation have been reported.

*Aryl amines:* The mutagenicity of 3-amino-1-methyl-5*H*-pyrido[4,3-*b*]indole (Trp-P-2) and 3-hydroxyamino-1-methyl-5*H*-pyrido[4,3-*b*]indole (N-OH-Trp-P-2), which are pyrolysis products of the amino acid tryptophan, in *S. typhimurium* TA98 is increased in the presence of glutathione, but the mechanism of the glutathione-dependent enhancement of mutagenicity is not understood (*45*, *46*). In contrast, glutathione blocks the mutagenicity of 2-acetylaminofluorene, aminofluorene, and *N*-hydroxy-2-acetylaminofluorene (*47*), indicating that the enhancing effect of glutathione is selective for certain aryl amines.

*Nitroimidazoles:* The binding of 1-methyl-4-phenyl-5-nitrosoimidazole, a metabolite of 1-methyl-4-phenyl-5-nitroimidazole, to DNA is increased markedly by physiological concentrations of glutathione (*48*). This interaction may involve the intermediacy of a thiol adduct that gives rise to an *N*-hydroxyiminoimidazole intermediate that reacts with DNA.

*Cancer chemotherapeutic agents:* DNA methylation by *N*-methyl-*N′*-nitro-*N*-nitrosoguanidine (MNNG) is dependent on a nonenzymatic, thiol-dependent reaction that gives rise to methyldiazohydroxide (*49*). The observation that MNNG-induced stomach tumors are localized in the glandular stomach, which has the highest glutathione concentration, is supportive of a role for thiols in MNNG action (*50*). The mutagenicity of MNNG is reduced in glutathione-deficient strains of *S. typhimurium* TA 1535 (*51*).

*N*-methylformamide, which exhibits antineoplastic activity and has been studied in clinical trials as an anticancer agent, is hepatotoxic. The conjugates *S*-(*N*-methylcarbamoyl)glutathione and *S*-(*N*-methylcarbamoyl)-*N*-acetylcysteine are cytotoxic in isolated mouse hepatocytes and are potent growth inhibitors of murine TLX5 lymphoma cells (*52*). Hence *N*-methylcarbamic acid thioester conjugates may be responsible for both the hepatotoxicity and antineoplastic activity of *N*-methylformamide and may act by releasing methyl isocyanate at cell membranes.

The mutagenicity of the cancer chemotherapeutic agent cyclophosphamide in *S. typhimurium* strain TA1535 is increased by low (0.1 to 1 mM) concentrations of glutathione and glutathione disulfide, whereas high (10 mM) concentrations of glutathione and glutathione disulfide decrease cyclophosphamide mutagenicity (*53*). The mechanism by which glutathione and glutathione disulfide enhance cyclophosphamide-induced mutagenicity has not been elucidated.

Glutathione enhances the cytotoxicity and mutagenicity of neocarzinostatin, apparently because neocarzinostatin requires the presence of a reducing agent to produce DNA damage (*54*). Similarly, glutathione may reduce a ferric iron-bleomycin complex and thereby stimulate DNA degradation by bleomycin (*55*).

Azathioprine, an immunosuppressant, is a prodrug of 6-mercaptopurine. 6-Mercaptopurine is formed from azathioprine by a glutathione *S*-transferase-catalyzed reaction (*56*).

Interestingly, glutathione itself is mutagenic in the Ames test (*57*). The formation of hydrogen peroxide or superoxide anion radical, or of active oxygen species derived from them, does not account for the observed mutagenicity of glutathione (*58*).

*Acknowledgment*

Work in the author's laboratory was supported by NIEHS grant ES03127. I thank Ms. Sandra E. Morgan for preparing the manuscript.

## REFERENCES

1. Coles, B. and Ketterer, B. The role of glutathione and glutathione transferases in chemical carcinogenesis. Crit. Rev. Biochem. Mol. Biol., *25*: 47–70, 1990.
2. Anders, M. W. Glutathione-dependent toxicity. Faseb J., in press.
3. Vamvakas, S. and Anders, M. W. Formation of reactive intermediates by Phase II enzymes: Glutathione-dependent bioactivation reactions. Adv. Exp. Med. Biol., *283*: 13–24, 1990.
4. Anders, M. W., Dekant, W., and Vamvakas, S. Glutathione-dependent toxicity. Xenobiotica, in press.
5. Kubic, V. L. and Anders, M. W. Metabolism of dihalomethanes to carbon monoxide. III. Studies on the mechanism of the reaction. Biochem. Pharmacol., *27*: 2349–2355, 1978.
6. Ahmed, A. E. and Anders, M. W. Metabolism of dihalomethanes to formaldehyde and inorganic halide. II. Studies on the mechanism of the reaction. Biochem. Pharmacol., *27*: 2021–2025, 1978.
7. van Bladeren, P. J., Breimer, D. D., Rotteveel-Smijs, G. M. T., and Mohn, G. R. Mutagenic activation of dibromomethane and diiodomethane by mammalian microsomes and glutathione *S*-transferases. Mutat. Res., *74*: 341–346, 1980.
8. Jongen, W. M. F., Harmsen, E. G. M., Alink, G. M., and Koeman, J. H. The effect of glutathione conjugation and microsomal oxidation on the mutagenicity of dichloromethane in *S. typhimurium*. Mutat. Res., *95*: 183–189, 1982.
9. Green, T. The metabolic activation of dichloromethane and chlorofluoromethane in a bacterial mutation assay using *Salmonella typhimurium*. Mutat. Res., *118*: 277–288, 1983.
10. Green, T., Provan, W. M., Collinge, D. C., and Guest, A. E. Macromolecular interactions of inhaled methylene chloride in rats and mice. Toxicol. Appl. Pharmacol., *93*: 1–10, 1988.
11. Huff, J. E. 1,2-Dibromoethane (ethylene dibromide). Environ. Health Perspect., *47*: 359–363, 1983.
12. Davidson, I. W. F., Sumner, D. D., and Parker, J. C. Ethylene dichloride: A review of its metabolism, mutagenic and carcinogenic potential. Drug Chem. Toxicol., *5*: 319–388, 1982.
13. Shih, T.-W. and Hill, D. L. Metabolic activation of 1,2-dibromoethane by glutathione transferase and by microsomal mixed function oxidase: Further evidence for formation

of two reactive metabolites. Res. Commun. Chem. Pathol. Pharmacol., *33*: 449–461, 1981.

14. van Bladeren, P. J., Breimer, D. D., van Huijgevoort, J.A.T.C.M., Vermeulen, N.P.E., and van der Gen, A. The metabolic formation of *N*-acetyl-*S*-2-hydroxyethyl-L-cysteine from tetradeutero-1,2-dibromoethane. Relative importance of oxidation and glutathione conjugation *in vivo*. Biochem. Pharmacol., *30*: 2499–2502, 1981.
15. van Bladeren, P. J., Breimer, D. D., Rotteveel-Smijs, G. M. T., de Jong, R. A. W., Buijs, W., van der Gen, A., and Mohn, G. R. The role of glutathione conjugation in the mutagenicity of 1,2-dibromoethane. Biochem. Pharmacol., *29*: 2975–2982, 1980.
16. Zoetemelk, C. E. M., Mohn, G. R., van der Gen, A., and Breimer, D. D. 1,2-Dibromo compounds. Their mutagenicity in *Salmonella* strains differing in glutathione content and their alkylating potential. Biochem. Pharmacol., *36*: 1829–1835, 1987.
17. White, R. D., Gandolfi, A. J., Bowden, G. T., and Sipes, I. G. Deuterium isotope effect on the metabolism and toxicity of 1,2-dibromoethane. Toxicol. Appl. Pharmacol., *69*: 170–178, 1983.
18. Ozawa, N. and Guengerich, F. P. Evidence for formation of an *S*-[2-($N^7$-guanyl)-ethyl]glutathione adduct in glutathione-mediated binding of the carcinogen 1,2-dibromoethane to DNA. Proc. Natl. Acad. Sci. U.S.A., *80*: 5266–5270, 1983.
19. Foureman, G. L. and Reed, D. J. Formation of *S*-[2-($N^7$-guanyl)ethyl]adducts by the postulated *S*-(2-chloroethyl)cysteinyl and *S*-(2-chloroethyl)glutathionyl conjugates of 1,2-dichloroethane. Biochemistry, *26*: 2028–2033, 1987.
20. Peterson, L. A., Harris, T. M., and Guengerich, F. P. Evidence for an episulfonium ion intermediate in the formation of *S*-[2-($N^7$-guanyl)ethyl]glutathione in DNA. J. Am. Chem. Soc., *110*: 3284–3291, 1988.
21. Whorton, M. D. and Foliart, D. E. Mutagenicity, carcinogenicity and reproductive effects of dibromochloropropane (DBCP). Mutat. Res., *123*: 13–30, 1983.
22. Omichinski, J. G., Søderlund, E. J., Dybing, E., Pearson, P. G., and Nelson, S. D. Detection and mechanism of formation of the potent direct-acting mutagen 2-bromoacrolein from 1,2-dibromo-3-chloropropane. Toxicol. Appl. Pharmacol., *92*: 286–294, 1988.
23. Holme, J. A., Søderlund, E. J., Brunborg, G., Omichinski, J. G., Bekkedal, K., Trygg, B., Nelson, S. D., and Dybing, E. Different mechanisms are involved in DNA damage, bacterial mutagenicity and cytotoxicity induced by 1,2-dibromo-3-chloropropane in suspensions of rat liver cells. Carcinogenesis, *10*: 49–54, 1989.
24. Omichinski, J. G., Brunborg, G., Holme, J. A., Søderlund, E. J., Nelson, S. D., and Dybing, E. The role of oxidative and conjugative pathways in activation of 1, 2-dibromo-3-chloropropane to DNA damaging products in rat testicular cells. Mol. Pharmacol., *34*: 74–79, 1988.
25. Omichinski, J. G., Brunborg, G., Søderlund, E. J., Dahl, J. E., Holme, J. A., Nelson, S. D., and Dybing, E. Renal necrosis and DNA damage caused by selectively deuterated and methylated analogs of 1, 2-dibromo-3-chloropropane. Toxicol. Appl. Pharmacol., *91*: 358–370, 1987.
26. Låg, M., Søderlund, E. J., Omichinski, J. G., Nelson, S. D., and Dybing, E. Metabolism of selectively methylated and deuterated analogs of 1,2-dibromo-3-chloropropane: Role in organ toxicity and mutagenicity. Chem. Biol. Interact., *69*: 33–44, 1989.
27. Pearson, P. G., Søderlund, E. J., Dybing, E., and Nelson, S. D. Metabolic activation of 1,2-dibromo-3-chloropropane: Evidence for the formation of reactive episulfonium ion intermediates. Biochemistry, *29*: 4971–4981, 1990.
28. Weber, G. L. and Sipes, I. G. Covalent interactions of 1,2,3-trichloropropane with hepatic macromolecules: Studies in the male F-344 rat. Toxicol. Appl. Pharmacol.,

*104*: 395–402, 1990.

29. Elfarra, A. A. and Anders, M. W. Renal processing of glutathione conjugates: Role in nephrotoxicity. Biochem. Pharmacol., *33*: 3729–3732, 1984.
30. Anders, M. W., Lash, L., Dekant, W., Elfarra, A. A., and Dohn, D. R. Biosynthesis and biotransformation of glutathione *S*-conjugates to toxic metabolites. CRC Crit. Rev. Toxicol., *18*: 311–341, 1988.
31. Dekant, W., Vamvakas, S., and Anders, M. W. Bioactivation of nephrotoxic haloalkenes by glutathione conjugation: Formation of toxic and mutagenic intermediates by cysteine conjugate $\beta$-lyase. Drug Metab. Rev., *20*: 43–83, 1989.
32. Dekant, W., Vamvakas, S., and Anders, M. W. Bioactivation of hexachlorobutadiene by glutathione conjugation. Drug Chem. Toxicol., *28*: 285–293, 1990.
33. Anders, M. W., Vamvakas, S., and Dekant, W. Bioactivation of haloalkenes through glutathione conjugation. *In;* J. D. Hayes, C. B. Pickett, and T. J. Mantle (eds.), Glutathione *S*-Transferases and Drug Resistance, pp. 121–130, Taylor & Francis, London, 1990.
34. Hargus, S. J., Fitzsimmons, M. E., Aniya, Y., and Anders, M. W. Stereochemistry of the microsomal glutathione *S*-transferase-catalyzed addition of glutathione to chlorotrifluoroethane. Biochemistry, *30*: 717–721, 1991.
35. Gietl, Y. and Anders, M. W. Biosynthesis and biliary excretion of *S*-conjugates of hexachlorobuta-1,3-diene in the perfused liver. Drug Metab. Dispos., *19*: 274–277, 1991.
36. Gietl, Y., Vamvakas, S., and Anders, M. W. Intestinal absorption of glutathione and cysteine *S*-conjugates of hexachlorobuta-1,3-diene. Unpublished.
37. Lash, L. H. and Anders, M. W. Uptake of nephrotoxic *S*-conjugates by isolated rat renal proximal tubular cells. J. Pharmacol. Exp. Ther., *248*: 531–537, 1989.
38. Elfarra, A. A., Jakobson, I., and Anders, M. W. Mechanism of *S*-(1,2-dichlorovinyl)-glutathione-induced nephrotoxicity. Biochem. Pharmacol., *35*: 283–288, 1986.
39. Lash, L. H. and Anders, M. W. Cytotoxicity of *S*-(1,2-dichlorovinyl)glutathione and *S*-(1,2-dichlorovinyl)-L-cysteine in isolated rat kidney cells. J. Biol. Chem., *261*: 13076–13081, 1986.
40. Vamvakas, S., Dekant, W., Berthold, K., Schmidt, S., Wild, D., and Henschler, D. Enzymatic transformation of mercapturic acids derived from halogenated alkenes to reactive and mutagenic intermediates. Biochem. Pharmacol., *36*: 2741–2748, 1987.
41. Cooper, A. J. L. and Anders, M. W. Glutamine transaminase K and cysteine conjugate $\beta$-lyase. Ann. N. Y. Acad. Sci., *585*: 118–127, 1990.
42. Lash, L. H. and Anders, M. W. Mechanism of *S*-(1,2-dichlorovinyl)-L-cysteine- and *S*-(1,2-dichlorovinyl)-L-homocysteine-induced renal mitochondrial toxicity. Mol. Pharmacol., *32*: 549–556, 1987.
43. Dekant, W., Urban, G., Görsmann, C., and Anders, M. W. Thioketene formation from $\alpha$-haloalkenyl 2-nitrophenyl disulfides: models for biological reactive intermediates of cytotoxic *S*-conjugates. J. Am. Chem. Soc., in press.
44. Vamvakas, S., Sharma, V. K., Sheu, S.-S., and Anders, M. W. Perturbations of intracellular calcium distribution in kidney cells by nephrotoxic haloalkenyl cysteine *S*-conjugates. Mol. Pharmacol., *38*: 455–461, 1990.
45. Saito, K., Yamazoe, Y., Kamataki, T., and Kato, R. Activation and detoxication of N-hydroxy-Trp-P-2 by glutathione and glutathione transferases. Carcinogenesis, *4*: 1551–1557, 1983.
46. de Waziers, I. and Decloître, F. Effect of glutathione and uridine-5′-diphosphoglucuronic acid on the mutagenicity of tryptophan pyrolysis products (Trp-P-1 and Trp-P-2) by rat-liver and -intestine S9 fraction. Mutat. Res., *139*: 15–19, 1984.

47. Hongslo, J., Haug, L. T., Wirth, P. J., Møller, M., Dybing, E., and Thorgeirsson, S. S. Influence of conjugation reactions on the mutagenicity of aromatic amines. Mutat. Res., *107*: 239–247, 1983.
48. Ehlhardt, W. J. and Goldman, P. Thiol-mediated incorporation of radiolabel from 1-[$^{14}$C]-methyl-4-phenyl-5-nitroimidazole into DNA. A model for the biological activity of 5-nitroimidazoles. Biochem. Pharmacol., *38*: 1175–1180, 1989.
49. Lawley, P. D. and Thatcher, C. J. Methylation of deoxyribonucleic acid in cultured mammalian cells by *N*-methyl-*N*′-nitro-*N*-nitrosoguanidine. The influence of cellular thiol concentrations on the extent of methylation and the 6-oxygen atom of guanine as a site of methylation. Biochem. J., *116*: 693–707, 1970.
50. Weistler, O., von Deimling, A., Kobori, O., and Kleihues, P. Location of *N*-methyl-*N*′-nitro-*N*-nitrosoguanidine-induced gastrointestinal tumors correlates with thiol distribution. Carcinogenesis, *4*: 879–883, 1983.
51. Kerklaan, P., Bouter, S., and Mohn, G. Isolation of a mutant of *Salmonella typhimurium* strain TA1535 with decreased levels of glutathione ($GSH^-$). Primary characterization and chemical mutagenesis studies. Mutat. Res., *122*: 257–266, 1983.
52. Han, D.-H., Pearson, P. G., Baillie, T. A., Dayal, R., Tsang, L. H., and Gescher, A. Chemical synthesis and cytotoxic properties of *N*-alkylcarbamic acid thioesters, metabolites of hepatotoxic formamides. Chem. Res. Toxicol., *3*: 118–124, 1990.
53. Hales, B. F. Modification of the teratogenicity and mutagenicity of cyclophosphamide with thiol compounds. Teratology, *23*: 373–381, 1981.
54. DeGraff, W. G. and Mitchell, J. B. Glutathione dependence of neocarzinostatin cytotoxicity and mutagenicity in Chinese hamster V-79 cells. Cancer Res., *45*: 4760–4762, 1985.
55. Caspary, W. J., Lanzo, D. A., and Niziak, C. Intermediates in the ferrous oxidase cycle of bleomycin. Biochemistry, *20*: 3868–3875, 1981.
56. Kaplowitz, N. Interaction of azathioprine and glutathione in the liver of the rat. J. Pharmacol. Exp. Ther., *200*: 479–486, 1977.
57. Glatt, H., Protić-Sabljić, M., and Oesch, F. Mutagenicity of glutathione and cysteine in the Ames test. Science, *220*: 961–963, 1983.
58. Glatt, H. Mutagenicity spectra in *Salmonella typhimurium* strains of glutathione, L-cysteine and active oxygen species. Mutagenesis, *4*: 221–227, 1989.

XENOBIOTICS AND CANCER, L. ERNSTER ET AL. (EDS.),
JAPAN SCI. SOC. PRESS, TOKYO/TAYLOR & FRANCIS LTD., LONDON, pp. 101–107, 1991

# DNA-glutathione Adducts Derived from *vic*-dihaloalkanes: Mechanisms of Mutagenesis

F. Peter GUENGERICH, W. Griffith HUMPHREYS, Dong-Hyun KIM, Tetsuya OIDA, and Joan L. CMARIK

*Department of Biochemistry and Center in Molecular Toxicology, Vanderbilt University School of Medicine, Nashville, Tennessee 37232-0146, U.S.A.*

*Abstract:* The conjugation of the prototype dihaloalkane ethylene dibromide (EDB) with glutathione (GSH) yields *S*-(2-bromoethyl)GSH, which gives rise to *S*-[2-($N^7$-guanyl)ethyl]GSH as the major DNA adduct ($\geq$95%). All reaction steps have $S_N2$ character. Another minor DNA and RNA adduct is *S*-[2-($N^1$-adenyl)ethyl] GSH, formed *in vitro* and *in vivo*. These adducts have similar half-lives *in vivo*. Enhancement of GSH conjugation or inhibition of cytochrome P-450 IIE1 oxidation enhances DNA adduct levels *in vivo* and GSH depletion lowers levels. The mercapturic acid *N*-acetyl-*S*-[2-($N^7$-guanyl)ethyl]cysteine is excreted in urine and may find use as a biomarker. A series of compounds of the general structure $RSCH_2CH_2Cl$ has been used to alkylate *Salmonella typhimurium* TA100. The ratio of (guanyl) base-pair mutations to $N^7$-guanyl adducts varies dramatically, with *S*-(2-chloroethyl)GSH apparently producing the most potent guanyl adduct. This mutagenicity is not due to SOS response or alkylation specificity. Physical studies with modified oligonucleotides indicate that the $N^7$-guanyl substitution weakens G-C pairing but does not in itself alter the selectivity of pairing to C in an isolated oligomer.

The bioactivation of chemicals to ultimate carcinogens *via* oxidation by cytochrome P-450 enzymes is well recognized. However, in some cases cytochrome P-450 oxidation is effectively a detoxication reaction and the so-called "Phase II" conjugative reactions are involved in bioactivation. An example that has been studied in this laboratory is ethylene dibromide (EDB)—this and other *vic*-dihaloalkanes are activated *via* conjugation with glutathione (GSH), and a number of lines of evidence indicate that this pathway is involved in tumor initiation by these chemicals. When considered together, *vic*-dihaloalkanes are used in high volume in industrial settings and their potential risk is of concern. Our own work in this field developed from our studies on the oxidation by cytochrome P-450 (*1–4*) [P-450 IIE1 now appears to be the major catalyst (*2*)] and the early reports from the groups of Rannug (*5*) and Breimer (*6*). Our results indicated that the binding of the analog ethylene dichloride (EDC) to DNA adducts was catalyzed by cytosolic GSH *S*-transferases and binding to protein was catalyzed by microsomal P-450s (*7*).

*Structures and Disposition of Adducts Derived from EDB*

The initial work of Rannug indicating that EDB mutations were GSH dependent suggested that an adduct should be formed which contains a DNA base, GSH, and an ethylene moiety derived from EDB (*5*). Such stoichiometry was established in *in vitro* radiolabeling experiments, even in isolated hepatocytes (*8*). Further, the major adduct formed *in vitro* was partially purified and then reduced with Raney Ni to form $N^7$-ethylguanine, which was characterized and postulated to arise from the adduct *S*-[2-($N^7$-guanyl)ethyl]GSH (*8*). Subsequently, the intact *S*-[2-($N^7$-guanyl)ethyl]GSH adduct was isolated and its structure was unambiguously identified by mass and NMR spectroscopy (*9*). Stereoisotopic deuterium labeling experiments and kinetic studies with models support a scheme in which an episulfonium ion is an obligatory intermediate and all of the reactions of interest in this pathway have $S_N2$ character (*i.e.*, proceed with inversion of configuration) (Fig. 1) (*10*). Another minor adduct has recently been characterized as *S*-[2-($N^1$-adenyl)ethyl]GSH, which exists in the tautomer shown in Fig. 1 at pH > 6.9 (*11*). No evidence for formation of an $N^6$-adenyl adduct, an $O^6$-guanyl adduct, or an imidazole ring-opened $N^7$-guanyl adduct could be found (all were synthesized).

The same adducts are formed *in vivo* in rat liver and account for > 98% of the DNA adducts derived from EDB. Although adducts resulting from the cytochrome P-450-catalyzed oxidation of EDB can be detected *in vitro* in RNA, none have been found in DNA *in vitro* or *in vivo* (*12, 13*). The structures of two very minor DNA adducts remain undefined but apparently do not contain purines (*11*). The half-lives of all of the DNA adducts are about 100 hr in rat liver (*11, 13*). The level of *S*-[2-($N^7$-guanyl)ethyl]GSH in rat liver can be decreased by depletion of GSH, and the level of the adduct can be increased by either (a) induction of GSH *S*-transferase or (b) inhibition of the cytochrome P-450 IIE1-catalyzed oxidation of EDB by disulfiram (*2*), a treatment known to dramatically increase the level of EDB-induced hepatocarcino-

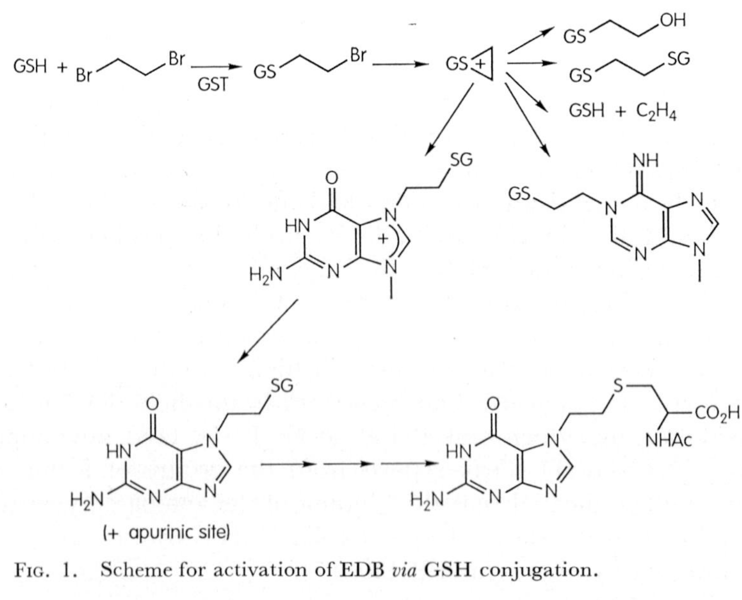


FIG. 1. Scheme for activation of EDB *via* GSH conjugation.

genesis (*1, 3, 14*). Repair of *S*-[2-($\mathcal{N}^7$-guanyl)ethyl]GSH DNA adducts appears to proceed primarily by excision repair in prokaryotes and eukaryotes (*15*), and the primary fate of the adduct appears to be urinary excretion as the mercapturic acid *N*-acetyl-*S*-[2-($\mathcal{N}^7$-guanyl)ethyl]cysteine (*16*).

Recently we have characterized the adducts formed from the analog 1,2-dibromo-3-chloropropane (DBCP), utilizing both cytosolic incubations and studies with two synthetic half-mustards (Fig. 2). All conjugates may be rationalized in terms of episulfonium ion intermediates. The methide GSH conjugate is apparently formed by rearrangement and, with the exception of the *S*-(3-chloro-2-hydroxypropyl)GSH adduct reported by Pearson *et al.* (*17*), all additions may be explained by nucleophilic attack at the unsubstituted methylene of each episulfonium ion. A considerable amount of the intra-strand crosslink of adjacent guanines is formed but we have been unable to detect inter-strand crosslinking in poly(G-C) or in a plasmid. The relevance of these adducts to the testicular and nephrotoxicity of DBCP remains to be established. It is of interest to note that DBCP is apparently not very mutagenic in bacterial systems, in contrast to EDB.

The approach of site-specific mutagenesis has not been applied in the case of

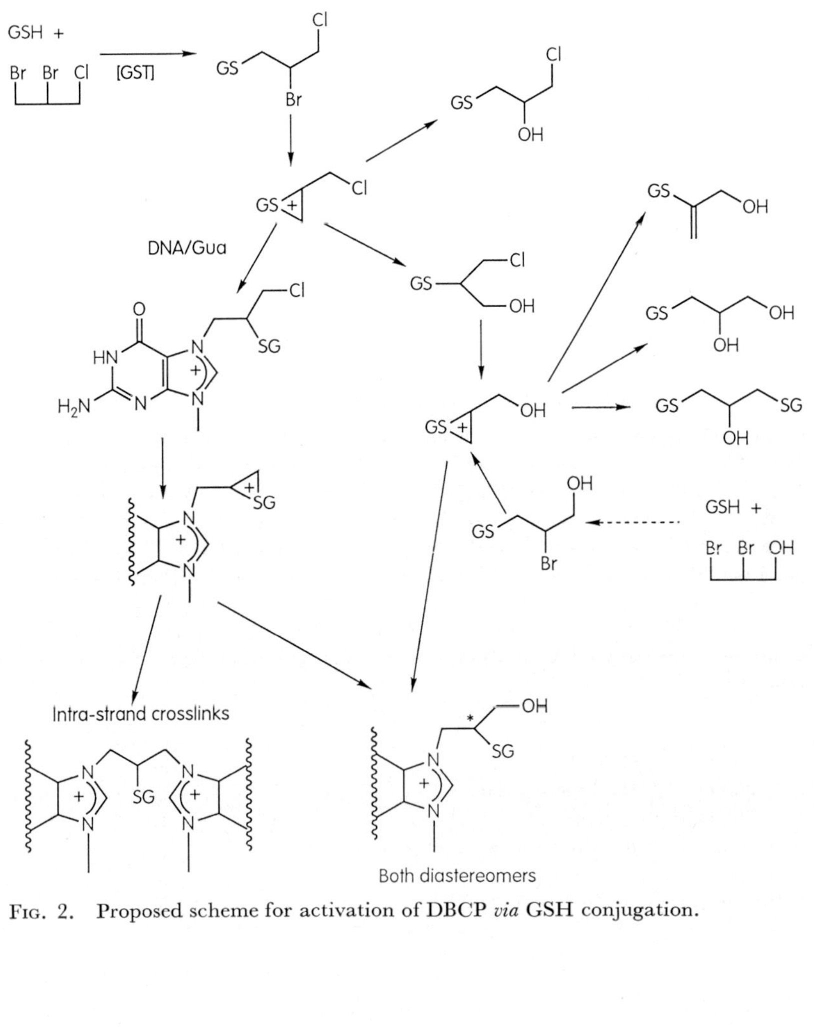


FIG. 2. Proposed scheme for activation of DBCP *via* GSH conjugation.

EDB-derived adducts because of the inherent instability of $N^7$-alkylguanine adducts to depurination. An alternate strategy was utilized in studies on the mechanisms of mutagenesis, where base-pair mutations were examined in *Salmonella typhimurium* TA100 at the two adjacent guanines known to lead to reversion. A series of half-mustard analogs of *S*-(2-bromoethyl)GSH was examined with regard to mutagenicity as a function of dose (Fig. 3) and the compounds were found to differ considerably (*4*). Bacteria were treated with a single concentration of each half-mustard; the $N^7$-alkylguanine adducts were released from bacterial DNA and quantified by HPLC with fluorescence detection, with reference to synthetic standards that were prepared for all adducts. The levels of alkylation varied considerably and are listed on the individual curves shown in Fig. 3. These values differ more than those estimated for the *in vitro* alkylation of calf thymus DNA for the same compounds, apparently being influenced by bacterial membrane permeability and transport. What is interesting is that the ratio of mutations/adducts varies considerably for these adducts, the major one formed from the half-mustards (Table 1) (*4*).

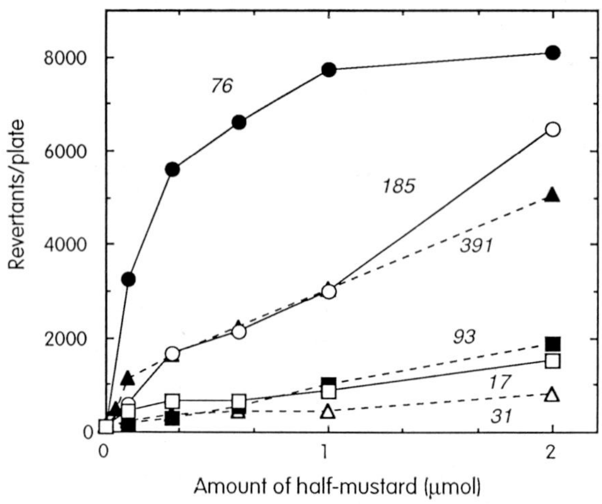


FIG. 3. His-independent *S. typhimurium* TA100 mutants formed by *S*-(2-haloethyl)thiol derivatives. The indicated amounts of the indicated compounds were used: *S*-(2-chloroethyl)cysteine (---△---), *S*-(2-chloroethyl)cysteine methyl ester (—□—), *N*-acetyl-*S*-(2-chloroethyl)cysteine (---■---), *N*-acetyl-*S*-(2-bromoethyl)cysteine methyl ester (—○—), *S*-(2-chloroethyl)GSH (—●—), and *S*-(2-chloroethyl)GSH dimethyl ester (---▲---). DNA $N^7$-guanyl adducts (numerals, pmol/mg DNA) are also presented in each case, measured at the 1 $\mu$mol dose (*4*).

TABLE 1. Radios of *S. typhimurium* TA100 Mutants to $N^7$-Guanyl Adduct Levels for Several *S*-(2-Haloethyl)-thiol Compounds (*4*)

| Compound | Relative ratio of mutants/adduct |
|---|---|
| *S*-(2-Chloroethyl)GSH | 13 |
| *S*-(Chloroethyl)GSH dimethyl ester | 1.0 |
| *S*-(2-Chloroethyl)cysteine | 1.8 |
| *N*-Acetyl-*S*-(2-bromoethyl)cysteine methyl ester | 2.0 |
| *N*-Acetyl-*S*-(2-chloroethyl)cysteine | 1.4 |
| *S*-(2-Chloroethyl)cysteine methyl ester | 6.5 |

Calculations can be made with assumptions about bacterial DNA concentration, *etc.* and indicate that 1 in every 3 *S*-[2-(*N*$^7$-guanyl)ethyl]GSH adducts gives rise to a mutation. However, this estimate might be biased if alkylation selectively occurs at the mutation target. A *Bam*HI/*Sal*I fragment of plasmid pBR322 was end-labeled with $^{32}$P and modified with each of the half-mustards under consideration (Table 1, Fig. 3). The plasmid was treated with hot piperidine to produce breaks at sites of modification, which were located using an electrophoretic method (*18*). Alkylation was found to occur selectively in runs of guanines and the differences among the patterns seen with the various half-mustards were not particularly dramatic. Further, the extent of alkylation at guanyl residues varied by less than an order of magnitude. Thus, the mutation frequency of an *S*-[2-(*N*$^7$-guanyl)ethyl]GSH adduct should still be regarded as being $>5\%$ in this model, even with adjustment for alkylation specificity—this level of mutation can probably only be explained in terms of *S*-[2-(*N*$^7$-guanyl)ethyl]GSH, since no evidence for other guanyl adducts exists, even at levels 1/10 of the mutation frequency (*vide supra*). Finally, the mutations are blocked by the presence of an excision repair system but are not dependent upon the SOS response. Mutations were observed at similar levels in *S. typhimurium* TA1535, devoid of the SOS response, and no positive response to these half-mustards was seen in an *S. typhimurium* TA1535/pSK1002 system, where a plasmid containing the *umuC* regulatory gene is fused to a *lacZ* structural reporter gene. The lack of SOS response argues against the involvement of apurinic sites as a factor in the mutagenesis seen with these compounds. No frameshift mutations have been seen (*4*).

What is the physical basis for the mutations? *N*$^7$-Guanyl alkylation of DNA occurs with many reagents, especially those that react *via* $S_N2$ reactions. However, in many cases evidence supports a more crucial role for alkylations at exocyclic heteroatoms (*e.g.*, *O*$^6$-alkylguanine). However, the bacterial studies cited above argue that *S*-[2-(*N*$^7$-guanyl)ethyl]GSH is relatively mutagenic, and in direct comparisons we have found that this adduct is apparently more mutagenic than the *N*$^7$-guanyl derivative of aflatoxin-8,9-oxide. Several oligomers have been prepared with a single derivatized guanine, including d(AT$\overset{*}{G}$CAT) and d(CAT$\overset{*}{G}$CCT), where $\overset{*}{G}$ indicates *S*-[2-(*N*$^7$-guanyl)ethyl]GSH (*19*). Pairing is weaker when the adduct is present, as indicated by UV, CD, and NMR spectroscopy. In the case of the palindrome d(ATGCAT) no pairing is seen even at 2°C (using NMR and CD spectra). Model building work indicates that the adducts should not sterically hinder pairing—the adduct itself is probably in the major groove and the NMR shifts are essentially unaffected by placement in the oligomer. The d(CAT$\overset{*}{G}$CCT) oligomer can pair with the complement d(AGGCATG) at low temperature. CD and NMR NOESY spectra indicate that d(CAT$\overset{*}{G}$CCT) is not so tightly paired to its complement, as judged by additional NMR studies where the H-bonds are observed in the presence of $H_2O$. The weakened pairing at the $\overset{*}{G}$C pair itself may be explained by the shift in p$K_a$ for formation of the enol tautomer due to the imposition of the positive charge in the imidazole ring, as demonstrated in titrations with model ribonucleosides in $H_2O$ and $(CH_3)_2SO$ (change of p$K_a$ from ~9 to ~7). However, changing the pH did not lead to further binding, at least as judged by UV and CD measurements.

The relevance of the alteration in the binding and structures of the olibonucleotides to mutagenesis remains unclear. More than 60 *S*-(2-chloroethyl)GSH-induced bacteriophage M13 mp18 mutants have been isolated with excision repair-deficient *S. typhimurium* TA100 and *Escherichia coli* and indicate a high proportion of GC/AT transitions, which could be evidence for pairing of a T opposite a guanyl adduct. Pairing to the oligonucleotide d(CAT$\overset{*}{G}$CCT) was considered with d(AGGXATG) heptamers, with X representing each of the four possible bases. However, although the binding with X=C was weaker than observed with (unmodified) d(CATGCCT), no evidence for binding of the other three potential complements was seen at 5°C [d(AGGXATG) where X=A, G, or T].

At the current time there are several potential explanations for the above results. One is that a guanyl adduct other than *S*-[2-($N^7$-guanyl)ethyl]GSH is the most mutagenic. However, several of the above results argue against this. The $O^6$-guanyl adduct was not found, imidazole ring opening was shown not to occur, and the lack of SOS response to *S*-(2-chloroethyl)GSH would argue that apurinic sites are not a factor in mutagenesis. Another possibility is that direct mispairing is seen only in the particular conformations of mutation-prone sequences. This hypothesis if being addressed experimentally. An alternate possibility is that the physical basis of mutation can be understood only in the context of the interaction of the replication fork containing the modified strand, the incoming base, and the polymerase.

*Acknowledgments*

We thank Drs. M. P. Stone, F-M. Chen, and D. Wilson for assistance in obtaining the oligonucleotide spectra. This work was supported in part by United States Public Health Service Grants CA44353, ES00267, and ES01590.

*Note Added in Proof*

The structure of the methide glutathione conjugate in Fig. 2 has been revised to *S*-(2-bromo-2-propenyl) glutathione (W, G, Humphreys, D-H. Kim, and F. P. Guengerich, Chem. Res. Toxicol., in press.

REFERENCES

1. Kim, D. H. and Guengerich, F. P. Formation of the DNA adduct *S*-[2-($N^7$-guanyl)-ethyl]glutathione from ethylene dibromide: effects of modulation of glutathione and glutathione *S*-transferase levels and lack of a role for sulfation. Carcinogenesis, *11*: 419–424, 1990.
2. Guengerich, F. P., Kim, D-H., and Iwasaki, M. Role of human cytochrome P-450 IIE1 in the oxidation of many low molecular weight cancer suspects. Chem. Res. Toxicol., *4*: 168–179, 1991.
3. van Bladeren, P. J., Hoogeterp, J. J., Breimer, D. D., and van der Gen, A. The influence of disulfiram and other inhibitors of oxidative metabolism on the formation of 2-hydroxyethyl-mercapturic acid from 1, 2-dibromoethane by the rat. Biochem. Pharmacol., *30*: 2983–2987, 1981.
4. Humphreys, W. G., Kim, D-H., Cmarik, J. L., Shimada, T., and Guengerich, F. P. Comparison of the DNA alkylating properties and mutagenic responses caused by a series of *S*-(2-haloethyl)-substituted cysteine and glutathione derivatives. Biochemistry, *29*: 10341–10350, 1990.

5. Rannug, U., Sundvall, A., and Ramel, C. The mutagenic effect of 1,2-dichloroethane on *Salmonella typhimurium*. I. Activation through conjugation with glutathione *in vitro*. Chem. Biol. Interact., *20*: 1–16, 1978.
6. van Bladeren, P. J., Breimer, D. D., Rotteveel-Smijs, G. M. T., de Jong, R. A. W., Buijs, W., van der Gen, A., and Mohn, G. R. The role of glutathione conjugation in the mutagenicity of 1,2-dibromoethane. Biochem. Pharmacol., *29*: 2975–2982, 1980.
7. Guengerich, F. P., Crawford, W. M., Jr., Domoradzki, J. Y., Macdonald, T. L., and Watanabe, P. G. *In vitro* activation of 1,2-dichloroethane by microsomal and cytosolic enzymes. Toxicol. Appl. Pharmacol., *55*: 303–317, 1980.
8. Ozawa, N. and Guengerich, F. P. Evidence for formation of an *S*-[2-($N^7$-guanyl)ethyl]-glutathione adduct in glutathione-mediated binding of 1,2-dibromoethane to DNA. Proc. Natl. Acad. Sci. U.S.A., *80*: 5266–5270, 1983.
9. Koga, N., Inskeep, P. B., Harris, T. M., and Guengerich, F. P. *S*-[2-($N^7$-Guanyl)-ethyl]glutathione, the major DNA adduct formed from 1,2-dibromethane. Biochemistry, *25*: 2192–2198, 1986.
10. Peterson, L. A., Harris, T. M., and Guengerich, F. P. Evidence for an episulfonium ion intermediate in the formation of *S*-[2-($N^7$-guanyl)ethyl]glutathione in DNA. J. Am. Chem. Soc., *110*: 3284–3291, 1988.
11. Kim, D.-H., Humphreys, W. G., and Guengerich, F. P. Characterization of *S*-[2-($N^1$-adenyl)ethyl]glutathione in RNA and DNA resulting from activation of 1,2-dibromoethane. Chem. Res. Toxicol., *3*: 587–594, 1990.
12. Inskeep, P. B. and Guengerich, F. P. Glutathione-mediated binding of dibromoalkanes to DNA: specificity of rat glutathione *S*-transferases and dibromoalkane structure. Carcinogenesis, *5*: 805–808, 1984.
13. Inskeep, P. B., Koga, N., Cmarik, J. L., and Guengerich, F. P. Covalent binding of 1,2-dihaloalkanes to DNA and stability of the major DNA adduct, *S*-[2-($N^7$-guanyl)-ethyl]glutathione. Cancer Res., *46*: 2839–2844, 1986.
14. Wong, L. C. K., Winston, J. M., Hong, C. B., and Plotnick, H. Carcinogenicity and toxicity of 1,2-dibromoethane in the rat. Toxicol. Appl. Pharmacol., *63*: 155–165, 1982.
15. Cmarik, J. L., Inskeep, P. B., Meredith, M. J., Meyer, D. J., Ketterer, B., and Guengerich, F. P. Selectivity of rat and human glutathione *S*-transferases in activation of ethylene dibromide by glutathione conjugation and DNA binding and induction of unscheduled DNA synthesis in human hepatocytes. Cancer Res., *50*: 2747–2752, 1990.
16. Kim, D. H. and Guengerich, F. P. Excretion of the mercapturic acid *S*-[2-($N^7$-guanyl)-ethyl]-*N*-acetylcysteine in urine following administration of ethylene dibromide to rats. Cancer Res., *49*: 5843–5851, 1989.
17. Pearson, P. G., Soderlund, E. J., Dybing, E., and Nelson, S. D. Metabolic activation of 1,2-dibromo-3-chloropropane: evidence for the formation of reactive episulfonium ion intermediates. Biochemistry, *29*: 4971–4981, 1990.
18. Maxam, A. M. and Gilbert, W. A new method for sequencing DNA. Proc. Natl. Acad. Sci. U.S.A., *74*: 560–564, 1977.
19. Oida, T., Humphreys, W. G., and Guengerich, F. P. Preparation of an oligonucleotide adducted with an ethylene dibromide glutathione conjugate. Biochemistry, *29*: 2189–2190, 1990.

XENOBIOTICS AND CANCER, L. ERNSTER ET AL. (EDS.),
JAPAN SCI. SOC. PRESS, TOKYO/TAYLOR & FRANCIS LTD., LONDON, pp. 109–117, 1991

# Acetyltransferase and Sulfotransferase Which Activate Mutagens and Carcinogens through O-esterification Mechanisms

Yasushi YAMAZOE, Medhat ABU-ZEID, Da-Wei GONG, Shogo OZAWA, Kiyoshi NAGATA, and Ryuichi KATO

*Department of Pharmacology, School of Medicine, Keio University, Tokyo 160, Japan*

*Abstract:* The regulatory mechanism of acetyltransferase and sulfotransferase, which are involved in the activation of carcinogenic arylamines and their N-hydroxy derivatives, has been studied. Cytosolic N-acetylation of 2-aminofluorene (2-AF) in hamster liver and skin showed tri-modal distribution in the presence of acetyl CoA, whereas no clear segregation was detected in the N-hydroxyarylacetamide-supported N-acetylation and acetyl CoA-dependent O-acetylation of N-hydroxy-Glu-P-1. From hamster livers, two forms of acetyltransferase, AT-I and AT-II, were purified and characterized to have different catalytic and chemical properties. AT-I was detectable in all the hamsters examined, but AT-II was detected only in the animals showing high rates of 2-AF N-acetylation. Cross-matings of the intra- and inter-phenotypes of three different acetylators (rapid, intermediate, and slow) indicate the genetic inheritance of the arylamine N-acetylation, which follows a Mendelian co-dominant trait. Cytosolic sulfotransferase catalyzes the activation of N-hydroxyarylamines and N-hydroxyarylacetamides through the enzymatic O-sulfonylation. The reaction often shows a sex-related difference in rats. Among three sulfotransferases isolated (HAST I, II, and PST I), the level of HASTs was correlated with the 3′-phosphoadenosine 5′-phosphosulfate (PAPS)-dependent activating capacity of N-hydroxy-2-acetylaminofluorene (N-hydroxy-AAF) in rat livers. In addition, hepatic content of HASTs was decreased by hypophysectomy and restored by the intermittent administration of growth hormone, which mimics the male secretory profile. These results indicate that the sex-related difference in secretory profile of pituitary growth hormone is a major determinant of the male-dominant sulfation in this species. The capacity of human liver to activate N-hydroxyarylamines is also discussed.

Living organisms are exposed daily to synthetic and natural chemicals as xenobiotics. These chemicals often contain primary arylamino-moiety in their molecules. Primary arylamines are also produced metabolically by reduction of azo-dyes, N-oxides and nitroarenes, and by dealkylation of N-substituted chemicals. Most primary arylamines are now known to undergo a two-step activation (N-oxidation and O-acylation) in the body to exert the carcinogenic effect. Several lines of evidence suggest that the level of O-esterification capacity is a major factor controlling the susceptibility to arylamine-induced carcinogenesis (*1, 2*). In mammalian cells, various conjugating enzymes exist and function as a so-called "second phase of drug metabolizing enzymes". Among them, cytosolic acetyltransferase and sulfotransferase often play key roles for the activation of arylamine and the N-hydroxy derivatives to cause the DNA damage necessary as the initial event to produce cancer (*3–6*). For the past years, we have been investigating factors regulating the expression of acetyltransferase and sulfotransferase, which may be important as modulators of arylamine-induced carcinogenesis. In this paper, we provide our recent data on genetic polymorphism of acetyltransferase in hamsters and on the mechanism of endocrine regulation of hepatic sulfotransferase in rats.

### *System for Assay of Acetylation and Sulfation*

*Chemicals:* Heterocyclic arylamines are supplied under the Research Resource Program for Cancer Research of the Ministry of Education, Science and Culture, Japan. N-hydroxy-2-acetylaminofluorene (N-hydroxy-AAF), N-hydroxy-4-acetylaminobiphenyl (N-hydroxy-AABP), and N-hydroxy-Glu-P-1 were synthesized as reported previously (*7, 8*). Other chemicals were obtained from local suppliers.

*Animal treatment:* Syrian golden hamsters were originally obtained from Tokyo Laboratory Animals Science, and matings were carried out in an animal care facility in our laboratory. Sprague-Dawley rats were obtained from Clea Japan. Hypophysectomy and treatment with human growth hormone (hGH) were performed as described previously (*9, 10*). Triiodothyronine was given to hypophysectomized rats as reported (*11*).

*Assay method:* Acetylations of arylamines and N-hydroxyarylamines were quantified as reported (*12, 13*). Sulfation of N-hydroxyarylamines and *p*-nitrophenol was respectively determined fluorometrically (*10*) and by HPLC-UV detection (*14*). Western blots were performed using 12.5% gels following the method of Towbin *et al.* (*15*) with some modification (*13*).

### *Acetylation of Arylamine and N-hydroxyarylamine in Hamster*

Cytosolic acetyltransferase is now known to catalyze five different-types of acetylating reactions, which are distinguished by the difference of acetyl donor and acetyl acceptor (substrate): 1) acetyl CoA-dependent N-acetylation of arylamines, 2) acetyl CoA-dependent O-acetylation of N-hydroxyarylamines, 3) N-hydroxyarylacetamide-dependent N-acetylation of arylamines, 4) N-hydroxyarylacetamide-dependent O-acetylation of N-hydroxyarylamines, and 5) N-hydroxyarylacetamide N,O-acetyltransfer (Fig. 1). In the hamster, cytosolic N-acetylation of 2-aminofluorene (2-AF) and *p*-aminobenzoic acid (PABA), which was measured in the presence of acetyl CoA, differed markedly among individual out-bred hamsters, and divided them into three groups as rapid, intermediate, and slow acetylators (Fig. 2). However, no clear segregation was observed on cytosolic N-acetylation of 2-AF and 4-aminoazobenzene, which was measured with N-hydroxyarylacetamide as the acetyl donor, and on acetyl CoA-dependent O-acetylation of N-hydroxy-Glu-P-1. These results suggest

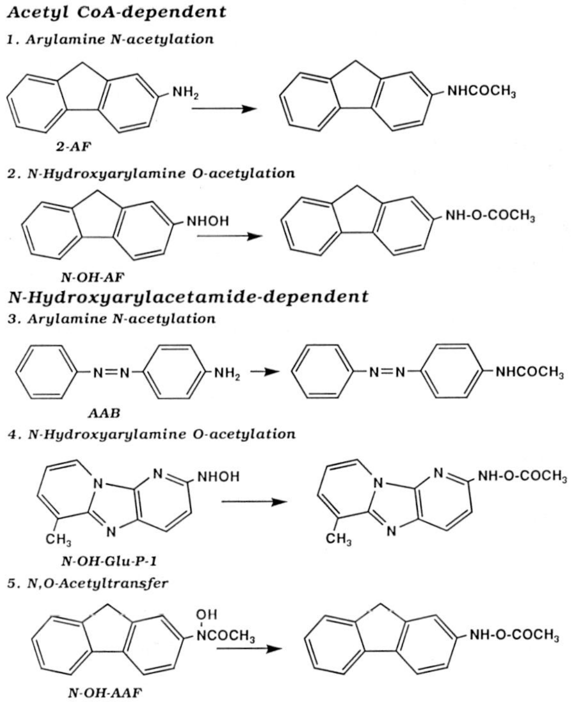


FIG. 1. Cytosolic acetyltransferase-catalyzed reactions. 2-AF, 2-aminofluorene; N-OH-AF, N-hydroxy-2-aminofluorene; AAB, 4-aminoazobenzene; N-OH-Glu-P-1, 2-hydroxyamino-6-methyldipyrido[1, 2-*a*: 3′, 2′-*d*]imidazole; N-OH-AAF, N-hydroxy-2-acetylaminofluorene.

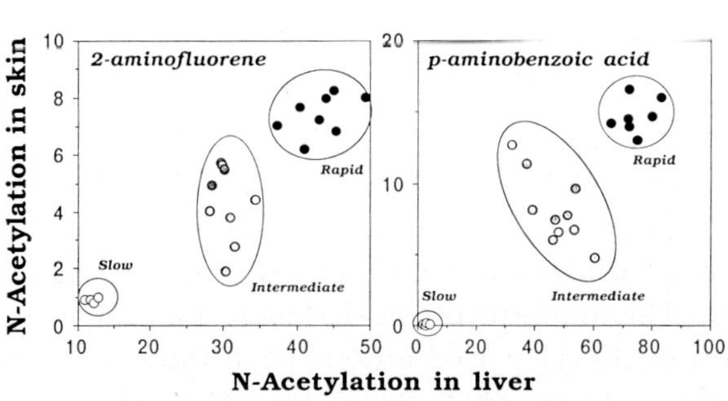


FIG. 2. Correlation of arylamine N-acetylation between liver and skin of out-bred Syrian hamster. Activity is shown as nmol/mg protein/min.

the existence of plural forms of acetyltransferases, which differ in their modes of expression in hamster livers. To understand the properties and mechanism of their expression, cytosolic acetyltransferases were purified from livers of out-bred hamsters. At the initial step, marker activities for respective tri-modal and mono-modal distribution, N-acetylation of *p*-aminobenzoic acid and 4-aminoazobenzene, were effectively separated: the former activity was precipitated by polyethylene glycol (PEG) treatment, while the latter remained in the supernatant. Using 4-aminoazobenzene-bound Sepharose affinity, gel filtration and Mono Q ion-exchange chromatography, two forms of acetyltransferase, AT-I and AT-II, were further purified from PEG super-

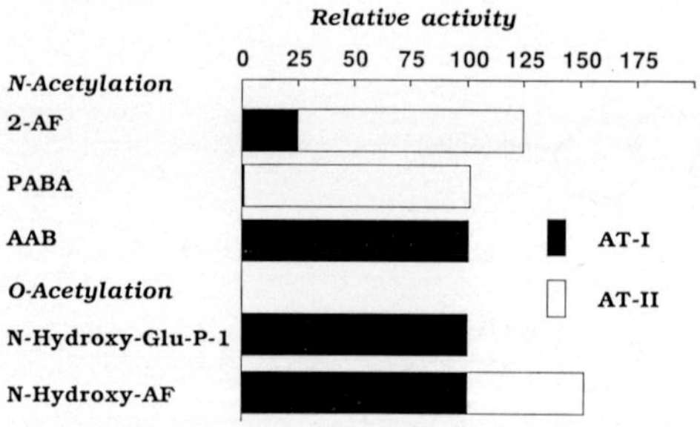


FIG. 3. Acetylation of arylamines and N-hydroxyarylamines by purified AT-I and AT-II. Activities of purified AT-I and AT-II are presented as relative values (expressed as 100 for the higher activity between two enzymes).

natant and precipitate, respectively. Homogeneous AT-I and AT-II showed 31 and 30 KDa, respectively, on sodium dodecyl sulfate-polyacrylamide gel electrophoresis, and catalyzed both N-acetylation of arylamides and O-acetylation of N-hydroxy-arylamines. The catalytic properties of AT-I and AT-II, however, differed in several points: 1) both AT-I and AT-II catalyzed N-acetylation of 2-AF, but AT-I had no activity for *p*-aminobenzoic acid N-acetylation; 2) AT-I used N-hydroxyarylacetamide as well as short chain acyl CoA, while AT-II did not utilize N-hydroxyarylacetamide; 3) therefore, N-acetylation of 4-aminoazobenzene was catalyzed only by AT-I; 4) AT-I and AT-II mediated the covalent binding to DNA of carcinogenic N-hydroxy-arylamines through O-acetylation, but AT-II showed strict substrate specificity, and thus catalyzed O-acetylation of N-hydroxy-AF, but not of N-hydroxy-Glu-P-1 (Fig. 3).

### *Genetic Polymorphism of Hamster Acetyltransferases*

To clarify the relationship between tri-modal segregation of arylamine N-acetylation and acetyltransferase expression, levels of AT-I and AT-II were quantified with Western blots using polyclonal antibodies raised against purified AT-I. Two protein bands were stained in hepatic cytosols, which corresponded to AT-I and AT-II (31 and 30 KDa), respectively. The amounts of AT-I stained had no clear individual difference, whereas the amount of AT-II varied among each individual. In addition, the cytosolic amounts of AT-II and rate of N-acetylation of 2-AF in hamster liver showed a clear correlation, indicating that trimodal segregation of 2-AF and *p*-aminobenzoic acid N-acetylation is determined by the difference in the level of AT-II expressed in hamster tissues. Therefore, rapid acetylators contained higher amounts of AT-II than intermediate phenotypes, and slow acetylator animals did not contain AT-II in their tissues. Cross-matings of intra- and inter-acetylation phenotypes were performed using a skin biopsy method (*12*, *16*). Cross-matings of intraphenotype animals with respective slow and rapid acetylators delivered only the same phenotype offspring, while all three phenotypes were detected in the progeny of intermediate × intermediate phenotypes (Fig. 4). The results obtained are consistent with the idea that the genetic trait is regulated by a Mendelian inheritance of two codominant alleles at a single gene locus.

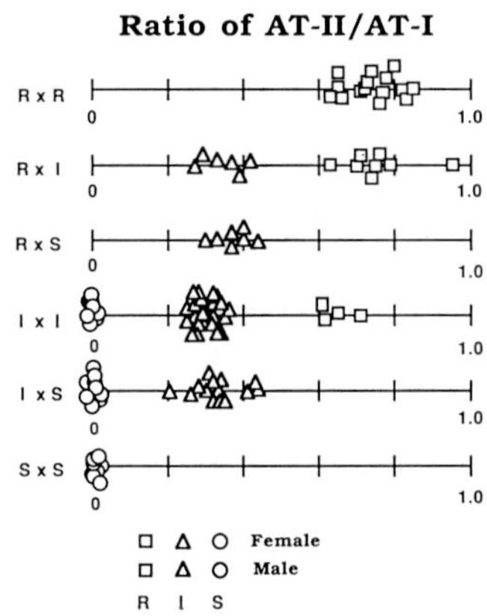


FIG. 4. Genetic inheritance of AT-II phenotype. R, rapid (high content of AT-II); I, intermediate (low content of AT-II); S, slow (contains no detectable amount of AT-II). Each symbol represents individual offspring from respective cross-matings.

TABLE 1. Activities of hamAT101-transfected COS-1 Cells and Purified Acetyltransferase AT-I and AT-II

| Substrate | Activity (nmol/mg protein/min) | | |
|---|---|---|---|
| | AT-I | AT-II | COS-1 (9,000 $\times g$ Sup.) |
| 2-AF | 4,700 | 19,400 | 9.1 |
| 4-AAB | 111,155 | ND | 13.5 |
| PABA | 300 | 46,000 | 3.1 |
| N-OH-Glu-P-1 | 3,460 | ND | 1.2 |

Sup., supernatant; 2-AF, 2-aminofluorene; 4-AAB, 4-aminoazobenzene; PABA, *p*-aminobenzoic acid; and N-OH-Glu-P-1, 2-hydroxyamino-6-methyldipyrido[1,2-*a*: 3′,2′-*d*]imidazole. N-acetylation of 2-AF and PABA, and O-acetylation of N-OH-Glu-P-1 were determined using acetyl CoA as the donor. N-acetylation of 4-AAB was quantified with N-hydroxy-AAF. Control COS-1 cell had no activities for acetylation of 2-AF, AAB, and N-OH-Glu-P-1, but showed PABA N-acetylating activity. Thus, N-acetylating activity of PABA in COS-1 cells is likely to be due to the basal activity of the cell.

### *cDNA Cloning and Expression of AT-I*

We have recently cloned a cDNA encoding an acetyltransferase from hamster λgt11 cDNA library using anti-AT-I antibodies. The cDNA (hamAT101) had 1.2 Kbp length and contained a coding region of 870 bp as well as 5′-untranslated region and 3′-polyA tail (*17*). To verify which protein is encoded by hamAT101 cDNA, the cDNA was inserted into a transfection vector and expressed in COS-1 cells. The 9,000 $\times g$ supernatant of the transfected cells showed N-acetylating activities of 2-AF and 4-aminoazobenzene, and also O-acetylating activity of N-hydroxy-Glu-P-1 in the presence of acetyl CoA, indicating that hamAT101 encodes AT-I isozyme (Table 1).

### *O-sulfation of N-hydroxyarylamine and N-hydroxyarylacetamide*

Since N-hydroxy-AAF was found to undergo activation in the presence of 3′-phosphoadenosine 5′-phosphosulfate (PAPS) generating system (*18*), sulfation is known as a major pathway of the activation of N-hydroxyarylamides. Recent studies from our and other laboratories (*4*, *10*, *14*, *19*) have shown that N-hydroxyarylamines also undergo O-sulfation to form the reactive species which binds to biological macromolecules. The activation was catalyzed by cytosolic PAPS-dependent sulfotransferase, and was often higher in the liver of male than female rats, although extents of the sex-related difference varied depending on the substrate used. Consistent with these results, multiple forms of sulfotransferase are now known to exist in rat livers (*20*, *21*). To identify the isozyme responsible for the male-dominant N-hydroxyarylamine(amide) sulfation, we tried to isolate sulfotransferases from the liver of male rats with N-hydroxy-AAF sulfation as the marker activity. Using ion-exchange, gel filtration, and ATP-bound affinity chromatography, three forms of arylsulfotransferase termed HAST I, HAST II, and PST I were purified. HAST I and HAST II showed high specific activities for O-sulfation of N-hydroxy-AAF. In addition, hepatic content of HAST I was $>4$ fold higher in the male adult rats than the female (*2*), while the content of PST I had no sex-related difference in Western blots. These results indicate that HAST I and HAST II are major isozymes responsible for the activation of N-hydroxyarylamines(amides).

### *Hormonal Regulation of N-hydroxyarylamine Sulfation*

To obtain an insight into the mechanism of the sex-related difference, the influence of endocrine hormone was investigated *in vivo*. As shown in Fig. 5, cytosolic content of HASTs was reduced by hypophysectomy to 40% of normal control male rats. Treatment of hypophysectomized rats with continuous infusion of hGH, which mimicked the secretion of growth hormone in female rats, slightly increased the content. A more effective increase was observed in both sexes of hypophysectomized rats given hGH intermittently, which mimicked the secretory profile of growth hormone in male rats. In addition, treatment of hypophysectomized rats with triiodothyronine was also effective to restore the level of HASTs in the male, and increased the content in female hypophysectomized rats to a level similar to normal male rats. Testosterone restored the hepatic level of HASTs in the liver of castrated rats, but sex-steroids had no clear effect on hypophysectomized rats (data not shown). These results indicate that sex-related differences in secretory profile of growth hormone caused the male-dominant expression of HASTs in rat livers. Sex-steroids also contribute to the

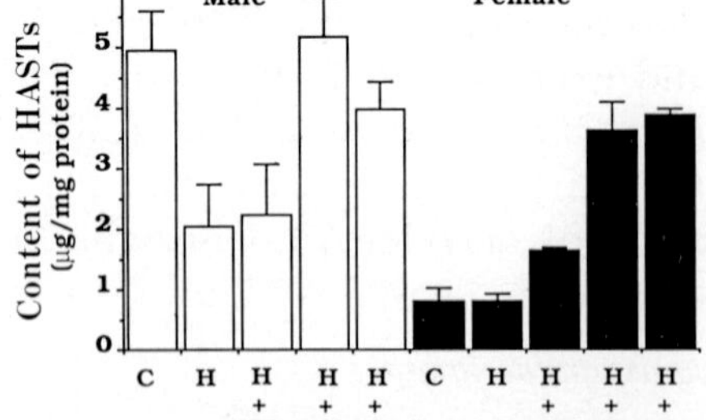


FIG. 5. Effects of growth hormone and triiodothyronine on hepatic content of HASTs in rats. C, untreated control; H, hypophysectomized; GH(i), continuous infusion of growth hormone; GH(s), intermittent injection of growth hormone; $T_3$, triiodothyronine-treated.

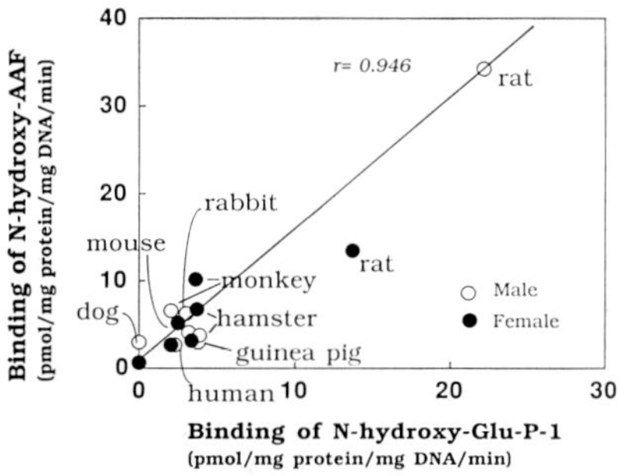


FIG. 6. Hepatic sulfotransferase-mediated activation of N-hydroxy-AAF and N-hydroxy-Glu-P-1.

difference, but are likely to function indirectly through the hypothalamus-pituitary axis by modulating growth hormone secretion. Interestingly, triiodothyronine was also effective in hypophysectomized rats to enhance HASTs content. Thus, thyroid hormone may have a direct action on the liver as well as the stimulation of growth hormone gene transcription at the pituitary.

*Species Difference in the PAPS-dependent Activation of N-hydroxyarylamine and N-hydroxyarylamide*

Sulfotransferase-mediated activation of N-hydroxy-AAF, N-hydroxy-Glu-P-1, and N-hydroxy-IQ was quantified with liver cytosol of eight different animal species including humans. Covalent bindings of N-hydroxy-AAF and N-hydroxy-Glu-P-1 to calf thymus DNA were stimulated by the addition of liver cytosol in all of the species examined, except that dogs showed no detectable activity for N-hydroxy-Glu-P-1 binding. Human livers showed a capacity comparable with other experimental animal species, except for rats, which showed the highest capacities for both chemicals. N-hydroxy-IQ was activated by rat cytosol, but the binding to DNA was not detected with cytosols of other species. Although no clear correlation exists between cytosolic *p*-nitrophenol sulfation and activation of N-hydroxy-AAF or of N-hydroxy-Glu-P-1, the extents of the binding of both N-hydroxy chemicals were correlated among these species (Fig. 6), suggesting that both chemicals are activated by the same or a closely related sulfotransferase in mammals.

REFERENCES


1. Cartwright, R. A., Glashan, R. W., Rogers, H. J., Ahmad, R. A., Barham-Hall, D., Higgins, E., and Kahn, M. A. Role of N-acetyltransferase phenotypes in bladder carcinogenesis: A pharmacogenetic epidemiological approach to bladder cancer. Lancet, *ii:* 842–845, 1982.
2. DeBaun, J. R., Miller, E. C., and Miller, J. A. N-hydroxy-2-acetylaminofluorene sulfotransferase: Its probable role in carcinogenesis and in protein-(methion-S-yl) binding in rat liver. Cancer Res., *30*: 577–595, 1970.
3. Yamazoe, Y., Shimada, M., Kamataki, T., and Kato, R. Covalent binding of N-hydroxy-Trp-P-2 to DNA by cytosolic proline-dependent system. Biochem. Biophys. Res. Commun., *107*: 165–172, 1982.

4. Lai, C. C., Miller, J. A., Miller, E. C., and Liem, A. N-sulfoöxy-2-aminofluorene is the major ultimate electrophilic and carcinogenic metabolite of N-hydroxy-2-acetylaminofluorene in the livers of infant male C57BL/6J × C3H/HeJ $F_1$ (B6C3$F_1$) mice. Carcinogenesis, *6*: 1037–1045, 1985.
5. Shinohara, A., Saito, K., Yamazoe, Y., Kamataki, T., and Kato, R. Acetyl coenzyme A-dependent activation of N-hydroxy derivative of carcinogenic arylamines: Mechanism of activation, species difference, tissue distribution and acetyl donor specificity. Cancer Res., *46*: 4362–4367, 1986.
6. Flammang, T. J. and Kadlubar, F. F. Acetyl coenzyme A-dependent metabolic activation and N-hydroxy-3,2′-dimethyl-4-aminobiphenyl and several carcinogenic *N*-hydroxyarylamines in relation to tissue and species differences, other acetyldonors, and arylhydroxamic acid-dependent acyltransferases. Carcinogenesis, *7*: 919–926, 1986.
7. Yamazoe, Y., Ishii, K., Yamaguchi, N., Kamataki, T., and Kato, R. Reduction of *N*-hydroxy-2-acetylaminofluorene by liver microsomes. Biochem. Pharmacol., *29*: 2183–2188, 1980.
8. Saito, K., Yamazoe, Y., Kamataki, T., and Kato, R. Syntheses of hydroxyamino, nitroso and nitro derivatives of Trp-P-2 and Glu-P-1, amino acid pyrolysate mutagens and their direct mutagenicities toward *Salmonella typhimurium* TA98 and TA98NR. Carcinogenesis, *4*: 1547–1550, 1983.
9. Yamazoe, Y., Shimada, M., Kamataki, T., and Kato, R. Effect of hypophysectomy and growth hormone treatment on sex-specific forms of cytochrome P-450 in relation to drug and steroid metabolism in rat liver microsomes. Jpn. J. Pharmacol., *42*: 371–382, 1986.
10. Yamazoe, Y., Manabe, S., Murayama, N., and Kato, R. Regulation of hepatic sulfotransferase catalyzing the activation of N-hydroxyarylamide and N-hydroxyarylamine by growth hormone. Mol. Pharmacol., *32*: 536–541, 1987.
11. Yamazoe, Y., Ling, X., Murayama, N., Gong, D., Nagata, K., and Kato, R. Modulation of hepatic level of microsomal testosterone 7$\alpha$-hydroxylase, P-450a (P450IIA), by thyroid hormone and growth hormone in rat liver. J. Biochem., *108*: 599–603, 1990.
12. Kawakubo, Y., Manabe, S., Yamazoe, Y., Nishikawa, T., and Kato, R. Properties of cutaneous acetyltransferase catalyzing N- and O-acetylation of carcinogenic arylamines and N-hydroxyarylamine. Biochem. Pharmacol., *37*: 265–270, 1988.
13. Ozawa, S., Abu-Zeid, M., Kawakubo, Y., Toyama, S., Yamazoe, Y., and Kato, R. Monomorphic and polymorphic isozymes of arylamine N-acetyltransferases in hamster liver: purification of the isozymes and genetic basis of N-acetylation polymorphism. Carcinogenesis, *11*: 2137–2144, 1990.
14. Yamazoe, Y., Abu-Zeid, M., Dawei, G., Staiano, N., and Kato, R. Enzymatic acetylation and sulfation of N-hydroxyarylamines in bacteria and rat livers. Carcinogenesis, *10*: 1675–1679, 1989.
15. Towbin, H., Staehelin, T., and Gordon, J. Electrophoretic transfer of proteins from polyacrylamide gels to nitrocellulose sheets; procedure and some applications. Proc. Natl. Acad. Sci. U.S.A., *76*: 4350–4354, 1979.
16. Kawakubo, Y., Yamazoe, Y., Kato, R., and Nishikawa, T. High capacity of human skin for N-acetylation of arylamines. Skin Pharmacol., *3*: 180–185, 1990.
17. Abu-Zeid, M., Nagata, K., Miyata, M., Ozawa, S., Fukuhara, M., Yamazoe, Y., and Kato, R. Arylamine N-acetyltransferase, AT-I, from Syrian golden hamster liver: Cloning, a complete nucleotide sequence and its expression in mammalian cells. Mol. Carcinogenesis, *4*: 81–88, 1991.

18. King, C. M. and Philips, B. Enzyme-catalyzed reactions of the carcinogen N-hydroxy-2-fluorenylacetamide with nucleic acid. Science, *159*: 1351–1353, 1968.
19. Snyderwine, E. G., Wirth, P. J., Roller, P. P., Adamson, R. H., Sato, S., and Thorgeirsson, S. S. Mutagenicity and *in vitro* covalent DNA binding of 2-hydroxyamino-3-methylimidazolo[4, 5-*f*]quinoline. Carcinogenesis, *9*: 411–418, 1988.
20. Jakoby, W. B., Sekura, R. D., Lyon, E. S., Marcus, C. J., and Wang, J. Sulfotransferases. *In;* W. B. Jakoby (ed.), Enzymatic Basis of Detoxication, Vol. 2, pp. 199–228, Academic Press, New York, 1980.
21. Singer, S. S. Preparation and characterization of different kinds of sulfotransferase. *In;* D. Zakim and D. A. Vessey (eds.), Biochemical Pharmacology and Toxicology. Methodological Aspects of Drug-Metabolizing Enzymes, Vol. 1, pp. 95–159, Wiley, Chichester, 1985.

XENOBIOTICS AND CANCER, L. ERNSTER ET AL. (EDS.),
JAPAN SCI. SOC. PRESS, TOKYO/TAYLOR & FRANCIS LTD., LONDON, pp. 119–126, 1991

# Polymorphic Acetylation of Arylamines and DNA-adduct Formation

Wendell W. WEBER, Gerald N. LEVY, and Karen J. MARTELL

*Department of Pharmacology, University of Michigan, Ann Arbor, Michigan 48109-0626, U.S.A.*

*Abstract:* Inbred mouse strains congenic for rapid and slow N-acetyltransferase (NAT) (A.B6, rapid and B6.A, slow) were used to separate the effect of the NAT polymorphism from the influence of other genetically polymorphic enzymes on DNA adduct formation induced by exposure to arylamine carcinogens. Adduct formation was measured by HPLC analysis of $^{32}$P-postlabeled nucleotides from DNA of the urinary bladder and liver. Acetylator phenotype was a significant determinant of DNA damage in females as slow acetylators had higher levels of bladder DNA adducts than rapids. This correlation was the reverse of that seen with liver DNA. Older mice (20–23 weeks) formed much higher bladder DNA adduct levels than young mice (7 week). The increase in bladder adduct formation with age was seen in both sexes of all mouse strains. The older male B6 mice showed a 26-fold increase in bladder adducts and the older females showed no more than a 2-fold increase. In addition, the older male B6 mice produced significant amounts of an unidentified, early eluting adduct peak. Biochemical studies of liver NAT and O-acetyltransferase (OAT) activities showed a direct correlation between the levels of liver 2-aminofluorene (AF) NAT activity and levels of liver DNA-adduct formation, but the role of OAT activity in adduct formation in the mouse remains unclear. These results indicate that the NAT phenotype, age and sex are all important determinants of arylamine-DNA adduct formation in mice.

Human hereditary differences in acetylation have been known for more than 30 years (*1*). The genetic difference in drug metabolizing N-acetyltransferases (NATs) in the liver and certain other organs allows classification of individuals as 'slow' and 'rapid' acetylators of amine and hydrazine drugs and arylamine carcinogens. We know from studies in humans and in genetic animal models of the human trait that the acetylator status has an important bearing on individual susceptibility to toxicity including cancer and other spontaneous disorders from these substances. The long range goals of our research on this genetic polymorphism in drug metabolism during the past 20 years have been to determine the molecular basis for the polymorphism, and to assess its pharmacological and toxicological significance.

In view of the proven value of inbred species as tools for the genetic analysis of hereditary traits, we felt the inbred mouse was potentially a valuable resource that would greatly facilitate our investigations. In 1976 we undertook the characterization of a mouse model for the human trait (*2–4*) and about 10 years ago the development of rapid and slow acetylator congenic mice (*5*). More recently, we have investigated the effect of the acetylator polymorphism on DNA damage induced by arylamine carcinogens, and are currently continuing this work. We are also engaged in the elucidation of the structural and quantitative differences in variant NATs involved in drug metabolism in the mouse model and humans through recombinant DNA and allied techniques.

### *The Development of Acetylator Congenic Mice*

Two inbred strains of acetylator congenic mice were produced from 'rapid' acetylator C57BL/6J (B6) and 'slow' A/J (A) inbred mouse strains by the backcross method using *p*-aminobenzoic acid (PABA) as the substrate to discriminate acetylator phenotypes (*5*). Mice were brother-sister mated at the 12th backcross generation ($N_{12}$) to establish the strains. By this technique, the slow *Nat* gene of the A mouse was incorporated into the genome of B6 mice replacing the B6 rapid *Nat* gene, producing the congenic strain designated B6.A-$Nat^{s}$ (B6.A). Conversely, in the congenic strain designated A.B6-$Nat^{r}$ (A.B6), the rapid *Nat* gene of B6 is incorporated into the genome of the A mice replacing the slow *Nat* gene.

Strain distribution analysis of 40 A$\times$B and B$\times$A recombinant inbred strains indicated linkage between the *Nat* gene and the *esterase 1* (*Es-1*) gene of chromosome 8. This information combined with additional information from a double backcross experiment indicated that the *Nat* and *Es-1* genes are $13 \pm 2.8$ cM apart (*5*). Analysis of our two acetylator congenic strains leads us to conclude that the length of the segment transferred to the B6.A strain extends less than about 13 cM in the direction of *Es-1* because the B6.A strain has the *Es-1* genotype of the B6 strain. The A.B6 strain has a differential segment at least 13 cM long, because A.B6 also has the *Es-1* genotype of the B6 strain.

The *Nat* and *Es-1* genes of the mouse are in a region of mouse chromosome 8 that has some homology with a region of human chromosome 8 (*6*). Our assignment of the *Nat* gene to mouse chromosome 8 appears to be consistent with observations of Blum and colleagues (*7*) who have recently assigned the human *NAT* gene(s) to the region designated 8pter-q11 of human chromosome 8.

### *Molecular Genetics of Drug Metabolizing Mouse N-acetyltransferases*

Work in progress shows that there are at least two genetic loci for drug metabolizing NATs in mice. We have evidence from genomic clones to show that these loci are on the same piece of DNA separated by no more than 20 kb. Structural analysis indicates that the coding region of one of the *NAT* genes is identical in the B6 and A strains, while the coding region of the other has a single nucleotide change that leads to a single amino acid difference in the deduced NAT sequence (*7a*). Expression studies to determine whether this amino acid change accounts for the murine acetylation polymorphism are in progress.

TABLE 1. AcCoA-dependent Acetyltransferase Activity in Inbred Mouse Liver Cytosol[a)]

| Mouse line | Acetylator genotype | $N$ | NAT activity PABA | AF | ABP | INH | OAT activity N-OH-DMABP |
|---|---|---|---|---|---|---|---|
| | | | (nmol/min/mg protein) | | | | (nmol bound/15 min/mg DNA/mg protein) |
| C57BL/6J | *Nat r/Nat r* | 5 | 7.35±0.21 | 2.80±0.30 | 1.01±0.03 | 0.34±0.06 | 0.96±0.15 |
| AC57F$_1$ | *Nat r/Nat s* | 5 | 4.18±0.49 | 1.79±0.12 | 0.75±0.09 | 0.28±0.02 | 1.30±0.10 |
| A/J | *Nat s/Nat s* | 5 | 3.88±0.37 | 1.45±0.15 | 0.65±0.06 | 0.31±0.04 | 1.58±0.44 |
| A.B6 | *Nat r/Nat r* | 9 | 14.5 ±2.69 | 4.09±0.58 | 2.25±0.46 | 0.24±0.04 | 0.50±0.16 |
| B6.A | *Nat s/Nat s* | 5 | 2.00±0.17 | 0.61±0.06 | 0.36±0.02 | 0.34±0.07 | 1.82±0.24 |

a) See ref. *8*.

*Arylamine N-acetyltransferase and O-acetyltransferase Activyty in Rapid and Slow Acetylator Parental and Congenic Inbred Mouse Strains*

Examination of AcCoA-dependent NAT and O-acetyltransferase (OAT) activities in mouse liver cytosols showed the presence of both polymorphic and monomorphic activity (*8*). The levels of NAT activity with PABA, 2-aminofluorene (AF), and 4-aminobiphenyl (ABP) of B6 mice were 1.5–2 times greater than those of A mice; intermediate levels were found in AC57F$_1$ mice (Table 1) (*8, 9*). Rapid acetylator congenic mice (A.B6) had PABA, AF, and ABP NAT activities that were approximately twice those in B6 mice. Also, slow acetylator congenic mice (B6.A) had PABA, AF, and ABP NAT activities that were about half those in A mice. Thus, there are modifier genes in the genetic background of the parental strains that influence the expression of NAT activity, a finding that is consistent with previous results obtained from studies of recombinant inbred mouse strains derived from B6 and A mice (*3*). Comparison of NAT activities with PABA, AF, and ABP as substrates show that A.B6 mice have approximately 7 times the activity of B6.A with these substrates.

The AcCoA-dependent binding of N-OH-dimethylaminobiphenyl (N-OH-DMABP), a substrate that has been used to show the presence of OAT activity in B6 and A mice (*4*), was also examined in liver cytosols of B6, A, AC57F$_1$, A.B6, and B6.A mice. Although the OAT activities obtained in the five mouse strains do not differ significantly between strains (*8*), the pattern across all strains is provocative because it suggests the OAT and NAT activities may be reciprocally related (Table 1). We have not investigated this phenomenon further.

Isoniazid (INH), a drug that is an important discriminator of rapid and slow acetylator human liver NATs, was also used as a substrate for NAT activity (*8*). Very low levels of AcCoA-dependent INH NAT activity were found in the liver cytosols and they did not differ between these five mouse strains. This observation is consistent with the results of *in vivo* studies of B6 and A mice dosed with INH (*10*).

Partial purification of the mouse liver cytosols by fast protein liquid chromatography (FPLC) yielded two peaks of NAT activity (*8*). One peak (eluting at 0.1 M KCl) exhibited specificity for PABA, AF, and ABP but not for INH while the other peak (eluting at 0.12 M KCl) exhibited specificity for INH but not for PABA, AF, and ABP. These findings indicate the presence of at least two NAT isozymes with different substrate specificities. The levels of activity of the INH NAT peak did not differ between the five mouse strains.

### Determination of Arylamine-induced DNA Damage

Since DNA-carcinogen adduct formation is considered a necessary step in arylamine-induced carcinogenesis (*11*), the measurement of DNA adducts affords a logical approach to determining susceptibility to carcinogens. Preliminary experiments with various rapid and sensitive methods of measuring adducts suggested that $^{32}$P-postlabeling was a method that we could use to greatest advantage in our studies. We adapted the methodology of Randerath (*12*) and Gupta (*13*) by substituting HPLC analysis of labeled products for four or five dimensional TLC commonly used (*14*). Separation requires about 60 min, and quantitation is achieved simultaneously, or nearly simultaneously by use of a flow through scintillation counter or collecting eluting fractions. Separation, detection, and measurement of AF- and AAF-DNA adducts is highly reproducible by our adaptation. We have found the method can also be used for detecting DNA adducted with polyaromatic hydrocarbons, alkenyl benzenes, and other arylamines.

Using this method (*14*) we have examined the role of differences in NAT activity on the formation of AF-adducts in liver and urinary bladder of mice of both sexes from four mouse strains with genetically defined differences in acetylation capacity. We have used the following procedure in most of these studies: unlabeled AF is injected into mice, hepatic (or urinary bladder) DNA is isolated and purified from individual mice, and nucleotides are produced by digestion with micrococcal nuclease and spleen phosphodiesterase II. The mixture obtained is extracted into butanol in the presence of tetrabutylammonium chloride, solvent is removed, and $^{32}$P-postlabeling of the 5′-OH of the nucleotides *via* polynucleotide kinase is carried out. An aliquot is injected into a reverse phase HPLC column which is eluted with potassium phosphate-acetonitrile and tetrabutylammonium phosphate. Fractions are collected for scintillation counting without addition of counting fluid.

### Aminofluorene—DNA Adduct Formation in Liver

At a high dose (60 mg/kg) of AF for a 3 hr exposure, we found that rapid (B6) mice accumulated twice the adducts of slow (A) mice (*15*). In acetylator congenic mice this difference increased so that rapid acetylators with the slow background (A.B6) had 5 to 7 times the DNA damage of the slow acetylator congenic with the rapid background (B6.A). Within each of the mouse lines examined, females had up to 3 times higher levels of DNA adducts compared to males (Table 2).

TABLE 2. 2-AF Hepatic DNA Adduct Formation in Rapid and Slow Acetylator Mice[a)]

| Mouse line | Acetylator genotype | Male | Female |
|---|---|---|---|
| | | (pmol adduct/mg DNA) | |
| B6 | RR | 0.14±0.01 (6) | 0.44±0.10 (7) |
| B6.A | rr | 0.10±0.03 (9) | 0.16±0.01 (5) |
| A | rr | 0.07±0.06 (6) | 0.21±0.04 (5) |
| A.B6 | RR | 0.72±0.10 (6) | 0.80±0.08 (5) |

[a)] See Ref. *15*.

TABLE 3. Comparison of Hepatic Cytosolic 2-AF Activity with Hepatic DNA-2-AF Adduct Formation[a)]

| Mouse line | Acetylator genotype | Relative to B6: 2-AF NAT activity | Adduct formation: Male | Adduct formation: Female |
|---|---|---|---|---|
| B6 | RR | 1.0 | 1.0 | 1.0 |
| B6.A | rr | 0.22 | 0.72 | 0.38 |
| A | rr | 0.52 | 0.52 | 0.47 |
| A.B6 | RR | 1.46 | 5.30 | 1.80 |

a) See Ref. *15*.

TABLE 4. 2-AF Urinary Bladder DNA Adducts in 7 and 20–23 Week Old Mice[a)]

| Mouse line | Acetylator genotype | 7 Weeks: Male (pmol adduct/mg DNA) | 7 Weeks: Female (pmol adduct/mg DNA) | 20–23 Weeks: Male (pmol adduct/mg DNA) | 20–23 Weeks: Female (pmol adduct/mg DNA) |
|---|---|---|---|---|---|
| B6 | RR | 0.51±0.11 (5) | 0.24±0.05 (6) | 13.4 ±5.61 (4) | 0.54±0.22 (3) |
| B6.A | rr | 0.41±0.27 (5) | 0.56±0.32 (4) | 2.06±0.70 (4) | 0.61±0.18 (4) |
| A | rr | 0.27±0.03 (4) | 0.92±0.17 (5) | 2.83±0.79 (4) | 1.12±0.31 (4) |
| A.B6 | RR | 0.39±0.09 (5) | 0.40±0.13 (4) | 2.63±0.66 (4) | 0.77±0.24 (4) |

a) See ref. *16*.

The NAT activity data from the isolated liver cytosols from the four strains of male mice in Table 1 compared to the adduct data in Table 2 shows that the activity data correlates very well with combined data for DNA adduct formation (Table 3). These results with liver demonstrate a correlation between high hepatic AF-NAT activity and increased hepatic AF-DNA adduct formation, and the rapid (RR) acetylator genotype.

*Aminofluorene—DNA Adduct Formation in Urinary Bladder*

The urinary bladder as well as the liver is a target organ of arylamines in mice. We found that male mice do not show a consistent relation between the acetylator phenotype and bladder DNA adduct formation (*16*). However, an effect of the acetylator phenotype on AF-bladder DNA adduct formation is seen in the female mice. Female slow acetylator mice exposed at 7 weeks of age and those exposed at 23 weeks of age formed greater levels of adducts than the corresponding rapid acetylators (Table 4). The difference is most pronounced on the A background (A *vs.* A.B6) but is also observed on the B6 background (B6.A *vs.* B6).

The wider difference in adduct levels between rapid and slow acetylators on the A background compared to the B6 background is similar to that observed for the liver adducts (Table 2). Comparing adduct formation in hepatic and bladder DNA in female mice shows a reciprocal relation with respect to the acetylator phenotype (*16*). In hepatic DNA, rapid acetylators have more DNA adducts than slow, whereas in bladder, show acetylators have more DNA adducts than rapids. This finding is consistent with rapid acetylators activating greater amounts of arylamines in the liver to form hepatic adducts while slow acetylators pass more unmetabolized carcinogen to

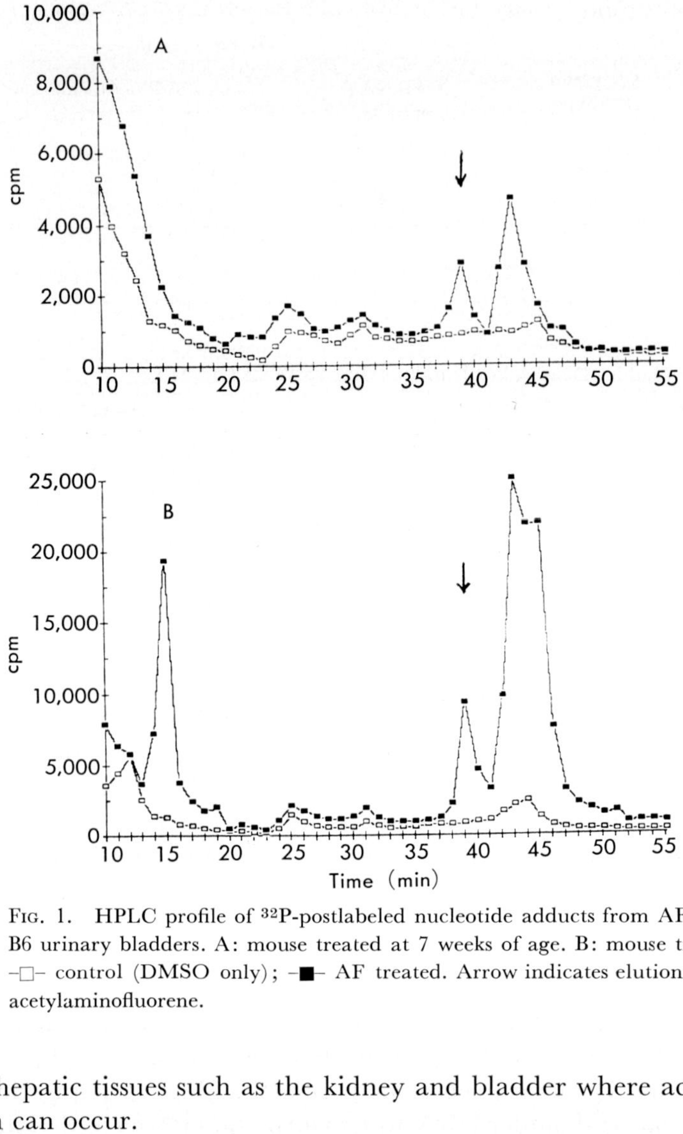


FIG. 1. HPLC profile of $^{32}P$-postlabeled nucleotide adducts from AF-treated and control male B6 urinary bladders. A: mouse treated at 7 weeks of age. B: mouse treated at 20 weeks of age. -□- control (DMSO only); -■- AF treated. Arrow indicates elution of a standard of dG-C8-acetylaminofluorene.

the extrahepatic tissues such as the kidney and bladder where activation and adduct formation can occur.

An age effect on bladder DNA adduct formation is apparent (*16*). Older mice (20–23 weeks) formed more bladder DNA adducts than young mice (7 week) (Table 4). The age-related increase in adducts was seen in both sexes of all mouse strains. Older male B6 mice showed a much larger increase than older females in bladder adduct levels (26-fold *vs.* 2-fold). Clearly, there is an important factor, as yet unidentified, in the B6 genetic background that increases bladder adduct formation in older B6 males. In addition, older male B6 mice produced an unidentified, early-eluting adduct peak (Fig. 1), possibly due to a peroxidative pathway of AF metabolism.

These results indicate that age, sex, and acetylator phenotype are all important determinants of aromatic amine-bladder DNA-adduct formation in mice.

*Concluding Remarks*

Acetylator phenotype, sex, and age each exert an influence on the levels of arylamine carcinogen-DNA adducts in tissues, and the level of adduct formation in a particular tissue may relate to the risk of tumorigenesis in that tissue. However, tumorigenesis studies are still required to interpret the importance of adduct levels because of differing repair capabilities, different rates of cell proliferation (*17*), cell death without replication or mutation in cells with high adduct levels, or whether the adduct present in high concentration is the adduct responsible for carcinogenesis. For these reasons we have begun tumorigenesis studies in both sexes of inbred mouse strains, including the acetylator congenic mouse strains.

## REFERENCES

1. Weber, W. The Acetylator Genes and Drug Response, Oxford, 1987.
2. Tannen, R. and Weber, W. Inheritance of acetylator phenotype in mice. J. Pharmacol. Exp. Ther., *213*: 480–484, 1980.
3. Glowinski, I. and Weber, W. Genetic regulation of aromatic amine N-acetylation in inbred mice. J. Biol. Chem., *257*: 1424–1430, 1982.
4. Mattano, S., Land, S., King, C. M., and Weber, W. Purification and biochemical characterization of hepatic arylamine N-acetyltransferase from rapid and slow acetylator mice: Identity with arylhydroxamic acid N,O-acyltransferase and N-hydroxyarylamine O-acetyltransferase. Mol. Pharmacol., *35*: 599–609, 1989.
5. Mattano, S., Erickson, R., Nesbitt, M., and Weber, W. Linkage of *Nat* and *Es-1* in the mouse and development of strains congenic for N-acetyltransferase. J. Hered., *79*: 430–433, 1988.
6. Lyon, M. and Kirby, M. Mouse chromosome atlas, in Mouse Genome, No. 87, 28–50, July, 1990.
7. Blum, M., Grant, D. M., McBride, W., Heim, M., and Meyer, U. Human arylamine N-acetyltransferase genes: Isolation, chromosomal localization, and functional expression. DNA and Cell Biol., *9*: 193–203, 1990.

7a. Martell, K., Vatsis, K., and Weber, W. The molecular genetic basis of rapid and slow acetylation in mice. Mol. Pharmacol., in press.

8. Hein, D., Trinidad, A., Yerokun, T., Ferguson, R., Kirlin, W., and Weber, W. Genetic control of acetylcoenzyme A-dependent arylamine N-acetyltransferase, hydrazine N-acetyltransferase, and N-hydroxy-arylamine O-acetyltransferase enzymes in C57BL/6J, A/J, AC57F1, and the rapid and slow acetylator A.B6 and B6.A congenic inbred mouse. Drug Metab. Disp., *16*: 341–347, 1988.
9. Mattano, S. and Weber, W. Kinetics of arylamine N-acetyltransferase in tissues from rapid and slow acetylator mice. Carcinogenesis, *8*: 133–137, 1987.
10. Tannen, R. and Weber, W. Antinuclear antibodies related to acetylator phenotype in mice. J. Pharmacol. Exp. Ther., *213*: 485–490, 1980.
11. Neumann, H. The role of DNA damage in chemical carcinogenesis of aromatic amines. J. Cancer Clin. Oncol., *112*: 100–106, 1986.
12. Randerath, K., Reddy, M., and Gupta, R. $^{32}$P-labeling test for DNA damage. Proc. Natl. Acad. Sci. U.S.A., *78*: 6126–6129, 1981.
13. Gupta, R., Reddy, M., and Randerath, K. $^{32}$P-postlabeling analysis of non-radioactive aromatic carcinogen-DNA adducts. Carcinogenesis, *3*: 1081–1092, 1982.

14. Levy, G. and Weber, W. High performance liquid chromatographic analysis of $^{32}$P-postlabeled DNA-aromatic carcinogen adducts. Anal. Biochem., *174*: 381–392, 1988.
15. Levy, G. and Weber, W. 2-Aminofluorene-DNA adduct formation in acetylator congenic mouse lines. Carcinogenesis, *10*: 705–710, 1989.
16. Levy, G. and Weber, W. 2-Aminofluorene-DNA adducts in mouse urinary bladder: Effect of age, sex, and acetylator phenotype. Carcinogenesis, unpublished.
17. Cohen, S. and Ellwein, L. Cell proliferation in carcinogenesis. Science, *249*: 1007–1011, 1990.

# XENOBIOTICS AND GENE REGULATION

XENOBIOTICS AND CANCER, L. ERNSTER ET AL. (EDS.),
JAPAN SCI. SOC. PRESS, TOKYO/TAYLOR & FRANCIS LTD., LONDON, pp. 129–136, 1991

# Altered Expression of Cytochrome P-450 Isozymes by Aromatic Amine Carcinogens in Experimental Animals: Correlation with Hepatocarcinogenesis

Yoshiyuki Hashimoto, Shinichi Miura, and Masakuni Degawa

*Department of Hygienic Chemistry, Faculty of Pharmaceutical Sciences, Tohoku University, Sendai 980, Japan*

*Abstract:* Carcinogenic aromatic amines such as amino acid and protein pyrolysate compounds and aminoazo dyes induced predominantly P450IA2, which is responsible for mutagenic activation of the aromatic amines, in rats and mice. The induction rate and total activity of this cytochrome P-450 isozyme were well correlated with sex, species, and target organ differences in hepatocarcinogenic susceptibility of animals to the aromatic amines. Preneoplastic liver cells induced by treatment with N, N-diethylnitrosamine and 2-acetylaminofluorene diminished the capacity for P450IA2 induction but retained that for P450IA1 induction. These findings confirm that P450IA2 has an important role in hepatocarcinogenesis by aromatic amines.

A large fraction of chemical carcinogens express the carcinogenic activity after undergoing metabolic activation *via* catalysis of cytochrome P-450 (P-450). P-450 consists of many isozymes that catalyze oxidation of various chemicals with broad but distinct substrate specificity (*1*). Therefore, the amount or activity of selected P-450 isozymes may be one of the key factors in chemical carcinogenesis. With regard to environmental carcinogens, protein or amino acid pyrolysates having heterocyclic amine or aromatic amine structure are activated to proximate carcinogenic or mutagenic metabolites by undergoing N-hydroxylation *via* catalysis of a cetain type of P-450 isozyme(s) (*2–6*).

In order to determine the correlation between carcinogenic susceptibility of animals or organs to aromatic amine carcinogens and the activity of P-450 in the course of carcinogenesis, we examined the effect of carcinogenic aromatic amines on the expression of P-450 isozymes in experimental animals. We focused on the change of these isozymes in the liver which is a major target organ of aromatic amines.

This review shows that carcinogenic aromatic amines can induce a P-450 isozyme responsible for mutagenic activation of the carcinogens, and that the induction rate is correlated with the susceptibility of animals to the carcinogens. We also report our recent findings on the characteristic change of P-450 isozymes in preneoplastic lesions induced in the rat liver.

### *Assays for P-450 Isozymes*

The activity and amount of P-450 isozymes were analyzed by a bacterial mutation test and immunochemical methods using monoclonal antibodies (mAbs) against the isozymes. The expression of P-450 mRNA was also analyzed by Northern blotting. For immunochemical assays of P-450, we prepared mAbs using several semi-purified P-450 isozymes as antigens; mAbs (APL-1, APL-2, APH-3, APH-8, and APF-1) showing characteristic antigen specificities were used for experiments (*7*, *8*). APL-1 and APH-3 are selective to P450IA1 and P450IA2, respectively. APL-2 and APH-8 are reactive with both isozymes, but react slightly with phenobarbital (PB)-inducible P-450 isozymes. In the mutation assay, we used *Salmonella typhimurium* TA98 together with aromatic amine substrates having different sensitivities to P-450 isozymes. 3-Amino-1-methyl-5*H*-pyrido[4, 3-*b*]indole acetate (Trp P-2) is sensitive to both P450IA1 and P450IA2, 2-amino-6-methyl-dipyrido[1,2-*a*; 3′,2′-*d*]imidazole hydrochloride (Glu P-1) to P450IA2 and 3-methoxy-4-aminoazobenzene (3-MeO-AAB) to PB-inducible P-450 isozymes (*4*, *9*).

### *Species, Sex, and Organ Differences in Induction of a Cytochrome P-450 Isozyme, P450IA2, Responsible for Carcinogen Activation*

Tryptophan pyrolysate compounds such as 3-amino-1,4-dimethyl-5*H*-pyrido-[4,3-*b*]indole acetate (Trp P-1) and Trp P-2 are found to be potent hepatocarcinogens in mice, and are more carcinogenic in females than in males (*10–12*). Trp P-2 is more active in mice than in rats (*10*, *12*). Based on these findings, we treated animals with a carcinogenic concentration of Trp P-1 or Trp P-2 in diet and examined the induction of P-450 isozymes responsible for mutagenic activation of these carcinogens (*13–15*). Representative results are depicted in Fig. 1.

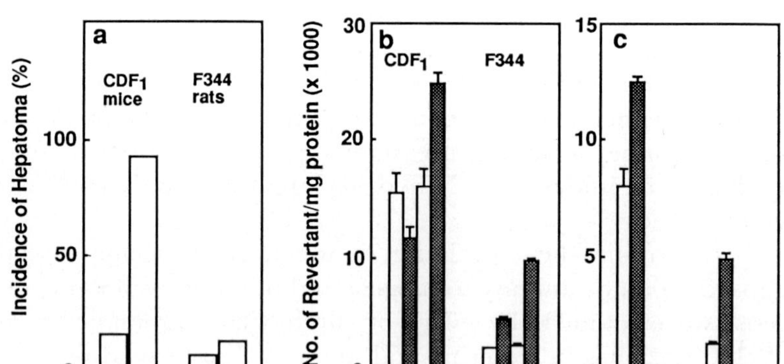


FIG. 1. Carcinogenic susceptibility of animals to Trp P-2, and species, sex, and target organ differences in activity and induction of P-450 isozyme responsible for mutagenic activation of Trp P-2. a: carcinogenic susceptibility of mice and rats to Trp P-2 (cited from refs. *10* and *11*). b: liver S-9 activity for mutagenesis of Trp P-2 before (open bar) and after (solid bar) treatment with Trp P-2 diet for 1 week. c: microsome activity of various organs for mutagenic activation of Trp P-2 before (open bar) and after (solid bar) treatment with Trp P-2 diet for 1 week. M, male; F, female; L, liver; O, extra-hepatic organs (lung, kidney, intestines).

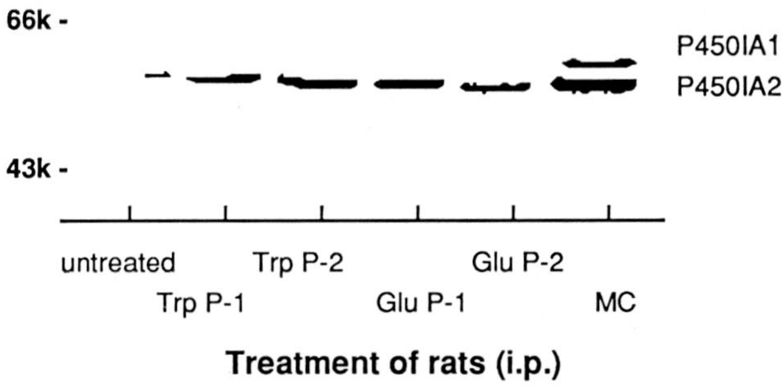


FIG. 2. Western blotting of liver microsomes of rats treated with an i.p. injection of the indicated compound.

*Sex difference in mice:* When BALB/c × DBA/2 $F_1$ ($CDF_1$) mice were treated with Trp P-1 diet (0.02%) for 1 week, the S-9 or microsomal activity in males for Trp P-1 mutagenesis was unchanged or slightly reduced, whereas that in females was markedly increased (*13*). Continuation of the feeding beyond 1 week resulted in increase of the S-9 or microsomal activity in both sexes, but the activity in female mice was consistently higher than in males. This increase by Trp P-1 feeding is due to the increase of a P-450 isozyme, probably P450IA2, responsible for the mutagenic activation or N-hydroxylation of Trp P-1, as determined by the response to P-450 inhibitors and immunological analyses (*13–16*). Castration of male mice afforded them female-like response to Trp P-1 and administration of testosterone to female mice inhibited the induction of P-450 by Trp P-1 feeding, indicating that suppressed response to the Trp P-1-mediated P-450 induction in males is dependent on their androgen level (*16*).

*Species difference:* Constitutive expression of microsomal enzyme activity for Trp P-2 mutagenesis in F344 rats was about 7 times lower than that in the sex-matched $CDF_1$ mice (*14*). When treated with Trp P-2 diet (0.02%) for 1 week, the enzyme activity was induced in both sexes of rats, however, the response was higher in female rats than in males. The enzyme activity in the induced stage was much lower in rats than in mice. The enzyme induced by Trp P-2 feeding was also identified to be mainly P450IA2 as determined by immunoblotting (Fig. 2), and substrate selectivity and response to P-450 inhibitors in mutagenicity assay (*14, 15*).

*Organ difference:* As described above, dietary Trp P-1 and Trp P-2 induced a P-450 isozyme responsible for mutagenic activation of aromatic amines in liver, whereas extra-hepatic organs such as lung, kidney, small and large intestines did not express such enzyme activity with or without Trp P-1 or Trp P-2 feeding (*14*). This is in accordance with our results that P450IA2 is solely induced in liver by treatment of animals with a selective inducer for P450IA2, 2-methoxy-4-aminoazobenzene (*17*).

*Expression and Induction of Cytochrome P-450 Isozymes in Preneoplastic Lesions in Rat Liver*

In general, chemical hepatocarcinogenesis proceeds through several steps: transformation of hepatocytes by an activated carcinogen to preneoplastic cells and progression of these cells to malignant cells by stimulation with a promoter. Certain chemical carcinogens such as 2-acetylaminofluorene (AAF) act as an initiator as well as a promoter after undergoing metabolic changes. Therefore, the metabolism of a carcinogen in liver will control its efficacy as an initiator or promoter. In the first part of this review, we demonstrated the principal role of P450IA2 in the early step of aromatic amine carcinogenesis. Here, we summarize the appearance of P-450 isozymes in preneoplastic hepatocytes induced by AAF-feeding and discuss their role in the promotion of hepatocarcinogenesis.

Although total content of P-450 is found to be lower in the preneoplastic cells (*18–20*), certain P-450 isozymes responsible for chemical carcinogens may be increased, as indicated by the early change of these isozymes in aromatic amine carcinogenesis (*13–20*). In this context, we examined the expression and induction of P-450 isozymes in preneoplastic hepatic lesions of rats treated by the method of Solt and Farber (*21*) (Fig. 3).

*1. Alteration of P-450 isozyme activity in carcinogen-treated rats*

Preneoplastic liver lesions, represented by multiple hyperplastic nodule formation, were induced in rats treated with N, N-diethylnitrosamine (DEN) plus AAF, but not in rats treated with DEN alone. The treatment with either DEN alone or DEN plus AAF reduced the total content of hepatic microsomal P-450 to 53% (DEN) or 32% (DEN plus AAF) of the untreated control. Treatment with DEN alone reduced the activity of liver microsomes (per protein) for mutagenesis of both Trp P-2 and Glu P-1. Although the treatment with DEN plus AAF decreased the microsomal activity for the Glu P-1 mutagenesis, it did not affect the activity for Trp P-2. If the microsomal activity is calculated as a fraction of P-450 amount, the microsomes from rats bearing hyperplastic nodules revealed more than 2 times greater activity than the controls in the mutagenesis of both Trp P-2 and Glu P-1, whereas the activity of the DEN-treated rat microsomes was the same as controls. These results indicate that expression of hepatic microsomal P-450 isozymes responsible for metabolic activation of the carcinogens is altered along with the development of preneoplastic lesions (hyperplastic nodules) in the liver.

In control rats, neither 3-MeO-AAB nor 3-methylcholanthrene (MC) significantly changed the total content of P-450 in liver microsomes. Although the content of microsomal P-450 was reduced by the pretreatment of rats with DEN or DEN plus AAF, the carcinogen-treated rats responded to the P-450 inducers and the overall content of microsomal P-450 was increased. In the mutagenicity assay, both MC and 3-MeO-AAB increased the microsomal activity in DEN-treated rats for Trp P-2 and Glu P-1 to the level of the control rats. Animals bearing hyperplastic nodules (DEN-AAF-treated rats) also responded to the P-450 inducers, but the induction rates of the microsomal activity were lower than those observed with other groups of rats.

The components reactive with APH-3 and APL-1 (corresponding to P450IA2 and P450IA1, respectively) were not detected in the liver microsomes from rats bearing hyperplastic nodules or those treated with DEN alone. The 3-MeO-AAB- or MC-treatment resulted in a definite increase of both P450IA2 and P450IA1, however, increase of the former was smaller in the hyperplastic nodule-bearing rats than in other groups. Immunoblotting analysis revealed that the amounts of P450IA2 in the microsomes were very small or undetectable in all groups, but that 3-MeO-AAB- or MC-treatment increased both P450IA1 and P450IA2. However, increase

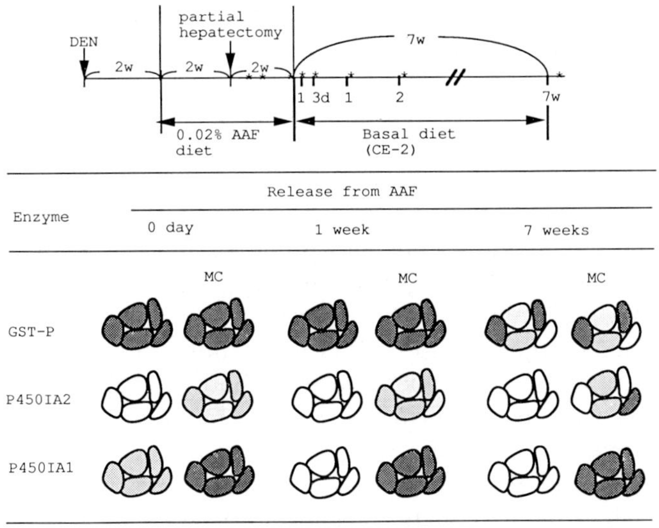


FIG. 3. Scheme of immunostaining profile of GST-P and P-450 isozymes expressed in hyperplastic nodules developed in F344 rat liver at the termination of AAF feeding (0 time) and after release from AAF feeding. Frozen sections were stained with anti-GST-P antibody, APL-1 MAb selective to P450IA1 or APH-3 MAb selective to P450IA2. The chart represents the apparent immunostaining profile of individual hyperplastic nodules. Dark to white indicates the grade of the staining.

of the P-450 isozymes, especially that of P450IA2, in rats with hyperplastic nodules was less than that in the untreated or DEN-treated rats.

*2. Immunohistochemical observation on the expression and induction of P-450 isozymes in hyperplastic nodules* (22)

The results are summarized in Fig. 3. At the termination of AAF-diet (2 weeks after partial hepatectomy), all hyperplastic nodules developed in the liver expressed a placental form of glutathione S-transferase (GST-P), a marker of preneoplastic lesion in rat liver. P450IA1 was detected in the hyperplastic nodules, however, the mode of P450IA1 expression was quite heterogeneous among individual cells in the islets; P450IA1-positive cells accumulated in the peripheral region of each islet. In contrast to P450IA1, P450IA2 was hardly detected in the liver sections. When MC was administered to the rats bearing hyperplastic nodules, P450IA1 was induced extensively in all GST-P-positive regions, whereas induction of P450IA2 was restricted to a portion of the GST-P-positive islets of hyperplastic nodules. In about 40% of islets, P450IA2 was expressed in all areas of each one, but in the remaining islets only a small number of cells expressed this isozyme.

After termination of the AAF diet, the rats bearing hyperplastic nodules were maintained on a normal diet and examined for the expression of P-450 isozymes and GST-P. Constitutive expression of P450IA1 in hyperplastic nodules became negative after 3 days, indicating that the expression of P450IA1 at the termination of the diet was due to the contribution of AAF. Observations at the 7th week after termination of the diet revealed that GST-P was lost in several foci of hyperplastic nodules. Constitutive expressions of both P450IA1 and P450IA2 were negative in all foci at this time. When the rats were treated with MC, P450IA1 was induced in all hyperplastic nodules as potently as in normal rat liver, whereas P450IA2 was induced only in whole or restricted area of hyperplastic nodules which were negative in the expression of GST-P.

These findings indicated that preneoplastic cells retained their response to P-450 inducers in terms of the induction of P-450IA1 but lost the response for the induction of P450IA2, and that preneoplastic cells in a portion of hyperplastic nodules normalize after cessation of carcinogen treatment in terms of the expression of GST-P and response to a P-450 inducer. It is notable that most preneoplastic cells could respond to MC for the induction of P450IA1 but only a small portion of the cells responded to the induction of P450IA2. This finding may suggest the presence of different MC-carrier proteins responsible for the induction of either P450IA1 or P450IA2.

With regard to the function of P-450 isozymes, both P450IA1 and P450IA2 catalyze the oxidations of various chemical carcinogens including polycyclic hydrocarbons and aromatic amines and convert these carcinogens to carcinogenic inactive and active metabolites. For aromatic amine carcinogens like AAF, major carcinogenic active metabolites are N-hydroxy derivatives which are yielded predominantly by a catalysis of P450IA2, while inactive metabolites are ring hydroxy derivatives yielded by a catalysis of P450IA1 (*23*). In general, carcinogenic active metabolites of chemicals are more cytotoxic than the original forms. Therefore, the retention of P450IA1 and reduction or loss of P450IA2 in preneoplastic cells might aid their escape from the contact with cytotoxic metabolities derived from an aromatic amine carcinogen and for their further growth and progression to cancer cells. As to strain differences in susceptibility to AAF in rats, Asamoto *et al.* (*24*) demonstrated the direct correlation between the susceptibility and capacity for the induction of P-450 isozymes in hyperplastic nodules and surrounding hepatocytes.

### *Conclusion*

Our work reveals the essential role of P450IA2 in hepatocarcinogenesis of rodent animals by aromatic amines. P450IA2, which is responsible for the activation (N-hydroxylation) of carcinogenic aromatic amines, is selectively induced in liver by treatment of animals with aromatic amines such as amino acid or protein pyrolysis products, aminoazo dyes and AAF. The total P450IA2 activity in induced state is well correlated with species, sex, and target organ differences in hepatocarcinogenesis. In preneoplastic cells, AAF treatment diminished the induction capacity for P450IA2 but not for P450IA1 which mainly catalyzes the detoxication metabolism (benzene ring hydroxylation) of aromatic amines.

### *Acknowledgments*

This work was supported in part by a Grant-in-Aid for Cancer Research from the Ministry of Education, Science and Culture of Japan. We thank Drs. T. Sugimura and M. Nagao, National Cancer Center, Tokyo, for their donation of amino acid pyrolysate compounds. We also thank Dr. N. Ito, Nagoya City Medical School, for his advice on carcinogenic experiments.

## REFERENCES


1. Nebert, D. W. and Gonzalez, F. J. P450 genes: structure, evolution and function. Annu. Rev. Biochem., *56*: 945–993, 1987.
2. Yamazoe, Y., Kamataki, T., and Kato, R. Species difference in N-hydroxylation of a tryptophan pyrolysis product in relation to mutagenic activation. Cancer Res., *41*: 4518–4522, 1981.
3. Degawa, M., Kanazawa, C., and Hashimoto, Y. *In vitro* metabolism of *o*-aminoazotoluene and mutagenesis of *Salmonella* by the metabolites. Carcinogenesis, *3*: 1113–1117, 1982.
4. Kamataki, T., Maeda, K., Yamazoe, Y., Matsuda, N., Ishii, K., and Kato, R. A high spin form of cytochrome P-450 highly purified from PCB-treated rats: catalytic characterization and immunochemical quantitation in liver microsomes. Mol. Pharmacol., *24*: 146–155, 1983.
5. Degawa, M., Miura, S., and Hashimoto, Y. Androgen-dependent renal microsomal cytochrome P-450 responsible for N-hydroxylation and mutagenic activation of 3-methoxy-4-aminoazobenzene in the BALB/c mouse. Cancer Res., *50*: 2729–2733, 1990.
6. Kimura, T., Kodama, M., Nagata, C., Kamataki, T., and Kato, R. Comparative study on the metabolism of N-methyl-4-aminoazobenzene by two forms of cytochrome P-448. Biochem. Pharmacol., *35*: 3375–3377, 1985.
7. Hashimoto, Y., Masuko, T., Itoh, K., Yagita, H., Hishinuma, T., Degawa, M., Kamataki, T., and Kato, R. Monoclonal antibodies against a high spin form of rat cytochrome P-448. Biochem. Biophys. Res. Commun., *131*: 600–606, 1985.
8. Degawa, M., Ohta, A., Namiki, M., Masuko, T., and Hashimoto, Y. *In vitro* selection of a low spin form of cytochrome P-448 from 3-methylcholanthrene-induced rat cytochrome P-450 isozymes by carbon tetrachloride. Biochem. Pharmacol., *36*: 3315–3317, 1987.
9. Degawa, M., Ueno, H., Miura, S., Ohta, A., and Namiki, M. A simple method for assessment of rat cytochrome P-448 isozymes responsible for the mutagenic activation of carcinogenic chemicals. Mutat. Res., *203*: 333–338, 1988.
10. Matsukura, N., Kawachi, T., Morino, K., Ohgaki, H., Sugimura, T., and Takayama, S. Carcinogenicity in mice of mutagenic compounds from a tryptophan pyrolysate. Science, *213*: 346–347, 1981.
11. Sugimura, T. Carcinogenicity of a mutagenic heterocyclic amines formed during the cooking process. Mutat. Res., *150*: 33–41, 1985.
12. Hosokawa, S., Matsushima, T., Hirono, I., and Sugimura, T. Carcinogenic activity of 3-amino-1-methyl-5*H*-pyrydo[4, 3-*b*]indole (Trp P-2), a pyrolysis product of tryptophan. Cancer Lett., *13*: 23–28, 1981.
13. Degawa, M., Kojima, M., Hishinuma, T., and Hashimoto, Y. Sex-dependent induction of hepatic enzymes for mutagenic activation of a tryptophan pyrolysate component, 3-amino-1, 4-dimethyl-5*H*-pyrido[4, 3-*b*]indole, by feeding in mice. Cancer Res., *45*: 96–102, 1985.
14. Degawa, M., Hishinuma, T., Yoshida, Y., and Hashimoto, Y. Species, sex and organ differences in induction of a cytochrome P-450 isozyme responsible for carcinogen activation: effect of dietary hepatocarcinogenic tryptophan pyrolysate components in mice and rats. Carcinogenesis, *8*: 1913–1918, 1987.
15. Degawa, M., Tanimura, S., Agatsuma, T., and Hashimoto, Y. Hepatocarcinogenic heterocyclic aromatic amines that induce cytochrome P-448 isozymes, mainly cytochrome P-448H (P450IA2), responsible for mutagenic activation of the carcinogens in

rat liver. Carcinogenesis, *10*: 1119–1122, 1989.

16. Degawa, M., Yamaya, C., and Hashimoto, Y. Hepatic cytochrome P-450 isozyme(s) induced by dietary carcinogenic aromatic amines preferentially in female mice of DBA/2 and other strains. Carcinogenesis, *9*: 567–571, 1988.
17. Degawa, M., Yamada, H., Hishinuma, T., Masuko, T., and Hashimoto, Y. Organ selective induction of cytochrome P-448 isozymes in rats by 2-methoxy-4-aminoazobenzene and 3-methylcholanthrene. J. Biochem., *101*: 1437–1445, 1987.
18. Okita, K., Fukumoto, Y., and Takemoto, T. Cytochrome P-450 in hyperplastic liver nodules during hepatocarcinogenesis with N-2-fluorenylacetamide in rats. Gann, *67*: 899–902, 1976.
19. Åström, A., DePierre, J. W., and Eriksson, L. Characterization of drug-metabolizing systems in hyperplastic nodules from the livers of rats receiving 2-acetylaminofluorene in their diet. Carcinogenesis, *4*: 577–581, 1983.
20. Sato, M., Yoshida, T., Suzuki, S., Degawa, M., and Hashimoto, Y. Selective induction of microsomal 2-acetylaminofluorene N-hydroxylation by dietary 2-acetylaminofluorene in rats. Carcinogenesis, *2*: 571–574, 1981.
21. Solt, D. and Farber, E. A new principle for the analysis of chemical carcinogenesis. Nature, *263*: 701–703, 1976.
22. Degawa, M., Miura, S., and Hashimoto, Y. Expression and induction of cytochrome P-450 isozymes in hyperplastic nodules of rat liver. Carcinogenesis, in press.
23. Goldstein, J. A., Weaver, R., and Sundheimer, D. W. Metabolism of 2-acetylaminofluorene by two 3-methylcholanthrene-inducible forms of rat liver cytochrome P-450. Cancer Res., *44*: 3768–3771, 1984.
24. Asamoto, M., Tsuda, H., Kato, T., Ito, N., Masuko, T., Hashimoto, Y., and Nagase, S. Strain differences in susceptibility to 2-acetylaminofluorene and phenobarbital promotion of hepatocarcinogenesis: immunohistochemical analysis of cytochrome P-450 isozyme induction by 2-acetylaminofluorene and phenobarbital. Jpn. J. Cancer Res., *80*: 1041–1046, 1989.

XENOBIOTICS AND CANCER, L. ERNSTER ET AL. (EDS.),
JAPAN SCI. SOC. PRESS, TOKYO/TAYLOR & FRANCIS LTD., LONDON, pp. 137–155, 1991

# Structure-function Aspects of the Glucocorticoid Receptor

Jan-Åke GUSTAFSSON, Karin DAHLMAN-WRIGHT, Per-Erik STRÖMSTEDT, Tony WRIGHT, and Jan CARLSTEDT-DUKE

*Department of Medical Nutrition and Centre for Biotechnology, Karolinska Institute, Novum, Huddinge University Hospital, S-141 86 Huddinge, Sweden*

*Abstract:* The glucocorticoid receptor belongs to a family of ligand activated nuclear receptors. In addition to steroid hormone receptors, this family also includes receptors for thyroid hormone, retinoic acid and 1,25-dihydroxyvitamin $D_3$ as well as some receptors with as yet unknown ligands, the so called orphan receptors. It is possible that the dioxin receptor is a member of this family as well although this cannot be definitely assessed until the receptor has been cloned. Interestingly, the clofibrate receptor, believed to be involved in clofibrate induction of certain isozymes of cytochrome P-450, has recently been shown to be a member of the steroid receptor supergene family and it is conceivable that other P-450 inducers might act *via* as yet uncharacterized receptors belonging to the same gene family.

Therefore, we should learn significantly about principles of P-450 regulation by considering basic mechanisms of glucocorticoid action; the glucocorticoid receptor probably represents the most extensively studied member of the nuclear receptor family. Our laboratory has been particularly interested in structural aspects of this receptor and has used gene technology to overexpress its different domains, particularly the DNA-binding domain, the structure of which has been resolved using NMR.

The steroid receptors are a family of intracellular soluble receptor proteins that act as ligand-dependent transcription factors (*1–4*). Their function is to transpose the hormone signal to the gene level, resulting in the regulation of transcription of a limited number of hormone-dependent genes. As well as the steroid receptor proteins, the superfamily of ligand-dependent transcription factors encompasses receptor proteins for thyroid hormone, 1,25-dihydroxy vitamin $D_3$ and retinoic acid as well as numerous related receptor proteins for which the ligand is as yet unknown. Within the superfamily, several sub-families can be identified based on similarities in structure as well as biological function of the individual receptor proteins. One such sub-family consists of the glucocorticoid receptor (GR), the progestin receptor (PR), the androgen receptor (AR) and the mineralocorticoid receptor (MR). The fifth classical steroid receptor protein, the estrogen receptor (ER), is markedly different and belongs to a different sub-family.

For each of the steroid receptors and the vitamin D receptor there is one single receptor protein, the product of a single gene, that is identical in all target cells. However, for thyroid hormone and retinoic acid there is a diversity at the receptor level, the result of multiple receptor genes for these ligands. The function of the various forms of these receptor proteins is unclear (*5–11*).

The particular interest of this group has focused on the mechanism of action of glucocorticoids. These hormones play a very important physiological role in the regulation of energy metabolism (gluconeogenesis) as well as modulation of the inflammatory and immune responses. Glucocorticoids play a central role in the response of an organism to stress.

The mechanism of action of each of the receptor proteins for which the ligand has been identified appears to be very similar. The basics for this mechanism were defined already 20 years ago when tritiated steroids with high specific activity became available. Radiolabelled estradiol was shown to be specifically retained by target tissues for estrogen (*12*) and the radioactivity was subsequently shown to be localised in the cell nucleus. Further studies showed that the radiolabelled steroids bound specifically to cytosolic proteins with high affinity in a saturable manner and that binding of the steroids to these proteins enabled the complex to be translocated to the nucleus. *In vitro*, the binding of steroids to these proteins enabled them to interact with DNA. However, this process required exposure to high ionic strength or increased temperature and it was concluded that it involved a conformational change in the receptor protein, induced by the binding of the steroid. The process has been called "activation" or "transformation" (*13*). These initial findings resulted in the general hypothesis for the mechanism of steroid hormone action shown in Fig. 1. This model holds true today, after further refinement. One particular aspect that has received considerable attention over the years and that has been discussed in the literature concerns the intracellular localisation of the receptor proteins.

In the initial studies following sub-cellular fractionation, the steroid receptor-binding activity was found in the cytosolic fraction and the nuclear translocation model was postulated. However, subsequent studies using immunocytochemistry or enucleation indicated that ER (*14*, *15*) and PR (*16–18*) were localised in the cell nucleus already prior to ligand-binding.

However, for GR numerous immunocytochemical and immunohistochemical

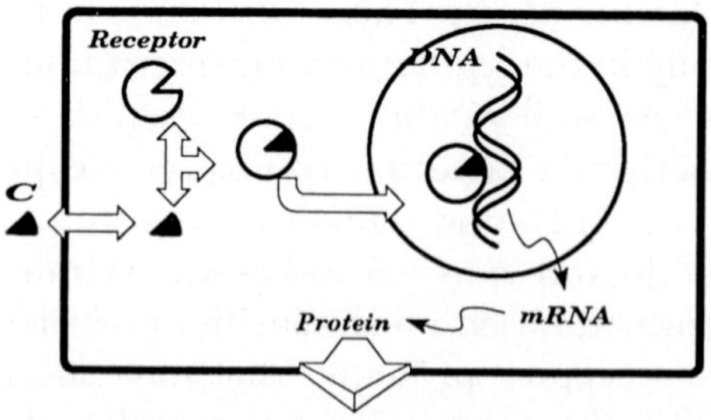


FIG. 1. Mechanism of action of the glucocorticoid receptor. The steroid (C) enters the cell by passive diffusion and binds to the cytoplasmic receptor protein. Binding of the steroid to the receptor enables the complex to enter the nucleus and bind to specific DNA sequences. The interaction with DNA results in changes in the rate of transcription of specific genes.

studies indicate a cytoplasmic localisation for non-liganded receptor and a hormone-dependent nuclear translocation (*19–22*). The receptor proteins for vitamin D, thyroid hormone and retinoic acid appear to be constantly localised in the target cell nucleus. Thus, it is entirely possible that the GR is exceptional in its intracellular localisation.

Further evidence for glucocorticoid-dependent nuclear translocation of the receptor has been obtained using chimaeric proteins containing various segments of GR. In this manner, two separate nuclear translocation signal sequences could be identified, one constitutive and one steroid-dependent (*23*). The constitutive nuclear localisation sequence consisted of a short basic segment adjacent to the DNA-binding domain. The hormone-dependent nuclear localisation signal could not be identified as a specific sequence but corresponded to the entire steroid-binding domain. The hormone-dependent signal sequence was dominant over the constitutive sequence. Both of these signal sequences could result in the nuclear translocation, either constitutively or in a hormone-dependent manner, of large cytoplasmic proteins such as transferrin or β-galactosidase.

As well as resulting in nuclear translocation of the receptor complex, the classical "activation" process also results in an increased affinity of the complex for DNA (*13*). This is also true for the receptor proteins that appear to reside constantly in the nucleus. Thus, independent of the question of whether hormone-dependent nuclear translocation occurs or not, there is clearly a hormone-dependent interaction of these receptor proteins with DNA (*24*). This interaction results in changes in the rate of transcription of specific genes. The consequent changes in protein levels result in the biological effects of these hormones.

Although there is one single GR, identical in all target cells, there is a multitude of different responses to glucocorticoids that vary considerably between target tissues. Each of these physiological responses can usually be related to specific effects at the gene level. Thus, the same receptor protein interacts with different genes in the various target cells. There is a limited gene network available for glucocorticoid regulation in each cell. The nature of the individual gene network available in a specific cell is the result of cellular differentiation. Furthermore, a specific gene frequently demonstrates multi-endocrine regulation, the result of the interaction of several different steroid receptors with one gene.

The specificity of response to a specific hormone is determined by the presence or absence of the corresponding receptor protein. The multiplicity of the response is determined at the gene level by differentiation.

### *Domain Structure of GR*

The nature of the role of the steroid receptor proteins entails multiple functions localised within the protein. Early studies of rat liver GR showed that a limited number of sites within the protein were highly susceptible to digestion with a variety of proteases (*25*). Following limited digestion of GR and isolation of the fragments, it was shown that various functions of the protein were recovered in specific fragments (*26, 27*). Based on the results of limited proteolysis of GR, at least three different functional domains could be identified: a steroid-binding domain, a DNA-binding

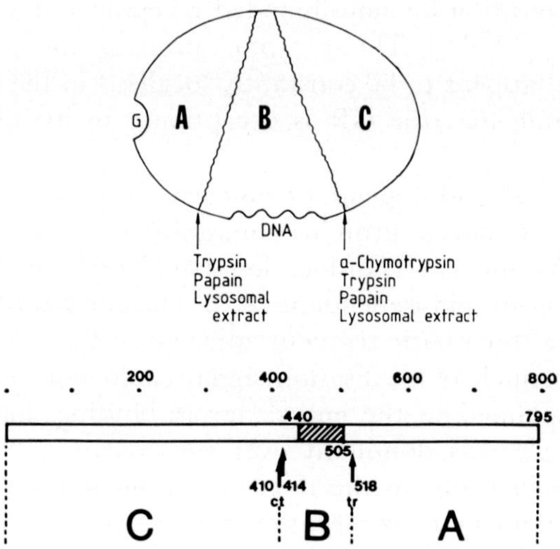


FIG. 2. Functional domains of the rat liver glucocorticoid receptor. Limited proteolysis of GR defined three different functional domains: A, steroid-binding domain; B, DNA-binding domain; C, transactivating modulatory domain (*27*). The domain borders were identified by N-terminal sequence analysis (*28*). The hatched region represents the highly conserved region characteristic for this family of proteins.

domain, and a third immunodominant domain that was a requirement for normal transcriptional regulatory function (*27*). Isolation of corresponding products of limited proteolytic digestion of the purified rat liver GR followed by N-terminal sequence analysis identified these domains at the primary structural level (*28*). The steroid-binding domain corresponds to one third of the protein and is localised at the C-terminus (Fig. 2). The DNA-binding domain is localised immediately N-terminal of the steroid-binding domain. The third domain corresponded to the N-terminal half of the protein.

The identification of the functional domains at the protein level has been confirmed by functional studies following expression of mutant or truncated GR cDNAs (*29–34*). Virtually all mutations reported within the C-terminal third of the protein have resulted in the loss of affinity for steroid. Deletion of only six residues at the C-terminus greatly reduces the affinity for steroid with subsequent loss of transcriptional regulation. Further deletion has even greater effect. However, deletion of almost the entire steroid-binding domain results in constitutive DNA-binding and transcriptional activation. Mutations within the DNA-binding domain resulted in the loss of both affinity for DNA as well as transcriptional regulation. In addition to the localisation of these two functions, mutational data also identified at least two regions that modulate the transcriptional response. A summary of the functional effects of mutation and deletion is shown in Fig. 3.

### *Interaction with Heat Shock Protein HSP90*

Under conditions of low ionic strength, the cytosolic GR was shown to occur in

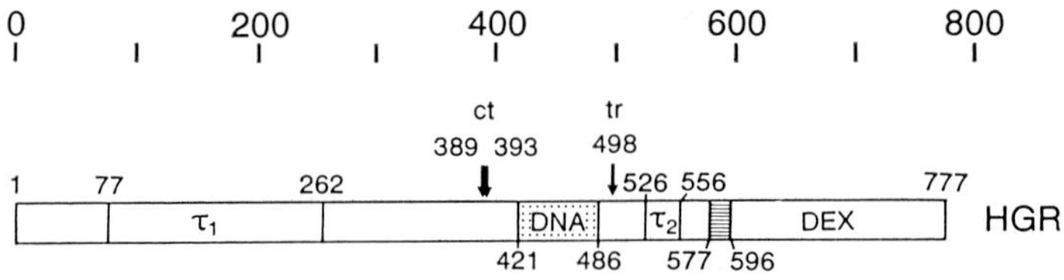


FIG. 3. Functional regions of the human glucocorticoid receptor. The location of the various functional regions of the protein relative to the primary structure are based on deletion and mutational studies using GR cDNA (*29–34*). DEX, hormone-binding function; DNA, DNA-binding function; $\tau$, transactivation modulatory function. The stippled region marks the highly conserved region within the DNA-binding domain. The hatched region marks a conserved region within the steroid-binding domain suggested as a putative contact site for HSP90. The hypersensitive proteolytic cleavage sites that define the domain border (Fig. 2) are also marked.

a larger multimeric form (8S form) (*35*). Following the binding of steroid and exposure to high ionic strength or increased temperature (*i.e.* "activation" conditions), the complex dissociated giving rise to monomeric GR (4S form). Although the 8S form occurs readily at low ionic strength, it could be greatly stabilised by the presence of molybdate (*35*). The addition of molybdate also inhibited the "activation" process. The 8S form of GR was shown to contain one molecule of GR in association with a dimer of HSP90 (*36*). The 4S form seen following "activation" consists of monomeric GR with no associated proteins. Thus, the dissociation of HSP90 from GR is related to "activation". However, the role of HSP90 in hormone action and its physiological significance remains unclear (*37, 38*). This association remains an *in vitro* phenomenon and has not yet been demonstrated to occur *in vivo*. Once dissociated from HSP90, GR cannot be reassociated with the protein to reform the 8S complex.

Expression of deleted forms of GR and analysis of their properties by sedimentation analysis showed that deletion of all or part of the steroid-binding domain interfered with the interaction with HSP90 (*39*). Analysis of the sequence of this segment of the steroid receptor proteins revealed a conserved region which has been proposed as a putative site for HSP90 interaction (Fig. 3).

### *DNA Binding*

The DNA-binding function is localised to a central segment of GR rich in Cys, Lys and Arg. The sequence of the region is very characteristic with pairs of Cys located within a short distance from each other. Comparison of the primary structure of the various members of this superfamily shows that this structure is highly conserved and is the characteristic feature for members of this superfamily (*3, 4*). As well as the nine conserved Cys residues, there are numerous other residues that are conserved in all members of this family. Expression of fragments of GR show that it is sufficient with just the DNA-binding domain for binding to DNA and for giving transcriptional regulation of specific genes (*32–34*). However, in the absence of the N-terminal domain, the transactivating function of the isolated DNA-binding domain is greatly reduced (*29, 30*). After deletion of the steroid-binding domain, the DNA-binding domain acts in a constitutive manner with regard to both interaction with DNA and transcriptional regulation. The DNA-binding function cannot be isolated from the transcriptional regulatory function.

In the intact GR, DNA-binding is entirely dependent on steroid-binding. These two functions are localised in separate domains and there must therefore be some form of interaction between the two domains that mediates the steroid-dependent effect. It has always been assumed that this effect is the result of a conformational change within GR although this has never been conclusively demonstrated. It has, however, been shown that the isolated steroid-binding domain of GR can confer steroid-dependence on other DNA binding proteins such as lex A or GAL4 (*40*). Chimaeric proteins consisting of the normally constitutive DNA-binding proteins with the GR steroid-binding domain no longer interact directly with DNA. It is only in the presence of glucocorticoids that the chimaeric proteins can bind to DNA. Thus, the steroid-binding domain exerts its effect by blocking the DNA-binding function and this effect is in turn inhibited by the binding of steroid.

### *Glucocorticoid Response Elements (GREs)*

The acquisition of affinity for DNA associated with "activation" in the early studies concerned a general affinity for DNA from any source (*13*). With access to purified receptor preparations as well as cloned fragments of glucocorticoid-regulated genes, it was possible to show that there also occurred a specific interaction with defined DNA sequences (*1, 2, 4, 41, 42*). The ability to interact with DNA, both specifically and non-specifically, was the result of the "activation" process. Affinity for non-specific DNA cannot be separated from the specific DNA-binding function.

The first studies of specific receptor-DNA interactions utilised the mouse mammary tumous virus which is induced by glucocorticoids. Sequences that specifically interacted with purified rat liver GR (*41, 42*) could be shown to confer glucocorticoid-dependent transcriptional regulation on heterologous promoters and these sequences act on the rate of transcriptional initiation at adjacent promoters, independent of orientation, distance or sequential order (*43*). Thus, GREs act as classical enhancer elements. The activity of GREs is entirely dependent on their occupancy by GR. Comparison of the sequence of a large number of GREs from a variety of glucocorticoid-regulated genes resulted in the definition of a partially palindromic consensus sequence GGTACANNNTGTTCT (*4, 44, 45*). The GRE consists of two hexanucleotides with three intervening nucleotides of indeterminate sequence but fixed number. The same consensus sequence also mediates the effects of androgens, progestins and mineralocorticoids, *via* the appropriate receptor. These four receptors are all members of the same sub-family. The estrogen response element (ERE) differs from the GRE at the two central nucleotides within each hexanucleotide. As with the GRE, there is a strict distance requirement between the two hexanucleotides in the ERE (*45–47*). In contrast, the thyroid hormone response element (TRE) consists of hexanucleotide sequences related to those of the ERE but without a strict distance requirement (*48*).

### *Synergistic Action of GREs*

The mechanism by which steroid receptors regulate gene transcription following binding to hormone response elements is unknown. The two properties, DNA-binding and transcriptional regulation, appear to be co-localised within GR (*29–34*). By combining various different response elements, synthetic promoters for studying hormone response have been constructed. The simplest promoter that will respond to glucocorticoids consists of a GRE in close proximity to a TATA box. However, as soon as the distance between the two elements is increased, it is not sufficient with just these two elements. When placed at a greater distance from the promoter, the GRE requires additional elements to mediate hormone response. Such elements can be either hormone response elements (GRE or ERE) or elements that bind other transcription factors such as Sp1 or NF1. Two hormone response elements or one GRE together with another element (*e.g.*, Sp1, NF1) act synergistically resulting in greatly enhanced hormone-dependent transcription (*49–52*).

In addition to potential protein-protein interactions between GR and other transcription factors based on the results described above, specific DNA-binding of GR can also affect the chromatin structure and thus regulate transcription. An example of this has been shown with the mouse mammary tumour virus promoter. If this region is reassembled in chromatin, there is a specific nucleosome phasing that results in the exposition of the GREs on the surface of the nucleosome. However, an adjacent NF1 site is blocked by the nucleosome. Binding of GR to the GREs results in the displacement of that particular nucleosome with exposition of the NF1 site as a result (*53*). This is a necessary step in transcriptional induction of the MTV promoter by glucocorticoids. Thus, DNA-binding alone cannot explain all the events involved in transcriptional regulation. The steroid receptors interact with other transcription factors and have therefore proven to be very useful instruments to study the mechanism of gene regulation in eukaryotic systems.

### *Aims of Our Study*

The primary aim of this study is to understand the mechanism of steroid hormone action, in particular glucocorticoid action. The key points that have been focused on are as follows: 1) Recognition of the steroid hormone by the hormone receptor. Determination of agonist/antagonist properties. 2) The "activation" process. How is the hormone signal transformed to a DNA-binding signal? 3) Receptor-DNA interaction—underlying mechanisms and recognition of specific sequences. 4) Transcriptional regulation. How does the interaction of a receptor protein with DNA result in changes in transcriptional activity?

Although purified preparations of rat liver GR have been available for more than 10 years, the quantities obtained have been insufficient for further structural studies. In order to understand the various functions of the receptor protein, the entire protein or isolated domains must be obtained in larger amounts for detailed structural analysis. Our aim was therefore to express GR and its individual domains in a functional form using various expression systems. The functions of the expressed products must be identical to that of the native protein to allow any conclusions concerning the relationship between structure and function. It is therefore of importance to develop functional assay systems in parallel with the expression systems. Further probing of the structure-function relationship is then possible using site-directed mutagenesis. Our aim has been to develop such systems and analyse the structure and function of the various products. A detailed knowledge of the structure of the receptor protein is of importance both for an understanding of the mechanism of steroid hormone action as well as a general understanding of the mechanism of gene regulation in eukaryotic cells.

*Summary of the Results of Our Study*

Characterisation of purified rat liver GR defined the two primary functional domains and their relationship to each other (*27, 28*). The availability of GR cDNA enabled the expression of the intact receptor as well as individual domains based on the borders defined at the protein level. At all stages, the characteristics of the proteins expressed have been related to their function in comparison with the intact native GR.

*1. Expression of GR*

Intact human GR or isolated domains of the protein, either individually or in combination, were expressed in bacteria (*Escherichia coli*) (*65–68*) or in yeast (*69*). Numerous expression systems have been tested resulting in both induced and constitutive expression at both high and low levels. The results of the expression varied considerably. The isolated DNA-binding domain was expressed as a fusion protein with protein A in bacteria in an inducible system (*66*). This resulted in high level expression of soluble functional protein. In contrast, expression of the intact GR in either yeast or bacteria resulted in either a product that underwent rapid proteolytic degradation or was denatured and insoluble. If expressed at a low level, it is possible to express functionally intact GR in yeast but not in bacteria. Expression of fragments of GR larger than the DNA-binding domain alone resulted in predominantly insoluble products with low levels of functional protein (*65, 67, 68*). In yeast, these problems could be overcome by lowering the expression levels (*69*).

*2. Reporter system*

The expressed proteins were characterised with respect to steroid-binding, DNA-binding and transcriptional activation. Steroid-binding was performed both *in vivo* (incubation of whole cells) or *in vitro* (incubation of cytosol or isolated cellular fractions). DNA-binding was characterised by DNase footprinting, gel shift analysis, methylation interference and missing base contact probing *in vitro*.

Transcriptional activation has been studied in yeast (*69*). A reporter system consisting of the *E. coli* Lac Z gene driven by the *CYC1* promoter stripped of its own activation sequences and replaced with GREs was stably maintained in yeast. This reporter could be used for studying either constitutive or steroid-dependent trans-activation. This system is better than transient transfection because stable levels of expression and reporter plasmids are the same in all cells. In order to make it more convenient to screen many GR mutants and variant hormone response elements, expression plasmids and reporter plasmids were maintained in different haploid strains which could be fused by mating to give diploid cells containing both plasmids.

*3. Steroid-binding domain (SBD)*

The isolated SBD was expressed in *E. coli* either alone or in combination with all or part of DBD either as a fusion protein with protein A or using the T7 polymerase expression system (*68*). The level of expression was inversely proportional to the size of the protein. The majority of protein expressed was recovered as an insoluble complex. Only a small percentage of the soluble fraction of expressed protein was found to be functional and bind steroid. However, the small fraction that was functional bound steroid with a specificity similar to that of native GR but with about 50-fold lower affinity. If the same constructions were instead used as templates for mRNA synthesis followed by *in vitro* translation in reticulocyte lysate, the product was found to bind steroid with normal affinity. The receptor fragments recovered from the reticulocyte lysate were found to form 8S complexes with HSP90 whereas no such complexes were formed in bacteria.

Exposure of rat liver GR to high ionic strength prior to steroid binding also resulted in the dissociation of GR from HSP90 (*70*). Concomitant with this dissociation, it was seen that the affinity for glucocorticoids was decreased 50-fold to levels equivalent to those found in the bacterial extracts. It was concluded that HSP90 plays a role in stabilising the structure of the SBD and maintaining a normal affinity for the hormone. Affinity labelling of the bacterial product showed that more than one Cys could be affinity labelled with dexamethasone mesylate. The structure of the SBD expressed in bacteria appeared to be more open than in the native protein. Attempts to reassociate the product with purified HSP90 or to coexpress the two proteins were unsuccessful.

### 4. *Identification of steroid-binding amino acid residues*

Amino acid residues occurring at the steroid-binding surface of GR SBD, and presumably active in the binding of steroid, were identified by affinity labelling with radio-labelled steroid followed by radiosequence analysis (*71, 72*). Cys 754 and Met-622 (rat GR) were affinity labelled *via* the A-ring of triamcinolone acetonide whereas Cys-656 (rat GR) was affinity labelled by the side chain of dexamethasone mesylate. Each of these residues occurs within a hydrophobic segment and presumably the protein folds to form a hydrophobic surface to which the steroid binds.

Similar studies of the rat and human GR and human PR were carried out using the synthetic progestin promegestone (*73*). In all three proteins, Met-622 (rat GR) and its equivalent was affinity labelled. Promegestone also labelled Cys-754 (rat GR) and its equivalent in human GR. However, in human PR, a residue 18 residues further C-terminal was labelled, Met-909 instead of the equivalent Cys. Thus, this method can detect subtle differences in the structure of the steroid-binding surfaces of the different receptors and how they distinguish between the different types of steroid.

Analysis of the recombinant GR SBD using this method resulted in labelling by dexamethasone mesylate of all Cys residues, more or less, although the residue equivalent to Cys-656 was the major site of labelling (*68*). Thus, this method seems to be a sensitive measure of the correct folding of the protein.

### 5. *DNA-binding domain (DBD)*

High level expression of the isolated GR DBD in *E. coli* as a fusion protein with protein A was far more successful than the expression of SBD (*66*). Using this system,

2–5 mg purified protein was recovered per litre bacterial culture. Purification was based on the affinity of protein A for IgG bound to Sepharose. After immobilisation of the fusion protein on the affinity matrix, GR DBD was separated from the rest of the fusion protein by cleavage with chymotrypsin, utilising the natural chymotrypsin cleavage site that defines the normal domain border (*28*). Finally DBD was separated from chymotrypsin by DNA-cellulose chromatography. The product thus obtained consisted of one single protein with an amino acid composition and sequence corresponding to the native DBD. The expression vector was constructed so that the GR sequence stopped at the C-terminal border of DBD. The initial construct also resulted in eight extra amino acids at the C-terminus of the fusion protein, derived from the polylinker. These were subsequently reduced to one extra residue in a later construction. The extra amino acids did not have any effect on the structure or function of the rest of the protein. Analysis of specific DNA-binding by DNase I and Exo III footprinting, gel shift analysis as well as methylation interference showed that the recombinant GR DBD bound to DNA with a specificity identical to that of native GR but with a 5–10-fold lower affinity (*66*, *74*).

Attempts to express larger fragments of GR containing the DBD in *E. coli* were less successful (*65*, *67*). Various expression vectors were used, including expression of protein A fusion proteins, but all the products were insoluble or degraded. Attempts to renature the recombinant proteins resulted in the restitution of affinity for non-specific DNA but not for specific sequences.

6. *Expression of GR fragments in yeast*

The equivalent fragments of GR that were expressed in *E. coli* were also expressed in yeast using both constitutive and inducible expression systems. Expression levels achieved were about the same as in bacteria, *i.e.* $\approx 1\%$ of soluble protein. However, there were similar problems with the solubility and in addition, it was more difficult to extract the protein from yeast without further degrading it. Expression of the combined DBD-SBD (human GR 415-777) gave a protein that could mediate steroid-dependent transactivation *in vivo* (*69*). The biological effect of different steroids corresponded to the normal specificity of GR. However, 100-fold higher concentrations of steroids were required to elicit full response compared to normal glucocorticoid target cells. No binding activity could be demonstrated in cytosol isolated from these yeast cells but this was probably due to problems with the extraction. The expressed protein occurred as a larger complex, $\approx$8S (*69*). Yeast contains HSP90 which is similar to mammalian HSP90 (*54*) so presumably this large complex represents interaction of GR with yeast HSP90. However, the biological efficiency of the different steroids was very similar to the binding affinity of the same GR fragment expressed in *E. coli*. Therefore, it seems likely that if the GR expressed in yeast is interacting with yeast HSP90, this forms a non-functional complex. Interestingly, expression of the intact GR in yeast at a low level results in a soluble protein that also mediates glucocorticoid-dependent transactivation *in vivo* but at concentrations equivalent to those required in normal eukaryotic target cells. However, the specificity of steroid effect in these yeast cells is changed with maximal effect induced by progesterone and deoxycorticosterone. Thus, care must be taken in the interpretation of steroid-dependent effects following GR expression in yeast.

Based on Ptashne's concept of squelching (*55*) in which limited transcription factors are titrated out by overexpressed activation domains, the effect of overexpression of the $\tau_1$ region in yeast has been tested. Using a galactose-inducible expression system and the reporter system described above, expression of *CYC1*-LacZ was reduced 10-fold in galactose media. Concomitantly, growth of the cells is severely impaired. We interpret this as a squelching effect of this region of GR, presumably due to interaction between $\tau_1$ and one or a few key transcription factors. Currently, work is in progress to characterise this effect in more detail and to identify the factor or factors involved.

*7. Interaction of GR DBD with DNA*

Comparison of the specificity of DNA-binding for the isolated recombinant DBD and native intact GR showed that the two proteins interact with exactly the same DNA sequence corresponding to the GRE (*66*). Thus, the recombinant DBD seems ideal for further structural analysis of this part of the GR in relation to its function. In contrast, the other constructions containing the GR DBD that were expressed in a denatured form proved to be unusable for this type of studies (*67*),

Having shown that DBD bound to DNA in an identical manner to intact GR, the interaction with non-specific DNA sequences was studied using flow linear dichroism and circular dichroism (*75*). These studies show that at saturation there is about one protein per 5 bp DNA. Binding to DNA does not lead to any observable structural changes in the protein but spectroscopically one does see that there is a stiffening of the DNA. At higher ionic strengths there is spectroscopic indication that the DNA forms a slight coil around the protein. The tyrosine residues do not participate by intercalation in the interaction with the DNA, but the protein associates to DNA mainly by electrostatic interactions. Attempts to study the specific interaction of DBD with GREs using these methods are in progress.

*8. Interaction of GR with glucocorticoid regulated genes*

In collaboration with various different groups, the specific interaction of GR with genes that are normally regulated by glucocorticoids has been studied. These studies have been carried out predominantly using purified rat liver GR, with some complementation using the recombinant GR DBD, and our specific contribution concerns the protein-DNA interaction. The genes studied each reflect a particular aspect of steroid-dependent gene regulation. Phosphoenolpyruvate carboxykinase (PEPCK) (*76*) is the rate determining step for gluconeogenesis, regulation of which is the primary function of glucocorticoids. This enzyme is under multiendocrine regulation including up-regulation by glucocorticoids and glucagon (*via* cAMP) and down-regulation by insulin. The insulin effect is dominant. Initial characterisation showed that the functional elements responsible for the glucocorticoid effect identified by deletion analysis did not correspond to the sequences to which GR bound. Further characterisation of this region showed that the glucocorticoid effect was mediated by a complex glucocorticoid regulatory unit which consisted of binding sites for both GR and other transcription factors, a total of at least five different binding sites. It is only when all five binding sites are intact that the full effect is achieved. Deletion of the accessory factor binding sites disrupts the glucocorticoid effect, even though the GR binding sites are intact.

The second gene studied is rat $\alpha_{2u}$-globulin which shows a delayed secondary response to glucocorticoids, dependent on active protein synthesis. Even though protein synthesis is required to mediate the glucocorticoid effect, which occurs first after a time lag of several hours, this effect seems to be dependent on a direct interaction of GR with the gene. Downstream sequences within the structural gene could be shown to confer delayed secondary response on a heterologous promoter. Multiple GR binding sites within this sequence could be demonstrated (*77*).

The third gene studied is the human osteocalcin gene. This is also a gene that is under multiendocrine regulation. Two of the most important hormones that regulate the activity of this gene are 1,25-dihydroxy vitamin $D_3$ (up-regulation) and glucocorticoids (down-regulation). The vitamin D response element has previously been delineated to a sequence at about −500 (*56*). The inhibitory effect of glucocorticoids is mediated by a fragment of the osteocalcin promoter encompassing −190/+30 but has not yet been localised more exactly (*57*). Analysis of GR interaction with this fragment, using intact GR and recombinant DBD, has been studied by DNase I and Exo III footprinting and gel shift analysis. Sequences overlapping the TATA box specifically interact with GR and we believe that the inhibitory effect of glucocorticoids on this gene is due to a competition between GR and transcription factor IID (TFIID) for the same DNA sequence. This hypothesis is now being tested.

### 9. *Cooperative interaction with DNA*

It was noted already at an early stage that the consensus GRE sequence was partially palindromic in nature (*cf.* above) and it was postulated that GR interacted with the GRE as a dimer. However, there was no direct evidence for this model. Although the recombinant DBD interacts with exactly the same sequence as the intact GR, *i.e.* the partially palindromic GRE, the affinity is slightly lower (*66*). This property has enabled us to dissect the interaction in more detail and it was noted that incubation of a GRE with increasing concentrations of DBD gave rise to two different complexes (*78*, *79*). Analysis by gel shift and methylation interference showed that there was binding of DBD first to one half of the GRE (TGTTCT) and then facilitated binding to the second half. Using mixtures of the protein A fusion protein and isolated DBD it could be shown that the larger complex contained two protein molecules. Measurement of the kinetics at equilibrium resulted in a cooperativity factor of about 1,000 (*80*). This study was carried out using a different GRE sequence than that used in the first studies (*78*, *79*) and measurement of GR binding by quenching of tyrosine fluorescence. The cooperativity factor for binding of the second DBD molecule to the GRE used in the first studies has also been measured by gel shift analysis. In this case a cooperativity factor of about 100 was obtained (*81*).

The facilitated binding of the second DBD molecule to the GRE could be the result of two possible mechanisms. Either the binding of the first molecule could modify the structure of the DNA, thus making the second site more readily available, or the facilitated binding of the second protein molecule could be the result of protein-protein interaction with the DBD molecule already bound to the GRE. These two possibilities were tested by studying the interaction of DBD with a variety of modified GREs (*81*). Variation in the distance between the two half-sites or inversion of the stronger half-site completely disrupted the facilitated binding of the second DBD molecule. On the other hand, the introduction of a nick in an intervening sequence between the two half-sites had no effect on the facilitated binding of the second DBD molecule. Thus, no change in DNA-structure was transmitted through the central part of the GRE sequence but there were very strict requirements concerning the relative orientation of the two DBD molecules. We conclude that the facilitated binding must be the result of protein-protein interaction.

*10. Identification of a protein-protein contact site within GR DBD*

Both the GRE and the ERE are characterised by a very strict distance relationship between the two half-sites of the response element (*44–47*). In contrast, the TRE contains half-sites similar to those of the ERE but without the same absolute distance requirement (*48*). It was previously reported that a mutant GR that recognised the ERE sequence could be changed to a form that recognised the TRE as well by changing a segment at the second zinc-binding site for the corresponding sequence from the thyroid hormone receptor (*58*). These effects were noted in a functional study using transient expression and a reporter gene. Having shown that the facilitated binding of GR DBD to the GRE was dependent on protein-protein interaction (*81*), the segment at the second zinc-binding site seemed a suitable candidate for such an interaction. The corresponding change was therefore introduced into the recombinant GR DBD (*81*). The mutant GR DBD bound to exactly the same GRE sequence but there was no longer any facilitated binding of the second DBD molecule. The cooperativity factor for the mutant DBD as measured by gel shift analysis was about 1.5 (*81*). The segment at the second zinc-binding site was therefore postulated to be the putative site of protein-protein interaction between GR molecules within this domain. This does not exclude other sites of interaction within other domains of the receptor.

*11. Identification of protein contact sites within the GRE*

In order to understand the mechanism by which the receptor protein recognises a specific DNA sequence it is necessary to identify the specific groups within the two molecules that participate in the interaction. Protein contact sites within the GRE were identified by missing base contact probing and ethylation interference (*82*). The former identifies nucleotides that are contacted by the protein and the latter identifies phosphate groups on the DNA backbone that participate in the interaction. These analyses show that the two receptor molecules interact with two consecutive major grooves of the DNA, binding to the same face of the DNA. The phosphate groups contacted, presumably representing non-specific interaction with DNA, flank the nucleotides recognised by the protein (Fig. 4).

*12. Mutant GR DBDs*

In addition to structural analysis of the native GR DBD, mutation of specific amino acids provides important complementary information on the function related to specific structures within the protein. One such mutation responsible for protein-protein interactions has already been described (*cf.* above). Recently three different groups have reported mutations of both GR and ER that change the specificity at the DNA level from a GRE to an ERE or *vice versa* in functional studies (*58–60*). By changing three amino acid residues in proximity of the first zinc-binding site to the corresponding sequence from the other receptor, the functional DNA specificity is

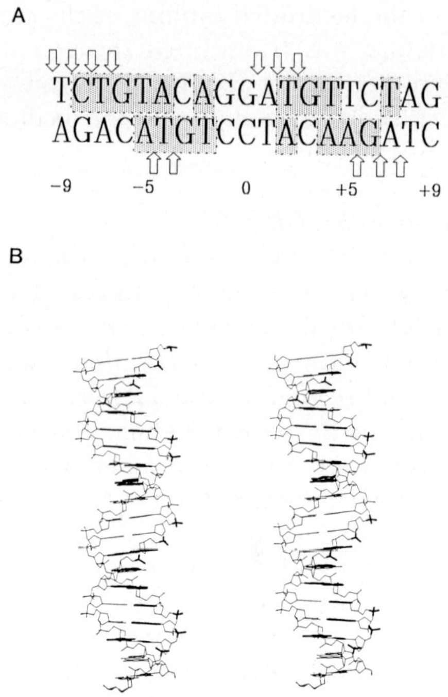


FIG. 4. Receptor contact sites within the glucocorticoid response element. Contacts between the GR DBD and the tyrosine aminotransferase $GRE_{II}$ were identified by missing base contact probing (shaded nucleotides) and ethylation interference (arrowed phosphates). In the lower part of the figure, a stereo diagram shows the contact sites marked with broader lines.

switched. Mutations of two or three of these residues have been introduced into the recombinant GR DBD and expressed as fusion proteins with protein A. The specificity of interaction with DNA using a GRE, an ERE and two response elements of intermediate sequence is now being studied by gel shift analysis. It is already apparent that the change in specificity with regard to DNA-binding as a result of the mutations is not nearly as clear cut as the results obtained by functional analysis. Further analysis of these proteins with the various response elements by missing base contact probing is now in progress. Also, *in vivo* assay of the function of the proteins in yeast using variant GREs and EREs is in progress.

Another set of mutations reported in the literature are mutations of the vitamin D receptor reported in families with vitamin D-resistant rickets (*61*). Two such families have been studied and each of them were found to contain a single point mutation within the loop region of one of the "zinc fingers". Each of the two mutations results in a change in charge within the affected region. The corresponding mutations have been introduced into the recombinant GR DBD. The mutant proteins were found to be expressed at the same level as native DBD and to fold correctly, based on the effect of limited proteolysis. Both of the mutations result in a greatly reduced affinity for non-specific DNA. Presumably this is a result of changes in interaction with the phosphate backbone of the DNA.

A final set of mutations concerns the last three conserved Cys residues of DBD as dicussed below.

*13. Metal binding*

Already when the first steroid receptor cDNA was cloned, the homology between this family of proteins and other zinc-binding transcription factors such as TFIIIA was noted (*62*). However, in contrast to TFIIIA, the DNA-binding properties of native GR and GR DBD were unaffected by high concentrations (50–100 mM) of various chelating reagents such as EDTA, dithiothreitol (DTT) and *o*-phenanthroline (*74*). Attempts to analyse the native intact GR for metal content were unsuccessful due to the low amounts of protein available. However, denaturation of GR DBD with 8 M urea or by reduced pH in the presence of EDTA completely destroyed the structure of the protein based on circular dichroism. Renaturation in the absence of divalent cations resulted in no change or restitution of DNA-binding properties. However, renaturation in the presence of $Zn^{2+}$, $Cd^{2+}$, $Ni^{2+}$, or $Mn^{2+}$ resulted in the restitution of specific DNA-binding properties (*74*). Further refinement of the denaturation/renaturation process has been carried out. Denaturation of the fusion protein to remove the $Zn^{2+}$ can be performed while the protein is bound to IgG Sepharose by reducing the pH to 4.5, without complete elution of the protein. Exchange of the metal ion or renaturation with $Zn^{2+}$ is then performed with the protein still bound to the matrix. The renatured DBD is then eluted by digestion with chymotrypsin as usual and purification on DNA cellulose. It is only protein that has renatured completely and folded correctly that survives the proteolysis and binds to DNA. This method enables the purification of DBD charged with specific metals for NMR as described below.

At the same time that these studies were performed, the zinc-content of GR DBD was reported in the literature (*63*). In that study it was shown that each molecule of GR DBD contained two zinc ions tetrahedrally coordinated with four Cys residues. However, there has been some debate in the literature which of the nine conserved Cys residues coordinate the zinc, particularly at the second zinc-binding site. In one study, transient expression of GR mutants in which several of the conserved Cys residues were each in turn mutated to Ser or Ala showed that it was only mutation of the ninth conserved Cys that gave rise to a functional receptor (*64*). In order to study the effect of these mutations on the structure of this domain, each of the last three conserved Cys residues was independently mutated to Ser. Mutation of Cys-473 or Cys-476 (human GR) to Ser resulted in a change of structure of this domain as judged by a greatly increased sensitivity to proteolysis. However, mutation of Cys-481 (human GR) had no apparent effect on the structure of the domain or on the interaction with DNA. Thus, we conclude that the second $Zn^{2+}$ is coordinated by Cys-457, Cys-463, Cys-473 and Cys-476 (human GR). The putative protein-protein contact surface is located at Ala-458-Asp-462 (*cf.* above).

*14. Structural analysis of GR DBD*

The high level of expression of GR DBD and purification of large amounts of functional protein have enabled studies of the three dimensional structure of the protein.

Attempts to crystallise the protein have not so far been successful. The protein has an exceptionally high pI ($>$10.5) and is not stable at low pH. After testing various conditions, microcrystals were obtained by salting out with ammonium sulphate.

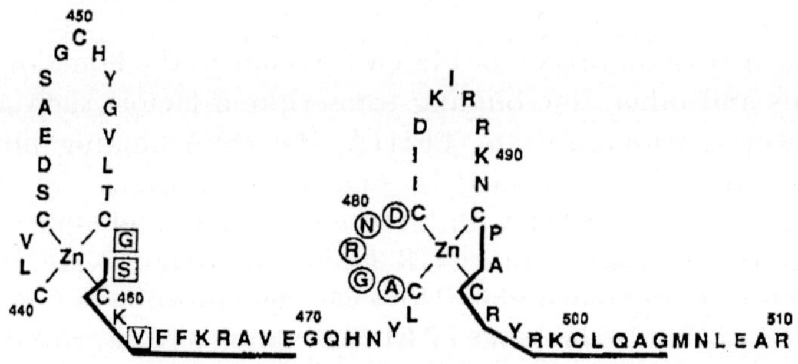


FIG. 5. Core sequence of the human glucocorticoid receptor DNA-binding domain. The figure shows the highly conserved sequence that characterises this family of transcription factors. Residues in boxes differentiate between a GRE and an ERE. Residues in circles mark the putative segment involved in DBD protein-protein interaction. The underlined sequences mark α-helices identified by NMR analysis.

However, refinement of the conditions did not improve the quality or size of the crystals. Analysis of the protein remaining in the wells after standing for one month under crystallisation conditions showed that the protein was proteolytically degraded. Presumably, there are still residual traces of chymotrypsin in the purified preparations that cannot be detected otherwise. Attempts to remove these traces of chymotrypsin have so far been unsuccessful.

An alternative method for studying protein tertiary structure is two dimensional NMR. The method has the advantage that the protein is studied in solution. Furthermore, the sample does not have to be homogeneous but can contain protein with heterogeneous ends without interfering with the analysis. Thus, slight proteolysis of the protein does not interfere. Analysis of our human GR DBD and rat GR DBD from Keith Yamamoto has enabled Robert Kaptein and his group at Utrecht to solve the solution structure of the overlapping sequences, the core DBD (*84, 85*). The domain contains two α-helices perpendicular to each other. One face of each helix is hydrophobic and makes up part of the hydrophobic core of the domain. The first helix starts at Ser-440 (human GR) and appears to be a recognition helix. The three residues that differentiate between the DNA-binding specificity of GR/ER (*cf.* above) lie on the outer face of this helix. Alignment of this helix in the major groove of a GRE half-site, taking into consideration the contact sites within the GRE (*83*) and the differences between a GRE and an ERE results in the orientation of the two DBD molecules so that the putative protein-protein contact surfaces are in contact with each other (*85*). Confirmation of the zinc coordination as discussed above is under progress using DBD charged with $^{113}$Cd. A summary of the structure of the core region of DBD is shown in Fig. 5.

REFERENCES

1. Yamamoto, K. R. Annu. Rev. Genet., *19*: 209–252, 1985.
2. Gustafsson, J.-Å., Carlstedt-Duke, J., Poellinger, L., Okret, S., Wikström, A.-C., Brönnegård, M., Gillner, M., Dong, Y., Fuxe, K., Cintra, A., Härfstrand, A., and Agnati, L. Endocrine Rev., *8*: 185–234, 1987.

3. Evans, R. M. Science, *240*: 883–895, 1988.
4. Beato, M. Cell, *56*: 334–344, 1989.
5. Thompson, C. C. and Evans, R. M. Proc. Natl. Acad. Sci. U.S.A., *86*: 3494–3498, 1989.
6. Murray, M. B., Zilz, N. D., McCreary, N. L., MacDonald, M., and Towle, H. C. J. Biol. Chem., *263*: 12770–12777, 1988.
7. Mitsuhashi, N. T., Tennyson, G. E., and Nikodem, V. M. Proc. Natl. Acad. Sci. U.S.A., *85*: 5804–5808, 1988.
8. Lazar, M. A., Hodin, R. A., Darling, D. S., and Chin, W. W. Mol. Cell. Biol., *9*: 1128–1236, 1989.
9. Hodin, R. A., Lazar, M. A., Wintman, B. I., Darling, D. S., Koenig, R. J., Larsen, P. R., Moore, D. D., and Chin, W. W. Science, *244*: 76–79, 1989.
10. Giguere, V., Ong, E. S., Segui, P., and Evans, R. M. Nature, *330*: 624–629, 1987.
11. Petkovich, M., Brand, J. J., Krust, A., and Chambon, P. Nature, *330*: 444–450, 1987.
12. Jensen, E. V. and Jacobson, H. I. Rec. Prog. Horm. Res., *18*: 387, 1962.
13. Schmidt, T. J. and Litwack, G. Physiol. Rev., *62*: 1131–1192, 1982.
14. Welshons, W. V., Lieberman, M. E., and Gorski, J. Nature, *307*: 747–749, 1984.
15. King, W. J. and Greene, G. L. Nature, *307*: 745–747, 1984.
16. Gasc, J. M., Renoir, J. M., Radanyi, C., Joab, I., Tuohimaa, P., and Baulieu, E.-E. J. Cell. Biol., *99*: 1193–1201, 1984.
17. Perrot-Applanat, M., Logeat, A., Groyer-Picard, M. T., and Milgrom, E. Endocrinology, *116*: 1473–1481, 1985.
18. Welshons, W. V., Krummel, B. M., and Gorski, J. Endocrinology, *117*: 2140–2147, 1985.
19. Papamichail, M., Tsokos, G., Tsawdaroglou, N., and Sekeris, C. E. Exp. Cell Res., *125*: 490–493, 1980.
20. Gustafsson, J.-Å., Carlstedt-Duke, J., Fuxe, K., Carlström, K., Okret, S., and Wrange, Ö. *In;* K. Fuxe, L. Wetterberg, and J.-Å. Gustafsson (eds.), Steroid Hormone Regulation of Brain, Pergamon Press, Oxford, pp. 31–39, 1981.
21. Antakly, T. and Eisen, H. J. Endocrinology, *115*: 1984–1989, 1984.
22. Wikström, A.-C., Bakke, O., Okret, S., Brönnegård, M., and Gustafsson, J.-Å. Endocrinology, *120*: 1232–1242, 1987.
23. Picard, D. and Yamamoto, K. R. EMBO J., *6*: 3333–3340, 1987.
24. Kalff, M., Gross, B., and Beato, M. Nature, *344*: 360–362, 1990.
25. Carlstedt-Duke, J., Gustafsson, J.-Å., and Wrange, Ö. Biochim. Biophys. Acta, *497*: 507–524, 1977.
26. Wrange, Ö. and Gustafsson, J.-Å. J. Biol. Chem., *253*: 856–865, 1978.
27. Carlstedt-Duke, J., Okret, S., Wrange, Ö., and Gustafsson, J.-Å. (1982) Proc. Natl. Acad. Sci. U.S.A., *79*: 4260–4264, 1982.
28. Carlstedt-Duke, J., Strömstedt, P.-E., Wrange, Ö., Bergman, T., Gustafsson, J.-Å., and Jörnvall, H. Proc. Natl. Acad. Sci. U.S.A., *84*: 4437–4440, 1987.
29. Giguere, V., Hollenberg, S. M., Rosenfeld, M. G., and Evans, R. M. Cell, *46*: 645–652, 1986.
30. Hollenberg, S. M., Giguere, V., Segui, P., and Evans, R. M. Cell, *49*: 39–46, 1987.
31. Danielsen, M., Northrop, J. P., and Ringold, G. M. EMBO J., *5*: 2513–2522, 1986.
32. Rusconi, S. and Yamamoto, K. R., EMBO J., *6*: 1309–1315, 1987.
33. Miesfeld, R., Godowski, P. J., Maler, B. A., and Yamamoto, K. R. Science, *236*: 423–427, 1987.
34. Godowski, P. J., Rusconi, S., Miesfield, R., and Yamamoto, K. R. Nature *325*: 365–368, 1987.

35. Sherman, M. R., Moran, M. C., Tuazon, F. B., and Stevens, Y.-W. J. Biol. Chem., *258*: 10366–10377, 1983.
36. Denis, M., Poellinger, L., Wikström, A.-C., and Gustafsson, J.-Å. Nature, *333*: 686–688, 1988.
37. Dalman, F. C., Bresnick, E. H., Patel, P. D., Perdew, G. H., Watson, S. J., and Pratt, W. B. J. Biol. Chem., *264*: 19815–19821, 1989.
38. Bresnick, E. H., Dalman, F. C., Sanchez, E. R., and Pratt, W. B. J. Biol. Chem., *264*: 4992–4997, 1989.
39. Pratt, W. B., Jolly, D. J., Pratt, D. V., Hollenberg, S. M., Giguere, V., Cadepond, F. M., Schweizer-Groyer, G., Catelli, M.-G., Evans, R. M., and Baulieu, E.-E. J. Biol. Chem., *263*: 267–273, 1988.
40. Godowski, P. J., Picard, D., and Yamamoto, K. R. Science, *241*: 812–816, 1988.
41. Payvar, F., Wrange, Ö., Carlstedt-Duke, J., Okret, S., Gustafsson, J.-Å., and Yamamoto, K. R. Proc. Natl. Acad. Sci. U.S.A., *78*: 6628–6632, 1981.
42. Payvar, F., DeFranco, D., Firestone, G. L., Edgar, B., Wrange, Ö., Okret, S., Gustafsson, J.-Å., and Yamamoto, K. R. Cell, *35*: 381–392, 1983.
43. Chandler, V. L., Maler, B. A., and Yamamoto, K. R. Cell, *33*: 489–499, 1983.
44. Jantzen, H.-M., Strähle, U., Glass, B., Stewart, F., Schmid, W., Boshart, M., Miksicek, R., and Schütz, G. Cell, *49*: 29–38, 1987.
45. Kloch, G., Strähle, U., and Schütz, G. Nature, *329*: 734–736, 1987.
46. Martinez, E., Givel, F., and Wahli, W. EMBO J., *6*: 3719–3727, 1987.
47. Green, S. and Chambon, P. Trends Genet., *4*: 309–314, 1988.
48. Glass, C. K., Holloway, J. M., Devary, O. V., and Rosenfeld, M. G. Cell, *54*: 313–323, 1988.
49. Schüle, R., Muller, M., Otsuka-Murakami, H., and Renkawitz, R. Nature, *332*: 87–90, 1988.
50. Schüle, R., Muller, M. Kaltschmidt, C., and Renkawitz, R. Science, *242*: 1418–1420, 1988.
51. Strähle, U., Schmid, W., and Schütz, G. EMBO J., *7*: 3389–3395, 1988.
52. Ankenbauer, W., Strähle, U., and Schütz, G. Proc. Natl. Acad. Sci U.S.A., *85*: 7526–7530, 1988.
53. Richard-Goy, H. and Hager, G. L. EMBO J., *6*: 2321–2328, 1987.
54. Borkovich, K. A., Farrelly, F. W., Finkelstein, D. B., Taulien, J., and Lindquist, S. Mol. Cell. Biol., *9*: 3919–3930, 1989.
55. Gill, G. and Ptashne, M. Nature, *334*: 721–724, 1988.
56. Kerner, S. A., Scott, R. A., and Pike, J. W. Proc. Natl. Acad. Sci. U.S.A., *86*: 4455–4459, 1989.
57. Morrison, N. A., Shine, J., Fragonas, J.-C., Verkest, V., McMenemy, M. L., and Eisman, J. A. Science, *246*: 1158–1161, 1989.
58. Umesono, K. and Evans, R. M. Cell, *57*: 1139–1146, 1989.
59. Mader, S., Kumar, V., de Verneuil, H., and Chambon, P. Nature, *338*: 271–274, 1989.
60. Danielsen, M., Hinck, L., and Ringold, G. M. Cell, *57*: 1131–1138, 1989.
61. Hughes, M. R., Malloy, P. J., Kieback, D. G., Kesterson, R. A., Pike, J. W., Feldman, D., and O'Malley, B. W. Science, *242*: 1702–1705, 1988.
62. Berg, J. M. Science, *232*: 485–487, 1986.
63. Freedman, L. P., Luisi, B. F., Korszun, Z. R., Basavappa, R., Sigler, P. B., and Yamamoto, K. R. Nature, *334*: 543–546, 1988.
64. Severne, Y., Wieland, S., Schaffner, W., and Rusconi, S. EMBO J., *7*: 2503–2508, 1988.
65. Bonifer, C., Dahlman, K., Lanzer, M., Bujard, H., Flock, J.-I., and Gustafsson, J.-Å. *In;* G. Ringold (ed.), Steroid Hormone Action, pp. 201–209, Alan R. Liss, Inc., New

York, 1988.
66. Dahlman, K., Strömstedt, P.-E., Rae, C., Jörnvall, H., Flock, J.-I., Carlstedt-Duke, J., and Gustafsson, J.-Å. J. Biol. Chem., *264*: 804–809, 1989.
67. Bonifer, C., Dahlman, K., Strömstedt, P.-E., Flock, J.-I., and Gustafsson, J.-Å. J. Steroid Biochem., *32*: 5–11, 1989.
68. Ohara-Nemoto, Y., Strömstedt, P.-E., Dahlman-Wright, K., Nemoto, T., Gustafsson, J.-Å., and Carlstedt-Duke, J. J. Steroid Biochem. Mol. Biol., *37*: 481–490, 1990.
69. Wright, A. P. H., Carlstedt-Duke, J., and Gustafsson, J.-Å. J. Biol. Chem., *265*: 14763–14769, 1990.
70. Nemoto, T., Ohara-Nemoto, Y., Denis, M., and Gustafsson, J.-Å. Biochemistry, *29*: 1880–1886, 1990.
71. Carlstedt-Duke, J. and Gustafsson, J.-Å. J. Steroid Biochem., *31*: 593–597, 1988.
72. Carlstedt-Duke, J., Strömstedt, P.-E., Persson, B., Cederlund, E., Gustafsson, J.-Å., and Jörnvall, H. J. Biol. Chem., *263*: 6842–6846, 1988.
73. Strömstedt, P.-E., Berkenstam, A., Jörnvall, H., Gustafsson, J.-Å., and Carlstedt-Duke, J. J. Biol. Chem., *265*: 12973–12977, 1990.
74. Carlstedt-Duke, J., Strömstedt, P.-E., Dahlman, K., Rae, C., Berkenstam, A., Hapgood, J., Jörnvall, H., and Gustafsson, J.-Å. *In;* J. Carlstedt-Duke, H. Eriksson, and J.-Å. Gustafsson (eds.), The Steroid/Thyroid Hormone Receptor Family and Gene Regulation, pp. 93–108, Birkhäuser-Verlag, Basel, 1989.
75. Hagmar, P., Dahlman, K., Takahashi, M., Carlstedt-Duke, J., Gustafsson, J.-Å., and Nordén, B. FEBS Lett., *253*: 28–32, 1989.
76. Imai, E., Strömstedt, P.-E., Quinn, P. G., Carlstedt-Duke, J., Gustafsson, J.-Å., and Granner, D. Mol. Cell. Biol., *10*: 4712–4719, 1990.
77. Hess, P., Meenakshi, T., Chan, G. C.-K., Carlstedt-Duke, J., Gustafsson, J.-Å., and Payvar, F. Proc. Natl. Acad. Sci. U.S.A., *87*: 2564–2568, 1990.
78. Tsai, S. Y., Carlstedt-Duke, J., Weigel, N. L., Dahlman, K., Gustafsson, J.-Å., Tsai, M.-J., and O'Malley, B. W. Cell, *55*: 361–369, 1988.
79. Tsai, M.-J., Tsai, S. Y., Klein-Hitpass, L., Bagchi, M., Elliston, J. F., Carlstedt-Duke, J., Gustafsson, J.-Å., and O'Malley, B. W. Cold Spring Harbor Symp. Quant. Biol., *53*: 829–833, 1988.
80. Härd, T., Dahlman, K., Carlstedt-Duke, J., Gustafsson, J.-Å., and Rigler, R. Biochemistry, *29*: 5358–5364, 1990.
81. Dahlman-Wright, K., Siltala-Roos, H., Carlstedt-Duke, J., and Gustafsson, J.-Å. J. Biol. Chem., *265*: 14030–14035, 1990.
82. Dahlman-Wright, K., Wright, A., Gustafsson, J.-Å., and Carlstedt-Duke, J. J. Biol. Chem., *266*: 3107–3112, 1991.
83. Cairns, C., Gustafsson, J.-Å., and Carlstedt-Duke, J. Mol. Endocrinol., *5*: 598–604, 1991.
84. Härd, T., Kellenbach, E., Kaptein, R., Dahlman, K., Carlstedt-Duke, J., Freedman, L. P., Maler, B. A., Hyde, E., Gustafsson, J.-Å., and Yamamoto, K. R. Biochemistry, *29*: 9015–9023, 1990.
85. Härd, T., Kellenbach, E., Boelens, R., Maler, B. A., Dahlman, K., Freedman, L. P., Carlstedt-Duke, J., Yamamoto, K. R., Gustafsson, J.-Å., and Kaptein, R. Science, *249*: 157–160, 1990.

XENOBIOTICS AND CANCER, L. ERNSTER ET AL. (EDS.),
JAPAN SCI. SOC. PRESS, TOKYO/TAYLOR & FRANCIS LTD., LONDON, pp. 157–164, 1991

# Transcriptional and Posttranscriptional Regulation of CYP2E1, an *N*-nitrosodimethylamine Demethylase

Frank J. GONZALEZ and Harry V. GELBOIN

*Laboratory of Molecular Carcinogenesis, National Cancer Institute, National Institutes of Health, Bethesda, Maryland 20892, U.S.A.*

*Abstract:* CYP2E1 is a cytochrome P-450 that is well conserved in many species and carries out oxidation of both endogenous and numerous foreign chemicals. This enzyme is the primary component of the methylglyoxal and propandiol pathways of gluconeogenesis. It is also the principal P-450 involved in metabolism of many small molecular weight chemicals that are found in solvents and in the environment. Among important drugs metabolized by CYP2E1 are anesthetic agents such as halothane, the analgesic acetaminophen, and the muscle relaxant chlorzoxazone. Most importantly CYP2E1 is capable of converting certain procarcinogenic nitrosamines to their active DNA-binding metabolites. The *CYP2E1* gene becomes transcriptionally active in the liver soon after birth. Although the physiological stimulus for this increase is still unknown, the molecular basis of *CYP2E1* gene activation is becoming clear. Transcription of the *CYP2E1* gene is primarily due to the binding of the hepatocyte-specific transcription factor HNF-1 to a segment of DNA just upstream of the start site for RNA synthesis. In adult animals, CYP2E1 is posttranscriptionally regulated through mRNA and protein stabilization. Stabilization of CYP2E1 protein is due to interaction of the enzyme with its own substrate.

Cytochrome P-450s (450) represent a superfamily of enzymes that are found in bacteria, fungi, plant, and animals. P-450s are intrinsic membrane proteins ranging from 46–60 KDa in size containing a noncovalently-bound heme molecule. These enzymes are classified into families and subfamilies on the basis of amino acid sequence similarities. Between families, P-450s display less than 36% sequence similarities and enzymes within a single subfamily display more than 65% sequence similarly with another member of that subfamily. Ten P-450 gene families have been found in mammals. Six families encode enzymes involved in crucial pathways of steroidogenesis and cholesterol metabolism. The steroidogenic P-450s play no role in foreign compound metabolism. Among the steroidogenic P-450 families are mitochondrial and microsomal P-450s. The former are found in the inner mitochondrial membranes and receive electrons from the iron sulfur protein adrenodoxin through NADPH-adrenodoxin oxidoreductase. The microsomal P-450s use NADPH-P-450 oxidoreductase as an electron source. The molecular biology of P-450s has been reviewed (*1*).

P-450 nomenclature is based entirely on sequence relatedness attained by global alignments of primary amino acid sequences (*2*). The superfamily is given the root CYP (Cytochrome P-450) followed by a gene family number, a letter designating the subfamily and a number designating the gene number. Thus CYP1A1 is the number 1 P-450 in family 1, subfamily A.

One family of P-450s, designated CYP4, carry out $\omega$ and $\omega$-1 oxidation of numerous fatty acids, both natural fatty acids and those foreign to mammals. The physiologic role of these oxidations, if any, are currently unknown although the oxidation of biologically active eicosanoids may play a role in their degradation.

The remaining three families, designated CYP1, CYP2, and CYP3 are the principal P-450s involved in foreign compound metabolism. These enzymes are responsible for oxidation of foreign chemicals so that they can easily be eliminated from the body. Typically, hydrophobic foreign compounds are oxidized by P-450 and then conjugated with glucuronic acid, sulfate, glutathione, and other hydrophilic chemicals; these reactions serve to render chemicals more water soluble so that they can be eliminated through the bile or kidney. In some cases, highly reactive metabolic intermediates escape from the P-450 active site and can react with cellular macromolecules producing cell toxicity and sometimes transformation. Thus P-450s are the primary means for activation of procarcinogens and promutagens.

The CYP2 family consists of eight known subfamilies in mammals, designated CYP2A through CYP2H. From one to eight individual genes are found in these subfamilies. The number of genes and the catalytic activities of their encoded P-450s can display marked species differences. Even within a species, polymorphisms in P-450 expression and activities are known. Polymorphisms in CYP2 P-450s have been well documented in rats, mice, rabbits, and humans. Inter- and intraspecies variabilities in P-450 expression and catalytic activities suggest that these enzymes evolved primarily to metabolize foreign compounds and not to carry out metabolic functions crucial to the organism such as those of intermediary metabolism. There may, however, be exceptions to this generalization as indicated below. The lack of a physiological role of many P-450s, under circumstances where animals are not exposed to foreign compounds, is suggested by the findings that animals lacking a particular P-450, due to a polymorphism, appear to have normal life spans and reproductive vigor.

P-450s are under complex regulation both during development and in adults by foreign compound inducing agents. In fact, some P-450s can be induced by their own substrates. A number of different P-450 inducers have been found. The most well studied are the dioxins and polycyclic aromatic hydrocarbons that induce the *CYP1A1* gene through action of a specific cytosolic receptor. The hypolipidemic drugs such as clofibrate also activate the *CYP4A* genes *via* a specific cytosolic receptor protein (*3*). A steroid receptor is involved in transcriptional activation of *CYP3A* genes by synthetic steroids. The mechanism of action of another class of inducers regulating the *CYP2B* and *CYP3A* genes, with phenobarbital as a prototype, is unknown.

*Catalytic Activities and Metabolic Role of CYP2E1*

In contrast to many other P-450s in the *CYP2* family, CYP2E1 expression and its associated activities are well conserved in mammals. It has been postulated that CYP2E1 functions in the methylglyoxal and propanediol pathway of gluconeogenesis (*4, 5*), a pathway that may be important in the brain during periods of starvation (*6*). This potentially crucial metabolic role for CYP2E1 may explain its evolutionary conservation.

In addition to its role in intermediary metabolism, CYP2E1 also oxidizes numerous foreign chemicals (*7*). These include drugs—acetaminophen, chlorzoxazone, enflurane, halothane, and pyrazole, solvents—benzene, carbon tetrachloride, dichloromethane, pentane, and pyridine; carcinogens—*N*-nitrosodimethylamine, *N*-nitrosodiethylamine, and *N*-nitrosopyridine. CYP2E1 also oxidizes ethanol to acetaldehyde, although this is not the major enzyme of ethanol metabolism. Thus CYP2E1 can serve a useful purpose in gluconeogenesis while it also is capable of activating procarcinogens to their ultimate DNA-binding metabolites.

*Developmental Regulation of the CYPE1 Gene*

The *CYP2E1* gene becomes transcriptionally activated within a few hours after birth (*8*). The timing of this expression may be related to acquiring of glucose metabolism capabilities by the neonate (*7*). Other enzymes involved in glucose metabolism are also induced in liver after birth, however, many of these are regulated by insulin and glucagon through cyclic AMP (*9, 10*). No evidence exists that the *CYP2E1* gene is regulated by insulin or glucagon. Indeed, a binding site for the cyclic AMP regulated enhancer binding protein (CREP) was not found in the vicinity of the *CYP2E1* gene's transcription start site.

Transcriptional regulation of the *CYP2E1* gene has been difficult to study since its expression is extinguished in hepatoma cells and in primary hepatocyte cultures (*11*). Therefore regulation of this gene must be studied in whole animals. To study *CYP2E1* gene regulation, *in vitro* experiments were performed using liver tissue taken from rats of various ages. The procedure used for *in vitro* transcription is diagramed in Fig. 1. In this experiment extracts are prepared from liver nuclei from either adult or newborn rats. These transcription extracts can be used to accurately transcribe cloned gene templates. The transcripts can be quantified by use of primer extension assays. To study regulation of a test genes promoter, a second independently regulated promoter, for example that controlling the murine sarcoma virus (Msv), is analyzed in the same transcription reaction. The ratios of the two transcripts are then compared using different extracts.

*In vitro* transcription extracts prepared from liver nuclei were found to accurately transcribe *CYP2E1* gene templates (*12*). The gene was not transcribed by extracts isolated from livers of fetal rats or 1-day-old rats. Activity was only detected when extracts from 3-day-old and adult rats were examined. These *in vitro* transcription results reflect the expression of the *CYP2E1* gene in the intact animal.

Further studies, using DNA deletion analysis, *in vitro* transcription and direct DNA-protein binding studies revealed that the Hepatocyte-Specific Nuclear Factor-1

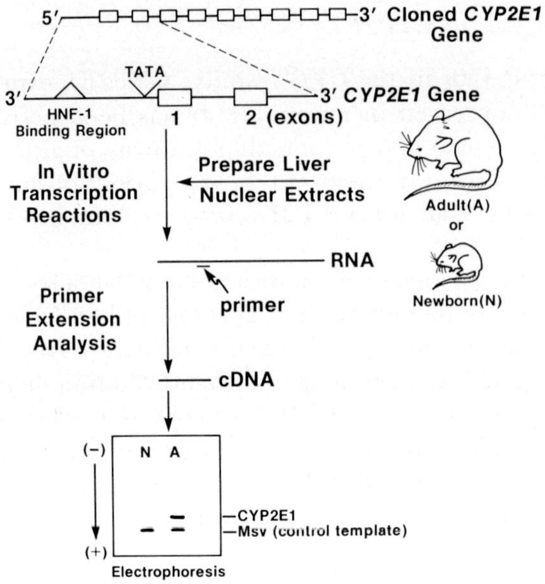


FIG. 1. *In vitro* transcription of the *CYP2E1* gene. Nuclear extracts are prepared from newborn or adult rat liver nuclei. A segment of the 5′ end of the cloned *CYP2E1* gene is used to direct transcription and RNA transcripts are isolated and quantified using primer extension analysis. The primer extended cDNA is then electrophoresed on high resolution DNA sequencing grade gels. A template containing the murine sarcoma virus (Msv) long terminal repeat promoter is analyzed in the same reaction tube as the *CYP2E1* gene and the ratio of *CYP2E1* to Msv gene-derived transcripts are determined.

(HNF-1) regulates transcription of the *CYP2E1* gene (*12*). This is one of many factors controlling transcription of liver genes (*13–15*).

The role of HNF-1 in regulation of the *CYP2E1* gene was also established *in vivo* using a strain of radiation deletion mice in which a 1.2 centiMorgan segment of chromosome 7 is deleted (*16*). Mice homozygous for this deletion die within a few days after birth. This premature death is due in part to liver disfunction. Heterozygous mice are phenotypically normal. Mutant mice can be identified by lack of eye pigment due to the deletion of the gene encoding tyrosinase. Heterozygous mice can also be distinguished on the basis of altered eye color.

Analysis of hepatic RNA from homozygous deletion mice revealed that expression of the *HNF-1* and *CYP2E1* genes were markedly reduced (*17*). Lack of significant expression is not due to their deletion in these animals since both genes are found in the mutant mouse genome. Expression of the β-actin gene in the mutant mouse livers was similar to that of heterozygous mice. These data indicate that HNF-1 controls expressions of the *CYP2E1* gene in the intact animal and further suggest that the deleted region of chromosome 7 encodes a gene controlling the *HNF-1* gene.

It is still unclear what signals or molecular events are responsible for *CYP2E1* gene activation soon after birth. The HNF-1 protein is found in nuclei of rats just before and immediately after birth at which time the *CYP2E1* gene is not expressed (*12*). The HNF-1 found in newborns is also able to bind to the *CYP2E1* gene regulatory sequence *in vitro*. However, gel mobility shift assays revealed that some of the HNF-1 protein in these livers has an altered gel mobility when bound to DNA as compared to that found in older animals having fully expressed *CYP2E1* gene. These data suggest that HNF-1 may be modified in livers of rats that do not express the *CYP2E1* gene. Alternatively, another protein may exists that interacts with HNF-1 and affects its ability to activate the *CYP2E1* gene. Another explanation is that HNF-1 does not bind to the *CYP2E1* regulatory region *in vivo*. These possibilities are currently being examined using DNase hypersensitivity assays and *in vivo* footprinting.

### *Induction of CYP2E1*

CYP2E1 was identified as an ethanol-inducible P-450 responsible for the microsomal ethanol oxidizing system, MEOS (*18*). This enzyme is induced by ethanol and a number of other small molecular weight compounds that are also substrates for the P-450. CYP2E1 is increased up to sixfold by giving rats ethanol or acetone but this increase is not accompanied by an elevation in its mRNA suggesting that it is posttranscriptionally regulated (*19*). When animals are made diabetic by treatment with streptozotocin or alloxan a marked increase in CYP2E1 mRNA is found in the absence of an increase in transcription (*20*). The mechanisms of mRNA stabilization is unknown. Substrate mediated induction, however, is beginning to be understood.

To examine the mechanism of CYP2E1 regulation by acetone, *in vivo* protein labeling was carried out using the protocol described in Fig. 2. Rats are given acetone in their drinking water for 1 week to maximally induce CYP2E1 protein. The animals are then injected with $^{14}C$-labeled sodium bicarbonate which is incorporated into several amino acids, most notable arginine. This amino acid is degraded in the urea cycle and thus is not reutilized for protein synthesis. Therefore, the rate of disappearance of the label from cellular CYP2E1 protein actually reflects the natural degradation rate of the enzyme. At various times after injection, the animals are killed and CYP2E1 is isolated using monoclonal antibody-based immunopurification. The specific radio activity of CYP2E1 protein at each time point after $^{14}C$-sodium bicarbonate injection is determined. Thus the turnover rates of degradation of the enzyme is measured in untreated and acetone-treated animals.

The rate of protein synthesis was found to be unaltered by acetone treatment indicating that the increase in protein accumulation in the absence of an mRNA increase was not due to an augmentation of translation rate. Analysis of the degradation rate of CYP2E1 protein revealed biphasic turnover with half-lives of about 7 hr and 36 hr in untreated rats (*21*). When rats are given acetone, the rapid turnover component is eliminated. These data indicate that acetone and probably other substrates stabilize the enzyme against degradation thus accounting for its elevation in treated animals.

The mechanism of substrate-induced stabilization may be due to phosphorylation by a cellular protein kinase. CYP2E1 can be phosphorylated *in vitro* at $Ser_{129}$ by the catalytic subunit of cyclic AMP-dependent protein kinase and this phosphorylation leads to its denaturation (*22*). Stimulation of cyclic AMP-dependent protein

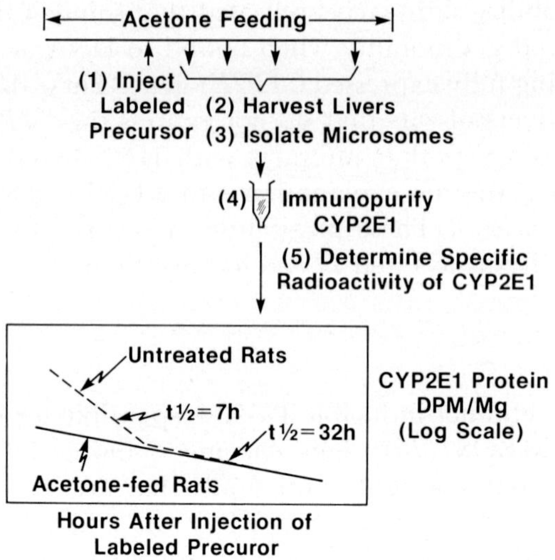


FIG. 2. Determination of the rate of degradation of CYP2E1 protein in untreated and acetone-fed rats. Rats are given acetone for 1 week prior to an injection of $^{14}$C-labeled sodium bicarbonate. Acetone treatment is continued throughout the course of the experiment. At various times after injection of the label, the rats are killed, livers excised and microsomes are isolated by differential centrifugation. The membrane proteins are made soluble with detergent and passed over a resin containing immobilized monoclonal antibody specific against CYP2E1. The purity of the preparations are ascertained using gel electrophoresis and the CYP2E1 protein from each time point is subjected to liquid scintillation counting to determine its specific radioactivity. The results are plotted Lot DPM/Mg CYP2E1 *vs.* time after administration of label. CYP2E1 in untreated rats is degraded with biphasic kinetics. In acetone treated rats, the rapid phase having a half-life ($t_{1/2}$) of 7 hr was eliminated leaving only the slow degradation phase of $t_{1/2}$ 32 hr. Thus, elimination of the rapid turnover component of CYP2E1 degradation by acetone treatment results in accumulation or induction of the enzyme.

kinase in isolated hepatocytes also leads to phosphorylation of CYP2E1. Most importantly, these phosphorylations are inhibited by the presence of various CYP2E1 substrates.

Phosphorylations of $Ser_{129}$ may destabilize the enzyme or otherwise serve as a tag for its degradation. Tagging or modification of proteins for degradation are known to play a general role in regulation of turnover (*23*). CYP2E1 and other P-450s can also be phosphorylated resulting in partial labilization *in vitro*, yet is unclear whether any enzyme is actually labelized by phosphorylation in intact cells. It is also uncertain whether phosphorylation plays a role in regulating CYP2E1 turnover in the intact animal.

*Conclusions*

CYP2E1 is an enzyme that is likely involved in an important endogenous pathway of gluconeogenesis in addition to playing a major role in oxidation of foreign compounds. This enzyme also has important toxicological and carcinogenic consequences since it can activated compounds such as carbon tetrachloride, acetaminophen, and low molecular weight nitrosamines to electrophilic metabolites. It is uncertain whether CYP2E1 is involved in nitrosamine-induced human cancers. However, levels of CYP2E1 can vary considerably in livers of different individuals (*24*). The drug chlorzoxazone may serve as a useful *in vivo* probe to measure levels of CYP2E1 in human populations to establish whether variable levels of the enzyme are genetically based or are due to induction and whether differences in *CYP2E1* gene expression are associated with susceptibility or risk to nitrosamine-induced human cancer.

The mechanism by which the *CYP2E1* gene is activated soon after birth is also not understood. More precise *in vivo* analysis of HNF-1 interaction with the CYP2E1 regulatory region in late gestation and newborn rats is required. The possibility of HNF-1 modification in the livers of these animals also needs to be evaluated.

The role of phosphorylation in substrate-induced stabilization must be confirmed *in vivo*. Indeed, this mechanism seems very attractive as a means for substrates to directly regulate levels of the enzyme. It also remains to be established whether CYP2E1 substrates act allosterically or whether they block phosphorylation of the protein by binding to the CYP2E1 active site.

Finally, the mechanism by which CYP2E1 mRNA is stabilized in diabetic animals remain a mystery. *In vivo* systems to measure RNA degradation must be designed in order to establish why the rate of CYP2E1 RNA degradation decreases under diabetic conditions.

## REFERENCES


1. Gonzalez, F. J. The molecular biology of cytochrome P450s. Pharmacol. Rev., *40*: 243, 1988.
2. Nebert, D. W., Nelson, D. R., Coon, M. J., Estabrook, D. W., Feyereisen, R., Fujii-Kuriyama, Y., Gonzalez, F. J., Guengerich, F. P., Gunsalus, I. C., Johnson, E. F., Loper, J. C., Sato, R., Waterman, M. R., and Waxman, D. J. The P450 superfamily: update on new sequences, gene mapping and recommended nomenclature. DNA and Cell Biol., *10*: 1, 1991.
3. Issemann, I. and Green, S. Activation of a member of the steroid hormone receptor superfamily by peroxysome proliferators. Nature, *347*: 645, 1990.
4. Casazza, J. P., Felver, M. E., and Veech, R. L. The metabolism of acetone in rat. J. Biol. Chem., *259*: 231, 1984.
5. Koop, D. R. and Casazza, J. P. Identification of ethanol-inducible P450 isozyme 3a as the acetone and acetol monooxygenase of rabbit microsomes. J. Biol. Chem., *260*: 13607, 1985.
6. Hansson, T., Tindberg, N., Ingelman-Sundberg, M., and Kohler, C. Regional distribution of ethanol-inducible cytochrome P450 IIE1 in the rat central nervous system. Neuroscience, *34*: 451, 1990.
7. Gonzalez, F. J., Ueno, T., Umeno, M., Song, B. J., Veech, R. L., and Gelboin, H. V. The microsomal ethanol oxidizing system: Transcriptional and post transcriptional regulation of cytochrome P450, CYP2E1. *In;* Proceedings of the International Society for Biomedical Research on Alcoholism, in press.
8. Umeno, M., Song, B. T., Kozak, C., Gelboin, H. V., and Gonzalez, F. T. The rat P450IIE1 gene: complete intron and exon sequences, chromosome mapping, and correlation of developmental expression with specific 5′ cytosine demethylation. J. Biol. Chem., *263*: 4956, 1988.

9. McKnight, S. L., Lane, S. D., and Gluecksohn-Waelsh, S. Is CCAAT/enhancer-binding protein a central regulator of energy metabolism? Genes Dev., *3*: 3021, 1989.
10. Granner, D. and Pilkis, S. The genes of hepatic glucose metabolism. J. Biol. Chem., *265*: 10173, 1990.
11. Schuetz, E. G., Li, D., Omiecinski, C. T., Muller-Eberhard, U., Kleinman, H. K., Elswick, B., and Guzelian, P. S. Regulation of gene expression in adult rat hepatocytes cultured on a basement membrane matrix. J. Cell Physiol., *134*: 309, 1988.
12. Ueno, T. and Gonzalez, F. T. Transcriptional control of the rat hepatic *CYP2E1* gene. Mol. Cell. Biol., *10*: 4495, 1990.
13. Johnson, P. F. Transcriptional activators in hepatocytes. Cell Growth Differ., *1*: 47, 1990.
14. Mueller, C. R., Maire, P., and Schibler, U. DBP, a liver enriched transcriptional activator is expressed late in ontogeny and its tissue specificity is determined post-transcriptionally. Cell, *61*: 279, 1990.
15. Descombes, P., Chojkier, M., Lichtsteiner, S., Falvey, E., and Schibler, U. LAP, as novel member of the C/EBP gene family, encodes as a liver-enriched transcription activator protein. Genes Dev., *4*: 1541, 1990.
16. Gluecksohn-Waelsch, S. Genetic control of morphogenic and biochemical differentiation: lethal albino deletions in the mouse. Cell, *16*: 225, 1979.
17. Gonzalez, F. J., Liu, S. Y., Kozak, C. A., and Nebert, D. W. Decreased Hnf-1 gene expression in mice homozygous for a 1.2-centiMorgan deletion chromosome 7. DNA and Cell Biol., *9*: 771, 1990.
18. Lieber, C. S. Mechanism of ethanol induced hepatic injury. Pharmacol. Ther., *46*: 1, 1990.
19. Song, B. J., Gelboin, H. V., Park, S. S., Yang, C. S., and Gonzalez, F. J. Complementary DNA and protein sequences of ethanol-inducible rat and human cytochrome P-450s: transcriptional and post-transcriptional regulation of the rat enzyme. J. Biol. Chem., *261*: 16689. 1987.
20. Song, B. J., Matsunaga, T., Hardwick, J. P., Park, S. S., Veech, R. L., Yang, C. S., Gelboin, H. V., and Gonzalez, F. J. Stabilization of cytochrome P450j messenger ribonucleic acid in the diabetic rat. Mol. Endocrinol., *1*: 542, 1987.
21. Song, B. J., Veech, R. L., Park, S. S., Gelboin, H. V., and Gonzalez, F. J. Induction of rat hepatic *N*-nitrosodimethylamine demethylase by acetone is due to protein stabilization. J. Biol. Chem., *264*: 3568, 1989.
22. Eliasson, E., Johansson, I., and Ingelman-Sundberg, M. Substrate-, hormone-, and cAMP-regulated cytochrome P450 degradation. Proc. Natl. Acad. Sci. U.S.A., *87*: 3225, 1990.
23. Stadtman, E. R. Covalent modification reactions are marking steps in protein turnover. Biochemistry, *29*: 6323, 1990.
24. Yoo, J.-S. H., Guengerich, F. P., and Yang, C. S. Metabolism of *N*-nitrosodialkylamines by human liver microsomes. Cancer Res., *88*: 1499, 1988.

XENOBIOTICS AND CANCER, L. ERNSTER ET AL. (EDS.),
JAPAN SCI. SOC. PRESS, TOKYO/TAYLOR & FRANCIS LTD., LONDON, pp. 165–175, 1991

# Transcriptional Regulation of 3-Methylcholanthrene-inducible P-450 Gene Responsible for Metabolic Activation of Aromatic Carcinogenes

Yoshiaki FUJII-KURIYAMA,*[1] Kazuhiro SOGAWA,*[1] Hiroaki IMATAKA,*[1] Ken-ichi YASUMOTO,*[1] Yasuo KIKUCHI,*[1] and Atsuko FUJISAWA-SEHARA*[2]

*Department of Chemistry, Faculty of Science, Tohoku University, Sendai 980, Japan*[1] *and National Center of Neurology and Psychiatry, Kodaira, Tokyo 187, Japan*[2]

*Abstract:* We have investigated the transcriptional regulation of 3-methylcholanthrene (3MC)-inducible P-450c gene which is involved in the metabolic activation of polycyclic aromatic carcinogens. Reverse genetic study using the fusion gene composed of the 5′ upstream sequence of P-450c gene and the structure gene for bacterial chloramphenicol acetyltransferase (CAT) and a cultured cell line of Hepa-1 cells localized two kinds of *cis*-acting regulatory DNA elements. One is designated XRE or xenobiotic responsive element which is responsible for the inducibility of the gene and is distributed 5 times in the region from −3.0 to −0.5 kb. The other is BTE or basal transcription element whose deletion reduces a low level of the constitutive CAT expression to a background level, and which is localized immediately upstream of the TATA sequence. Both kinds of regulatory elements are necessary for a high level of inducible expression. Gel mobility shift assay strongly suggests that the binding protein to the XRE is an Ah receptor with a specific affinity for 3MC or 2,3,7,8,tetrachlorodibenzo-*p*-dioxin (TCDD). Without inducer treatment, cryptic form of the binding protein occurs only in the cytoplasm of the Hepa-1 cells. Upon treatment with the inducer, the cryptic form of the binding protein exhibits binding activity to XRE and, at the same time, translocates to the nuclei. The BTE-binding protein is an ubiquitous nuclear factor and its cDNA cloning reveals the DNA-binding feature with zinc finger motifs.

Some forms of the P-450 superfamily are called drug-metabolizing enzymes and catalyze the first phase reaction in drug metabolism or monooxygenase reaction of various xenobiotics (*1*). Most of the oxidized compounds are detoxicated, but some others are activated to form unfavorable products to the host animals. More than 90% of the so-called chemical carcinogens are not carcinogenic in themselves, but acquire ultimate carcinogenicity upon oxidation by the action of these forms of P-450 (*2*). It has been suggested, therefore, that there is some relation between phenotypic expression of drug metabolizing P-450s and susceptibility to chemical carcinogenesis in human individuals as well as experimental animals (*3, 4*).

We have been interested in the regulatory mechanism of expression of 3-methylcholanthrene (3MC) or 2,3,7,8,tetrachlorodibenzo-*p*-dioxin (TCDD)-inducible

P-450c and d which are involved in the metabolic activation of polycyclic aromatic carcinogens and arylamines or heterocyclic amines, respectively. The two species of P-450 belong to the same superfamily and their genes are structurally related to each other (*5, 6*). Although these two genes have many inducers in common, distinct differences between them are recognized in transcriptional regulation. When a host animal is treated with the inducer, P-450c is not only expressed inducibly in liver, but also many extrahepatic tissues such as lung, skin, kidney, and others, while the expression of P-450d is limited to liver (*1, 7*). Isosafrole is a potent inducer for P-450d, but not for P-450c (*7, 8*). Primary cultures of hepatocytes maintain the inducibility of P-450c for a long time, but easily lose that of P-450d.

We have been studying the molecular mechanisms underlying the inducible expression of P-450c gene with the method of reverse genetics using a cell culture system of Hepa-1 and a chimeric gene of the chloramphenicol acetyltransferase (CAT) structural gene and the putative P-450c upstream regulatory sequence. We summarize here recent progress in our study on the regulatory expression of P-450c gene in response to the treatment with inducers.

Although studies on the regulatory mechanism of the P-450d gene have been hampered by the lack of a cultured cell line system suitable for its expression, a cultured HepG2 cell line has very recently been found to express the CAT activity from the transfected chimeric gene of the CAT gene and the P-450d upstream regulatory sequence (*9*). This expression system will open a way to approach the molecular mechanism of the transcriptional regulation of the P-450d gene, and will also provide an insight into the regulatory mechanisms common and specific to the P-450c and d genes.

## *Cis-acting Regulatory DNA Elements*

To investigate *cis*-acting regulatory elements in the P-450c gene, we constructed a fusion gene by placing the 5′ upstream flanking sequence (up to −6.3 kb) of this gene on the 5′ end of the bacterial CAT gene and then transfected it into cultured cell lines such as Hepa-1, H4IIE, and HeLa cells. These transfected cells were found to express the CAT activity in response to treatment with 3MC or TCDD. The induced CAT activity attained a maximal level of about 40 fold activity over the constitutive expression at 1 $\mu$M concentration of the inducer. It was therefore considered that the upstream sequence contained most, if not all, of the regulatory DNA elements of the P-450c gene (*10–12*).

To locate the regulatory elements of the P-450 gene, various external deletions were introduced into the upstream sequence of the fusion gene, and the mutated fusion genes were transfected into the Hepa-1 cells. The transfected cells were treated with 3MC for assay of the inducible expression of the CAT activity.

As shown in Fig. 1, there are about 3 regions whose deletion caused marked reduction in the induced CAT activity. These regions are between −3674 and −3067 bp, −1682 and −1429 bp, and −1139 and −1029 bp relative to the transcription start site. A small region between −1139 and −1029 bp appears to be especially important for the transcriptional regulation of the gene, because deletion of this region greatly reduced the inducibility expressed by the ratio of the induced to

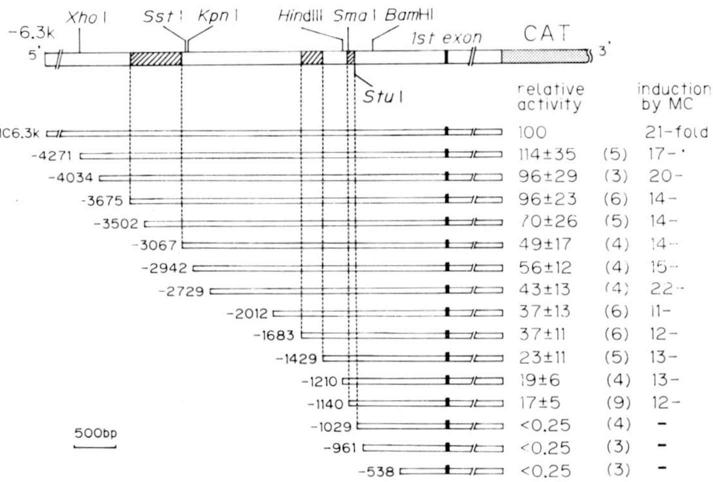


FIG. 1. Regulatory activity of the upstream sequence of P-450c gene. The upstream sequence of P-450c gene was placed on the 5′ end of the CAT structural gene (indicated by a stippled bar) to construct a fusion gene. Various external deletions were introduced into the upstream sequence and the deletion mutants in the fusion gene were transfected into Hepa-1 cells for expression of the CAT activity. The 5′ end of the upstream sequence is numbered in negative from the transcription start site. Relative activity indicates the CAT activity from each of the mutated fusion genes in the presence of 3MC relative to that of the original fusion gene, pMC6.3k. The number of experiments with each deletion plasmid is shown in parenthesis. The extent of induction by 3MC is shown by the ratio of the induced activity to the non-induced activity. The DNA sequences whose deletion caused marked reduction in the induced CAT activity are indicated by hatched areas.

the non-induced CAT activity as well as the level of the fully induced activity (*12*).

We isolated the small region −1140 to −844 bp and placed it in both directions on the 5′ or 3′ end of the fusion gene consisting of SV40 promoter and the CAT structural gene. The Hepa-1 cells transfected with these fusion genes expressed the CAT activity in response to treatment with 3MC, thus suggesting location of inducible enhancer sequences in this fragment. To define a core sequence of the inducible enhancer, we divided the regulatory sequence of −1140 to −844 bp into various short fragments and placed them separately on the 5′ end of the SV40 promoter of the fusion gene. The two halves of the sequence (SmSt and StBm) retained the enhancer activity in response to 3MC as shown in Fig. 2. Further subdivision of these fragments allowed us to define the core sequences essential for the inducible enhancer activity. Two fragments (StBn from −1029 to −997 bp and NhGn from −1092 to −1069 bp) as small as 33 and 24 bp, respectively, were found to express the enhancer activity in response to the inducer. Eventually, the 24 bp fragment generated an active fragment of the indicible enhancer of 15 bp by further subdivision. Further deletion of 4 bp from the 5′ end of the N15 fragment abolished the inducible enhancer activity and may suggest that this fragment contains the minimal requirement for the activity (*13*).

Comparison of the DNA sequence between the two active subfragments (StBn and NhFn) in both orientations revealed the presence of a common sequence of TCACGC with some common nucleotides intermittently distributed in its flanking

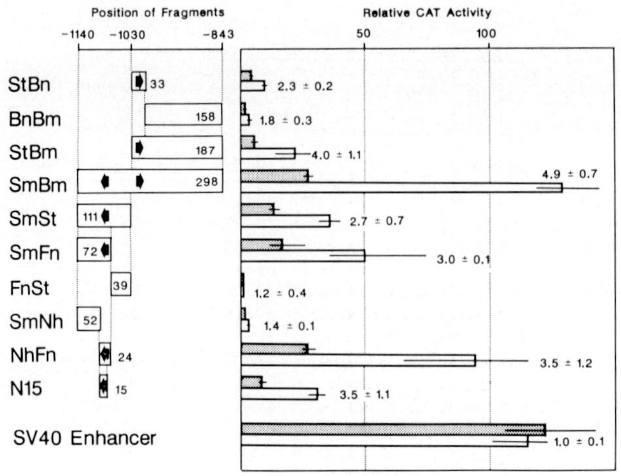


FIG. 2. Inducible enhancer activity of DNA fragments in the upstream sequence of P-450c gene. Various subfragments of the sequence of −1140 to −844 bp were placed on the 5′ end of the fusion gene consisting of SV40 promoter sequence and the CAT structural gene, and the constructed fusion genes were transfected into Hepa-1 cells. Open boxes to the right of the fragment names indicate their lengths and positions in the original gene. Arrows in the boxes indicate the position and orientation of XREs. The length of bars on the left side indicates the corrected activity which is expressed as the ratio of the CAT activity from the subfragment-containing fusion gene to that of the fusion gene consisting of SV40 promoter and the CAT gene. Open and stippled bars represent the corrected CAT activities in the presence and absence of 3MC, respectively, and the figures show the inducibility of the chimeric genes expressed in the ratio of the induced to the non-induced CAT activity with standard deviation.

```
ggatcCCTCCAGGCTCTTCTCACGCAACTCCGGGCACgatc     XRE1 (-1029/-997)
          I    I  I IIIIIII I
gatcCGGGTCCCAGTGCTCTCACGCTAGgatccccgggtacc    XRE2 (-1069/-1092)
```

FIG. 3. Comparison of nucleotide sequence of XRE1 and XRE2. XRE1 and XRE2 correspond to the DNA fragments of StBn and NhFn (see Fig. 2), respectively. Sequences of the plus and minus strands of XRE1 and XRE2 were compared. Small letters indicate flanking polylinker sequences.

region (Fig. 3). The two homologous sequences are inversely oriented with each other in the original regulatory fragment (SmBm). These observations led us to designate the homologous sequences xenobiotic responsive elements or XRE. The sequences derived from StBm and NhFn were denoted XRE1 and XRE2, respectively. Survey of the upstream sequence of the P-450c gene localized other XRE-homologous sequences at the −537, −1233, and −3586 bp positions. Interestingly, these XRE-homologous sequences are localized in the regions whose deletion caused marked reduction in the induced CAT activity, and were proved to bind the XRE-binding factor or Ah-receptor by the competitive gel mobility shift assay, as will be described (*14*).

When the external deletion from the 5′ end of the upstream regulatory sequence in the fusion gene further proceeded to the region proximal to the TATA sequence, the fusion gene had already lost substantial inducibility in response to the inducers, but retained the constitutive expression. The progressive deletion beyond −53 bp in

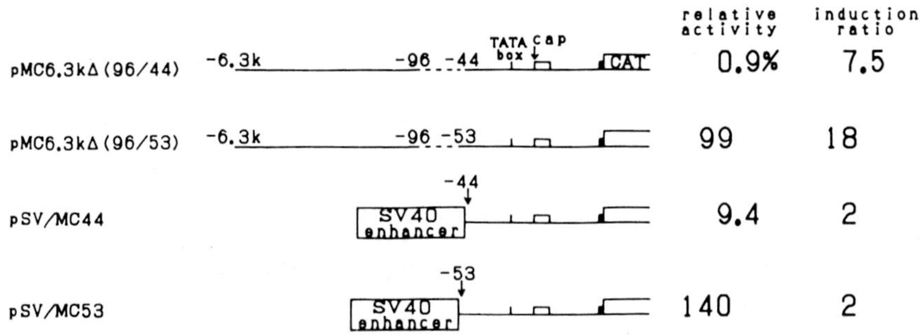


FIG. 4. Effect of the BTE region on expression of the CAT fusion gene. Relative activity is expressed as the percentage of the CAT activity relative to that of the original plasmid pMC6.3 k in the presence of 3MC. The inducibility of the gene is shown by induction ratios as described in the legend to Fig. 2.

the upstream sequence of the gene lost the constitutive expression of the fusion gene. The CAT activities expressed from small internal deletion mutants from −96 to −53 bp and from −96 to −44 bp also suggested the presence of another DNA element of transcriptional regulation (Fig. 4). This reduced CAT activity from the deletion mutant from −96 to −44 bp appeared to be due to lowered basal expression rather than to decreased inducibility, because the induction ratio was not so much influenced in the deletion mutant. The reduced CAT expression by the deletion from −53 to −44 bp was also clearly demonstrated by the augmented constitutive expression when the SV40 enhancer was placed at the 5′ end of the −44 bp and −53 bp fusion genes.

The SV40 enhancer sequence placed on the 5′ end of the −53 bp fusion gene constitutively expressed enhanced CAT activity, while less than 1/10 of the activity was expressed from the −44 bp fusion gene with the SV40 enhancer sequence placed on its 5′ end. Thus, we concluded that another *cis*-acting DNA element involved in the transcriptional regulation is present in the region −53 to −44 bp and designated this sequence basic transcription element or BTE (*15*, *16*).

### *Trans-acting Factors Binding to the XRE Sequence*

To detect factors that interact with the XRE sequence, we performed gel mobility shift assay using nuclear extracts from Hepa-1 cells with or without 3MC treatment for 10 hr. When the DNA fragment containing XRE-1 was used as a probe, a specific retarded band was observed with the nuclear extract from the 3MC-treated cells. It was found that not only 3MC but also TCDD could induce the band with the same mobility. This band could not be detected, however, with the nuclear extract from non-treated Hepa-1 cells, 3MC-treated C4 (a mutant of Hepa-1 defective in the xenobiotic receptor function), L929 fibroblast or HTC cells which are rather insensitive to the inducer for the expression of the P-450c gene. Thus, the presence of the nuclear factor specifically interacting with the XRE is intimately correlated with the inducible expression of the XRE-driven CAT or endogenous P-450c (*14*).

We next asked whether or not this DNA-binding factor was liganded with the inducer, 3MC or TCDD. Hepa-1 cells were cultured in the presence of [$^3$H]-TCDD (0.1 $\mu$M) for 10 hr and then nuclear extracts were prepared from the cells. These extracts were incubated with unlabeled XRE and applied to gel electrophoresis together with the nuclear extracts incubated with $^{32}$P-labeled XRE probe in parallel The prominent peak of [$^{3}$H]-TCDD coincided exactly with the position of the $^{32}$P-labeled XRE bound with the cognate DNA-binding factor (data not shown), while such a peak of [$^{3}$H]-radioactivity could not be detected when the extract was incubated in the absence of the XRE; this suggests that the XRE-binding factor is an xenobiotic receptor itself or includes the receptor as a component of the XRE-binding complex. On the other hand, no radioactive peak of [$^{3}$H]-TCDD was observed when the cytoprasmic fraction of the treated cells was incubated with the XRE, showing the nuclear localization of the ligand-bound receptors with the XRE-binding activity in the treated cells (*14*).

From the suggestion that the XRE-binding factor was associated with the xenobiotic inducer in the treated nuclei, it was reasonable to suppose that induction of the XRE-binding factor in nuclei is triggered by binding of the ligands to the receptor. In our investigation of the induction of the XRE-binding factor in the cell-free system, the cytoplasmic fraction and nuclear extract prepared from non-treated Hepa-1 cells were separately incubated with 3MC to examine the induction of the XRE-binding activity. Although the activity was absent in the non-treated cytoplasmic fraction *per se*, incubation of the cytoplasmic fraction with 3MC resulted in induction of this activity that gave a retarded band of the XRE with the same mobility as the nuclear factor from the inducer-treated cells (Fig. 5A, lanes 3 and 4). More than 2 hr of incubation was necessary to induce maximal DNA-binding activity at 25°C (Fig. 5C), and the concentration of 3MC necessary for this maximal level was 1 $\mu$M (Fig. 5B), roughly the same as the optimal concentration for the transcriptional activation of P-450c gene in Hepa-1 cells. On the other hand, the XRE-binding factor was absent in the nuclei from non-treated cells, because the retarded band was undetectable even after incubation with 3MC. In contrast to the case of the non-treated cells, the XRE-binding factor was dramatically decreased in the cytoplasmic fraction upon treatment of the cells, and concomitantly appeared in the nuclear extract. The XRE-binding factor, a small amount of which remained in the cytoplasm, was not increased at all by incubation with 3MC. Thus, the results show that 3MC induces the XRE-binding activity in the preexisting cryptic factor and suggest that, at the same time, the activated factor-ligand complex is translocated to the nuclei (*14, 17*). This cryptic XRE-binding factor in the cytoplasm has been found associated with a heat shock protein, HSP90 (*18, 19*), as reported with steroid hormone receptors (*20, 21*).

*Trans-acting Factor Binding to the BTE Sequence*

To investigate the regulatory factor(s) binding to the BTE sequence, gel mobility shift assay was performed using the synthetic oligonucleotide containing the −59 to −40 bp sequence as a probe. The BTE-containing DNA fragment gave approximately three retarded bands in the gel electrophoresis, when incubated with the nuclear extracts from Hepa-1 cells. Although the molecular mechanism giving rise to these three bands has not yet been determined, it is clear that all were retarded in the gel electrophoresis by the sequence-specific interactions between the BTE sequence

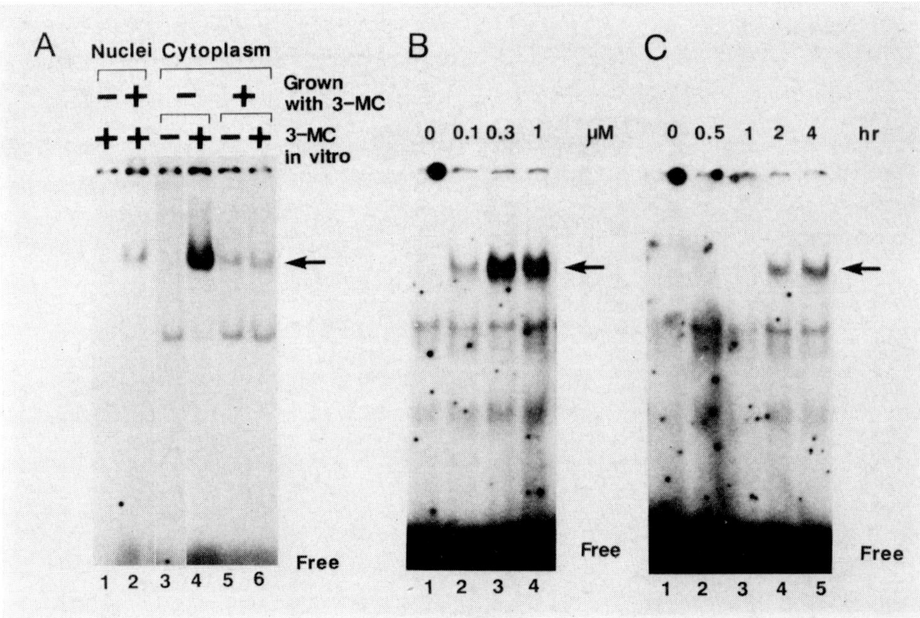


FIG. 5. Gel mobility shift assay of XRE and the XRE-binding factor. (A) Induction of XRE-binding factor *in vitro*. Nuclear extracts (lanes 1 and 2) or cytoplasmic fractions (lanes 3–6) prepared from Hepa-1 cells grown in the absence (lanes 1, 3, and 4) or presence (lanes 2, 5, and 6) of 3MC were incubated with (lanes 1, 2, 4, and 6) or without (lanes 3 and 5) 3MC *in vitro*. An arrow indicates inducible bands. (B) Concentration of 3MC required for induction of XRE-binding factor *in vitro*. Cytoplasmic fraction prepared from non-treated Hepa-1 cells was incubated for 2 hr with 0 to 1 μM of 3MC. An arrow indicates inducible bands. (C) Time course of induction of XRE-binding factor *in vitro*. Cytoplasmic fraction prepared from non-treated Hepa-1 cells was incubated with 1 μM of 3MC *in vitro* for the indicated time periods at 20°C.

and the binding factor(s), because excess amounts of the cold BTE probe competed efficiently with the labeled probe for the DNA-binding factor(s), while two base substitutions (GGAGGCGTGGCCAAC) to (GGAGGCCTCGCCAAC) in the BTE sequence were not competitive (*16*).

Figure 6 shows the result of the DNase I footprint analysis using $^{32}$P-end labeled DNA fragment (−162 to +44 bp) containing the BTE sequence and nuclear extract from Hepa-1 cells. The $^{32}$P-labeled DNA fragment was incubated with the nuclear extract and then the reaction mixture was digested by addition of DNase I. The digested DNA fragment was applied to gel electrophoresis. DNase protection was clearly observed in the regions containing the BTE sequence from −61 to −41 bp in the plus strand and from −56 to −41 bp in the minus strand (Fig. 6). The nuclear extracts from the cells with or without inducer treatment gave the same DNase I footprinting pattern. Both strands in another region from −147 to −122 bp were also protected from DNase I digestion, suggesting the presence of another DNA-binding factor interacting with the sequences; the role of this region in the transcriptional regulation of the P-450c gene, however, remains to be determined.

We investigated the distribution of the DNA-binding factor(s) in nuclear extracts from various cells, not only liver cells and hepatocyte cell lines but also lymphocyte-

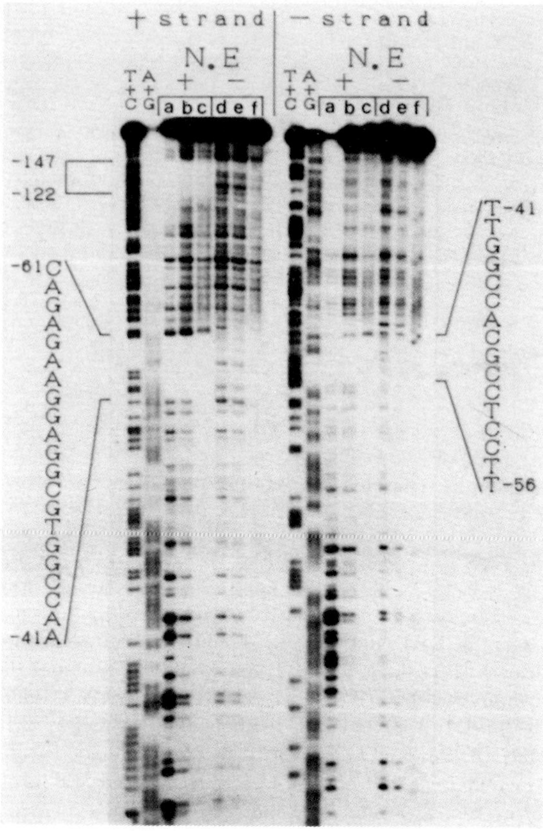


FIG. 6. DNase I footprint analysis of the promoter region of P-450c gene. $^{32}P$ end-labeled DNA fragment from −166 to +42 bp of P-450c gene was incubated with nuclear extracts from non-treated Hepa-1 cells and then digested by various concentrations of DNase I. Lanes a to c show digestion by 0.6, 0.3, and 0.15U of DNase I, respectively, and lanes d to f, digestion by 0.6, 0.3, and 0.15U of DNase I without nuclear extracts.

derived EL4, EC cell line P19 and L929 cells which do not express P-450c. These nuclear extracts were found to give retarded bands of the BTE sequence with the same mobility as those observed with nuclear extracts from Hepa-1 cells (data not shown). It is suggested, therefore, that the BTE-binding factor(s) is not unique to the cells expressing the endogenous P-450c gene, but may function as a sort of ubiquitous transcriptional regulatory factor for other genes as well (*16*).

In searching for homologous sequences to the BTE in the region proximal to the TATA sequence of other genes, we found several such sequences in equivalent positions on various genes, most prominently genes belonging to the P-450 superfamily which show different modes of gene regulation (Fig. 7); they are inducible by phenobarbital (P-450b and P-450e), ethanol (P-450j), and an endogenous effector, cyclic AMP (P-450SCC and P-450C21).

To investigate its properties in detail, we attempted to purify the BTE-binding factor(s) from the nuclei of rat livers or to isolate the cDNA clone for the BTE-binding factor mRNA. Although purification of the factor has not yet been successful because

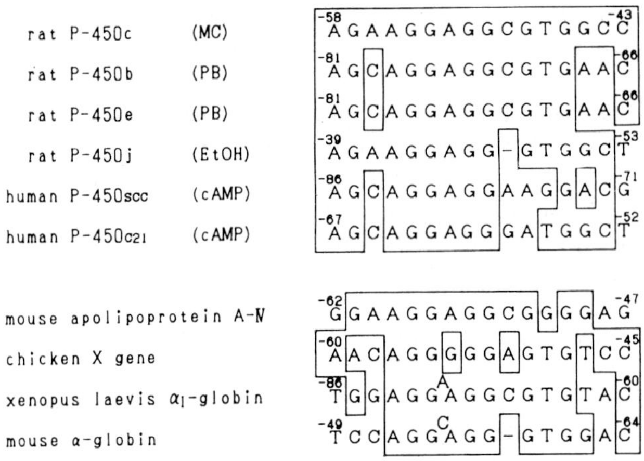


FIG. 7. Analogous sequences to BTE in the region proximal to the TATA sequence of other genes. Minus numbers are the positions of nucleotides counted from the transcription initiation site. Nucleotides identical to those in the BTE are enclosed by solid lines.

of its unusual lability, two kinds of cDNA clones were isolated from a cDNA library of rat liver mRNA in λgt11 vector using the BTE sequence as a probe. One is considered to be a cDNA clone for rat Sp1, because the amino acid sequence encoded by the cDNA shows about 95% sequence similarity to the sequence of human Sp1. The reason why Sp1 cDNA clone was isolated by this method is that the BTE sequence shows some similarity to the GC-box sequence. The other clone is tentatively designated a cDNA for the BTE-binding protein, because the bacterially expressed protein from the latter cDNA in an expression vector bound the BTE sequence with high affinity and gave the same DNase 1 footprinting as the liver nuclear extracts (data not shown). Sequence analysis of the cDNA shows that a motif of 3-time repeated zinc finger structure features the BTE-binding protein (*22*). It remains of interest to see whether this factor acts as an activator or repressor to expression of the P-450c gene. The detailed mechanism of the BTE binding protein in the transcriptional regulation of P-450c gene (especially its cooperation with the XRE-binding factor and the significance of its sharing the same DNA sequence with the Sp1) will be elucidated in future.

*Acknowledgments*

This work was initiated in the Department of Biochemistry, Cancer Institute, Japanese Foundation for Cancer Research, when Y. Fujii-Kuriyama, K. Sogawa, and A. Fujisawa-Sehara worked there during 1985–1987, and was supported in part by Grants in Aid of Scientific Research from the Ministry of Education, Science and Culture of Japan, and Research Grants from the Ministry of Health and Welfare of Japan and the Princess Takamatsu Cancer Research Fund.

REFERENCES

1. Gonzalez, F. J. Molecular genetics of the P-450 superfamily. Pharmacol. Ther., *45*: 1–38, 1989.
2. Kato, R. Metabolic activation of mutagenic heterocyclic aromatic amines from protein pyrolysates. CRC Crit. Rev. Toxicol., *16*: 307–348, 1986.

3. Legraverend, C., Mansour, B., Nebert, D. W., and Holland, J. M. Genetic differences in benzo[a]pyrene-initiated tumorigenesis in mouse skin. Pharmacology, *20*: 242–255, 1980.
4. Ayesh, R., Idle, J. R., Ritchie, J. C., Crothers, M. J., and Hetzel, M. R. Metabolic oxidation phenotypes as markers for susceptibility to lung cancer. Nature, *312*: 169–170, 1984.
5. Sogawa, K., Gotoh, O., Kawajiri, K., and Fujii-Kuriyama, Y. Complete nucleotide sequence of a methylcholanthrene inducible cytochrome P-450 (P-450d) gene in the rat. J. Biol. Chem., *260*: 5026–5032, 1985.
6. Gonzalez, F. J., Kimura, S., and Nebert, D. W. Comparison of the flanking regions and introns of the 2, 3, 7, 8-tetrachlorodibenzo-*p*-dioxin inducible cytochrome $P_1$-450 and $P_3$-450 genes. J. Biol. Chem., *260*: 5040–5049, 1985.
7. Whitlock, J. P., Jr. The regulation of cytochrome P-450 gene expression. Annu. Rev. Pharmacol. Toxicol., *26*: 333–369, 1986.
8. Ryan, D. E., Thomas, P. E., and Levin, W. Hepatic microsomal cytochrome P-450 from rats treated with isosafrol: purification and characterization of four forms. J. Biol. Chem., *255*: 7941–7955, 1980.
9. Quattrochi, L. C. and Tukey, R. H. The human cytochrome CypIA2 gene contains regulatory elements responsive to 3-methylcholanthrene. Mol. Pharmacol., *36*: 66–71, 1989.
10. Jones, P. B. G., Galeazzi, D. R., Fisher, J. M., and Whitlock, J. P., Jr. Control of cytochrome P1-450 gene expression by dioxin. Science, *227*: 1499–1502, 1985.
11. Fujisawa-Sehara, A., Sogawa, K., Nishi, C., and Fujii-Kuriyama, Y. Regulatory DNA elements localized remotely upstream from the drug-metabolizing cytochrome P-450 gene. Nucl. Acids Res., *14*: 1465–1477, 1986.
12. Sogawa, K., Fujisawa-Sehara, A., Yamane, M., and Fujii-Kuriyama, Y. Location of regulatory elements responsible for drug induction in the rat cytochrome P-450c gene. Proc. Natl. Acad. Sci. U.S.A., *83*: 8044–8048, 1986.
13. Fujisawa-Sehara, A., Sogawa, K., Yamane, M., and Fujii-Kuriyama, Y. Characterization of xenobiotic responsive elements upstream from the drug-metabolizing cytochrome P-450c gene; a similarity to glucocorticoid regulatory element. Nucl. Acids Res., *15*: 4179–4191, 1987.
14. Fujisawa-Sehara, A., Yamane, M., and Fujii-Kuriyama, Y. A DNA-binding factor specific for xenobiotic responsive elements of P-450c gene exists as a cryptic form in cytoplasm: its possible translocation to nucleus. Proc. Natl. Acad. Sci. U.S.A., *85*: 5859–5863, 1988.
15. Neuhold, L. A., Shirayoshi, Y., Ozato, K., Jones, J. J., and Nebert, D. W. Regulation of mouse CYP1A1 gene expression by dioxin: requirement of two *cis*-acting elements during induction. Mol. Cell. Biol., *9*: 2378–2386, 1989.
16. Yanagida, A., Sogawa, K., Yasumoto, K., and Fujii-Kuriyama, Y. A novel *cis*-acting DNA element required for a high level of inducible expression of the rat P-450c gene. Mol. Cell. Biol., *10*: 1470–1475, 1990.
17. Wilhelmsson, A., Cuthill, S., Denis, M., Wikström, A.-C., Gustafsson, J.-Å., and Poellinger, L. The specific DNA binding activity of the dioxin receptor is modulated by the 90 kd heat shock protein. EMBO J., *9*: 69–76, 1990.
18. Denis, M., Cuthill, S., Wikström, A.-C., Poellinger, L., and Gustafsson, J.-Å. Association of the dioxin receptor with the Mr 90,000 heat shock protein: a structural kinship with the glucocorticoid receptor. Biochem. Biophys. Res. Commun., *155*: 801–807, 1988.
19. Perdew, G. H. Association of the Ah receptor with the 90-kDa heat shock protein. J.

Biol. Chem., *263*: 13802–13805, 1988.
20. Denis, M., Poellinger, L., Wikström, A.-C., and Gustafsson, J.-Å. Requirement of hormone for thermal conversion of the glucocorticoid receptor to a DNA-binding state. Nature, *333*: 686–688, 1988.
21. Tienaungroj, W., Meohinchi, S., Sanchez, E. R., Pratt, S. E., Grippo, J. F., Holmgren, A., and Pratt, W. B. The role of sulfhydryl groups in permitting transformation and DNA binding of the glucocorticoid receptor. J. Biol. Chem., *262*: 6992–7000, 1987.
22. Imataka, H., Sogawa, K., and Fujii-Kuriyama, Y. Unpublished observation.

XENOBIOTICS AND CANCER, L. ERNSTER ET AL. (EDS.),
JAPAN SCI. SOC. PRESS, TOKYO/TAYLOR & FRANCIS LTD., LONDON, pp. 177–187, 1991

# Regulation of Enzymes that Detoxify the Electrophilic Forms of Chemical Carcinogens

Paul TALALAY, Hans J. PROCHASKA, and Sharon R. SPENCER

*Department of Pharmacology and Molecular Sciences, School of Medicine, The Johns Hopkins University, Baltimore, Maryland 21205, U.S.A.*

*Abstract:* Most chemical carcinogens require activation to reactive electrophilic forms by Phase 1 enzymes (cytochromes P-450) in order to exert their toxic and neoplastic effects. The resultant electrophiles are susceptible to metabolic conjugation and other types of detoxications by Phase 2 enzymes (glutathione transferases, NAD(P)H: quinone reductase, glucuronosyltransferases). The balance between Phase 1 and Phase 2 enzymes is an important determinant of whether exposure to carcinogens will result in toxicity and neoplasia. Measurements of the activity of quinone reductase (QR) provide an efficient method for studying the potency and mechanism of Phase 2 enzyme induction. QR can be measured easily in murine hepatoma cells (Hepa lclc7) grown in microtiter plate wells, and the inductive response of these cells closely parallels the behavior of rodent tissues *in vivo*. Some inducers (such as large planar aromatics) are bifunctional; they induce both Phase 1 and Phase 2 enzymes and require binding to the *Ah* receptor and enhanced transcription of the cytochrome $P_1$-450 system. Other inducers (*e.g.*, phenolic antioxidants, 1, 2-dithiole-3-thiones, coumarins, thiocarbamates) are monofunctional and are independent of *Ah* receptor function. Monofunctional enzyme induction protects against carcinogens. The induction of Phase 2 enzymes by monofunctional inducers depends on the presence, or acquisition by metabolism, of electrophilic centers, and many of these inducers are Michael reaction acceptors. Our search for chemoprotective enzyme inducers for potential use as chemoprotectors in man is currently focused on fumarate derivatives, as well as on the identification of other monofunctional inducers in extracts of vegetables.

Despite much recent progress in our understanding of the fundamental nature of malignancy and advances in early diagnosis and management of human cancer, it is difficult to demonstrate significant progress in reducing the incidence or prolonging the survival of patients with most common types of cancer. Since, however, the majority of human neoplasms are related causally to extrinsic ("extra-constitutional") factors, much human cancer is, in principle, avoidable (*1*). Furthermore, experiments in animals document that a variety of chemical agents block the effects of many different types of carcinogens (*2–4*), a process designated *chemoprotection*. Hence, we believe that human cancer risk can be reduced by two approaches: reduction, and if possible elimination, of exposure to extrinsic carcinogens, *i.e.*, *prevention*; and administration of chemical agents that lower the susceptibility of tissues to the toxic and neoplastic effects of carcinogens, *i.e.*, *chemoprotection.* Protective measures are especially important because, apart from well-defined risk factors such as cigarette smoking, the unequivocal identification of most extrinsic carcinogens is complex and controversial (*5–7*).

Chemical carcinogenesis comprises multiple events that may be operationally dissected into initiation, promotion, conversion, and progression. These processes require considerable time and involve genetic damage, cell proliferation, and clonal selection and expansion. It is therefore not surprising that there are multiple opportunities for blocking carcinogenesis, and that a number of strategies for achieving protection are being pursued. Our laboratory has focused on the modulation of carcinogenesis by modification of the metabolism of carcinogens.

The great majority of chemical carcinogens require metabolic activation by Phase 1 enzymes (mostly certain cytochromes P-450) to their ultimate (electrophilic) carcinogenic forms that damage DNA and initiate tumor formation. However, these ultimate electrophiles are subject to metabolic disposal by Phase 2 enzymes (glutathione transferases, NAD(P)H: quinone reductase, glucuronosyltransferases, *etc.*) which bring about detoxication because their products are less reactive and more easily excreted. Consequently, whether most carcinogens manifest their toxic and/or neoplastic effects is in part dependent upon the balance between Phase 1 and Phase 2 enzymes. These conclusions are supported by the finding that genetically defined mice lacking certain cytochromes P-450 show reduced susceptibility to carcinogens (*8*), and that elevation of Phase 2 enzymes generally results in protection (*4*).

*Role of Phase 2 Enzyme Induction in Protection against Chemical Carcinogenesis*

Administration of an extraordinary variety of chemical compounds to animals protects against the toxic and neoplastic effects of an equally diverse group of chemical carcinogens. These chemoprotectors include not only small doses of polycyclic aromatics (many of which are also carcinogens), but also azo dyes, phenolic antioxidants (*e.g.*, [2(3)-*tert*-butyl-4-hydroxyanisole] (BHA)), naturally occurring lactones such as coumarins and α-methylenebutyrolactone, flavonoids, organic isothiocyanates, thiocarbamates (*e.g.*, disulfiram, diethyldithiocarbamate, bisethylxanthogen), 1,2-dithiole-3-thiones, indoles, and cinnamates (*2–3*). Thus chemoprotectors appear to be structurally quite dissimilar and include both synthetic and natural products. Notably, some are already intrinsic minor constituents of the human diet, or have been added as preservatives or as condiments.

Many experiments performed in the last decade have shown that the abovementioned types of chemoprotectors have one common property: they are inducers of enzymes of xenobiotic metabolism, and much evidence is accumulating that this biological property is central to the mechanisms of their chemoprotective activities (*4, 9*).

Chemoprotective enzyme inducers belong to two families which we have designated as *monofunctional* and *bifunctional* (*10*). Monofunctional inducers, such as phenolic antioxidants, 1,2-dithiole-3-thiones, aromatic isothiocyanates, and thiocarbamates, elevate Phase 2 enzymes selectively without major effects on tissue levels of Phase 1 enzymes (*e.g.*, aryl hydrocarbon hydroxylase). Moreover, monofunctional inducers act independently of the *Ah* receptor. In contrast, bifunctional inducers, such as 2,3,7,8-tetrachlorodibenzo-*p*-dioxin (TCDD), polycyclic aromatic hydrocarbons, azo dyes, and flavonoids, are ligands for the *Ah* receptor, and cause increases in the activities of both Phase 1 and Phase 2 enzymes. Since certain cytochromes P-450 play an important role in the activation of carcinogens, whereas elevation of Phase 2 enzymes alone is a sufficient condition for chemoprotection, it is desirable that chemoprotectors be monofunctional rather than bifunctional inducers.

*Experimental Systems for Study of Phase 2 Enzyme Induction*

Since there is compelling evidence that selective Phase 2 enzyme induction results in a chemoprotected state, our laboratory has focused on the molecular mechanisms by which the above-mentioned compounds induce Phase 2 enzymes with the goal of designing effective, potent, and nontoxic anticarcinogens. Elucidation of the mechanisms of induction of Phase 2 enzymes and their role in protection against toxic electrophiles required the development of suitable cell culture systems and an appropriate and easily-measurable enzyme to serve as a representative marker for Phase 2 enzyme activity.

*1. NAD(P)H: (quinone-acceptor) oxidoreductase*

This enzyme, here designated quinone reductase (QR; EC 1.6.99.2)* and also known as DT-diaphorase, is a widely-distributed, cytosolic, FAD-containing protein that promotes the nicotinamide nucleotide-dependent reduction of many quinones to hydroquinones (*11, 12*). Notable properties of this enzyme are that: (1) NADH and NADPH are equally efficient electron donors; (b) the reduction of quinones is an obligatory two-electron process; (c) the enzyme is potently inhibited by dicoumarol and other anticoagulants; (d) QR is induced in many cells and tissues by a variety of xenobiotics, including the various above-mentioned chemoprotectors (*12*).

Although the functions of QR are not fully established, much evidence indicates that this enzyme plays a protective role against the toxicity of quinones and perhaps also certain high valency metals such as chromium (VI). The evidence for a protective function of QR may be summarized as follows (*12*): (a) induction of QR is often associated with decreased toxicity of a wide variety of quinones (*13, 14*); (b) the toxicity of quinones and of quinone precursors is enhanced by dicoumarol (*14, 15*); (c) chemiluminescence due to singlet oxygen generated by oxidative cycling of quinones is lowered by induction of QR, or by direct addition of pure QR to cell-free systems (*16, 17*); (d) binding of radioactive phenol to microsomal proteins (which is considered a manifestation of benzene toxicity) is depressed by direct addition of QR (*18*); and (e) cell lines with high QR levels appear to be more resistant to quinones and their metabolic precursors (*19, 20*).

The protective effects of QR have been attributed to the unusual obligatory two-

* Abbreviations: QR, NAD(P)H: (quinone-acceptor) oxidoreductase (EC1.6.99.2), also known as DT-diaphorase, menadione reductase, and referred to in this chapter as quinone reductase.

electron reduction of quinones by this enzyme (*21*), thereby promoting the metabolic disposal of the resulting relatively stable hydroquinones by conjugation with glucuronic acid. More recently, Cadenas and colleagues (*22, 23*) have made the interesting and potentially important observation that QR may act in concert with superoxide dismutase to protect against the toxicity of quinones. Although the mechanisms of this partnership are not entirely clear, quinone-mediated redox cycling (resulting in depletion of pools of reduced nicotinamide nucleotides and glutathione, as well as generation of superoxide radicals) can be much more efficiently suppressed by the combined action of QR and superoxide dismutase than by the action of each enzyme alone. This synergism is particularly striking since in some systems each enzyme alone *enhances* redox cycling.

Although it is very likely (but not certain) that QR protects against the toxicities of quinones, and perhaps other electrophiles, it clearly can serve as an important marker enzyme for the chemoprotection of cells and tissues since it is induced by many chemoprotective agents (*24*).

2. *Hepa 1c1c7 murine hepatoma cells*

This cell line is ideally suited for measuring the potency of chemoprotective agents to induce QR and to study the mechanism of induction. QR activity is easily and reproducibly measurable in Hepa 1c1c7 cells, and is induced in this cell line by nearly all known chemoprotectors that induce Phase 2 enzymes *in vivo* (*25–27*). Hepa 1c1c7 cells retain many of the enzymes of their tissue of origin, including *Ah*-receptor mediated cytochromes P-450. Moreover, mutant lines defective in either *Ah* receptor function or in cytochrome $P_1$-450 transcription are available (*28, 29*). It has therefore been possible to analyze not only the induction of QR as representative of Phase 2 enzymes, but also to elucidate the relation between Phase 1 and Phase 2 enzyme induction (*10, 30*).

3. *Microtiter plate assay for quinone reductase*

The measurement of QR in Hepa 1c1c7 cells has been further simplified by carrying out the inductions on cells grown in 96-well microtiter plates (*31*). Measurements of QR specific activities are carried out by means of a microtiter plate optical scanner which is interfaced with a computer for data analysis. This method permits many more assays to be performed in a much shorter time, and has substantially extended the utility of the system.

### *Identification of the Chemical Signal Responsible for the Induction of Phase 2 Enzymes*

Since monofunctional inducers elevate Phase 2 enzyme levels without appreciably inducing Phase 1 enzymes (which may activate carcinogens), we have examined the structural features necessary for selective Phase 2 enzyme induction. Monofunctional inducers belong to many different chemical classes and superficially show very little structural similarity. Although the idea that a single chemical signal might be responsible for these inductions initially seemed quite unpromising, such a chemical signal was identified by structure-activity studies. Our studies revealed that all of the inducers contain or acquire by metabolism electrophilic centers, and many are Michael reaction acceptors (*25, 27*).

It was first shown that the induction of QR and glutathione transferases by a series of monoalkyl and dialkyl ethers of *tert*-butylhydroquinone appeared to depend on conversion to the diphenol (*32*). Since all of the compounds tested were 1, 4-diphenols, the issue arose whether this orientation of the phenolic hydroxyl groups was a requirement for inducer activity. In a subsequent study (*25*) involving comparison of the potencies of induction of a series of 1, 2-diphenols (catechols), 1, 3-diphenols (resorcinols), and 1, 4-diphenols (hydroquinones), it was observed that only the catechols and hydroquinones were inducers whereas the resorcinols were not. The presence of other substituents was of minor importance in controlling inductive potency. This observation, in combination with the parallel finding that only *ortho*- and *para*-phenylenediamines were inducers, whereas *meta*-phenylenediamine was inactive, strongly suggested that oxidative lability was essential for inducer activity, since the *ortho*- and *para*-derivatives can undergo oxidation to quinones or quinoneimines, whereas the *meta*-substituted compounds are resistant to such oxidations. These studies did not, however, settle the question whether the oxidation products of the diphenols and phenylenediamines were the actual inducers, or whether the easily reversible redox process that led to the formation of the quinones and quinoneimines generated a secondary signal (*e.g.*, an active oxygen species), which was responsible for the induction.

More precise insight into the nature of the inducer signal was obtained by structural dissection of a series of coumarins into their component substructures (*9, 27*). It was concluded that inducer activity was associated with the $\alpha$, $\beta$-unsaturated lactone function of coumarin, and that $\alpha,\beta$-unsaturated ketones were even more potent inducers than the lactones (esters) (*27*). These findings immediately suggested that the critical structural feature for induction was the electrophilic olefin activated by conjugation with an electron-withdrawing group. The reactivity of such electrophilic olefins is well-recognized and forms the basis of the Michael reaction which is widely used in synthetic chemistry (*33*). Consequently, the induction of oxidizable diphenols and phenylenediamines could be ascribed to their oxidation to quinones and quinoneimines, which are excellent Michael reaction acceptors.

Michael reaction acceptors have the following generic structures: R–CH=CH–Z, Z′–CH=CH–Z (which include quinones), or R–C≡C–Z (acetylenes), in which Z and Z′ are electron-withdrawing substituents. The Michael acceptor reactivity of these compounds depends upon the power of the electron-withdrawing function. The inducer potency of a series of cyclic and acyclic olefins was likewise closely related to the electron-withdrawing power of the Z group(s). For instance, ketones and aldehydes were more potent inducers than esters, and nitro groups were among the most potent inducers (*27*). These generalizations were in part based on studies with vinyl ($CH_2$=CH–), propenyl ($CH_3$–CH=CH–), and styryl ($C_6H_5$–CH=CH–) derivatives, related to acrylates, crotonates, and cinnamates, respectively. Among these compounds also, potency of enzyme induction correlated with Michael acceptor reactivity. We concluded that in both cyclic and acyclic olefins conjugated with a variety of electron-withdrawing groups, potency of induction of Phase 2 enzymes was a function of the reactivity of the double bond with nucleophiles (*27, 34*).

These generalizations not only provided a logical explanation for the activity of many known enzyme inducers, but also led to the identification of several new classes of Phase 2 enzyme inducers, including $\alpha,\beta$-unsaturated aldehydes, ketones, thioketones, sulfones, esters, nitriles, and nitro-olefins (*27*). Furthermore, among a series of *trans*-methyl cinnamates the potency of induction was controlled by the efficacy of electron-withdrawing or electron-donating properties of substituents on the aromatic ring (*34*).

Not all inducers of Phase 2 enzymes are Michael reaction acceptors. Notable exceptions are the aromatic isothiocyanates, thiocarbamates, and halogenated aromatics such as 1-chloro-2, 4-dinitrobenzene (CDNB) and 1, 4-dichloro-2-nitrobenzene (DCNB). Nevertheless, these compounds all contain electrophilic centers and are substrates (like the above-mentioned Michael reaction acceptors) for glutathione transferases (*27, 34, 35*).

### *Search for Novel Chemoprotectors*

Based on the belief that induction of Phase 2 enzymes is a major and effective strategy for achieving protection against the toxic and neoplastic effects of carcinogens, we are pursuing two avenues in searching for chemoprotective enzyme inducers for potential use in human populations: (a) development of novel chemical structures based on knowledge of the chemical nature of the induction signal (electrophilic center or Michael reaction acceptor function), with the proviso that such inducers should be monofunctional and have low toxicity; and (b) survey of components of the human diet, especially vegetables, for inducer activity, with the objective of identifying new chemoprotective components and formulating dietary recommendations for reducing the risk of cancer.

#### *1. Chemoprotective potential of fumarate derivatives*

Among the many types of Michael acceptors and other types of electrophiles identified as Phase 2 enzyme inducers (*9, 27*), rather few are natural constituents of animal tissues. Although the endogenous presence of a compound in animal tissues is no guarantee of lack of toxicity, introduction of modest doses of such compounds into human populations at high risk for cancer is likely to engender fewer difficulties than the use of synthetic chemical entities as chemoprotectors. Among the many inducers thus far identified, fumarate, an essential intermediate in the tricarboxylic acid cycle, stands out as one of the few compounds that is an endogenous constituent of animal tissues. Although fumarate is a weak inducer (presumably because it is a poor Michael reaction acceptor), several fumarate derivatives are excellent inducers of QR in cell lines and of QR and glutathione S-transferase (GST) in rodent tissues (*36*).

In particular, dimethyl fumarate (DIMEFU) and several related compounds induce QR in Hepa 1c1c7 murine hepatoma cells. Furthermore, DIMEFU is a monofunctional inducer since it raises these enzymes in both the $BP^{r}c1$ and c1 mutants of this cell line, which are defective in cytochrome $P_1$-450 function. The former mutant has a normal *Ah* receptor but fails to translocate the liganded receptor to the nucleus, whereas the latter mutant produces an inactive (truncated) gene product. Both mutants have no detectable cytochrome $P_1$-450 activity (*28, 29*). Low doses (0.2–0.5%) of dietary DIMEFU were well-tolerated by outbred strains of mice and rats and elevated the cytosolic activities of QR and glutathione transferases (measured with CDNB and DCNB) in many organs (*36*). Thus 0.5% DIMEFU fed for 14 days (although a shorter period might have sufficed) to female CD-1 mice and Sprague-Dawley rats raised the specific activities of Phase 2 enzymes in the cytosols of liver, forestomach, glandular stomach, and proximal small intestine by a factor of 2 to 10, and to a lesser but significant extent in colon, lung, and kidney.

Experiments to assess the ability of DIMEFU to protect animals against chemical carcinogenesis are currently in progress, but the correlation between induction of Phase 2 enzymes and chemoprotection in other systems is excellent. For example, certain chemoprotective diterpenes were isolated from green coffee beans by monitoring the induction of glutathione transferases in mice (*37*), and the chemoprotective functions of 1, 2-dithiole-3-thiones were deduced from their ability to induce Phase 2 enzymes (*38*). We therefore anticipate that DIMEFU will display chemoprotective activity *in vivo*.

Several considerations make the development of DIMEFU as a chemoprotector an interesting objective: (a) as already mentioned, DIMEFU is a monofunctional inducer and therefore unlikely to induce *Ah* receptor-dependent cytochromes P-450; (b) fumaric acid, the parent acid of DIMEFU is widely distributed in plants, is used as an additive to impart tartness to jello and other foods, has very low acute and chronic toxicity at high doses, and is "Generally Recognized As Safe" (GRAS); (c) fumaric acid salts and esters are used as systemic therapeutic agents in man, *e.g.*, ferrous fumarate for iron deficiency anemia, and fumarate esters, including DIMEFU, for psoriasis (see *39*, and references therein); (d) high doses of fumaric acid protect against the development of forestomach and lung tumors induced by a nitrofuran (*40*), and against azo dye-induced hepatic tumors in rats (*41*); (e) fumaric acid, as well as the related anhydrides of $\alpha,\beta$-unsaturated dicarboxylic acids, protect against hydrocarbon-induced skin tumors in mice, as shown almost 50 years ago by Crabtree (*42, 43*); (f) fumaric acid protects animal cells against the toxicity of mitomycin C apparently without abolishing its anti-neoplastic effects (*44*).

The pharmacological and possible therapeutic (diuretic, oxytocic, anti-inflammatory, antiulcer, and tumor growth-inhibitory) effects of fumaric acid were uncovered by Kuroda and her colleagues in studies on the reputed medicinal properties of shepherd's purse (*Capsella bursa-pastoris*), a cruciferous weed that has been widely used as a traditional herbal and homeopathic remedy. The active principle of shepherd's purse responsible for these activities was isolated and identified as fumaric acid (*45*). Fumaric acid was then shown to exert some of the pharmacological and therapeutic properties described above (for references see *36*).

2. *Presence of Phase 2 enzyme inducers in vegetables*

Another approach to the development of chemoprotectors is the survey of inducer activity in the human diet. Epidemiological studies have shown that consumption of fruits and certain vegetables, and especially of crucifers, is associated with a lower risk of development of a number of epithelial malignancies such as those of the colon and breast (for references see *46*). Furthermore, feeding of dried vegetables and of some of their known components induces certain Phase 2 enzymes in animal tissues (*47*). In light of these observations, and the availability of the rapid microtiter plate cell culture system for measuring the potencies of inducer activities for QR (*31*), we have recently initiated a systematic survey of solvent extracts of organically-grown vegetables as inducers of QR in Hepa 1c1c7 murine hepatoma cells.* Considerable variations in the inducer potency of such organic solvent extracts were noted. Thus, for instance, extracts of many members of the family *Cruciferae* (*e.g.*, cauliflower, bok choi, brussels sprouts, broccoli) were especially potent inducers, whereas extracts obtained from *Rosaceae* (apples) and *Solanaceae* (potatoes, tomatoes) were much less active. Furthermore, different varieties of the species *Brassica oleracea*, which includes broccoli, brussels sprouts, and green cabbage, varied considerably in their ability to induce QR in murine hepatoma cells. Effects to isolate and characterize the compounds responsible for inducer activity are now in progress. The rapid microtiter plate assay should make it possible to identify the inducers and to examine the effects of food preparation on such inducer activity.

*Acknowledgments*

Studies performed in the laboratories of the authors were supported by grants from the National Cancer Institute and the American Cancer Society.

## REFERENCES

1. Doll, R. and Peto, R. The causes of cancer. Quantitative estimates of avoidable risks of cancer in the United States today. J. Natl. Cancer Inst., *66*: 1196–1308, 1981.
2. Wattenberg, L. W. Inhibition of neoplasia by minor dietary constituents. Cancer Res., *43*: 2448s–2453s, 1983.
3. Wattenberg, L. W. Chemoprevention of cancer. Cancer Res., *45*: 1–8, 1985.
4. Talalay, P., De Long, M. J., and Prochaska, H. J. Molecular mechanisms in protection against carcinogenesis. *In;* J. G. Cory and A. Szentivanyi (eds.), Cancer Biology and Therapeutics, pp. 197–216, Plenum Press, New York, 1987.
5. Ames, B. N. and Gold, L. S. Chemical carcinogenesis: Too many rodent carcinogens. Proc. Natl. Acad. Sci. U.S.A., *87*: 7772–7776, 1990.
6. Ames, B. N., Profet, M., and Gold, L. S. Dietary pesticides (99.99% all natural). Proc. Natl. Acad. Sci. U.S.A., *87*: 7777–7781, 1990.
7. Ames, B. N., Profet, M., and Gold, L. S. Nature's chemicals and synthetic chemicals: Comparative toxicology. Proc. Natl. Acad. Sci. U.S.A., *87*: 7782–7786, 1990.
8. Kouri, R. E. and Nebert, D. W. Genetic regulation of susceptibility to polycyclic-hydrocarbon-induced tumors in the mouse. *In;* H. H. Hiatt, J. D. Watson, and J. A. Winsten (eds.), Origins of Human Cancer. Book B. Mechanisms of Carcinogenesis, pp. 811–835, Cold Spring Harbor Laboratory, Cold Spring Harbor, New York, 1977.
9. Talalay, P. Mechanisms of induction of enzymes that protect against chemical carcinogenesis. Adv. Enzyme Reg., *28*: 237–250, 1989.
10. Prochaska, H. J. and Talalay, P. Regulatory mechanisms of monofunctional and bifunctional anticarcinogenic enzyme inducers in murine liver. Cancer Res., *48*: 4776–4782, 1988.
11. Ernster, L., Estabrook, R. W., Hochstein, P., and Orrenius, S. (eds.). DT Diaphorase: A quinone reductase with special functions in cell metabolism and detoxication. Chemica Scripta, *27A*: 1–207, 1987.
12. Prochaska, H. J. and Talalay, P. Role of NAD(P)H: quinone reductase in protection

* Santamaria, A.B., Prochaska, H.J., and Talalay, P. Rapid identification of anticarcinogenic enzyme inducers in vegetable extracts, unpublished observation.

against the toxicity of quinones and related agents. *In;* H. Sies (ed.), Oxidative Stress: Oxidants and Antioxidants, pp. 195–211, Academic Press, London, 1991.

13. Lind, C., Vadi, H., and Ernster, L. Metabolism of benzo(a)pyrene-3,6-quinone and 3-hydroxybenzo(a)pyrene in liver microsomes from 3-methylcholanthrene-treated rats. Arch. Biochem. Biophys., *190*: 97–108, 1978.
14. Lind, C., Hochstein, P., and Ernster, L. DT-diaphorase as a quinone reductase: A cellular control device against semiquinone and superoxide radical formation. Arch. Biochem. Biophys., *216*: 178–185, 1982.
15. Thor, H., Smith, M. T., Hartzell, P., Bellomo, G., Jewell, S. A., and Orrenius, S. The metabolism of menadione (2-methyl-1,4-naphthoquinone) by isolated hepatocytes. J. Biol. Chem., *257*: 12419–12425, 1982.
16. Wefers, H. and Sies, H. Hepatic low-level chemiluminescence during redox cycling of menadione and the menadione-glutathione conjugate: Relation to glutathione and NAD(P)H: quinone reductase (DT-diaphorase) activity. Arch. Biochem. Biophys., *224*: 568–578, 1983.
17. Prochaska, H. J., Talalay, P., and Sies, H. Direct protective effect of NAD(P)H: quinone reductase against menadione-induced chemiluminescence of postmitochondrial fractions of mouse liver. J. Biol. Chem., *262*: 1931–1934, 1987.
18. Smart, R. C. and Zannoni, V. G. DT-diaphorase and peroxidase influence the covalent binding of the metabolites of phenol, the major metabolite of benzene. Mol. Pharmacol., *26*: 105–111, 1984.
19. Thomas, D. J., Sadler, A., Subrahmanyam, V. V., Siegel, D., Reasor, M. J., Wierda, D., and Ross, D. Bone marrow stromal cell bioactivation and detoxification of the benzene metabolite hydroquinone: Comparison of macrophages and fibroblastoid cells. Mol. Pharmacol., *37*: 255–262, 1990.
20. Twerdok, L. E. and Trush, M. A. Differences in quinone reductase activity in primary bone marrow stromal cells derived from C57BL/6 and DBA/2 mice. Res. Commun. Chem. Path. Pharmacol., *67*: 375–386, 1990.
21. Iyanagi, T. and Yamazaki, I. One-electron-transfer reactions in biochemical systems. V. Differences in the mechanism of quinone reduction by the NADH dehydrogenase and the NAD(P)H dehydrogenase (DT-diaphorase). Biochim. Biophys. Acta, *216*: 282–294, 1970.
22. Cadenas, E., Mira, A., Lind, C., Segura-Aguilar, J., and Ernster, L. Effect of superoxide dismutase on the autooxidation of various hydroquinones—a possible role of superoxide dismutase as a superoxide: semiquinone oxidoreductase. Free Radical Biol. Med., *5*: 71–79, 1988.
23. Öllinger, K., Buffinton, G. D., Ernster, L., and Cadenas, E. Effect of superoxide dismutase on the autooxidation of substituted hydro- and semi-naphthoquinones. Chem.-Biol. Interact., *73*: 53–76, 1990.
24. Talalay, P. and Prochaska, H. J. Mechanisms of induction of NAD(P)H: quinone reductase. Chemica Scripta *27A*: 61–66, 1987.
25. Prochaska, H. J., De Long, M. J., and Talalay, P. On the mechanism of induction of cancer protective enzymes: A unifying proposal. Proc. Natl. Acad. Sci. U.S.A., *82*: 8232–8236, 1985.
26. De Long, M. J., Prochaska, H. J., and Talalay, P. Induction of NAD(P)H: quinone reductase in murine hepatoma cells by phenolic antioxidants, azo dyes and other chemoprotectors: A model system for the study of anticarcinogens. Proc. Natl. Acad. Sci. U.S.A., *83*: 787–791, 1986.
27. Talalay, P., De Long, M. J., and Prochaska, H. J. Identification of a common chemical

signal regulating the induction of enzymes that protect against chemical carcinogenesis. Proc. Natl. Acad. Sci. U.S.A., *85*: 8261–8265, 1988.

28. Miller, A. G., Israel, D., and Whitlock, Jr., J. P. Biochemical and genetic analysis of variant mouse hepatoma cells defective in the induction of benzo(a)pyrene-metabolizing enzyme activity. J. Biol. Chem., *258*: 3523–3527, 1983.
29. Hankinson, O., Andersen, R. D., Birren, B. W., Sander, F., Negishi, M., and Nebert, D. W. Mutations affecting the regulation of transcription of the cytochrome $P_1$-450 gene in the mouse hepa-1 cell line. J. Biol. Chem., *260*: 1790–1795, 1985.
30. De Long, M. J., Santamaria, A. B., and Talalay, P. Role of cytochrome $P_1$-450 in the induction of NAD(P)H: quinone reductase in a murine hepatoma line and its mutants. Carcinogenesis, *8*: 1549–1553, 1987.
31. Prochaska, H. J. and Santamaria, A. B. Direct measurement of NAD(P)H: quinone reductase from cells cultured in microtiter wells: A screening assay for anticarcinogenic enzyme inducers. Anal. Biochem., *169*: 328–336, 1988.
32. Prochaska, H. J., Bregman, H. S., De Long, M. J., and Talalay, P. Specificity of induction of cancer protective enzymes by analogues of *tert*-butyl-4-hydroxyanisole (BHA). Biochem. Pharmacol., *34*: 3909–3914, 1985.
33. March, J. Advanced organic chemistry: Reactions, mechanisms and structure. Wiley, New York, 1985.
34. Spencer, S. R., Xue, L., Klenz, E. M., and Talalay, P. The potency of inducers of NAD(P)H: (quinone-acceptor) oxidoreductase parallels their efficiency as substrates for glutathione transferases. Structural and electronic correlations. Biochem. J., *273*: 711–717, 1991.
35. Talalay, P. and Spencer, S. R. Regulation of the induction of glutathione transferases and NAD(P)H: quinone reductase by glutathione transferase substrates. *In;* J. D. Hayes, C. B. Pickett, and T. J. Mantle (eds.), Glutathione *S*-Transferases and Drug Resistance, pp. 176–185, Taylor and Francis, London, 1990.
36. Spencer, S. R., Wilczak, C. A., and Talalay, P. Induction of glutathione transferase and NAD(P)H: quinone reductase by fumaric acid derivatives in rodent cells and tissues. Cancer Res., *50*: 7871–7875, 1990.
37. Lam, L. K. T., Sparnins, V. L., and Wattenberg, L. W. Isolation and identification of kahweol palmitate and cafestol palmitate as active constituents of green coffee beans that enhance glutathione *S*-transferase in the mouse. Cancer Res., *42*: 1193–1198, 1982.
38. Wattenberg, L. W. and Bueding, E. Inhibitory effects of 5-(2-pyrazinyl)-4-methyl-1, 2-dithiol-3-thione (oltipraz) on carcinogenesis induced by benzo[a]pyrene, diethylnitrosamine and uracil mustard. Carcinogenesis, *7*: 1379–1381, 1986.
39. Nieboer, C., de Hoop, D., van Leonen, A. C., Langendijk, P. N. J., and van Dijk, E. Systemic therapy with fumaric acid derivatives: New possibilities in the treatment of psoriasis. J. Am. Acad. Dermatol., *20*: 601–608, 1989.
40. Kuroda, K., Kanisawa, M., and Akao, M. Inhibitory effect of fumaric acid on forestomach and lung carcinogenesis by a 5-nitrofuran naphthyridine derivative in mice. J. Natl. Cancer Inst., *69*: 1317–1319, 1982.
41. Kuroda, K., Terao, K., and Akao, M. Inhibitory effect of fumaric acid on 3-methyl-4′-(dimethylamino)azobenzene induced hepatocarcinogenesis in rats. J. Natl. Cancer Inst., *71*: 855–857, 1983.
42. Crabtree, H. G. Influence of unsaturated dibasic acids on the induction of skin tumors by chemical carcinogens. Cancer Res., *5*: 346–351, 1945.
43. Crabtree, H. G. Anti-carcinogenesis. Br. Med. Bull., *4*: 345–348, 1947.
44. Kuroda, K. and Akao, M. Reduction by fumaric acid of the side effects of mitomycin C. Biochem. Pharmacol., *29*: 2839–2844, 1980.

45. Kuroda, K. and Akao, M. Inhibitory effect of fumaric acid and dicarboxylic acids on gastric ulceration in rats. Arch. Int. Pharmacodyn. Ther., *226*: 324–330, 1977.
46. National Research Council. Diet and Health. Implications for Reducing Chronic Disease Risk. National Academy Press, Washington, 1989.
47. Bradfield, C. A., Chang, Y., and Bjeldanes, L. F. Effects of commonly-consumed vegetables on hepatic xenobiotic metabolizing enzymes in the mouse. Fd. Chem. Toxicol., *23*: 899–904, 1985.

XENOBIOTICS AND CANCER, L. ERNSTER ET AL. (EDS.), JAPAN SCI. SOC. PRESS, TOKYO/TAYLOR & FRANCIS LTD., LONDON, pp. 189–198, 1991

# Mechanism of Specific Expression of Glutathione Transferase P Gene during Hepatocarcinogenesis

Masami Muramatsu, Akihiko Okuda, Shigeru Morimura, Shigehiro Osada, Mitchell B. Diccianni, and Masayoshi Imagawa

*Department of Biochemistry, The University of Tokyo Faculty of Medicine, Tokyo 113, Japan*

*Abstract:* The mechanism of specific expression of glutathione transferase P gene during hepatocarcinogenesis of the rat has been investigated by cloning the gene and determining the upstream regulatory sequences. Two enhancers and a silencer are located within 3 kb upstream of the promoter. The stronger enhancer designated GPEI has two TPA (12-O-tetradecanoyl phorbol 13-acetate)-response element (TRE)-like sequences arranged in a palindrome at a 3 base pairs spacing. This special combination was found to form a very strong enhancer which could act efficiently even in F9 cells where the collagenase enhancer with a singlet TRE cannot work due to the low c-jun content. Whether this structure is operating with a very low concentration of c-jun/c-fos heterodimer or with any other proteins remains to be determined. These findings suggest that new and more efficient enhancers evolve by a combination of basic enhancer elements. The silencer region consists of several sequences that can bind specific protein(s) and works cooperatively.

During the course of carcinogenesis, some specific genes are known to be expressed at a high frequency. They are sometimes called tumor markers. Elucidation of the mechanism by which those genes are activated during the course of malignant transformation may shed some light on the specific alteration of gene expression in these cells leading to malignant phenotype. As a model system, we have examined the expression of specific marker proteins during the course of hepatocarcinogenesis of the rat using two dimensional gel electrophoresis (*1*). Among several newly appearing spots, glutathione transferase P (GST-P) was the most conspicuous. This protein which was present in normal liver in only a trace amount increased 50–100 times in a hyperplastic nodule (a precancerous lesion) and in hepatocellular carcinoma to comprise a few percent of the soluble protein. Because it was highly expressed in all the specimens of hyperplastic nodules and hepatocellular carcinomas induced by various carcinogens including acetylaminofluorene, diethylnitrosamine, and dimethyl-aminoazobenzene with the sole exception of peroxisome-proliferating agents such as clofibrate but not in regenerating or fetal liver, it seemed specifically related to hepatocarcinogenesis but not to cell growth itself or to undifferentiated states (*1–3*). In fact, GST-P is expressed only at low levels (less than one-tenth of the chemically-induced hepatocellular carcinoma) in lung, kidney, and testis among normal tissues. We therefore proceeded to investigate the molecular mechanism by which this gene became highly expressed during the course of chemical hepatocarcinogenesis. Here, we describe the special nature of an enhancer that was found in the upstream regulatory region of the GST-P gene.

### *Cloning and Structure of the GST-P Gene*

We first purified the GST-P protein from the rat hepatocellular carcinoma induced with acetylaminofluorene by repeated two dimensional gel electrophoresis and determined N-terminal 25 amino acids using a gas-phase protein sequencer. Then, three sets of deoxyoligonucleotides corresponding to two sites of this sequence were synthesized and used for screening a cDNA library constructed from the poly$(A)^+$ RNA of chemically induced hepatocellular carcinoma (*4*).

A cDNA clone obtained in this manner contained the complete amino acid sequence of GST-P and the enzyme was found to situate in the phylogenetic tree at a site separated from other GST's. Next, we isolated the genomic clone of GST-P from a rat genomic library and determined the whole structure (*5*). Active GST-P gene existed in only one, though several processed-type pseudogenes were present. The active gene was composed of seven exons split by six introns spanning over about 3 kb (*5*).

### *Upstream Regulatory Sequences of GST-P Gene*

The regulatory regions of the GST-P gene were surveyed by ligating the bacterial chloramphenicol acetyltransferase (CAT) structural gene to the first exon of the GST-P gene. Various deletions from upstream were made and tested for their gene activating abilities by introducing the constructs into a hepatoma cell line, dRLh84, which was actively expressing GST-P endogenously. Figure 1 summarizes the data which show that the GST-P gene has at least two enhancer regions and a silencer-like region (*6*). A TATA-box and a GC-box (SP1 binding site) were present in the promoter region. In addition, a TPA (12-O-teradecanoyl phorbol 13-acetate)responsive element (TRE, TGACTCA) was present just upstream of the promoter. The transcription activation up to this point, however, was relatively low as compared with the construct having more upstream regions. The upstream DNA fragment between −2.5 and −2.2 kb (SA fragment) contained a strong enhancing activity in a distance- and orientation-independent manner, which was characteristic of an enhancer (*6*). This region could be divided into two enhancer activities designated GPEI and GPEII, but the former was subsequently found to be much stronger in every cell line tested including dRLh84, HeLa, and 3Y1 cells. We therefore, studied GPEI in more detail.

### *Characteristic Structure of the GPEI*

To delimit the region having the enhancer activity in the GPEI fragment, we made a series of 5′- and 3′-deletion mutants and the enhancer activity was determined by CAT assay after ligating the mutants directly to the GST-P gene promoter connec-

A

| Transfected DNA | % Acetylated | Fold stimulation |
|---|---|---|
| Experiment I | | |
| 5CAT | 9.1 | 1.0 |
| EA-5CAT | 92.2 | 10.0 |
| AE-5CAT | 72.3 | 7.9 |
| EA-5CATbam | 58.3 | 6.4 |
| ES-5CAT | 9.6 | 1.1 |
| SA-5CAT | 96.4 | 10.6 |
| SA5-5CAT | 89.4 | 9.8 |
| SA3-5CAT | 84.1 | 9.2 |
| Experiment II | | |
| Δ56CAT | 38.4 | 1.0 |
| BP-Δ56CAT | 16.3 | 0.44 |
| PB-Δ56CAT | 8.9 | 0.23 |
| PB-Δ56CATbam | 11.1 | 0.29 |
| 4CAT | 7.2 | 0.19 |

B

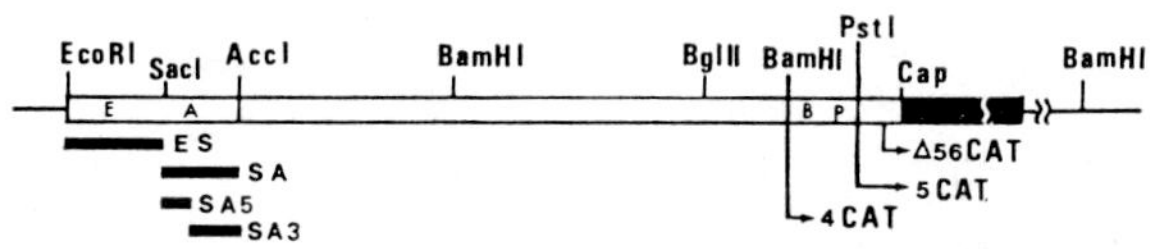


FIG. 1. Identification of enhancer and silencer elements in the upstream of GST-P gene. A. Each construct was introduced into dRLh84 cells and CAT activity was determined. B. Restriction map of the 5′ flanking region of GST-P gene. Positions of the fragments used are shown by bold bars.

ted to a CAT gene (*Δ*-56 CAT). At the same time, a gel-shift assay was carried out to learn the possible factor-binding to the enhancer elements. The results indicated that GPEI contained a TRE-like sequence (TGATTCA), but required a dozen additional base-pairs just upstream of the TRE-like sequence for its enhancer activity. A protein, probably of the Jun-family, was shown to bind to the TRE-like sequence even without the upstream region. A close look at the upstream sequence revealed the presence of two TRE-like sequences arranged palindromically to the first (downstream) TRE-like sequence (*7*). The relationship of these sequences for the enhancer activity of GPEI was investigated by introducing various mutations in each sequence. The single-point mutation which destroyed the downstream TRE-like sequence abolished the whole GPEI activity, indicating that this sequence was essential in GPEI (data not shown, see ref. *7*). Next, we introduced consecutive triple point mutations in the upstream region and examined how the activity of GPEI was affected .The data indicated that, although the destruction of the most upstream TRE-like sequence (also arranged palindromically to the downstream TRE-like sequence) did not affect the enhancer activity of GPEI, that of the next upstream TRE-like sequence severely inhibited the GPEI activity (*7*). Therefore, these two TRE-like sequences arranged in a palindrome at a three base-pairs distance forms a strong enhancer which works in dRLh84 cells.

### *GPEI Works in F9 Cells That Have a Very Low c-jun Activity*

It has been demonstrated that an oncoprotein dimer c-jun/c-fos binds to the TRE for its activation (*8*, *9*). To analyze the mode of function of GPEI enhancer having two palindromic TRE-like sequences, we introduced the GPEI into an embryonic carcinoma cell line, F9. F9 cells are known to have such a low level of c-jun that the collagenase gene enhancer having an authentic TRE cannot work. Unex-

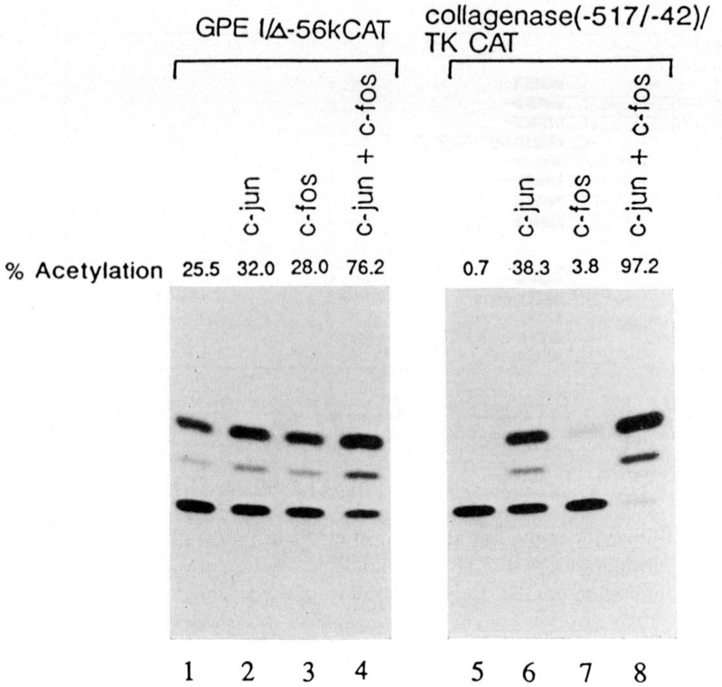


FIG. 2. Activity of GPEI and collagenase enhancers in F9 cells. Effects of c-jun and c-fos co-expression.

pectedly, however, the GPEI showed a relatively high activity in F9 cells even without co-transfection of the c-jun expression vector (Fig. 2). The collagenase enhancer required the co-expression of c-jun for its activity. These results indicate either that GPEI can work under a very low level of c-jun or that it is working with some other protein which is relatively abundant in F9 cells.

To confirm the cooperativity of the two TRE-like sequences under these conditions, we tested the effect of mutations of each component in F9 cells. Figure 3a depicts the GPEI enhancer sequence and the mutations introduced. As shown in Fig. 3b, the destructive single-point mutation on the downstream (3′-side) TRE-like sequence completely abolished the enhancer activity of GPEI in F9 cells and it was not recovered by co-transfection of the c-jun expression vector (lanes 7 and 8). The loss of GPEI activity by the triple point mutations was the same in F9 cells as in dRLh84 (*7, 10*). However, it was remarkable that the loss of the enhancer activity by triple point mutations at the upstream (5′-side) TRE-like sequence could be recovered by co-expressing the c-jun protein (Fig. 3C, lanes 8 and 10). This clearly indicates that the downstream TRE-like sequence is indeed the major and dominant element and the upper TRE-like sequence is required for this complex to work efficiently in F9 cells, probably under low c-jun conditions (*10*).

### *A Specific Combination of Two TREs Can Form an Extremely Efficient Enhancer*

To define more precisely the structural requirements of the GPEI, we first

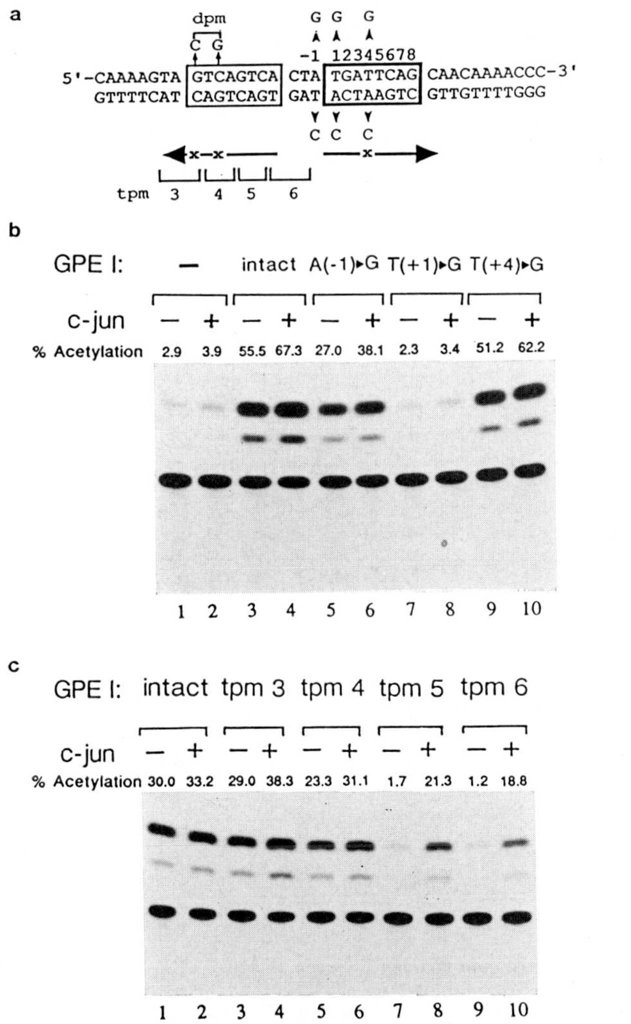


FIG. 3. Cooperative function of two TRE-like sequences of GPEI in F9 cells. a. Structure of GPEI mutants used. b. Examination of the downstream TRE-like sequences by single point mutants. c. Examination of the upstream TRE-like sequence by triple-point mutants.

examined the effects of changes in the spacing of the two TRE-like sequences. Figure 4 shows that the removal of two base pairs from the linker region (three bp) of the two TRE-like sequences decreased the enhancing activity in F9 cells to less than one-third (28%). Insertion of two, four, and ten additional base pairs in the linker sequence decreased the activity to 33, 17, and 7% of the wild-type. Next, we tested the effect of orientation of the two TRE sequences. In these experiments, we used the consensus TREs in order to confirm that the cooperativity holds true not only for the TRE-like sequences found in GPEI but also for consensus TREs. The data shown in Fig. 5 indicate that the palindromic arrangement found in GPEI is the most potent combination and other orientations are much less effective for eliciting cooperativity between the two TREs. It is also evident that this palindromic structure works much better not only in F9 cells but also in HeLa cells having a sufficient amount of c-jun product.

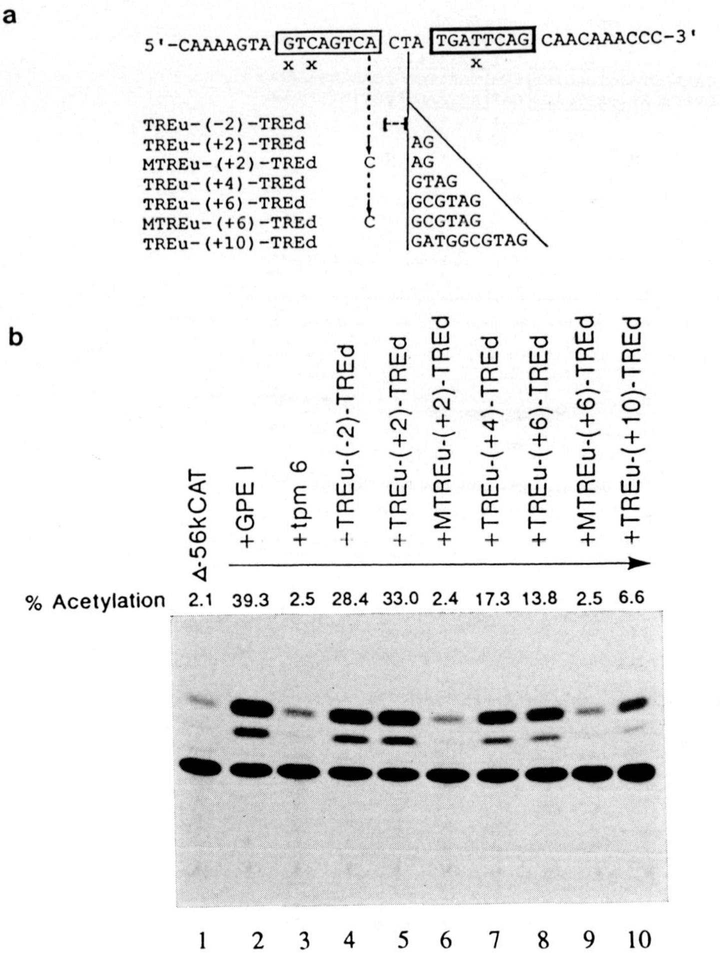


FIG. 4. Requirement of a stringent spacing between the two TRE-like sequences for the GPEI activity. a. Diagram of deletion and insertion constructs at the spacer. b. CAT assays with the mutants shown above.

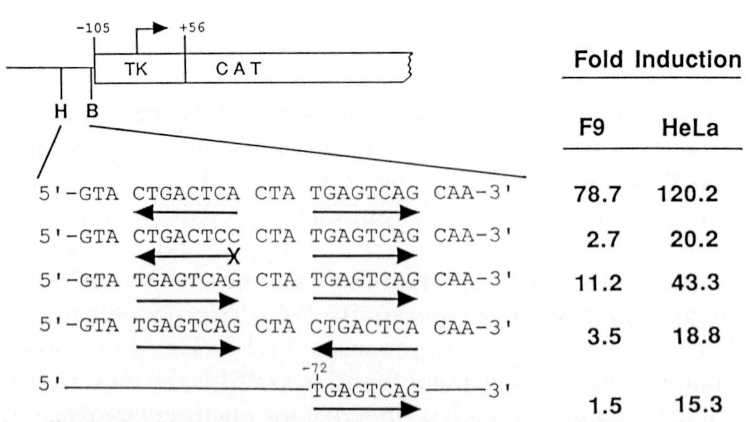


FIG. 5. Requirement of a certain palindromic orientation for the proper cooperativity of the two TREs. Synthetic DNAs shown are connected to the HSV thymidine kinase promoter and CAT activity assayed in respective cells.

TABLE 1. Silencing Effects of Negative Fragment in GST-P Gene on Activities of Heterologous Promoters and Enhancer in Non-hepatoma and Hepatoma cells

| Construct | Relative CAT activity | |
|---|---|---|
| | Non-hepatoma (3Y1) | Hepatoma (dRLh84) |
| A. GST-P promoter | | |
| Δ-106CAT | 1.00 | 1.00 |
| BPΔ-106CAT | 0.45 | 0.44 |
| PBΔ-106CAT | 0.17 | 0.23 |
| Δ-106CATBP | 0.27 | 0.29 |
| B. SV40 promoter and enhancer | | |
| pSV2CAT | 1.00 | 1.00 |
| BPpSV2CAT | 0.44 | 0.35 |
| PBpSV2CAT | 0.38 | 0.35 |
| C. TK promoter | | |
| TKCAT | 1.00 | 1.00 |
| BPTKCAT | 0.33 | 0.43 |

BP (BamHI-Pstl) fragment located from −396 to −140 in GST-P 5′ flanking region was introduced just upstream of heterologous promoters including the GST-P promoter itself in normal (BP) or reverse orientation (PB). In Δ-106CATBP, BP fragment was joined to BamHI site located 0.8 kilobase downstream from the end of CAT structural gene, and was 2 kilobase away from the cap site. Each construct was transfected into 3Y1 and dRLh84 cells and CAT activities were determined.

### *Silencer Region Consists of Several Elements That Bind Specific Proteins*

To evaluate the involvement of the silencer region in the specific expression of GST-P gene during hepatocarcinogenesis, we began to analyze the structure and function of the silencer (*11*). This region as a whole revealed a silencing activity when introduced in either dRLh84 or in 3YI (fibroblast) cells (Table 1). Figure 6 shows a DNase I footprinting pattern of this region (from cap site to −300) with a nuclear extract of rat liver. Several stretches of the DNA are clearly protected from the DNase I. These regions are designated GPS1 to 5. These five elements had partial homology to each other (*11*). None of their homopolymers showed silencing activity; however, when each region was separately deleted, all the promoter (plus enhancer) constructs showed two to three times higher activity, suggesting that they really had a silencing effect, albeit not very strong (data not shown).

The purification and cloning of the factors that bind to these regions are now under way and one cDNA clone coding for a silencer factor that binds to region 1 (Fig. 6) has recently been obtained (manuscript in preparation).

### *Conclusion*

We have described here our recent investigation into the nature of an enhancer that is present in the upstream region of the rat GST-P gene. We have shown that a new enhancer (GPEI) could be formed by a specific combination of known enhancer elements (TREs). This must have been a way for genes to develop new regulatory apparatuses and circuits during evolution. The mechanism which allows this new complex enhancer to function much more efficiently than the prototype sequence is an intriguing subject of future study. It is of particular interest that a gene with this

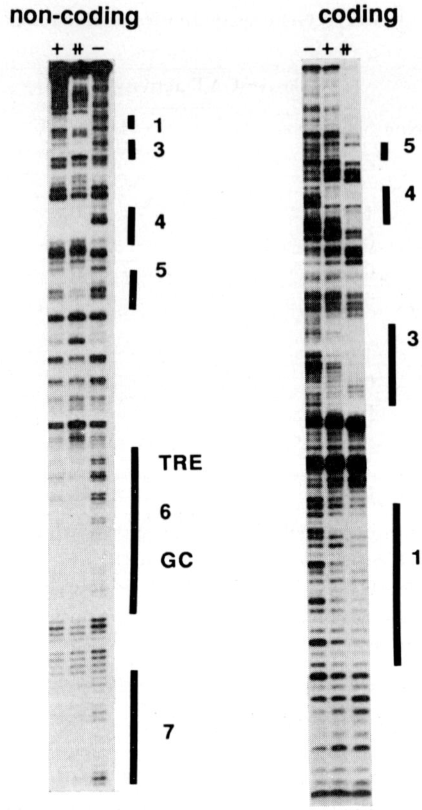


FIG. 6. DNase I footprint analysis of rat liver nuclear extract on promoter and silencer of GST-P gene. The DNA probes consist of a BamHI-HindIII fragment (−396 to +59) labeled at the HindIII end of the non-coding strand and a SalI-HindIII fragment (−305 to +59) labeled at the SalI end of the coding strand by Klenow fragment. The probe was incubated without (−) or with 12 μg (+) or 24 μg (++) of nuclear extract heated at 55°C for 5 min. The boundaries of several protected regions are indicated by vertical bars. TRE and GC box are indicated.

special enhancer complex is specifically expressed at a certain stage of hepatocarcinogenesis and is also elevated in some tumors with drug resistance (*12–15*). However, the mechanism of specific expression of GST-P gene during chemical hepatocarcinogenesis is yet to be solved. We found that c-jun was induced in precancerous lesions during this carcinogenesis (*16*). The obvious question is whether the elevation of c-jun protein is the major cause of the high expression of GST-P. We have recently succeeded in introducing GST-P-CAT gene into the primary culture of normal rat liver cells. As expected, the expression of this gene was low mimicking the situation of normal liver cells. However, the co-expression of c-jun protein alone could not induce the GST-P-CAT expression (in preparation). Meanwhile, we identified proteins which bound to the silencer region of the GST-P gene as described here. Thus, this gene appears to be regulated in a complex manner by different elements and factors. The real cause of the deregulation of GST-P gene at the early stages of hepatocarcinogenesis is now being pursued using isolated gene elements and transacting factors in primary culture hepatocytes and hepatocellular carcinoma cells.

## REFERENCES


1. Sugioka, Y., Fujii-Kuriyama, Y., Kitagawa, T., and Muramatsu, M. Changes in polypeptide pattern of rat liver cells during chemical hepatocarcinogenesis. Cancer Res., *45*: 365–378, 1985.
2. Sato, K., Kitahara, A., Soma, Y., Inaba, Y., Hatayama, I., and Sato, K. Purification, induction, and distribution of placental glutathione transferase: A new marker enzyme for preneoplastic cells in the rat chemical hepatocarcinogenesis. Proc. Natl. Acad. Sci. U.S.A., *82*: 3964–3968, 1985.
3. Sato, K. Glutathione S-transferase and hepatocarcinogenesis. Jpn. J. Cancer Res., *79*: 556–572, 1988.
4. Sugioka, Y., Kano, T., Okuda, A., Sakai, M., Kitagawa, T., and Muramatsu, M. Cloning and the nucleotide sequence of rat glutathione S-transferase P cDNA. Nucl. Acids Res., *13*: 6049–6057, 1985.
5. Okuda, A., Sakai, M., and Muramatsu, M. The structure of the rat glutathione S-transferase P gene and related pseudogenes. J. Biol. Chem., *262*: 3858–3863, 1987.
6. Sakai, M., Okuda, A., and Muramatsu, M. Multiple regulatory elements and phorbol 12-O-tetradecanoate 13-acetate responsiveness of the rat placental glutathione transferase gene. Proc. Natl. Acad. Sci. U.S.A., *85*: 9456–9460, 1988.
7. Okuda, A., Imagawa, M., Maeda, Y., Sakai, M., and Muramatsu, M. Structure and functional analysis of an enhancer GPEI having a phorbol 12-O-tetradecanoate 13-acetate responsive element-like sequence found in the rat glutathione transferase P gene. J. Biol. Chem., *264*: 16919–16926, 1989.
8. Chieu, R., Boyle, W. J., Meek, J., Smeal, T., Hunter, T., and Karin, M. The c-fos protein interacts with c-jun/AP-1 to stimulate transcription of AP-1 responsive gene. Cell, *54*: 541–552, 1988.
9. Sassone-Corsi, P., Lamph, W. W., Kamps, M., and Verma, I. M. fos-associated cellular p39 is related to nuclear transcription factor AP-1. Cell, *54*: 553–560, 1988.
10. Okuda, A., Imagawa, M., Sakai, M., and Muramatsu, M. Functional cooperativity between two TPA responsive elements in undifferentiated F9 embryonic stem cells. EMBO J., *9*: 1131–1135, 1990.
11. Imagawa, M., Osada, S., Okuda, A., and Muramatsu, M., Silencer binding proteins function on multiple *cis*-elements in the glutathione transferase P gene. Nucleic Acids Res., *19*: 5–10, 1991.
12. Cowan, K. H., Batist, G., Tulpule, A., Shinha, B. K., and Myers, C. E. Similar biochemical changes associated with multidrug resistance in human breast cancer cell and carcinogen-induced resistance to xenobiotics in rats. Proc. Natl. Acad. Sci. U.S.A., *83*: 9328–9332, 1986.
13. Nakagawa, K., Yokota, J., Wada, M., Sasaki, Y., Fujiwara, Y., Sakai, M., Muramatsu, M., Terasaki, T., Tsunokawa, Y., Terada, M., and Saijo, N. Levels of glutathione S-transferase mRNA in human lung cancer cell lines correlate with the resistance to cisplatin and carboplatin. Jpn. J. Cancer Res. (Gann)., *79*: 301–304, 1988.
14. Nakagawa, K., Saijo, N., Tsuchida, S., Sakai, M., Tsunokawa, Y., Yokota, J., Muramatsu, M., Sato, K., Terada, M., and Tew, K. Glutathione S-transferase as a determinant of drug resistance in transfectant cell lines. J. Biol. Chem., *265*: 4296–4301, 1990.
15. Miyazaki, M., Kohno, K., Saburi, Y., Matsuo, K., Ono, M., Kuwano, M., Tsuchida, S., Sato, K., Sakai, M., and Muramatsu, M. Drug resistance to *cis*-diaminedichloro platinum (II) Chinese hamster ovary cell lines transfected with glutathione S-transferase Pi gene. Cancer Res., *166*: 1358–1364, 1990.

16. Sakai, M., Okuda, A., Hatayama, I., Sato, K., Nishi, S., and Muramatsu, M. Structure and expression of the rat c-jun messenger RNA: Tissue distribution and increase during chemical hepatocarcinogenesis. Cancer Res., *49*: 5633–5637, 1989.

XENOBIOTICS AND CANCER, L. ERNSTER ET AL. (EDS.),
JAPAN SCI. SOC. PRESS, TOKYO/TAYLOR & FRANCIS LTD., LONDON, pp. 199–211, 1991

# Molecular Genetics of the Human Glutathione S-transferase

Philip G. Board, Peter N. Johnston, Veronica L. Ross, Graham C. Webb, Marjorie Coggan, and Takashige Suzuki

*Molecular Genetics Group, John Curtin School of Medical Research, Australian National University, Canberra ACT 2601, Australia*

*Abstract:* Multiple human cytosolic glutathione transferases have been described. These enzymes are the products of multiple genes that can be classified into at least four evolutionary classes. The genes encoding each class appear to be clustered on distinct chromosomes. Over-expression of glutathione S-transferase (GST) isoenzymes has been implicated in drug resistance and, conversely, deficiency of GST isoenzymes has been implicated in susceptibility to carcinogens. Some GST genes are expressed at varying levels in different individuals, and there is a frequent deficiency of the Mu class GST1 isoenzyme in all the racial groups studied so far. This deficiency is due to a deletion of the *GST 1* gene.

The Alpha class genes are located on the short arm of chromosome 6 and are closely linked, with less than 2 kb separating some genes. There is evidence for the existence of several pseudogenes in this cluster. A complete Alpha class gene has 7 exons and extends over 13 kb. The 5′ flanking region of the gene encoding the GST2 type 1 isoenzyme has been cloned and sequenced. This region contains a number of putative promoter and enhancer elements that are similar to those found in rat and mouse Alpha class genes.

The glutathione *S*-transferases (GSTs) are a family of multifunctional proteins. One of their major roles is to catalyze the conjugation of reduced glutathione to a variety of hydrophobic and electrophilic compounds. Many of these substrates are xenobiotic in origin and include many known carcinogens in addition to a number of therapeutic compounds (*1–4*). Some endogenous substrates have been identified. For example, the products of lipid peroxidation such as the 4-hydroxyalkenals have been shown to be good substrates for a particular GST isoenzyme (*5*). Furthermore, some GSTs have been shown to have glutathione peroxidase activity (*6, 7*); this activity has been implicated in the prostaglandin endoperoxidase conversion pathway and suggests a significant role for GSTs in prostaglandin biosynthesis (*8*), as well as protecting against oxidative damage from lipid peroxides. Leukotriene $C_4$ has been shown to be a glutathione conjugate, suggesting that a GST isoenzyme may be involved in its synthesis from leukotriene $A_4$ (*9*). The synthesis of fatty acid ethyl esters (FAEEs) in human heart has been shown to be catalyzed by an enzyme that has GST activity and sequence homology with a well characterized GST isoenzyme (*10*). Our recent studies have shown that FAEE synthesis is not, however, a general property of all human GSTs (*11*).

In addition to their catalytic role, the GSTs are known to bind a number of hydrophobic compounds including, for example, haeme, bilirubin, and steroids (*12–14*). As a result of this binding function, the most abundant GST isoenzyme from rat liver was originally termed ligandin (*15, 16*). The abundance of GST in both rat and human liver suggests that the binding function may be of even greater significance than its catalytic role and it has been suggested (*17–20*) that the GSTs may function as intracellular ligand storage proteins or for the transport of organic compounds with limited solubility in aqueous solution.

The GSTs therefore appear to make a significant contribution to the protection of the cell from a variety of exogenous and endogenous challenges. Elevated levels of GST expression have been reported in tumors (*21–23*) and increased expression of GSTs in cell lines selected for resistance to cytotoxic drugs has been reported (*24–28*). In addition, expression of recombinant GSTs in yeast and cultured cell lines results in increased resistance to several anti-cancer drugs and potential therapeutic agents including chlorambucil, adriamycin, and ethacrynic acid (*29–31*). These studies suggest that over-expression of GSTs in tumours may be a significant factor in the emergence of resistance to anti-cancer drugs. In contrast, we have discovered a genetically determined deficiency of a GST isoenzyme in some individuals and have suggested that deficient individuals may be at a greater risk and have increased sensitivity to particular carcinogenic compounds (*32, 33*).

It has been evident from the earliest studies that the GSTs are quite heterogeneous and there is clearly variation between tissues, between individuals, and between different stages of development. In order to understand this variation and the mechanisms of over-expression and deficiency it is useful to have a genetic model and to understand the relationships between the various isoenzymes. We have therefore focussed much of our attention on gaining a greater understanding of the genetic factors regulating the heterogeneity of the human GSTs.

### *Genetic Relationships between Human GST Isoenzymes*

In our original studies (*32, 34*), we developed a specific non-denaturing electrophoretic technique that could be used to detect charge differences in GST isoenzymes from different tissues and different individuals in the same experiment under identical conditions. This technique therefore had several advantages over ion exchange chromatographic techniques. From these studies, we deduced that the human cytosolic GSTs could be divided into groups that appeared to be genetically distinct. These were termed GST1, GST2, and GST3. Subsequent studies in our own and other laboratories have largely confirmed this arrangement (*7, 35–38*) and have expanded the basic model to include additional isoenzymes encoded by genes that appear to be related to one of the three groups.

On the basis of a comparative study of the amino terminal sequences and immunological cross-reactivity together with substrate and inhibitor specificities, Mannervik and co-workers (*39*) suggested that the mammalian cytosolic GSTs could be subdivided into three classes termed Mu, Alpha, and Pi. These classes correspond broadly with the loci termed GST1, GST2, and GST3 in humans. Because these classes appear to cross species boundaries and are present in humans, rats and mice, it is apparent that they have some evolutionary significance and appear to have differentiated before the divergence of these mammalian species.

A survey of the literature will provide references to a large number of GST isoenzymes isolated from a variety of human tissues that have been given an equally large variety of names. Many of these isoenzymes are identical, but it is not possible to make concise and meaningful comparisons of all the available data. The relationships between many of the well characterized isoenzymes are shown in Fig. 1. As a minimum, all of the isoenzymes included have known amino terminal sequences, have been purified, and have been immunologically screened. In some cases where a particular isoenzyme is also well known by alternate names we have included all these names or symbols. The characterization of the isoenzymes described in Fig. 1 has been presented in detail elsewhere (*7, 37, 40–44*).

A GST from microsomes has also been well characterized (*45*) and its amino acid

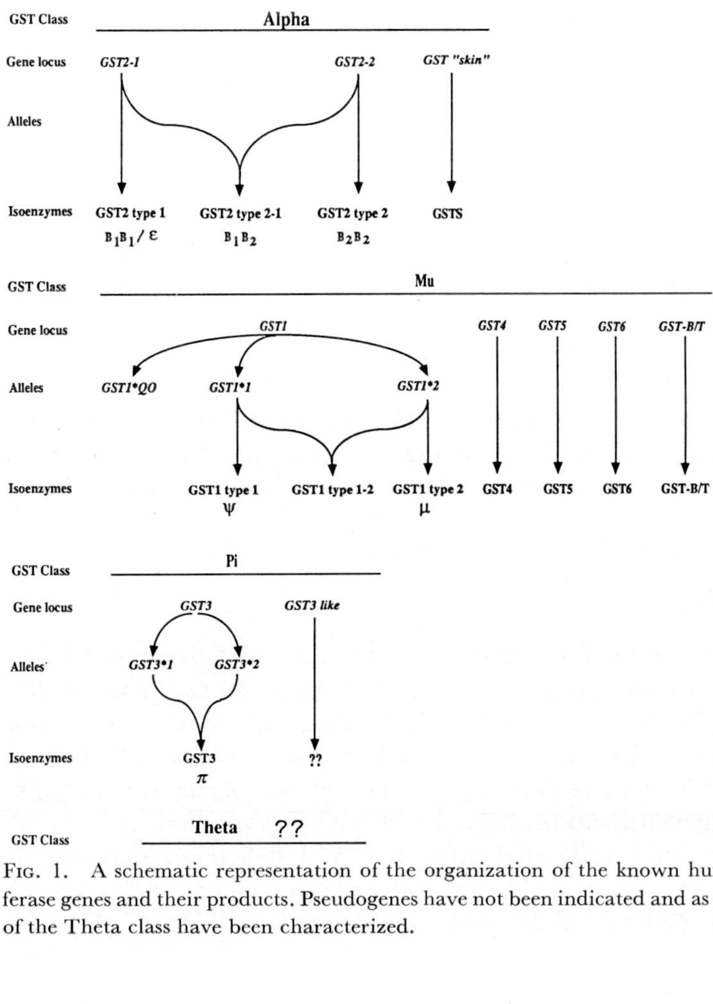


FIG. 1. A schematic representation of the organization of the known human glutathione transferase genes and their products. Pseudogenes have not been indicated and as yet no human members of the Theta class have been characterized.

sequence and functional properties suggest that it has evolved *via* a separate pathway and is quite distinct from the cytosolic GSTs.

All the known human cytosolic GSTs are dimeric proteins, thus some heterogeneity can arise from the presence of heterodimers. There is some evidence that heterodimers can form between the products of allelic genes and also between the products of genes that are from different but closely related loci. For example, as shown in Fig. 1, the GST1 type 1 and GST1 type 2 subunits are thought to be allelic products of the *GST1* locus, and can combine to form a heterodimer. In comparison, the two forms of GST2 are thought to be the products of distinct gene loci and also combine to form a heterodimer. So far, the only well-characterized heterodimers have been formed from subunits within the same evolutionary class. There are considerable differences in the amino acid sequences between isoenzymes of different classes and these differences probably result in sufficient modifications in tertiary structure to preclude the formation of interclass heterodimers.

Many of the studies carried out to date have identified glutathione transferases by their ability to utilize the model substrate 1-choloro-2, 4-dinitro benzene (CDNB) and their ability to bind to either a glutathione agarose or hexylglutathione agarose affinity matrix. It therefore remains possible that there are additional members of the GST family that have only one or neither of these properties. In this respect, it is of interest that rat GST isoenzymes have recently been identified that have high activity with DNA hydroperoxides and reactive sulphate esters, do not utilize CDNB, and do not bind to glutathione affinity columns (*46, 47*). It is suggested that these enzymes may represent an additional evolutionary class termed Theta. It is highly likely that equivalent human isoenzymes of this class will be identified and characterized in the near future.

While some parasite species such as *Schistosoma japonicum* have GST sequences that have regions of homology with the mammalian classes (*48*), it is striking that the GSTs so far identified in insects such as *Drosophila melanogaster* (*49*) and *Lucilia cuprina* (Board and Russell, unpublished data) fail to show any significant similarity with any of the mammalian GSTs, despite the fact that they utilize CDNB and bind to glutathione affinity columns. It remains to be determined if there are related isoenzymes whose function has been modified in higher mammals. So far, we have not been able to detect any cross-hybridization between a *L. cuprina* GST cDNA and human genomic DNA.

### *Quantitative Variation*

We previously reported a genetically determined deficiency of GST1 isoenzymes and attributed this to the existence of a null allele at the *GST1* locus (*32*). This null allele has a gene frequency of $\simeq$0.7 in Europeans and is the most common allele in all racial groups studied so far (*50, 51*). In some small Pacific island populations, where founder effects and population bottlenecks can occur, we have found that the null allele has achieved fixation (*51*).

We have previously suggested that the GST1 deficiency may increase an individual's sensitivity to certain environmentally derived compounds (*33*). The Mu class isoenzymes have a relatively high specific activity for epoxides (*41, 52*) compared with isoenzymes from the other classes. For example, trans-stilbene oxide is readily utilized by the Mu class isoenzyme known as GST$\mu$ GST1 type 2 but is not a significant substrate for GST2 (Alpha class) or GST3 (Pi class) (*53*; Board, unpublished observation). This high substrate selectivity may leave GST1 deficient individuals susceptible to cellular and genetic damage by a range of such compounds and there is some evidence supporting this hypothesis. In a study of the occurrence of lung cancer in smokers, Seidegärd and colleagues (*54*) have found an increased frequency of GST1 deficiency in smokers with lung cancer compared with smokers without lung cancer. This apparent differential sensitivity of GST1 deficient individuals may be relevant to a wider range of cancers and it remains to be determined if it is relevant to the metabolism of some therapeutically administered agents.

GST1 deficiency appears to result from the deletion of the *GST1* gene as it correlates with the absence of cross-hybridizing fragments on "Southern" blots of genomic DNA digested with a variety of restriction enzymes (*50, 51, 55*).

The methods available to determine the presence of the deficiency include the electrophoretic phenotyping of tissue extracts (*32*), the determination of GST activity with trans-stilbene oxide (*56*), and the Southern blotting of genomic DNA (*50, 51, 55*). In order to obtain a relatively rapid and reliable method to identify deficient individuals, we have utilized the polymerase chain reaction (PCR) to amplify a region predicted to include exons 4 and 5 and the intervening intron. We have previously reported the amplification of exon 5 or the 3′ non-translated region and found difficulty in differentiating the products of related Mu class genes (*50*). The incorporation of the intron region allows the differentiation of the *GST1* gene. In Fig. 2, the 180 bp

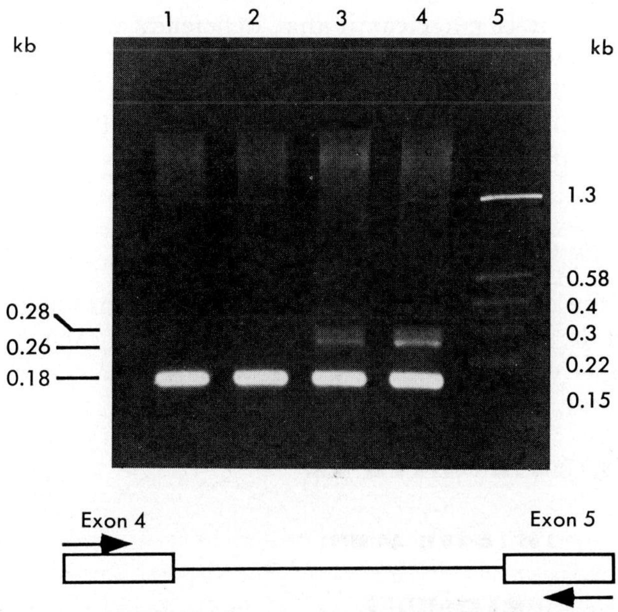


FIG. 2. Amplification of the *GST1* gene by the polymerase chain reaction. Lanes 1 and 2 are GST1 deficient subjects, lanes 3, and 4 from subjects expressing the GST1 isoenzyme. Lane 5 contains size markers. The schematic diagram indicates the relative position of the primers.
Exon 4, 5′-TGCCCTACTTGATTGATGGGG.
Exon 5, 5′-AATTCTGGATTGTAGCAGACTATG.

product is amplified in all individuals and is the size of a product that contains exons 4 and 5 without the intervening intron, and so may indicate the presence of a Mu class intronless pseudogene. The 260 bp and 280 bp fragments are only amplified from DNA obtained from individuals known to express GST1. The observation that two fragments have been differentially amplified in the GST1 positive individuals suggests that the deletion may actually encompass more than one Mu class gene. The PCR amplification of the region between exons 4 and 5 therefore appears to be able to identify individuals who are homozygous for the *GST1* gene deletion.

We have characterized an acidic Mu class isoenzyme termed GST6 (*7*, *38*). This isoenzyme was detected in many tissues but was not present in all individuals studied (*7*). At this stage it is not clear if the absence of GST6 was due to underlying genetic factors or if its expression is regulated by other environmental factors.

As reviewed by us elsewhere (*51*), deficiency of the human Alpha class isoenzymes appears to be relatively rare. However, we have previously reported large individual variations in the relative expression of GST2 type 1 and GST2 type 2 in the liver (*32*). These two isoenzymes were originally thought to be allelic products of a single locus and the variation was attributed to the homozygous and heterozygous expression of the two alleles. Since the two isoenzymes are now known to be the products of closely linked independent gene loci, it is evident that there must be additional factors that differentially regulate their expression. Whether these factors are genetic or environmental remains to be determined.

Large variations in the activity of GST3, the major human Pi class isoenzyme, have been reported on several occasions (*57*, *58*) and there is some evidence that this variation may be inherited (*57*). A single case of erythrocyte GST3 deficiency has been reported (*59*), however, it is not clear if that deficiency was genetically determined. Secondary deficiency of erythrocyte GST3 occurs in glutathione deficiency (*60*) and it appears that GST3 is susceptible to oxidative stress. Recent studies have suggested that a reactive cysteine residue is required for activity in Pi class isoenzymes (*61*). Genetically determined deficiency of GST3 therefore appears to be a relatively rare event.

### *The Chromosomal Location of the GST Genes*

We have determined the chromosomal locations of several cytosolic GST genes by *in situ* hybridization and the data suggest that the genes encoding each evolutionary class are clustered on distinct chromosomes as shown in Fig. 3 (*62*, *63*; Webb, Ross and Board, unpublished data).

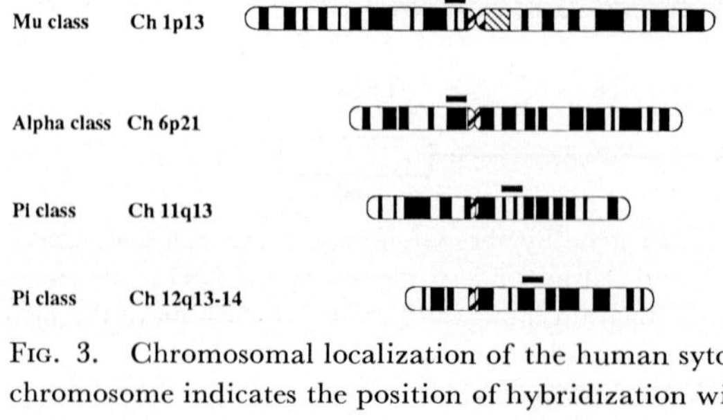


FIG. 3. Chromosomal localization of the human sytosolic *GST* genes. The heavy bar over each chromosome indicates the position of hybridization with class specific cDNA probes.

There appears to be some question over the location of the Mu class genes. Previous studies by *in situ* hybridization (*64*) have suggested that the gene for the *GST1* gene is located at band p31 of chromosome 1. In contrast, other studies (*65*) using a rat Mu class probe on somatic cell hybrid DNA have suggested that there is a Mu class gene on chromosome 3. Our own *in situ* hybridization studies (Webb, Ross and Board, unpublished data) using a human Mu class probe isolated from a testis cDNA library have identified band 1p13 as the most likely location of the Mu class gene cluster; our studies have included individuals with and without the *GST1* gene deletion and have not identified any significant hybridization on chromosome 3.

The Alpha class genes appear to be clustered at band p12 on chromosome 6 (*62*). "Southern" blots show a number of hybridizing bands suggesting that there are multiple Alpha class genes in this region.

In contrast to the Mu and Alpha class genes, Pi class genes have been mapped to more than one chromosome. Previous studies using somatic cell hybrids and an electrophoretic zymogram technique mapped the Pi class *GST3* gene to chromosome 11 (*66*). Subsequent *in situ* hybridization studies have refined this location to 11q13 (*63*). In the course of those studies we have identified an additional area of hybridization on chromosome 12 at bands q13–14. Further studies are in progress to determine if this additional locus encodes an active gene.

The gene encoding the microsomal GST has been mapped broadly to chromosome 12 by the use of a panel of somatic cell hybrids (*67*).

### *The Structure of the GST Genes*

The *GST3* gene has been cloned and sequenced by two groups (*68, 69*). It is encoded by 7 exons and is contained within approximately 3 kb. While the structure of the *GST3* gene is similar to the Pi class *GSTP* gene in rats, their regulation appears to be quite distinct (*70, 71*).

The complete structure of a human Mu class gene has not been published, however, preliminary data (*72*) suggests that they have similar exon-intron structures to those found in the rat.

We have recently cloned and sequenced part or all of seven human Alpha class genes. Many of these genes appear to be pseudogenes because of the presence of a range of exon deletions, point mutations, and frame shift mutations. The human Alpha class genes have a similar structure to those of rats and mice and include 7 exons with similar exon-intron boundaries and conservation of exon sequence (*73, 74*). A complete human Alpha class gene extends over 13 kb, thus the Alpha class genes appear to be the largest of all the known GST genes.

The human Alpha class genes appear to be closely linked, and we have isolated several $\lambda$ phage genomic clones that incorporate parts of more than one gene. For example, the gene encoding the GST2 type 1 isoenzyme lies 1.74 kb downstream of a pseudogene. We have sequenced the entire intergenic region which should contain many of the elements regulating expression of this major liver isoenzyme. The regulatory elements in the 5′ flanking regions of the rat and mouse Ya (Alpha class) genes have been studied in some detail (*75–77*) and alignment of this region shows large areas of homology. Despite this similarity, there appear to be differences in the regula-

TABLE 1. Putative Regulatory Elements from the GST2 1 Gene

| Response element | Sequence | Position |
|---|---|---|
| Heat shock (HSE) | CAAGAATTGTCCTG | −1,494 |
| | CCTGCGTCTTCTAG | −990 |
| | CTTCTAGCTTCTGG | −983 |
| | TCTGGACTTTCATG | −955 |
| consensus (78) | CNNGAANNTTCNNG | |
| Drug response (DRE) | CCTGGCTGCG | −1,114 |
| | CATAGCTGGG | −334 |
| consensus (77) | $^{C}_{G}$N$^{TA}_{GG}$GCTGGG | |
| Xenobiotic response (XRE) | TTGAGTGacgcaaa | −600 |
| | AACtcaGTGCGTTT | |
| consensus (75) | TNGCGTG | |
| Antioxidant response (ARE) | | |
| | GCCCTAGTCTTTGCACCCAACTCATGAAAAAAAGCATCTTT | −287 |
| | GTGAGGACAATTGTCATTGGATTTGGGGCCTATCCAGATAT | −996 |
| rat (74) | GAGCTTGGAAATGGCATTGCTAATGGTGACAAAGCAACTTT | |

tion of these two rodent genes. The rat gene has a functional xenobiotic response element (XRE) and a so-called antioxidant response element (ARE) (*75*). In contrast, the mouse gene appears to respond only to an element equivalent to the rat ARE (*76*).

Alignment and comparison of the 5′ flanking sequence of the *GST2* type 1 gene with the equivalent region of the rat and mouse Ya genes (*75, 77*) reveals very few areas of homology, suggesting there has been little conservation or that these genes are not orthologues. The sequence of the 5′ flanking region of the *GST2 type 1* gene has been scanned for regions of homology to known regulatory elements and a summary of those identified is shown in Table 1. Although a direct alignment of 5′ flanking sequences is not informative, there appear to be two regions with weak homology to the rat ARE (*75*). The putative ARE at −287 bp appears to have a good match over the last 11 base pairs. As the essential components of an ARE have not yet been determined, it is difficult to predict if either or both of these elements are functional in the human gene.

A complex of two XREs occurs between −610 bp and −576 bp. These elements are on different strands and form an almost perfect palindrome. Two possible drug response elements (DREs) (*78*) have been identified. These elements do not appear to be present in the regions of the rat and mouse genes studied so far. The DRE at −334 bp is an exact match of the previously reported consensus (*78*) but occurs on the complimentary strand.

Four possible heat shock elements (HSEs) (*79*) have been detected in the 5′ flanking region of the human *GST2 type 1* gene. In contrast, we have only detected one in the rat and mouse genes. HSEs can confer heat or stress inducibility on heterologous promoters and frequently occur in overlapping configurations (*79*). The presence of several possible HSEs suggests that the human gene may respond to environmental stress.

Although the enhancer motifs identified in the 5′ flanking region of the human *GST2 type 1* gene suggest that it may be subjected to regulation by xenobiotics and other environmental factors, the absolute function of these elements in the regulation of transcriptions needs to be confirmed experimentally. These studies are currently in progress.

### *Conclusion*

The glutathione transferases are a large family of multifunctional proteins. The high degree of heterogeneity of the human GSTs appears to be largely genetically determined and results from the differential expression of multiple genes between tissues, stages of development, and individuals.

The glutathione transferase gene family can be subdivided into at least five classes, each comprised of varying numbers of genes. To a large extent, the genes of a particular class are clustered in distinct chromosomal regions.

There are clearly large differences in the factors regulating the expression of the various GST genes. These differences in expression presumably reflect the differences in catalytic activity and function of the various isoenzymes.

*Acknowledgment*

The authors are grateful to S. Smith for technical assistance.

## REFERENCES

1. Jakoby, W. B. The glutathione S-transferases: a group of multifunctional detoxification proteins. Adv. Enzymol., *46*: 383–414, 1978.
2. Chasseaud, L. F. The role of glutathione and glutathione S-transferases in the metabolism of chemical carcinogens and other electrophilic agents. Adv. Cancer Res., *29*: 175–274, 1979.
3. Dulik, D. M., Fenselau, C., and Hilton, J. Characterization of melphalan-glutathione adducts whose formation is catalysed by glutathione transferases. Biochem. Pharmacol., *35*: 3405–3409, 1986.
4. Ciaccio, P. J., Tew, K. D., and La Creta, F. P. The spontaneous and glutathione S-transferase-mediated reaction of chlorambucil and glutathione. Cancer Commun., *2*: 279–286, 1990.
5. Jensson, H., Guthenberg, C., Alin, P., and Mannervik, B. Rat glutathione transferases 8–8, an enzyme efficiently detoxifying 4-hydroxyalk-2-enals. FEBS Lett., *203*: 207–209, 1986.
6. Prohaska, J. R. and Ganther, H. F. Glutathione peroxidase activity of glutathione S-transferases purified from rat liver. Biochem. Biophys. Res. Commun., *76*: 437–445, 1977.
7. Suzuki, T., Coggan, M., Shaw, D. C., and Board, P. G. Electrophoretic and immunological analysis of human glutathione S-transferase isoenzymes. Ann. Hum. Genet., *51*: 95–106, 1987.
8. Burgess, J. R., Chow, N. W. I., Reddy, C., and Tu, C.-P. D. Amino acid substitutions in the human glutathione S-transferases confer different specificities in the prostaglandin endoperoxide conversion pathway. Biochem. Biophys. Res. Commun., *158*: 497–502, 1989.
9. Samuelson, B. Leukotrienes: mediators of immediate hypersensitivity reactions and inflammation. Science, *220*: 568–575, 1983.

10. Bora, P. S., Spilburg, C. A., and Lange, L. G. Metabolism of ethanol and carcinogens by glutathione transferases. Proc. Natl. Acad. Sci. U.S.A., *86*: 4470–4473, 1989.

11. Suzuki, T., Kovacs, M., and Board, P. G. Do the major human glutathione S-transferases have fatty acid ethylester synthase activity? FEBS Lett., 1990, in press.

12. Homma, H. and Listowsky, I. Identification of Yb-glutathione S-transferase as a major rat liver protein labelled with dexamethasone 21-methanesulfonate. Proc. Natl. Acad. Sci. U.S.A., *82*: 7165–7169, 1985.

13. Bhargava, M. M., Listowsky, I., and Arias, I. M. Ligandin. Bilirubin binding and glutathione-S-transferase activity are independent processes. J. Biol. Chem., *253*: 4112–4115, 1978.

14. Vander Jagt, D. L., Hunsaker, L. A., Garcia, K. B., and Royer, R. E. Isolation and characterization of the multiple glutathione S-transferases from human liver. J. Biol. Chem., *260*: 11603–11610, 1985.

15. Litwack, G., Ketterer, B., and Arias, I. M. Ligandin: a hepatic protein which binds steroids, bilirubin, carcinogens and a number of exogenous organic anions. Nature, *234*: 466–467, 1971.

16. Habig, W. H., Pabst, M. J., Fleischner, G., Gatmaitan, Z., Arias, I. M., and Jakoby, W. B. The identity of glutathione S-transferase B with ligandin, a major binding protein of liver. Proc. Natl. Acad. Sci. U.S.A., *71*: 3879–3882, 1974.

17. Wolkoff, A. W., Goresky, C. A., Sellin, J., Gatmaitan, Z., and Arias, I. M. Role of ligandin in transfer of bilirubin from plasma into liver. Am. J. Physiol., *236*: E638–E648, 1979.

18. Tipping, E. and Ketterer, B. The influence of soluble binding proteins on lipophile transport and metabolism in hepatocytes. Biochem. J., *195*: 441–442, 1981.

19. Harvey, J. W. and Beutler, E. Binding of heme by glutathione S-transferase: a possible role for the erythrocyte enzyme. Blood, *60*: 1227–1230, 1982.

20. Senjo, M., Ishibashi, T., and Imai, Y. Purification and characterization of cytosolic liver protein facilitating heme transport into apocytochrome $b_5$ from mitochondria. J. Biol. Chem., *260*: 9191–9196, 1985.

21. Dahlöf, B., Martinsson, T., Mannervik, B., Jensson, H., and Levan, G. Characterization of multidrug resistance in SEWA mouse tumor cells: increased glutathione transferase activity and reversal of resistance with verapamil. Anticancer Res., *7*: 65–69, 1987.

22. Shea, T. C., Kelley, S. L., and Henner, W. D. Identification of an anionic form of glutathione transferase present in many human tumours and human tumour cell lines. Cancer Res., *48*: 527–533, 1988.

23. Moscow, J. A., Fairchild, C. R., Madden, M. J., Ransom, D. T., Wieand, H. S., O'Brien, E. E., Poplack, D. G., Cossman, J., Myers, C. E., and Cowan, K. Y. Expression of anionic glutathione S-transferase and P glycoprotein genes in human tissues and tumors. Cancer Res., *49*: 1322–1428, 1989.

24. Wang, A. L. and Tew, K. D. Increased glutathione S-transferase activity in a cell line with acquired resistance to nitrogen mustards. Cancer Treatment Reports, *69*: 677–682, 1985.

25. Buller, A. L., Clapper, M. L., and Tew, K. D. Glutathione S-transferases in nitrogen mustard-resistant and sensitive cell lines. Mol. Pharmacol., *31*: 575–578, 1987.

26. Lewis, A. D., Hickson, I. D., Robson, C. N., Harris, A. L., Hayes, J. D., Griffith, S. A., Manson, A. M., Hall, A. E., Moss, J. E., and Wolf, C. R. Amplification and increased expression of alpha class glutathione S-transferase-encoding genes associated with resistance to nitrogen mustards. Proc. Natl. Acad. Sci. U.S.A., *85*: 8511–8515, 1988.

27. Batist, G., Tupule, A., Sinha, B., Katki, A. G., Myers, E. E., and Cowan, K. H. Overexpression of a novel anionic glutathione S-transferase in multi-drug resistant human

breast cancer cells. J. Biol. Chem., *261*: 15544–15549, 1986.

28. Smith, M. T., Evans, C. G., Doane-Setzer, P., Castro, V. M., Tahir, M. K., and Mannervik, B. Denitrosation of 1, 3-bis(2-chloroethyl)-1-nitrosourea by class Mu glutathione transferases and its role in cellular resistance in rat brain tumor cells. Cancer Res., *49*: 2621–2625, 1989.
29. Nakagawa, K., Saijo, N., Tsuchida, S., Sakai, M., Tsunokawa, Y., Yokota, J., Muramatsu, M., Sato, K., Terada, M., and Tew, K. Glutathione S-transferase $\pi$ as a determinant of drug resistance in transfectant cell lines. J. Biol. Chem., *265*: 4296–4301, 1990.
30. Puchalski, R. B. and Fahl, W. E. Expression of recombinant glutathione S-transferase P, Ya Yb1 confers resistance to alkylating agents. Proc. Natl. Acad. Sci. U.S.A., *87*: 2443–2447, 1990.
31. Black, S. M., Beggs, J. D., Hayes, J. D., Bartoszek, A., Muramatsu, M., Sakai, M., and Wolf, C. R. Expression of human glutathione S-transferases in *Saccharomyces cerevisiae* confers resistance to the anticancer drugs adriamycin and chlorambucil. Biochem. J., *268*: 309–315, 1990.
32. Board, P. G. Biochemical genetics of glutathione S-transferase in man. Am. J. Hum. Genet., *33*: 36–43, 1981.
33. Board, P. G. Gene deletion and partial deficiency of the glutathione S-transferase (ligandin) system in man. FEBS Lett., *135*: 12–14, 1981.
34. Board, P. G. A method for the localization of glutathione S-transferase isoenzymes after starch gel electrophoresis. Anal. Biochem., *105*: 147–149, 1980.
35. Strange, R. C., Faulder, C. G., Davis, B. A., Hume, R., Brown, J. A. H., Cotton, W., and Hopkinson, D. A. The human glutathione S-transferases: studies on the distribution and genetic variation of GST-1, GST-2, and GST-3 isozymes. Ann. Hum. Genet., *48*: 11–20, 1984.
36. Laisney, V., Van Cong, N., Cross, M. S., and Frezal, J. Human genes for glutathione S-transferases. Hum. Genet., *68*: 221–227, 1984.
37. Board, P. G., Suzuki, T., and Shaw, D. C. Human muscle glutathione S-transferase (GST4) shows close homology to human liver GST1. Biochim. Biophys. Acta, *953*: 214–217, 1988.
38. Suzuki, T., Shaw, D. C., and Board, P. G. Purification and characterization of acidic glutathione transferase GST6 from human brain. Biochem. J., *274*: 405–408, 1991.
39. Mannervik, B., Ålin, P., Guthenberg, C., Jensson, H., Tahir, M. K., Warholm, M., and Jörnvall, H. Identification of three classes of cytosolic glutathione transferase common to several mammalian species: correlation between structural data and enzymatic properties. Proc. Natl. Acad. Sci. U.S.A., *82*: 7202–7206, 1985.
40. Stockman, P. K., McLellan, L. I., and Hayes, J. D. Characterization of the basic glutathione S-transferase B1 and B2 subunits from human liver. Biochem. J., *244*: 55–61, 1987.
41. Warholm, M., Guthenberg, C., and Mannervik, B. Molecular and catalytic properties of glutathione transferase mu from human liver: an enzyme efficiently conjugating epoxides. Biochemistry, *22*: 3610–3617, 1983.
42. Del Boccio, G., Di Ilio, C., Ålin, P., Jörnvall, H., and Mannervik, B. Identification of a novel glutathione transferase in human skin homologous with class alpha glutathione transferase 2–2 in the rat. Biochem. J., *244*: 21–25, 1987.
43. Campbell, E., Takahashi, Y., Abramovitz, M., Peretz, M., and Listowsky, I. A distinct human testis and brain class m glutathione S-transferase; molecular cloning and characterization of a form present even in individuals lacking hepatic type mu isoenzymes. J. Biol. Chem., *265*: 9188–9193, 1990.

44. Singh, S. V., Kurosky, A., and Awasthi, Y. C. Human liver glutathione S-transferase $\psi$. Chemical characterization and secondary structure comparison with other mammalian glutathione S-transferases. Biochem. J., *243*: 61–67, 1987.
45. Morgenstern, R., De Pierre, J. W., and Jörnvall, H. Microsomal glutathione transferase: primary structure. J. Biol. Chem., *260*: 13976–13983, 1985.
46. Tan, K. H., Meyer, D. J., Gillies, N., and Ketterer, B. Detoxification of DNA hydroperoxide by glutathione transferases and the purification and characterization of glutathione transferases of the rat liver nucleus. Biochem. J., *254*: 841–845, 1988.
47. Hiratsuka, A., Sebata, N., Kawashima, K., Okuda, H., Ogura, K., Watabe, T., Satoh, K., Hatayama, I., Tsuchida, S., Ishikawa, T., and Sato, K. A new class of rat glutathione S-transferases Yrs-Yrs inactivating reactive sulphate esters as metabolites of carcinogenic arylmethanols. J. Biol. Chem., *265*: 11973–11981, 1990.
48. Smith, D. B., Dayern, K. M., Board, P. G., Tiu, W. U., Garcia, E. G., and Mitchell, G. F. Mr26,000 antigen of *Schistosoma japonicum* recognised by resistant WEHI 129/j mice in a parasite glutathione S-transferase. Proc. Natl. Acad. Sci. U.S.A., *83*: 8703–8707, 1986.
49. Toung, Y-P. S., Hsieh, T-S., and Tu, C-P. D. *Drosophila* glutathione S-transferase 1–1 shares a region of sequence homology with maize glutathione S-transferase III. Proc. Natl. Acad. Sci. U.S.A., *87*: 31–35, 1990.
50. Board, P. G. Genetic polymorphism of glutathione S-transferase in man. *In;* J. D. Hayes, C. B. Pickett, and T. J. Mantle (eds.), Glutathione S-Transferases and Drug Resistance, pp. 232–241, Taylor and Francis, London, 1990.
51. Board, P. G., Coggan, M., Johnston, P., Ross, V., Suzuki, T., and Webb, G. Genetic heterogeneity of the human glutathione transferases. A complex of gene families. Pharmacol. Ther., *48*: 357–369, 1990.
52. Mannervik, B. and Danielson, H. Glutathione transferases—structure and catalytic activity. CRC Crit. Rev. Biochem., *23*: 283–337, 1988.
53. Seidegärd, J., Guthenberg, C., Pero, R. W., and Mannervik, B. The trans-stilbene oxide-active glutathione transferase in human mononuclear leucocytes is identical with the hepatic glutathione transferase $\mu$. Biochem. J., *246*: 783–785, 1987.
54. Seidegärd, J., Pero, R. W., Miller, D. G., and Beattie, E. J. A glutathione transferase in human leukocytes as a marker for the susceptibility to lung cancer. Carcinogenesis, *7*: 751–753, 1987.
55. Seidegärd, J., Varachek, W. R., Pero, R. W., and Pearson, W. R. Hereditary differences in the expression of the human glutathione transferase active on trans-stilbene oxide are due to a gene deletion. Proc. Natl. Acad. Sci. U.S.A., *85*: 7293–7297, 1988.
56. Seidegärd, J., De Pierre, J. W., Birberg, W., Plotti, A., and Pero, R. W. Characterization of soluble glutathione transferase activity in resting mononuclear leukocytes from human blood. Biochem. Pharmacol., *19*: 3053–3058, 1984.
57. Scott, E. M. and Wright, R. C. Variability of glutathione S-transferase of human erythrocytes. Am. J. Hum. Genet., *32*: 115–116, 1980.
58. Strange, R. C., Johnson, P. H., Lawton, A., Moult, J. A., Tector, M. J., Tyminski, R. J., and Cotton, W. Studies on the variability of glutathione S-transferase from human erythrocytes. Clin. Chim. Acta, *120*: 251–260, 1982.
59. Beutler, E., Dunning, D., Dabe, I. B., and Forman, L. Erythrocyte glutathione S-transferase deficiency and hemolytic anemia. Blood, *72*: 73–77, 1988.
60. Beutler, E., Gelbart, T., and Pegelow, C. Erythrocyte glutathione synthetase deficiency leads not only to glutathione but also glutathione S-transferase deficiency. J. Clin. Invest., *77*: 38–41, 1986.
61. Katsuto, T., Santoh, K., Tsuchida, S., Hatayama, I., Maki, T., and Sato, K. Specific inactivation of glutathione S-transferases in class Pi by SH-modifiers. Biochem. Biophys.

Res. Commun., *167*: 331–338, 1990.

62. Board, P. G. and Webb, G. C. Isolation of a cDNA clone and localization of glutathione S-transferase 2 genes to chromosome band 6p12. Proc. Natl. Acad. Sci. U.S.A., *84*: 2377–2381, 1987.
63. Board, P. G., Webb, G. C., and Coggan, M. C. Isolation of a cDNA clone and localization of the human glutathione S-transferase 3 genes to chromosome bands 11q13 and 12q13–14. Ann. Hum. Genet., *53*: 205–213, 1989.
64. De Jong, J. L., Chang, C.-M., Whang-Peng, J., Knutsen, T., and Tu, C.-P. D. The human liver glutathione S-transferase gene superfamily: expression and chromosome mapping of an Hb subunit cDNA. Nucl. Acids Res., *16*: 8541–8554, 1989.
65. Islam, M. Q., Platz, A., Szpirer, J., Szpirer, C., Levan, G., and Mannervik, B. Chromosomal localization of human glutathione transferase genes of classes alpha, mu and pi. Hum. Genet., *82*: 338–342, 1989.
66. Suzuki, T. and Board, P. G. The gene for glutathione S-transferase 3 (GST3) is on chromosome 11. Som. Cell Gen., *10*: 319–320, 1984.
67. De Jong, J. L., Mohandas, T., and Tu, C-P. D. The gene for the microsomal glutathione S-transferase is on human chromosome 12. Genomics, *6*: 379–382, 1990.
68. Cowell, I. G., Dixon, K. H., Pemble, S. E., Ketterer, B., and Taylor, J. B. The structure of the human glutathione S-transferase $\pi$ gene. Biochem. J., *255*: 79–83, 1988.
69. Morrow, C. S. Cowan, K. H., and Goldsmith, M. E. Structure of the human genomic glutathione S-transferase-$\pi$ gene. Gene, *75*: 3–11, 1989.
70. Sakai, M., Okuda, A., and Muramatsu, M. Multiple regulatory elements and phorbol 12-O-tetradecanoate 13-acetate responsiveness of rat placental glutathione transferase gene. Proc. Natl. Acad. Sci. U.S.A., *85*: 9456–9460, 1988.
71. Dixon, K. H., Cowell, I. G., Xia, C. L., Pemble, S. E., Ketterer, B., and Taylor, J. B. Control of expression of the human glutathione S-transferase $\pi$ gene differs from its rat orthologue. Biochem. Biophys. Res. Commun., *163*: 815–822, 1989.
72. Taylor, J. B., Oliver, J., Pemble, S. E., and Ketterer, B. Structural relationships of human class mu glutathione S-transferase genes: Evidence for gene conversion and for a subdivision of the class. *In;* J. D. Hayes, C. B. Pickett, and T. J. Mantle (eds.), Glutathione S-Transferases and Drug Resistance, pp. 242–249, Taylor and Francis, London, 1990.
73. Telakowski-Hopkins, C. A., Rothkopf, G. S., and Pickett, C. B. Structural analysis of a rat liver glutathione S-transferase Ya gene. Proc. Natl. Acad. Sci. U.S.A., *83*: 9393–9397, 1986.
74. Daniel, V., Sharon, R., Tichauer, Y., and Sarid, S. Mouse glutathione S-transferase Ya subunit: Gene structure and sequence. DNA, *6*: 317–324, 1987.
75. Rushmore, T. H., King, R. G., Paulson, K. E., and Pickett, C. B. Regulation of glutathione S-transferase Ya subunit gene expression: Identification of a unique xenobiotic-response element controlling inducible expression by planar aromatic compounds. Proc. Natl. Acad. Sci. U.S.A., *87*: 3826–3830, 1990.
76. Rushmore, T. H. and Pickett, C. B. Transcriptional regulation of the rat glutathione S-transferase Ya subunit gene. J. Biol. Chem., *265*: 14648–14653, 1990.
77. Daniel, V., Tichauer, Y., and Sharon, R. 5′ flanking sequence of mouse glutathione transferase Ya gene. Nucleic Acids Res., *16*: 351, 1988.
78. Sogawa, K., Fujisawa-Sehara, A., Yamaue, M., and Fuji-Kuriyama, Y. Location of regulatory elements responsible for drug induction in the rat cytochrome P-450c gene. Proc. Natl. Acad. Sci. U.S.A., *83*: 8044–8048, 1986.
79. Bienz, M. and Pelham, H. R. B. Mechanisms of heat-shock gene activation in higher eukaryotes. Adv. Genet., *24*: 31–72, 1987.

XENOBIOTICS AND CANCER, L. ERNSTER ET AL. (EDS.),
JAPAN SCI. SOC. PRESS, TOKYO/TAYLOR & FRANCIS LTD., LONDON, pp. 213–226, 1991

# Effects of Xenobiotics on Signal Transduction and $Ca^{2+}$ Mediated Processes in Mammalian Cells

George E. N. KASS, Pierluigi NICOTERA, and Sten ORRENIUS

*Department of Toxicology, Karolinska Institutet, S-104 01 Stockholm, Sweden*

*Abstract:* Cellular responses to hormones and growth factors that act through the hydrolysis of membrane-bound inositol phospholipid are mediated by at least two second messengers—diacylglycerol and inositol 1, 4, 5-trisphosphate. While diacylglycerol stimulates protein kinase C activity, inositol 1, 4, 5-trisphosphate mobilizes intracellular $Ca^{2+}$.

Studies in our laboratory have demonstrated that xenobiotics can interfere with signal transduction at different levels with a resulting loss of normal $Ca^{2+}$ responses to hormones and growth factors. Effects of toxicants on ion channels, receptors, G proteins, and other enzymes involved in cell signalling have been investigated. Our recent studies have shown that mild oxidative stress can activate protein kinase C which may in turn stimulate cell proliferation. In addition, toxic agents can directly affect intracellular $Ca^{2+}$ homeostasis by interfering with $Ca^{2+}$ pumps and $Ca^{2+}$ channels. This can compromise the ability of the cell to buffer $Ca^{2+}$ changes and result in a sustained elevation of the cytosolic $Ca^{2+}$ concentration with the subsequent activation of various $Ca^{2+}$-dependent degradative processes. Thus, the alteration of cell signalling by toxicants may affect several important cell functions, including cell differentiation and proliferation, and may ultimately lead to cell death.

The involvement of $Ca^{2+}$ in the regulation of a large number of physiological processes, such as cell differentiation and proliferation, secretion, and control of metabolic reactions is now well established (*1*). Along with this knowledge has come the understanding that $Ca^{2+}$ can also play a determinant role in a variety of pathological and toxicological processes. It has long been recognized that $Ca^{2+}$ accumulates in necrotic tissue (*2, 3*), and subsequent work has revealed that a disruption of intracellular $Ca^{2+}$ homeostasis is frequently associated with the early development of cell injury (*3–5*). This led to the formulation of the $Ca^{2+}$ hypothesis of cell injury, proposing that disruption of the intracellular $Ca^{2+}$ homeostasis may be a common step in the development of cytotoxicity (*4*).

During the past several years it has become progressively clear that sustained increases in intracellular $Ca^{2+}$ can activate cytotoxic mechanisms associated with irreversible injury in various cell systems and organs. Thus, $Ca^{2+}$ appears to mediate the neurotoxicity of cyanide, chlordecone and heavy metals, including lead, mercury and organotin compounds (*6*). In addition, intracellular $Ca^{2+}$ accumulation due to excessive stimulation of excitatory amino acid receptors and enhanced $Ca^{2+}$ influx through membrane channels appears to play an important role in brain ischemia (*7*). An elevation of intracellular $Ca^{2+}$ also seems to contribute to cell killing by several hepatotoxic agents, such as acetaminophen (*8–10*), diquat and $CCl_4$ (*10*), quinones (*11*), cyanide (*12*), and N-methyl-4-phenylpyridine (*13*). An increased intracellular $Ca^{2+}$ level has also been reported to be the determinant factor in the development of thymocyte killing by 2,3,7,8-tetrachlorodibenzo-*p*-dioxin (TCDD) and tributyltin (*14, 15*), and in the development of reperfusion injury in the heart (*16*) and oxidative damage to kidney membranes during cold ischemia (*17*). There is also increasing evidence that $Ca^{2+}$ plays an important role in cell killing in the immune system. Finally, recent studies have suggested that both bacterial toxins (*18*) and viral components such as the HIV envelope glycoprotein gp 120 (*19*) can promote killing of infected cells by increasing intracellular $Ca^{2+}$ levels.

### *Regulation of Intracellular $Ca^{2+}$ Homeostasis*

Recent studies using selective indicators have shown that the $Ca^{2+}$ concentration in the cytosol ($[Ca^{2+}]_i$) of unstimulated cells is maintained between 0.1 and 0.2 $\mu$M (see ref. *20* for review). Consequently, there is a concentration difference of about four orders of magnitude between the extracellular $Ca^{2+}$ level (approximately 1.3 mM) and the cytosolic $Ca^{2+}$ concentration. This produces a large electrochemical driving force which is balanced primarily by active $Ca^{2+}$ extrusion through the plasma membrane and by the coordinated activity of $Ca^{2+}$ sequestering systems located in the endoplasmic reticular, mitochondrial, and nuclear membranes.

#### *1. $Ca^{2+}$ transport by the plasma membrane*

The cellular influx of $Ca^{2+}$ is driven by its electrochemical gradient. In excitable tissue, at least three types of voltage-dependent $Ca^{2+}$ channels (VDC) with different pharmacological properties have been identified (*21*). In contrast, there is no clear evidence for the existence of voltage-operated $Ca^{2+}$ channels in most non-excitable cells. Recent studies in this and other laboratories have shown that $Ca^{2+}$ inflow during agonist stimulation in hepatocytes occurs *via* receptor-operated $Ca^{2+}$ channels (ROC) (*22*). However, it is not yet clear whether $Ca^{2+}$ influx under resting conditions involves these channels or others yet to be identified.

The continuous inflow of $Ca^{2+}$ through the plasma membrane is balanced by specific $Ca^{2+}$-ATPases which extrude $Ca^{2+}$ from cells. In addition, in excitable tissues various ion exchangers can function in a coordinated fashion to extrude calcium ions (*20*). In hepatocytes, the plasma membrane $Ca^{2+}$-ATPase is the predominant $Ca^{2+}$ extrusion system (*23*). It is located in the sinusoidal region of the plasma membrane and has a molecular mass of around 140 kDa (*24*) and a very high affinity for $Ca^{2+}$ ($K_{0.5}=14$ nM) (*25*). In contrast with the erythrocyte enzyme, the liver plasma membrane $Ca^{2+}$-ATPase does not appear to be stimulated by calmodulin, although recent evidence from our laboratory suggests that this $Ca^{2+}$ transporter may be activated by second messenger(s) generated in response to $Ca^{2+}$-mobilizing hormones (*26*).

*2. $Ca^{2+}$ sequestration by the endoplasmic reticulum*

The endoplasmic reticulum sequesters $Ca^{2+}$ through a $Ca^{2+}$-ATPase with a molecular weight of about 125 kDa (*27*). This enzyme has a high affinity for $Ca^{2+}$ ($K_{0.5}=0.2$–$1$ μM), and isolated liver microsomes can accumulate 10–20 nmoles of $Ca^{2+}$ per mg protein in the presence of ATP. We have recently reported that the antioxidant, 2,5-di-(*tert*-butyl)-1,4-benzohydroquinone (tBuBHQ), is a potent ($K_i=350$ nM) and selective inhibitor of the liver endoplasmic reticular $Ca^{2+}$-ATPase (*28–30*). The regulation of $Ca^{2+}$ sequestration by the hepatic endoplasmic reticulum is still poorly understood. Although the involvement of calmodulin in this process has been suggested (*31*), convincing evidence for this assumption is still missing. More recently, a role for glucose-6-phosphatase in the regulation of $Ca^{2+}$ sequestration by the hepatic endoplasmic reticulum has been proposed in an attempt to couple the hydrolysis of glucose-6-phosphate to the termination of the $Ca^{2+}$ transient by enhancing $Ca^{2+}$ sequestration through the intraluminal accumulation of inorganic phosphate (*32*).

*3. $Ca^{2+}$ sequestration by mitochondria*

The inner mitochondrial membrane possesses a uniport carrier which allows the electrogenic entry of $Ca^{2+}$ in response to the negative transmembrane potential (*33*). This $Ca^{2+}$ uniporter has a low affinity for $Ca^{2+}$ ($K_{0.5}=5$–$10$ μM), and it is inhibited by ruthenium red, a hexavalent ammonium complex of Ru. Mitochondria also exhibit a pathway for $Ca^{2+}$ efflux which is separate from the uniporter. In heart and brain, $Ca^{2+}$ efflux from mitochondria is $Na^+$-dependent, whereas in liver mitochondria the predominant $Ca^{2+}$ efflux pathway is a $Na^+$-independent and electroneutral $Ca^{2+}/H^+$ antiporter (*20*), which appears to be regulated by protein mono (ADP-ribosylation) (*34*).

*4. $Ca^{2+}$ sequestration by liver nuclei*

The existence of relatively large pores in the nuclear envelope has generally been taken as evidence for the free diffusion of ions and small molecules in and out of the nucleus. However, using a suspension of isolated liver nuclei we have recently identified and partially characterized an ATP-stimulated $Ca^{2+}$ uptake system which promotes an increase in the intranuclear free $Ca^{2+}$ concentration (*35*). The $Ca^{2+}$ uptake is coupled to ATP hydrolysis and it appears to be regulated by calmodulin. Additional studies have shown that liver nuclei can sequester about 2 nmoles of $Ca^{2+}$ per mg protein and have suggested a potential role for the nucleus in the regulation of the cytosolic free $Ca^{2+}$ concentration (*36*). We have also found that the intracellular messenger, inositol 1, 4, 5-trisphosphate, stimulates the release of a fraction of the nuclear $Ca^{2+}$ and transiently lowers the intranuclear free $Ca^{2+}$ concentration.

## *Control of $Ca^{2+}$ Homeostasis in Hepatocytes and Role of $Ca^{2+}$ in Cell Signalling*

As described above, the low sub-micromolar $[Ca^{2+}]_i$ is achieved by the concerted action of the plasma membrane $Ca^{2+}$ pump and active $Ca^{2+}$ sequestration by the mitochondria, endoplasmic reticulum, and nucleus. Although isolated mitochondria can accumulate large amounts of $Ca^{2+}$, the affinity for $Ca^{2+}$ of the uniport carrier is low, which implies that under resting conditions mitochondria play a minor role in buffering cytosolic $Ca^{2+}$. In addition, electron probe X-ray microanalysis of rapidly frozen liver sections has demonstrated that mitochondria contain little $Ca^{2+}$ *in situ* (about 1 nmol $Ca^{2+}$ per mg protein), whereas the endoplasmic reticulum represents the major intracellular $Ca^{2+}$ store (*37*). Our recent finding that the nucleus has a high $Ca^{2+}$-buffering capacity opens the possibility that this compartment may also be involved in the regulation of the cytosolic free $Ca^{2+}$ concentration.

Stimulation of hepatocytes with $Ca^{2+}$-mobilizing hormones such as vasopressin, angiotensin II, or phenylephrine produces a transient elevation of $[Ca^{2+}]_i$ to 0.4–1 $\mu$M (*38*). Such hormone-induced $[Ca^{2+}]_i$ transients in populations of hepatocytes are comprised of two separate phases, an initial rapid increase in $[Ca^{2+}]_i$ followed by a slow return to basal, or near basal, levels. With the recent development of digital imaging techniques, it has become possible to study $[Ca^{2+}]_i$ transients in individual cells and this has led to the observation that at low, close to threshold concentrations of $Ca^{2+}$-mobilizing hormones, the hepatocytes respond to these agents with oscillating $[Ca^{2+}]_i$ spikes (*39*). The mechanisms by which $Ca^{2+}$-mobilizing hormones produce $[Ca^{2+}]_i$ transients have been extensively studied in recent years (*40*). The signal transduction pathway leading to the elevation of $[Ca^{2+}]_i$ can be summarized as follows. Upon binding of the hormone to its plasma membrane receptor, a specific phospholipase C becomes activated *via* stimulation of a G protein, and hydrolyzes phosphatidylinositol 4,5-bisphosphate to generate two second messengers, inositol 1,4,5-trisphosphate and diacylglycerol. Diacylglycerol is a potent activator of protein kinase C (*41*) and inositol 1,4,5-trisphosphate is the mediator for $Ca^{2+}$ release from a non-mitochondrial intracellular store; this release of $Ca^{2+}$ is responsible for the initial rapid elevation of $[Ca^{2+}]_i$ (*40*). The $Ca^{2+}$ mobilization sequence is schematically illustrated in Fig. 1.

The precise location of the inositol 1,4,5-trisphosphate-sensitive $Ca^{2+}$ pool is not known. Subcellular fractionation and immunocytochemical studies on the localization of the specific receptor for inositol 1, 4, 5-trisphosphate are suggesting that part of this pool is located within the endoplasmic reticulum (*42, 43*). The $Ca^{2+}$ content of this pool is largely controlled by the endoplasmic reticular $Ca^{2+}$ translocase and is releasable by the specific inhibitor of the latter enzyme, tBuBHQ (*30*). In addition,

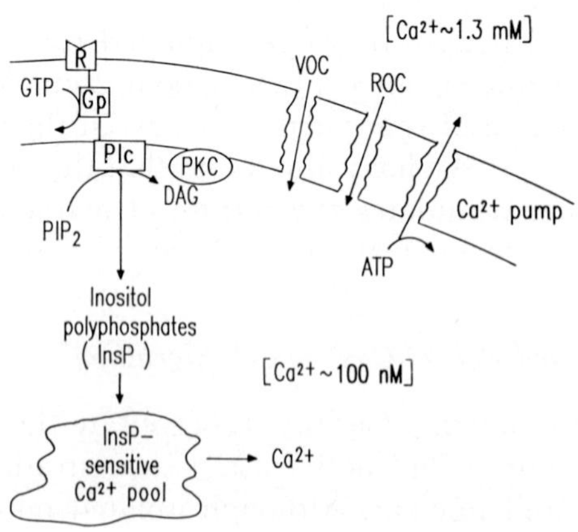


FIG. 1. Schematic illustration of $Ca^{2+}$ signalling pathways in non-muscle cells.

as discussed above, recent work from our laboratory has produced evidence for the existence of a second inositol 1,4,5-trisphosphate-sensitive, but tBuBHQ-insensitive, $Ca^{2+}$ store that is located within the hepatocyte nucleus (*36*). The contribution of this pool to the agonist-induced elevation of cytosolic $Ca^{2+}$ is yet to be elucidated.

An intriguing observation is that GTP can potentiate inositol 1, 4, 5-trisphosphate-mediated $Ca^{2+}$ release and also release $Ca^{2+}$ by itself from liver microsomes (*44*) and from permeabilized hepatocytes (*45*). The mechanism by which the GTP-mediated $Ca^{2+}$ release occurs and its physiological significance are still a matter of debate.

### *Hormonal Stimulation of $Ca^{2+}$ Fluxes across the Hepatic Plasma Membrane*

The addition of tBuBHQ to isolated hepatocytes results in a rapid release of the inositol 1,4,5-trisphosphate-sensitive $Ca^{2+}$ store; however, in contrast with $Ca^{2+}$-mobilizing hormones, the release of this $Ca^{2+}$ pool results in sustained elevation of $[Ca^{2+}]_i$ instead of a $[Ca^{2+}]_i$ transient (*30*). Furthermore, addition of a $Ca^{2+}$-mobilizing hormone after tBuBHQ produces a rapid return of $[Ca^{2+}]_i$ to basal levels by stimulating $Ca^{2+}$ efflux (*26*), and, when added after a hormone-induced $[Ca^{2+}]_i$ transient, tBuBHQ also produces a $[Ca^{2+}]_i$ transient rather than the sustained elevation observed in the absence of hormones. These findings led us to conclude that $Ca^{2+}$-mobilizing hormones, in addition to releasing $Ca^{2+}$ from intracellular stores *via* the generation of inositol 1,4,5-trisphosphate, also regulate the termination of the $[Ca^{2+}]_i$ signal by activating a specific $Ca^{2+}$ efflux pathway.

The duration of the second phase of the $[Ca^{2+}]_i$ transient evoked by $Ca^{2+}$-mobilizing hormones depends on the presence of extracellular $Ca^{2+}$ and has been shown in liver cells to involve the stimulation of $Ca^{2+}$ influx (*46*), partly through specific receptor-operated $Ca^{2+}$ channels (*22*). Opening of these channels requires the transduction of the receptor activation signal *via* a pertussis toxin-insensitive G protein, and the rate of cation influx is independently controlled by the intracellular levels of cyclic AMP and the $Ca^{2+}$ content of an intracellular $Ca^{2+}$ store (*22*).

### *Alteration of Cell Signalling and $Ca^{2+}$ Responses by Toxicants*

#### 1. *Importance of cell signalling for cell survival*

Given the many physiological functions that are attributed to calcium and which are under tight hormonal or growth factor control, it is not surprising that hormone- and growth factor-dependent signal transduction pathways may be the targets for a number of toxicants. Indeed, normal growth of cells requires the continuous presence of various growth factors, and removal of such factors will not only deprive these cells of a trophic stimulus but, as recent evidence clearly indicates (*47*), it may also result in the activation of a suicide process referred to as "programmed cell death" or "apoptosis" (*48*). Apoptosis is a physiological process of self-destruction that is involved in embryo morphogenesis as well as in clonal deletion during thymic development (*48*). Several early morphological changes occur in apoptotic cells, including widespread plasma and nuclear membrane blebbing, compacting of organelles, and chromatin condensation. The most reliable and characteristic marker for this process is the activation of a $Ca^{2+}$-dependent endonuclease which cleaves DNA at the internucleosomal linker regions, producing oligonucleosome-sized fragments (*49*). Apoptosis can be induced *in vitro* by interleukin 3 deprivation of hemopoietic precursor cells (*52*) and fibroblast growth factor deprivation of endothelial cells (*51*). Several *in vivo* cases are also known where removal of certain trophic stimuli results in apoptosis of, for example, adenocarcinoma cells (*52, 53*). Consequently, perturbation of hormonal signalling by toxins could generate an inability of the target cells to properly respond to the physiological stimuli necessary for their survival. In addition, a number of toxins have been identified that inappropriately activate or markedly modify cellular signalling, and this may contribute to the mechanism of cell killing by these agents.

*2. Toxins act at different levels of the signal transduction cascade*

Among the best described examples of cytotoxins that act at the receptor level are the neurotoxic organophosphorus drugs. This family of compounds which includes soman and malaoxon act by inhibiting cholinesterases, thereby producing cholinergic receptor overstimulation, increased phosphoinositide turnover (*54, 55*) and cell death, probably as a consequence of a pathological elevation of intracellular calcium levels (*54*). In contrast, many toxins have been reported to inhibit hormone-stimulated inositol phosphate release (Table 1). For instance, exposure of hepatocytes to oxidative stress has been shown to inhibit the generation of inositol phosphates, possibly by inactivating the transducing G protein (*56*). Interestingly, mild oxidative stress can, under certain conditions, promote the activation of protein kinase C in hepatocytes (*57*), and this may result in stimulation of cell proliferation. Thus, the exposure level to prooxidants may be critical to stimulate either lethal processes or proliferative responses.

Table 2 lists a number of toxins that have been shown to alter protein kinase C activity. While it is not clear yet what detrimental effects inhibition or stimulation can have on cell survival (see also below), the lethal effects of excessive protein phos-

TABLE 1. Toxicants Affecting Phosphoinositide Turnover

| Stimulators of inositol phosphate formation | | |
|---|---|---|
| | Postulated mechanism | Reference |
| Maitotoxin | Elevation of $[Ca^{2+}]_i$ | (*74*) |
| Calcium ionophore | $PLA_2$-dependent arachidonate metabolism | (*75*) |
| Malaoxon | Inhibition of cholinesterase | (*54*) |
| Soman | Inhibition of cholinesterase | (*55*) |
| Pumliotoxin B | Activation of $Na^+$ channels | (*76*) |
| Mastoparan | Activation of G protein | (*77*) |
| Hydroxyalkenals | Activation of PLC | (*78*) |
| Ethanol | Membrane perturbation | (*79*) |
| Gliotoxin | ? | (*80*) |
| **Inhibitors of agonist-stimulated inositol phosphate formation** | | |
| | Postulated mechanism | Reference |
| Prooxidants | Inhibition of G protein | (*56*) |
| Mercury | Interaction with thiol groups | (*81*) |
| Antimycin A | Depletion of cellular ATP | (*62*) |
| Antitumor ether lipids | ? | (*82*) |

TABLE 2. Toxins Affecting Protein Kinase C Activity

| Activators of protein kinase C | Reference |
|---|---|
| Prooxidants | (*57*) |
| Lead | (*66*) |
| Bistratene A & B | (*83*) |
| Endotoxic lipid A | (*84*) |
| Halothane | (*85*) |
| Chloroform | (*86*) |
| **Inhibitors of protein kinase C** | **Reference** |
| Ebselen | (*87*) |
| Suramin | (*88*) |
| Endotoxic lipid X | (*84*) |
| Mercury | (*66*) |

phorylation have become apparent with the discovery that the potent cyanobacterial hepatotoxin microcystin-LR (*58*) is a specific inhibitor of mammalian protein phosphatases 1 and 2A (*59*).

Inability of cells to respond to $Ca^{2+}$-mobilizing hormones can also result from the selective depletion of the intracellular agonist-sensitive $Ca^{2+}$ pool by compounds such as tBuBHQ (*30*) or bromotrichloromethane (*60*). A further possible target are the $Ca^{2+}$ channels, as recently demonstrated with maitotoxin (*61*). This potent dinoflagellate toxin opens verapamil-sensitive $Ca^{2+}$ channels in the plasma membrane and causes cell death by inducing a sustained elevation of $[Ca^{2+}]_i$. Perturbation of signal transduction can also be induced by mitochondrial poisons, including antimycin A and the uncoupler FCCP. These agents have been found, probably as a result of their ATP-depleting effect, to inhibit inositol triphosphate ($InsP_3$) formation (*62*), to deplete the agonist-sensitive intracellular $Ca^{2+}$ store and to inhibit $Ca^{2+}$ fluxes in and out of cells (*63*).

### 3. *Disruption of $Ca^{2+}$ homeostasis and cell signalling by heavy metals*

A perturbation of cell signalling can occur during heavy metal intoxication. For instance, Schöfl *et al.* (*64*) have recently reported that aluminium salts disrupt $Ca^{2+}$ oscillations in hepatocytes exposed to $Ca^{2+}$-mobilizing hormones, producing broad $Ca^{2+}$ spikes lasting several minutes. Protein kinase C may act as a target for heavy metals and their interaction with this enzyme generally results in the inhibition of its activity (*65*). Surprising, however, is the effect of lead which at extremely low concentration ($10^{-15}$M) has been found to activate rather than inhibit protein kinase C (*66*).

Recent work in our laboratory has focused on the mechanism of inorganic mercury neurotoxicity and has revealed that exposure of neuroadrenergic Pc-12 cells to $Hg^{2+}$ at concentrations between 0.1 $\mu$M and 2 $\mu$M modified the ability of the cells to respond to agonist stimulation. Interestingly, at lower $Hg^{2+}$ concentrations (0.1–0.5 $\mu$M), we observed a stimulation of agonist-induced increase in cytosolic $Ca^{2+}$. At these concentrations, $Hg^{2+}$ did not stimulate $InsP_3$ formation by itself, nor did the heavy metal modify the resting cytosolic $Ca^{2+}$ level. In contrast, at higher concentrations of mercury (0.5–2 $\mu$M), agonist-stimulated $InsP_3$ production was markedly reduced and the $Ca^{2+}$ transient associated with hormone stimulation was decreased. At these higher concentrations, $Hg^{2+}$ caused a rapid increase in $[Ca^{2+}]_i$ which was concentration-dependent. This increase was prevented by the $Ca^{2+}$ channel blocker verapamil, suggesting that $Hg^{2+}$ facilitates $Ca^{2+}$ influx by a modification of verapamil-sensitive, voltage-dependent $Ca^{2+}$ channels. Since verapamil pretreatment did not modify the agonist-induced increase in cytosolic $Ca^{2+}$ concentration, we investigated whether the addition of $Hg^{2+}$ after verapamil pretreatment could still inhibit the $Ca^{2+}$ changes induced by agonist stimulation. We found that even in the presence of verapamil agonist-dependent $Ca^{2+}$ increase was depressed. This indicated that at least two effects are involved in the modification of the agonist-stimulated signal in Pc-12 cells at higher $Hg^{2+}$ concentrations, *i.e.*, enhanced $Ca^{2+}$ influx through voltage-regulated $Ca^{2+}$ channels and inhibition of $InsP_3$ production caused by interference with one or more proteins in the signal transduction pathway.

Tributyltin, an organometal pollutant known to cause thymic atrophy, induces a rapid increase in $[Ca^{2+}]_i$ when added to immature rat thymocytes (*15*). The elevation of $[Ca^{2+}]_i$ was followed by extensive DNA fragmentation, with a pattern that was characteristic of that produced by agents that activate the above described $Ca^{2+}$-dependent endogenous endonuclease during apoptosis. Buffering the elevation of $[Ca^{2+}]_i$ with intracellular $Ca^{2+}$ chelators prevented DNA fragmentation and tributyltin-induced cell killing. Interestingly, other organotin compounds, including trimethyltin, triphenyltin, and dibutyltin had minimal effects on cytosolic $Ca^{2+}$, DNA fragmentation and thymocyte viability (*67*). These observations are consistent with the hypothesis that $Ca^{2+}$-mediated DNA fragmentation can contribute to tributyltin toxicity *in vivo*. A schematic representation of the events involved in tributyltin-induced thymocyte killing is illustrated in Fig. 2.

### 4. *Effect of cell signalling stimulation on toxic cell injury*

Whereas a variety of cytotoxins have been reported to alter signal transduction

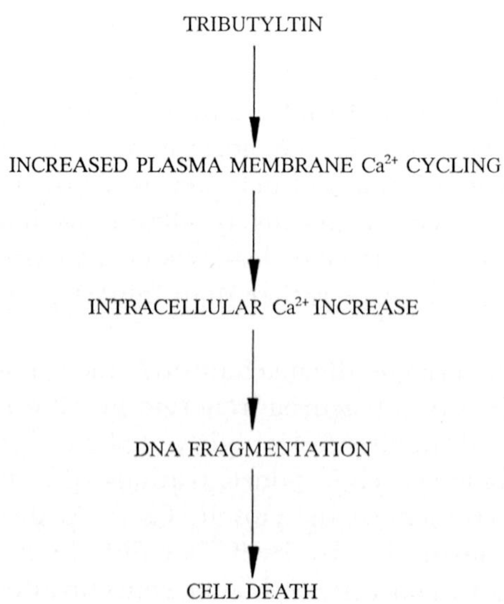


FIG. 2. Proposed mechanism of thymocyte killing by tributyltin.

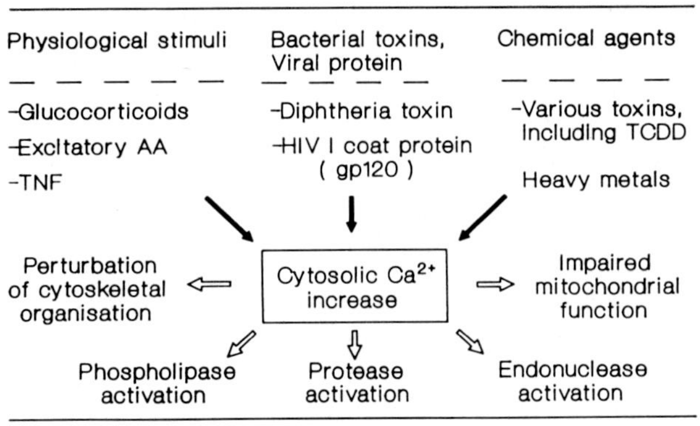


FIG. 3. Mechanisms of $Ca^{2+}$ -mediated cell killing.

pathways, evidence is slowly emerging that turning on the cell signalling machinery can dramatically alter the outcome of exposure to chemical toxins both *in vivo* and *in vitro*. For example, acetaminophen toxicity can be prevented by prostacyclin treatment (*67*), and interleukin 1 pretreatment has recently been reported to protect from ischemia-reperfusion injury (*68*). Activators of protein kinase C, such as phorbol ester tumor promoters, have also been shown to prevent apoptosis induced by serum deprivation (*69*), radiation (*70*), glucocorticoid hormones, and $Ca^{2+}$ ionophore (*71*). The exact mechanism by which protein kinase C activation counteracts programmed cell death is presently unknown, but may involve modification of intracellular $Ca^{2+}$ fluxes (*72*), alteration of chromatin structure, or increased intracellular polyamine levels (*73*).

## *Conclusion*

It is apparent that the calcium ion is important both in physiological and toxicological processes. A perturbation of intracellular $Ca^{2+}$ homeostasis by toxins can lead to a sustained increase in cytosolic $Ca^{2+}$ levels. This can result in the alteration of cell signalling as well as the activation of several degradative processes that can precipitate cell injury and death (Fig. 3). Further studies are required to expand our current knowledge of $Ca^{2+}$ signals in cell physiology and their involvement in cytotoxic processes.

## REFERENCES

1. Campbell, A. K. Intracellular Calcium: Its Universal Role as Regulator, Wiley, New York, 1983.
2. Fleckenstein, A., Frey, M., and Fleckenstein-Grün, G. Cellular injury by cytosolic calcium overload and its prevention by calcium antagonists—a new principle of tissue protection. *In;* D. Keppler, H. Popper, L. Bianchi, and W. Reutter (eds.), Mechanisms of Hepatocyte Injury and Death, pp. 321–335, MTP Press Limited, Lancaster, 1983.
3. Trump, B. F., Berezesky, I. K., Smith, M. W., Phelps, P. C., and Elliget, K. A. The relationship between cellular ion deregulation and acute and chronic toxicity. Toxicol. Appl. Pharmacol., *97*: 6–22, 1989.

4. Jewell, S. A., Bellomo, G., Thor, H., Orrenius, S., and Smith, M. T. Bleb formation in hepatocytes during drug metabolism is associated with alterations in intracellular thiol and calcium ion homeostasis. Science, *217*: 1257–1259, 1982.
5. Pounds, J. G. and Rosen, J. F. Cellular $Ca^{2+}$ homeostasis and $Ca^{2+}$-mediated cell processes as critical targets for toxicant action: conceptual and methodological pitfalls. Toxicol. Appl. Pharmacol., *94*: 331–341, 1988.
6. Komulainen, H. and Bondy, S. C. Increased free intracellular $Ca^{2+}$ by toxic agents: an index of potential neurotoxicity? Trends Pharmacol. Sci., *9*: 154–156, 1988.
7. Manev, H., Costa, E., Wroblewski, J. T., and Guidotti, A. Abusive stimulation of excitatory amino acid receptors: a strategy to limit neurotoxicity. FASEB J., *4*: 2789–2797, 1990.
8. Moore, M., Thor, H., Moore, G., Nelson, S., Moldéus P., and Orrenius, S. The toxicity of acetaminophen and N-acetyl-*p*-benzoquinoneimine in isolated hepatocytes is associated with thiol depletion and increased cytosolic $Ca^{2+}$. J. Biol. Chem., *260*: 13035–13040, 1985.
9. Boobis, A. R., Seddon, C. E., Nasseri-Sina, P., and Davies, D. S. Evidence for a direct role of intracellular $Ca^{2+}$ in paracetamol toxicity. Biochem. Pharmacol., *39*: 1277–1281, 1990.
10. Tsokos-Kuhn, J. O. Evidence *in vivo* for elevation of intracellular $Ca^{2+}$ in the liver after diquat, acetaminophen and $CCl_4$. Biochem.Pharmacol., *38*: 3061–3065, 1989.
11. Dypbukt, J. M., Thor, H., and Nicotera, P. Intracellular $Ca^{2+}$ chelators prevent DNA damage and protect hepatoma 1c1c7 cells from quinone-induced cell killing. Free Radical Res. Commun., *18*: 347–354, 1990.
12. Nicotera, P., Thor, H., and Orrenius, S. Cytosolic free $Ca^{2+}$ and cell killing in hepatoma 1c1c7 cells exposed to chemical anoxia. FASEB J., *3*: 59–64, 1989.
13. Kass, G. E. N., Wright, J. M., Nicotera, P., and Orrenius, S. The mechanism of 1-methyl-4-phenyl-1,2,3,6-tetrahydropyridine toxicity. Role of intracellular calcium. Arch. Biochem. Biophys., *260*: 789–797, 1988.
14. McConkey, D. J., Hartzell, P., Duddy, S. K., Håkansson, H., and Orrenius, S. 2,3,7,8-tetrachlorodibenzo-*p*-dioxin kills immature thymocytes by $Ca^{2+}$-mediated endonuclease activation. Science, *242*: 256–259, 1988.
15. Aw, T. Y., Nicotera, P., Manzo, L., and Orrenius, S. Tributyltin stimulates apoptosis in rat thymocytes. Arch. Biochem. Biophys., *283*: 46–50, 1990.
16. Tani, M. Mechanisms of $Ca^{2+}$ overload in reperfused ischemic myocardium. Annu. Rev. Physiol., *52*: 543–559, 1990.
17. Cotterill, L. A., Gower, J. D., Fuller, B. J., and Green, C. J. Oxidative damage to kidney membranes during cold ischemia: evidence of a role for calcium. Transplantation, *48*: 745–751, 1989.
18. Caspar, M., Florin, I., and Thelestam, M. Calcium and calmodulin in cellular intoxication with clostridium difficile toxin B. J. Cell. Physiol., *132*: 168–172, 1987.
19. Dreyer, E. B., Kaiser, P. K., Offerman, J. T., and Lipton, S. A. HIV-1 coat protein neurotoxicity prevented by calcium channel antagonists. Science, *248*: 364–367, 1990.
20. Carafoli, E. Intracellular $Ca^{2+}$ homeostasis. Annu. Rev. Biochem., *56*: 395–433, 1987.
21. Hosey, M. M. and Lazdunski, M. Calcium channels. Molecular pharmacology, structure and regulation. J. Membrane Biol., *104*: 81–105, 1988.
22. Kass, G. E. N., Llopis, J., Chow, S. C., Duddy, S. K., and Orrenius, S. Receptor-operated $Ca^{2+}$ influx in rat hepatocytes: identification and characterization using manganese. J. Biol. Chem., *265*: 17486–17492, 1990.
23. Lotersztajn, S., Hanoune, D., and Pecker, F. A high affinity calcium stimulated magnesium-dependent ATPase in rat liver plasma membranes: dependence on an endo-

genous protein activator distinct from calmodulin. J. Biol. Chem., *256*: 11209–11215, 1981.

24. Kessler, F., Bennardini, F., Bachs, O., Serratosa, J., James, P., Caride, A. J., Gazzotti, P., Penniston, J. T., and Carafoli, E. Partial purification and characterization of the $Ca^{2+}$-pumping ATPase of the liver plasma membrane. J. Biol. Chem., *265*: 16012–16019, 1990.
25. Pavoine, C., Lotersztajn, S., Mallat, A., and Pecker, F. The high affinity ($Ca^{2+}$-$Mg^{2+}$)-ATPase in liver plasma membrane is a $Ca^{2+}$ pump: reconstitution of the purified enzyme into phospholipid vesicles. J. Biol. Chem., *262*: 5113–5117, 1987.
26. Duddy, S. K., Kass, G. E. N., and Orrenius, S. $Ca^{2+}$-mobilizing hormones stimulate $Ca^{2+}$ efflux from hepatocytes. J. Biol. Chem., *264*: 20863–20866, 1989.
27. Kraus-Friedmann, N., Fleschner, C. R., Zimniak, P., and Moore, P. B. The hepatic microsomal $Ca^{2+}$ sequestering system. *In;* D. R. Pfeiffer, J. B. McMillan, and S. Little (eds.), Cellular $Ca^{2+}$ Regulation, pp. 59–68, Plenum Press, New York, 1988.
28. Moore, G. A., McConkey, D. J., Kass, G. E. N., O'Brian, P. J., and Orrenius, S. 2, 5-Di(*tert*-butyl)-1,4-benzohydroquinone—a novel inhibitor of liver microsomal $Ca^{2+}$ sequestration. FEBS Lett., *224*: 331–336, 1987.
29. Moore, G. A., Kass, G. E. N., Duddy, S. K., Farrell, G. C., Llopis, J., and Orrenius, S. 2, 5-Di(*tert*-butyl)-1, 4-benzohydroquinone—A novel mobilizer of the inositol 1,4,5-trisphosphate-sensitive $Ca^{2+}$ pool. Free Rad. Res. Commun., *8*: 337–345, 1990.
30. Kass, G. E. N., Duddy, S. K., Moore, G. A., and Orrenius, S. Di-(*tert*-butyl)-1, 4-benzohydroquinone rapidly elevates cytosolic $Ca^{2+}$ concentration by mobilizing the inositol 1,4,5-tris-phosphate-sensitive $Ca^{2+}$ pool. J. Biol. Chem., *264*: 15192–15198, 1989.
31. Moore, P. B. and Kraus-Friedman, N. Hepatic microsomal $Ca^{2+}$-ATPase. Biochem. J., *214*: 61–75, 1983.
32. Benedetti, A., Fulceri, R., Ferro, M., and Comporti, M. On a possible role of glucose-6-phosphatase in the regulation of liver cell $Ca^{2+}$ concentration. Trends Biochem. Sci., *11*: 284–285, 1986.
33. Nicholls, D. J. Intracellular $Ca^{2+}$ homeostasis. British Med. Bull., *43*: 353–358, 1986.
34. Richter, C. and Kass, G. E. N. Oxidative stress in mitochondria: its relationship to cellular $Ca^{2+}$ homeostasis, cell death, proliferation, and differentiation. Chem.-Biol. Interactions, *77*: 1–23, 1991.
35. Nicotera, P., McConkey, D. J., Jones, D. P., and Orrenius, S. ATP stimulates $Ca^{2+}$ uptake and increases the free $Ca^{2+}$ concentration in isolated liver nuclei. Proc. Natl. Acad. Sci. U.S.A., *86*: 453–457, 1989.
36. Nicotera, P., Orrenius, S., Nilsson, T., and Berggren, P. O. An inositol (1,4,5,)-trisphosphate-sensitive $Ca^{2+}$ pool in liver nuclei. Proc. Natl. Acad. Sci. U.S.A., *87*: 6858–6862, 1990.
37. Somlyo, A. P., Bond, M., and Somlyo, A. V. Calcium content of mitochondria and endoplasmic reticulum in liver frozen rapidly *in vivo*. Nature, *314*: 622–625, 1985.
38. Charest, R., Blackmore, P. F., Berthon, B., and Exton J. H. Changes in free cytosolic $Ca^{2+}$ in hepatocytes following adrenergic stimulation. Studies on quin-2-loaded hepatocytes. J. Biol. Chem., *258*: 8769–8773, 1983.
39. Woods, N. M., Cuthbertson, K. S. R., and Cobbold, P. E. Repetitive transient rises in cytoplasmic free calcium in hormone stimulated hepatocytes. Nature, *319*: 600–602, 1986.
40. Berridge, M. J. Inositol trisphosphate and diacylglycerol: two interacting second messengers. Annu. Rev. Biochem., *56*: 159–193, 1987.
41. Nishizuka, Y. The role of protein kinase C in cell surface signal transduction and tumor

promotion. Nature, *308*: 693–698, 1984.

42. Guillemette, G., Balla, T., Baukal, A. J., and Catt, K. J. Characterization of inositol 1, 4, 5-trisphosphate receptors and calcium mobilization in a hepatic plasma membrane fraction. J. Biol. Chem., *263*: 4541–4548, 1988.
43. Ross, C. A., Meldolesi, J., Milner, T. A., Satoh, T., Supattapone, S., and Snyder, S. H. Inositol 1,4,5-triphosphate receptor localized to endoplasmic reticulum in cerebellar Purkinje neurons. Nature, *339*: 468–470, 1989.
44. Dawson, A. P. GTP enhances inositol triphosphate-stimulated $Ca^{2+}$ release from rat liver microsomes. FEBS Lett., *185*: 147–150, 1985.
45. Thomas, A. P. Potentiation by GTP of Ins (1,4,5)$P_3$-induced $Ca^{2+}$ mobilization in permeabilized hepatocytes. *In;* D. R. Pfeiffer, J. B. McMillin, S. Little (eds.), Cellular $Ca^{2+}$ Regulation, pp. 197–201, Plenum Press, New York, 1988.
46. Barritt, G. J., Parker, J. C., and Wadsworth, J. C. A kinetic analysis of the effects of adrenaline on calcium distribution in isolated rat liver parenchymal cells. J. Physiol. (London), *312*: 29–55, 1981.
47. Barnes, D. S. Cells without growth factor commit suicide. Science, *242*: 1510–1511, 1988.
48. Arends, M. J., Morris, R. G., and Wyllie, A. H. Apoptosis—The role of the endonuclease. Am. J. Pathol., *136*: 593–608, 1990.
49. Wyllie, A. H. Glucocorticoid-induced thymocyte apoptosis is associated with endogenous endonuclease activation. Nature, *280*: 555–556, 1980.
50. Williams, G. T., Smith, C. A., Spooncer, E., Dexter, T. M., and Taylor, D. R. Haemopoietic colony stimulating factors promote cell survival by suppressing apoptosis. Nature, *343*: 76–79, 1990.
51. Araki, S., Shimada, Y., Kaji, K., and Hayashi, H. Apoptosis of vascular endothelial cells by fibroblast growth factor deprivation. Biochem. Biophys. Res. Commun., *168*: 1194–1200, 1990.
52. Szende, B., Srkalovic, G., Groot, K., Lapis, K., and Schally, A. V. Growth inhibition of mouse MXT mammary tumor by the luteinizing hormone-releasing hormone antagonist SB-75. J. Natl. Cancer Inst., *82*: 513–517, 1990.
53. Kyprianou, N., English, H. F., and Isaacs, J. T. Programmed cell death during regression of PC-82 human prostate cancer following androgen ablation. Cancer Res., *50*: 3748–3753, 1990.
54. Hirvonen, M.-R., Paljärvi, L. Naukkarinen, A., Komulainen, H., and Savolainen, K. Potentiation of malaoxon-induced convulsions by lithium: early neuronal injury, phosphoinositide signaling, and calcium. Toxicol. Appl. Pharmacol., *104*: 276–289, 1990.
55. Mobley, P. L. The cholinesterase inhibitor soman increases inositol trisphosphate in rat brain. Neuropharmacology, *29*: 189–191, 1990.
56. Bellomo, G., Thor, H., and Orrenius, S. Alterations in inositol phosphate production during oxidative stress in isolated hepatocytes. J. Biol. Chem., *262*: 1530–1534, 1987.
57. Kass, G. E. N., Duddy, S. K., and Orrenius, S. Activation of protein kinase C by redox cycling quinones. Biochem. J., *260*: 490–507, 1989.
58. Eriksson, J., E. Paatero, G. I. L., Meriluoto, J. A. O., Codd, G. A., Kass, G. E. N., Nicotera, P., and Orrenius, S. Rapid microfilament reorganization induced in isolated rat hepatocytes by microcystin-LR, a cyclic peptide toxin. Exp. Cell Res., *185*: 86–100, 1989.
59. MacKintosh, C., Beattie, K. A., Klumpp, S., Cohen, P., and Codd, G. A. Cyanobacterial microcystin-LR is a potent and specific inhibitor of protein phosphatases 1 and 2A from both mammals and higher plants. FEBS Lett., *264*: 187–192, 1990.

60. Benedetti, A., Graf, P., Fulceri, R., Romani, A., and Sies, H. $Ca^{2+}$ mobilization by vasopressin and glucagon in perfused livers: effect of prior intoxication with bromotrichloromethane. Biochem. Pharmacol., *38*: 1799–1805, 1989.
61. Kutty, K. R., Singh, Y., Santostasi, G., and Krishna, G. Maitotoxin-induced liver cell death involving loss of ATP following influx of calcium. Toxicol. Appl. Pharmacol., *101*: 1–10, 1989.
62. Lo, T. N., Saul, W., and Beaven, M. A. The actions of $Ca^{2+}$ ionophores on rat basophilic (2H3) cells are dependent on cellular ATP and hydrolysis of inositol phospholipids: a comparison with antigen stimulation. J. Biol. Chem., *262*: 4141–4145, 1987.
63. Mohr, F. C. and Fewtrell, C. The effect of mitochondrial inhibitors on calcium homeostasis in tumor mast cells. Am. J. Physiol., *258*: C217–C226, 1990.
64. Schöfl, C., Sanchez-Bueno, A., Dixon, C. J., Woods, N. M., Lee, J. A. C., Cuthbertson, K. S. R., Cobbold, P. H., and Birchall, J. D. Aluminium perturbs oscillatory phosphoinositide-mediated calcium signalling in hormone-stimulated hepatocytes. Biochem. J., *269*: 547–550, 1990.
65. Saijoh, K., Inoue, Y., Katsuyama, H., and Sumino, K. The interactions of cations with activity of soluble protein kinase C from mouse brain. Pharmacol. Toxicol., *63*: 221–224, 1988.
66. Markovac, J. and Goldstein, G. W. Picomolar concentrations of lead stimulate brain protein kinase C. Nature, *334*: 71–73, 1988.
67. Guarner, F., Boughton-Smith, N. K., Blackwell, G. J., and Moncada, S. Reduction by prostacyclin of acetaminophen-induced liver toxicity in the mouse. Hepatology, *8*: 248–253, 1988.
68. Brown, J. M., White, C. W., Terada, L. S., Grosso, M. A., Shanley, P. F., Mulvin, D. W., Bauergee, A., Whitman, G. J. R., Harken, A. H., and Repine, J. E. Interleukin 1 pretreatment decreases ischemia/reperfusion injury. Proc. Natl. Acad. Sci. U.S.A., *87*: 5026–5030, 1990.
69. Kanter, P., Leister, K. J., Tomei, L. D., Wenner, P. A., and Wenner, C. E. Epidermal growth factor and tumor promoters prevent DNA fragmentation by different mechanisms. Biochem. Biophys. Res. Commun., *118*: 392–399, 1984.
70. Tomei, L. D., Kanter, P., and Wenner, C. E. Inhibition of radiation-induced apoptosis *in vitro* by tumor promoters. Biochem. Biophys. Res. Commun., *155*: 324–331, 1988.
71. McConkey, D. J. Hartzell, P., Jondal, M., and Orrenius, S. Inhibition of DNA fragmentation in thymocytes and isolated thymocyte nuclei by agents that stimulate protein kinase C. J. Biol. Chem., *264*: 13399–13402, 1989.
72. McCarthy, S. A., Hallam, T. J., and Merritt, J. E. Activation of protein kinase C in human neutrophils attenuates agonist-stimulated rises in cytosolic free $Ca^{2+}$-concentration by inhibiting bivalent-cation influx and intracellular $Ca^{2+}$ release in addition to stimulating $Ca^{2+}$ efflux. Biochem. J., *264*: 357–364, 1989.
73. Brüne, B., Hartzell, P., Nicotera, P., and Orrenius, S. Spermine prevents endonuclease activation and apoptosis in thymocytes. Exp. Cell Res., in press.
74. Gusovsky, F., Bitrau, J. A., Yasumoto, T., and Daly, J. W. Mechanism of maitotoxin-stimulated phosphoinositide breakdown in HL-60 cells. J. Pharmacol. Exp. Ther., *252*: 466–473, 1990.
75. Rittenhouse, S. E. Activation of human platelet phospholipase C by ionophore A 23187 is totally dependent upon cyclo-oxygenase products and ADP. Biochem. J., *222*: 103–110, 1984.
76. Daly, J. W., Gusowsky, F., McNeal, E. T., Secunda, S., Bell, M., Creveling, C. R., Nishigawa, Y., Overman, L. E., Sharp, M. J., and Rossignol, D. P. Pumiliotoxin alkaloids: a new class of sodium channel agents. Biochem. Pharmacol., *40*: 315–326,

1990.

77. Tohkin, M., Yagami, T., and Matsubara, T. Mastoparan, a peptide toxin from wasp venom, stimulates glycogenolysis mediated by an increase of the cytosolic free $Ca^{2+}$ concentration but not by an increase of cAMP in rat hepatocytes. FEBS Lett., *260*: 179–182, 1990.
78. Rossi, M. A., Fidale, F., Garramone, A., Esterbauer, H., and Dianzani, M. V. Effect of 4-hydroxyalkenals on hepatic phosphatidylinositol-4,5-bisphosphate-phospholipase C. Biochem. Pharmacol., *39*: 1715–1719, 1990.
79. Hoek, J. B., Rubin, R., and Thomas, A. P. Ethanol-induced phospholipase C activation is inhibited by phorbol esters in isolated hepatocytes. Biochem. J., *252*: 865–871, 1988.
80. Waring, P. DNA fragmentation induced in macrophages by gliotoxin does not require protein synthesis and is preceded by raised inositol trisphosphate levels. J. Biol. Chem., *265*: 14476–14480, 1990.
81. Guiramand, J., Lenoir, M., Pujol, R., and Récaseus, M. Ototoxic and nephrotoxic drugs inhibit agonist-induced inositol phosphate formation in rat brain synaptoneurosomes. Toxicol. Lett., *251*: 331–338, 1990.
82. Seewald, M. J., Olsen, R. A., Sehgal, I., Melder, D. C., Moobst, E. J., and Powis, G. Inhibition of growth factor-dependent inositol phosphate $Ca^{2+}$ signaling by antitumor ether lipid analogues. Cancer Res., *50*: 4458–4463, 1990.
83. Watters, D., Marshall, K., Hamilton, S., Michael, J., McArthur, M., Seymour, G., Hawkins, C., Gardiner, R., and Lavin, M. The bistratenes: new cytotoxic marine macrolides which induce some properties indicative of differentiation in HL-60 cells. Biochem. Pharmacol., *39*: 1609–1614, 1990.
84. Romano, M. and Hawiger, J. Interaction of endotoxic lipid A and lipid X with purified human platelet protein kinase C. J. Biol. Chem., *265*: 1765–1770, 1990.
85. Tsuchiya, M., Okimasu, E., Veda, W., Hirakawa, M., and Utsumi, K. Halothane, an inhalation anesthetic, activates protein kinase C and superoxide generation by neutrophils. FEBS Lett., *242*: 101–105, 1988.
86. Roghani, M., DaSilva, C., and Castagna, M. Tumor promoter chloroform is a potent protein kinase C activator. Biochem. Biophys. Res. Commun., *142*: 738–744, 1987.
87. Cotgreave, I. A., Duddy, S. K., Kass, G. E. N., Thompson, D., and Moldéus, P. Studies on the anti-inflammatory activity of ebselen: ebselen interferes with granulocyte oxidative burst by dual inhibition of NADPH oxidase and protein kinase C? Biochem. Pharmacol., *38*: 649–656, 1989.
88. Mahoney, C. W., Azzi, A., and Huang, K.-P. Effects of suramin, an anti-human immunodeficiency virus reverse transcriptase agent, on protein kinase C: differential activation and inhibition of protein kinase C isozymes. J. Biol. Chem., *265*: 5424–5428, 1990.

# DRUG RESISTANCE

XENOBIOTICS AND CANCER, L. ERNSTER ET AL. (EDS.),
JAPAN SCI. SOC. PRESS, TOKYO/TAYLOR & FRANCIS LTD., LONDON, pp. 229–239, 1991

# Structure and Function of P-glycoprotein in the Normal Liver and Intestine

Irwin M. ARIAS, Zenaida GATMAITAN, Roberto MAZZANTI, Hsing SHU, and Yukio KUMAMOTO

*Department of Physiology, Tufts University School of Medicine, Boston, Massaschusetts 02111, U.S.A.*

*Abstract:* Multidrug resistance (MDR) genes encode a family of membrane glycoproteins of approximately 170 kD (P-glycoproteins). In man and mouse, the MDR 1 (mdr 1) genes confer resistance to relatively hydrophobic cationic anti-cancer drugs (*i.e.*, vinblastin, adriamycin). Anti-cancer drug sensitivity is restored by addition of other drugs (*i.e.*, verapamil, reserpine) which are also P-glycoprotein substrates. Transfection of MDR 1 genes produces the resistance phenotype and overexpression of P-glycoprotein. Parenchymal cells in several normal tissues express P-glycoprotein in the secretory domain of the plasma membrane (*i.e.*, bile canaliculus of hepatocytes, brush border of proximal tubular, and small intestinal cells).

Studies using plasma membrane vesicles of different sidedness derived from the bile canaliculus and small intestinal brush border permit characterization of P-glycoprotein as a unidirectional, temperature dependent, saturable, ATP-dependent transporter which is competitively inhibited by various anti-cancer drugs and other compounds. Transport studies using single cell fluorescence microscopy with image analysis confirm observations in vesicles. No natural substrate has been identified. Structural studies indicate that the requirements for substrates are molecular weight of 350 to 100, hydrophobicity, two planar rings, and a weak cationic charge. Alternative mechanisms of transport function are considered.

The identity of P-glycoproteins in normal rat and human tissues has not been established. Antibody reactions suggest that they may belong to the MDR 2 or 3 class. Studies using everted gut sacs suggest that inhibition of P-glycoprotein may facilitate accumulation of anti-cancer drugs in the tissue.

Treatment with one anticancer drug can produce resistance to that drug and to other anticancer drugs which have seemingly different structures and mechanisms of action. This is the multidrug resistance (MDR) phenomenon which commonly occurs in the absence of prior chemotherapy in primary cancer of the liver, kidney, colon, and other organs, and after chemotherapy in virtually any malignant disease (*1, 2*). In addition, cell lines which acquire resistance to anticancer drugs often have cross-resistance to other anticancer drugs. The MDR phenotype in these cell lines correlates with expression of a 170 kD glycoprotein in the plasma membrane. The gene responsible for the MDR phenomenon in these cells was cloned and sequenced after morphological studies of resistant cells revealed many double minute chromosomes (*3*). As described by Schimke *et al.* (*4*), these structures contain amplified genes. Genomic DNA for the amplified DNA in resistant cell lines was identified using in-gel renaturation (*5*). Two closely related human genomic sequences, designated MDR 1 and MDR 2, were identified and mapped to chromosome 7q. A 4.5 kb m RNA was identified in multi-drug resistant cells and, using the genomic MDR 1 probe, overlapping cDNA segments for the entire MDR 1 RNA were obtained and sequenced. The murine equivalents, mdr 1, 2, and 3, were similarly identified (*6*). The human MDR 1 cDNA encodes a protein of 1,280 amino acids. Analysis of hydrophobic sequences and their assignment to transmembrane domains resulted in a model with 12 transmembrane spanning regions. The two halves of the molecule have 43% sequence identity, suggesting that they result from gene duplication. The regions of greatest identity involve two putative nucleotide binding domains. These sequences have high homology to membrane proteins in other species, which include peptide and sugar transporters in bacteria (*7*) and the a-mating factor in yeast (*8*). Genes expressing substantial sequence identity have also been cloned from drosophila, plasmodia, amoebae, and leishmania (*9, 10*). The cystic fibrosis gene product also has nucleotide binding site homology with MDR genes (*11*).

The following evidence supports the view that P-glycoprotein is related to the MDR phenomenon: (a) transfection of drug-sensitive cells with full-length cDNA for MDR 1 (or the murine form, mdr 1) results in expression of P-glycoprotein in the plasma membrane and a drug-resistant phenotype (*12*). (b) Point mutations in MDR 1 affect different expression of drug resistance. (c) There is a positive correlation between the degree of expression of P-glycoprotein and drug resistance in various cell lines and malignant tumors (*13, 14*). (d) The transport of various anticancer drugs is inhibited by compounds which also bind to P-glycoprotein and the resistance phenotype is reversed.

There is multiplicity of MDR-like genes in various species; however, only some produce the MDR phenomenon after transfection into drug sensitive cells. For example, in man and mouse, transfection with the corresponding MDR 1 genes confers drug resistance. The function of the MDR (mdr) 2 and 3 gene products is not known. Type specific antibodies and cDNA probes are not available with which to investigate this problem in rats, which is the species best studied with respect to the functional mechanism of P-glycoproteins.

### *Expression of MDR Gene Product in Normal Tissues*

MDR genes are expressed not only in MDR tumor cells but in normal tissues as well (*13–15*). These include kidney, liver, small intestine, and colon. Immunomorphological studies using monoclonal antibodies which recognize all three MDR gene products in human and rodent liver reveal that Gp170 is localized to the apical plasma membrane domain in these cells. Localization in liver is to the bile canaliculus, in kidney to the brush border of the proximal convoluted tubule, in small intestine to the brush border and in colon to the superficial apical membrane. In others, such as adrenal cortical cells, Gp170 is present in the plasma membrane in a nonpolarized distribution. These observations suggest that Gp170 may be physiologically important in normal tissues. However, its functional role and natural substrates are unknown.

### *P-glycoprotein-mediated Transport in Hepatocellular and Intestinal Plasma Membrane Vesicles*

We previously developed methods to separate the basal-lateral and apical domains of the plasma membrane of rat hepatocytes (*16–18*). This method has proven valuable in determining the polar distribution of transport systems and their function. Canalicular membrane vesicles are prepared from rat liver after perfusion, Dounce homogenization, nitrogen cavitation, and $Ca^{2+}$ precipitation. They are 80% right-side out and vesicles of different sidedness can be separated based on affinity perturbation centrifugation (*18*). We prepared right-side in and right-side out basal lateral and canalicular membrane vesicles from rat liver. Only canalicular membrane vesicles contained P-glycoprotein as determined by immunoblotting. Daunomycin and other P-glycoprotein substrates were transported in canalicular but not basal lateral membrane vesicles by an ATP-dependent process (Fig. 1) (*19*). Uptake followed Michael-Menten kinetics with an apparent $K_m$ of 49 $\mu$M and $V_{max}$ of 1.7 nmol/mg protein/min. ATP-dependent daunomycin transport was temperature dependent, osmotically sensitive and saturable. Among several nucleotides, only ATP facilitated

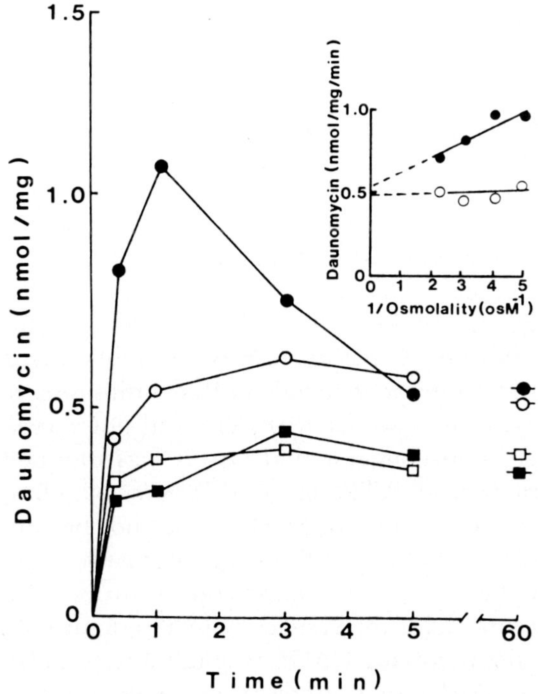


FIG. 1. Time course of daunomycin transport in liver membrane vesicles. Daunomycin transport in canalicular membrane vesicles (CMV) (circles) and basal lateral membrane vesicles (SMV) (squares) was measured as described (*19*) and included an ATP-regenerating system with ATP (closed symbols) or without ATP (open symbols). At appropriate times, aliquots were removed and filtered. Radioactivity associated with vesicles was measured. Inset shows the effect of medium osmolarity on daunomycin transport by CMV.

TABLE 1. The Effect of Various Inhibitors on ATP-dependent Daunomycin Transport in CMV (*21*)

| Inhibitor | Concentration | Relative transport (%) |
|---|---|---|
| Control | | 100 |
| Amiloride | 1 mM | 100±19 |
| DIDS | 0.2 mM | 97±7 |
| Strophanthidin | 1 mM | 100±12 |
| Ouabain | 1 mM | 100±2 |
| Vanadate | 30 μM | 80±36 |
| | 100 μM | 31±2 |
| NBD-Cl | 18 μM | 68±3 |
| N-ethylmaleimide | 18 μM | 125±6 |
| Oligomycin | 9 μg/ml | 11±5 |
| Sodium azide | 1 mM | 81±5 |
| Venturicidin | 2 μg/ml | 90±5 |

transport, whereas non- or slowly hydrolyzable analogues (adenosin-5-O-(3-thiotriphosphate, adenyl-5-yl-imidodiphosphate) were ineffective. ATP-dependent daunomycin transport was inhibited by cytotoxic drugs (vinblastine, vincristine, and adriamycin) and other drugs, such as verapamil and quinidine, which restore anticancer drug sensitivity in resistant cells. Only inside-out canalicular membrane vesicles manifested ATP-dependent daunomycin transport.

The mechanism whereby P-glycoprotein functions as a transporter was studied using inhibitors which affect other well-defined transport systems (Table 1) (*19*). ATP-daunomycin transport was not inhibited by amiloride which inhibits $Na^+H^+$ exchange, 4,4′-diisothiocyanostilbene-2,2′-disulfonate (DIDS), which is an anion transport inhibitor, ouabain or strophthantidin. Orthovanadate, which acts as a transition state analogue for phosphate release from $Na^+K^+$ ATPase and $Ca^{2+}$ ATPase and inhibits their activities at micromolar concentrations, had little effect at 30 μM. NBD-Cl, which reacts with nucleophiles and inhibits coated vesicle $H^+$-ATPase at 18 μM slightly inhibited daunomycin uptake but N-ethylmaleimide, which also inhibits coated vesicle $H^+$-ATPase, did not. Oligomycin was inhibitory whereas sodium azide and venturicidin, which are also mitochondrial ATPase inhibitors, had little or no effect. Pulse-chase experiments using gamma 32-P-ATP did not reveal active site phosphorylation of Gp170. These results suggest that Gp170 has unique features as compared with other well-characterized ATPases. Gp170 can be phosphorylated *in vitro* by several kinases; however, *in vivo* phosphorylation has not been observed.

Unlike canalicular membrane vesicles, small intestinal brush border vesicles cannot be made to be inside-out. Presumably the large concentration of actin which forms the brush border prevents inversion of vesicles which remain entirely right-side out. Therefore, transport studies involving Gp170 in small intestinal brush border vesicles were performed by loading vesicles after osmotic shock with an ATP-generating system, labeled daunomycin and other ligands (*20*, *21*). ATP-dependent transport of daunomycin was demonstrated in small intestinal brush border vesicles (Fig. 2). Transport followed Michaelis-Menten kinetics with an apparent $K_m$ of 39 μM and $V_{max}$ of 2.0 nmol/mg protein/min. Only hydrolyzable ATP facilitated daunomycin transport which was inhibited by 100–200 μM vinblastin, verapamil, and colchicine.

Western blot analysis using C219 antibody revealed a band at approximately 160 kD in solubilized brush border vesicle preparations from rat ileum and jejunum. Thus, the small intestinal brush border has a similar P-glycoprotein-mediated transport system to that observed in the liver.

These transport studies were performed using rat tissues. Unfortunately, there are no peptide-specific antibodies or mRNA probes for different mdr genes in rat tissue. The only antibody which crossreacts with rat tissues is C219, which was developed by Ling and reacts with the products of the mdr 1, 2, and 3 genes. In mouse tissues, all three mdr genes are expressed at the mRNA level in liver and small intestine (*22*). Thus, we do not know which gene products are responsible for the P-glycoprotein which is expressed in the brush border or bile canaliculus of normal animals and man.

Evidence that P-glycoprotein in the brush border may function as an efflux pump *in vivo* was obtained by studying the transport of rhodamine 123 (Rho) in inverted gut sacs from rats (*22*). Rho is a substrate for P-glycoprotein and is easily measured by fluorescence. Incubation of everted gut sacs with Rho was followed by its secretion into the lumen after its addition on the serosal surface (Fig. 3). Addition of Rho to

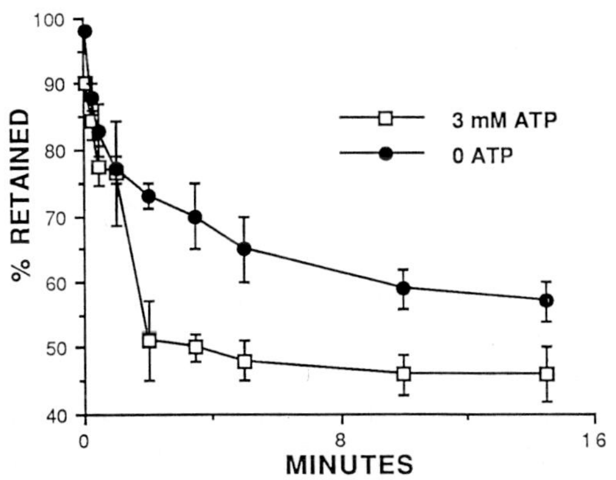


FIG. 2. Daunomycin transport in rat intestinal brush border vesicles (*21*). Vesicles were preloaded with ATP, daunomycin and an ATP-generating system using a freeze-thaw technique (*20*). Details are provided in ref. *21*.

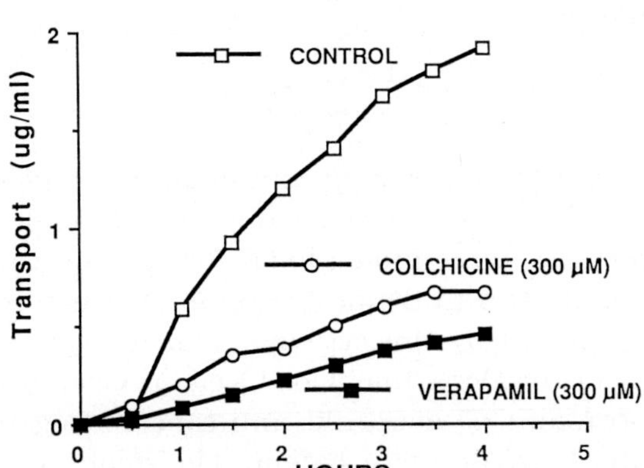


FIG. 3. Time course of Rho transport in everted rat small intestine and the effect of addition of 300 $\mu$M verapamil or colchicine. See ref. *21* for further details.

the mucosal surface was not followed by transport through the serosal surface. Addition of verapamil or colchicine to the medium reduced Rho transport in the everted gut sacs (Fig. 3). These observations suggest that P-glycoprotein in the intestinal brush border is capable of secreting Rho by a verapamil and colchicine inhibitable process, presumably Gp170. Inhibition of this process, as well as that observed in canalicular membrane vesicles, by verapamil suggests that cytotoxicity may result from anticancer agents if they are given with P-glycoprotein inhibitors as chemotherapy agents for drug-resistant cancer. The possibility that P-glycoprotein inhibitors may block normal transporters *in vivo* requires careful examination as it may facilitate tissue injury.

### *P-glycoprotein Functions as an Efflux Pump in Intact Cells*

Further evidence that P-glycoprotein functions as an efflux pump in intact cells was provided using drug sensitive and resistant nonpolarized cells (NIH3T3) and polarized (human hepatocellular cancer Alexander) cells (*22*). These cells were made resistant either by transfection with the MDR 1 gene (for NIH3T3 cells) or establishment of stable adriamycin resistant (0.5 $\mu$g/ml) Alexander cell line. Resistance is associated with abundance of P-glycoprotein in the plasma membrane, expression of MDR 1 mRNA and drug resistance in culture. NIH 3T3 cells express P-glycoprotein on their entire plasma membrane, whereas the resistant Alexander cells express P-glycoprotein only on the bile canaliculus. Using Rho as a P-glycoprotein substrate, we incubated cells in a temperature controlled, oxygenated chamber and quantitated fluorescence uptake, concentration and efflux using a single cell fluorescence microscope connected to an image analysis system and on-line computer software for analysis (*22*). In drug sensive cells, Rho was rapidly taken up but did not efflux from the cell after perfusion with medium alone. In resistant cells, dye accumulation was similar to that in sensitive cells for the first 10 min but thereafter attained a plateau because of increased efflux from the cell. After cessation of Rho perfusion, resistant cells rapidly lost fluorescence. This latter process was blocked by addition of verapamil and other P-glycoprotein inhibitors to the medium. Rho excretion by Alexander cells is into the bile canaliculus, whereas the resistant NIH3T3 cells excrete the dye into the medium. This method is quantitative and can be performed within an hour. It is ideally suited to examine the following major questions.

### *Is There a Naturally Occurring Substrate for P-glycoprotein?*

From the tissue and cellular distribution of P-glycoprotein, it is difficult to propose a single substrate that might be functionally restricted to the cells under question. One approach has been to examine the three dimensional structure of various anticancer drugs and P-glycoprotein inhibitors to define the limiting structural requirements for a compound to be transported by this system. With the collaboration of Professor T. Kishi, Harvard University Department of Organic Chemistry, we examined the three dimensional structure of over 120 anti-cancer drugs and other compounds which interact with the P-glycoprotein system. The results are consistent with those reported by other investigators who studied various analogs inhibiting compounds (*23, 24*). The common denominator for a P-glycoprotein substrate is hydrophobicity, at least two planar rings, molecular weight of 400 to 1,000 and usually a cationic charge. Consideration of naturally occurring substrates based upon these structural requirements has not been productive. Cationic hydrophobic molecules of 400–1,000 daltons are not abundant in human biology and, to date, we have not detected any.

Another approach is to consider what compounds are normally secreted by the particular tissues. The intestine, colon, and kidney are not known for their ability to secrete hydrophobic molecules by a transmembrane process. Using canalicular membrane vesicles and cells which overexpress P-glycoprotein, we have examined a large number of putative substrates. Sterols, steroids and their available metabolites, GSH, GSSG, epinephrine and metabolites, tryptophan, serotonin, prostaglandins E1, B1, and E2, various amines and sphingosine have been studied without effect. A detailed study has been made of the effect of bile acids and their conjugates on ATP-dependent daunomycin transport by canalicular membrane vesicles and on Rho efflux in transfected cells (*25*). There is a direct relationship between the hydrophobicity of individual bile acids and their ability to inhibit P-glycoprotein-mediated transport. Monohydroxy bile acids are good inhibitors whereas trihydroxy and dihydroxy bile acids are not. Kinetic analysis reveals that the observed inhibition is noncompetitive. It is highly unlikely that bile acids are transported by P-glycoproteins because bile acid transport by canalicular membrane requires an electrochemical gradient and a 100 kD membrane transporter (*26*). Furthermore, bile acid transport is not ATP-dependent. Horwitz and her colleagues have presented evidence supporting the view that progesterone is a natural substrate (*27*); however, progesterone did not inhibit ATP-dependent daunomycin transport by canalicular membrane vesicles or Rho transport in resistant NIH3T3 or Alexander cells. Inhibition was only observed at concentrations well beyond physiological limits.

### *Speculations Regarding the Mechanism of P-glycoprotein Function*

The presence of this system in primitive organisms suggests that it may have developed to secrete hydrophobic compounds, such as plant products, which might produce cellular injury. According to this concept, the P-glycoprotein system resembles the P-450, GSH transferase, and UDP glucuronyl transferase systems which are families of enzymes with overlapping substrate specificity, high capacity, and varying affinity. According to this hypothesis, P-glycoprotein functions as part of a detoxification mechanism.

There is another important consideration. Namely, that our current views about the transport function of P-glycoprotein may be incorrect. The normal P-glycoprotein may interact with hydrophobic molecules and facilitate their efflux; however, there are important thermodynamic constraints. The transported species are not biologically altered during transfer across the plasma membrane; there is no detoxification or conjugation which would render the ligands hydrophilic. Furthermore, there are no downstream "sinks" in the bile and renal tubular or intestinal lumen which bind hydrophobic molecules and thereby prevent their cellular reentry. "Conventional wisdom" (which is invariably wrong) suggests that cells are not likely to use ATP for transport of hydrophobic molecules which are capable of cellular reentry. Estimated energy consumption during canalicular transport of 1.7 nm daunomycin per mg per min when extrapolated to the entire liver per day and assuming one mole of ATP consumed per mole of daunomycin transport is $\simeq$1,000 cal. Daunomycin thus transported can readily diffuse into the cell membrane as demonstrated *in vitro*.

Studies in yeast suggest other possibilities (*8*). Yeasts require the product of the STE gene to transport the a-mating factor across the plasma membrane; otherwise they are sterile. The a-factor is a peptide which becomes farnesylated and methylated prior to attachment to an MDR-like protein which is the product of the STE gene. Similarly, bacteria transport other peptides, hemolysin, by an ATP-dependent membrane transporter which has substantial homology to the product of other MDR genes. It may be important that each of the normal cells which contain P-glycoprotein has an abundance of ectoenzymes on its plasma membrane. The retinue includes $Ca^{2+}$ $Mg^{2+}$ ATPase and AMPase, which degrade extracellular ATP to adenosine which, in liver, is conserved by a unidirectional purine transport system (*28*): gammaglutamyl transpeptidase and dipeptidyl peptidase which degrade extracellular GSH to substituent amino acids which can be conserved by unidirectional amino acid transporters, as well as many carboxy and amino peptidases (*29*). Why are these ectoenzymes abundant in the secretory domain of hepatocytes, proximal tubular cells, and intestinal mucosal cells? In each instance in which it has been studied, these enzymes are ectoenzymes; that is, they are intrinsic membrane proteins whose active site faces outside of the cell.

If we consider all of the above observations, a novel hypothesis can be generated regarding the possible transport mechanism of P-glycoproteins. We postulate that small peptides are the natural substrates for the normal P-glycoprotein system and that, following their transmembrane transport, the peptides are rapidly hydrolyzed by ectoenzymes with conservation of the substituent amino acids. During normal protein turnover, many hydrophobic peptides are formed intracellularly and some are rapidly secreted.

We have tested the peptides indicated in Table 2 for their ability to inhibit ATP-

TABLE 2. Peptides Which Did Not Inhibit ATP-dependent Daunomycin Transport in Rat Liver CMV or Rho Transport in Wild Type and MDR-expressing NIH3T3 and Alexander Cells

| Peptide |
|---|
| Lysine-tyrosine-glutamine |
| Arginine-glutamine |
| Lysine-arginine-glutamic-phenylalanine-alanine |
| Lysine-arginine-glutamic-phenylalanine-glutamine |
| Neurokinin A |
| Substance P |
| GSH (2.5 mM) |
| GSSG (1 mM) |
| RNAse-S-peptide |
| Insulin beta chain |
| Neurotensin-like peptide |
| CCK tetrapeptides I through X |
| Prostaglandin E1, B1, E2 |
| Sphingosine |

Peptides were added at 100–200 $\mu$M unless otherwise stated; see text for further details.

dependent daunomycin transport in canalicular membrane vesicles or Rho efflux in cells overexpressing P-glycoprotein. The results with each compound have been negative with both systems.

Thus, we do not know a natural substrate; however, we suspect that current concepts about how P-glycoprotein works are incorrect or, at least, incomplete. The functional association of P-glycoprotein with ectoenzymes in the plasma membrane requires further study.

### *Can the MDR System Be Utilized in the Treatment of Malignant Disease?*

In theory, inhibition of the transport activity of P-glycoprotein should permit resistant cells to temporarily regain sensitivity to anticancer drugs. Knowledge of the expression of MDR genes in various cancers is essential in addition to development of P-glycoprotein inhibitors lacking pharmacologic effects on other systems which may limit their clinical use. For example, quinidine and verapamil, which are being used in clinical trials for treatment of colon and renal cancer, are potent pharmacologic agents. Their effects on the heart and other tissues may limit their use as P-glycoprotein inhibitors in cancer cells. Compounds which retain affinity for P-glycoprotein but do not have substantial pharmacologic actions need to be developed and tested. Verapamil and other calcium channel blockers which inhibit P-glycoprotein were developed with a specific goal in mind. Compounds which were rejected as calcium channel blockers but retain P-glycoprotein inhibitory activity may prove to be more clinically useful. The situation is reminiscent of Paul Ehrlich and the development of Neosalvarsan which was the 606th organic arsenical developed for the treatment of syphilis. It would be interesting to study the comparable "six hundred and five" other compounds which were rejected as poor calcium channel blockers.

Recent studies by the National Cancer Institute utilized slot blot analysis of MDR 1 gene mRNA and observed that cancers of the colon, kidney, and liver frequently showed high levels of P-glycoprotein mRNA even though the patients had not been previously treated with anticancer drugs (*29*). Worldwide, primary cancer of the liver is the most common lethal malignant disease. There are few *in vivo* animal models in which the MDR has been studied in terms of pharmacologic therapy based on P-glycoprotein inhibition. Recently, we have been successful in injecting wild type and MDR 1 transfected human hepatocellular carcinoma (Alexander) cells into the spleen of mice with severe combined immunodeficiency (scid). Hepatic cancers rapidly develop and the tumor mass was estimated by serial measurement of HBsAg, the gene of which is integrated into each Alexander cell. In addition, MDR 1 with a hepatocyte-specific probe confirmed location and tumor mass. Resistant cells showed no response to adriamycin treatment unless a P-glycoprotein inhibitor was added to the regimen. Sensitive cells showed transient response to adriamycin. This model is useful for study of P-glycoprotein inhibition *in vivo*.

*Acknowledgment*

Research in the authors' laboratory was supported in part by a research grant from the National Institutes of Health (DK 35653).

## REFERENCES

1. Kartner, N. and Ling, V. Multidrug Resistance in Cancer. Sci. Am., March: 44–51, 1989.
2. Gottesman, M. M. and Pastan, I. The multidrug transporter, a double-edged sword. J. Biol. Chem., *263*: 12163–12166, 1988.
3. Baskin, F., Rosenberg, R. N., and Dev., V. Correlation of double-minute chromosomes with unstable multidrug resistance in uptake mutants of neuroblastoma cells. Proc. Natl. Acad. Sci. U.S.A., *78*: 3654–3658, 1981.
4. Schimke, R. T., Kaufman, R. J., Alt, F. W., and Kellem, R. F. Gene amplification and drug resistance in cultured murine cells. Science, *202*: 1051–1055, 1978.
5. Roninson, I. B., Chin, J. E., Choi, K., Gros, P., and Housman, D., Isolation of human mdr DNA sequences amplified in multidrug-resistant KB carcinoma cells. Proc. Natl. Acad. Sci. U.S.A., *83*: 4538–4542, 1986.
6. Gros, P., Ben-Neriah Y., Croop, J., and Houseman, D. E.: Isolation and expression of a complementary DNA that confers multidrug resistance. Nature, *323*: 728–731, 1986.
7. Gros, P., Croop, J., and Housman, D. Mammalian multidrug resistance gene: complete cDNA sequence indicates strong homology to bacterial transport proteins. Cell, *47*: 371–389, 1986.
8. McGrath, J. P. and Varshavsky, A. The yeast STE6 gene encodes a homologue of the mammalian multidrug resistance P-glycoprotein. Nature, *340*: 400–404, 1989.
9. Foote, S. J., Thompson, J. K., Cowman, A. F., and Kempt, D. J. Amplification of the multidrug resistance gene in some chloroquine-resistant isolates of *P. falciparum*. Cell, *57*: 921–930, 1989.
10. Raymond, M. and Gros, P. Mammalian multidrug-resistance gene: correlation of exon organization with structure and duplication of an ancestral gene. Proc. Natl. Acad. Sci. U.S.A., *86*: 6488–6492, 1989.
11. Riordan, J. R., Rommens, J. M., Kerem, S.-S., Alon, N., Rosmahel, R., Grzelczak, J., and Zielenski, J. Identification of the cystic fibrosis gene: cloning and characterization of complementary DNA. Science, *245*: 1066–1073, 1989.
12. Ueda, K., Cardarelli, C., Gottesman, M. M., and Pastan, I. Expression of a full-length cDNA for the human "MDR1" gene confers resistance to colchicine, doxorubicin, and vinblastine. Proc. Natl. Acad. Sci. U.S.A., *84*: 3004–3008, 1987.
13. Fojo, A. T., Ueda, K., Slamon, D. J., Poplack, D. G., Gottesman, M. M., and Pastan, I. Expression of a multidrug-resistance gene in human tumors and tissues. Proc. Natl. Acad. Sci. U.S.A., *84*: 265–269, 1987.
14. Thiebault, F., Tsuruo, T., Hamada, H., Gottesman, M. M., Pastan, I., and Willingham, M. C. Cellular localization of the multidrug-resistance gene product P-glycoprotein in normal human tissues. Proc. Natl. Acad. Sci. U.S.A., *84*: 7735–7738, 1987.
15. Willingham, M. C., Richert, N. D., Cornwell, M. M., Tsuruo, T., Hamada, H., Gottesman, M. M., and Pastan, I. Immunocytochemical localization of P170 at the plasma membrane of multidrug-resistant human cells. J. Histochem. Cytochem., *35*: 1451–1456, 1987.
16. Inoue, M., Kinne, R., Tran, T., and Arias, I. M. Taurocholate transport by liver sinusoidal membrane vesicles: evidence of sodium co-transport. Hepatology, *2*: 572–579, 1982.
17. Inoue, M., Kinne, R., Tran, T., and Arias, I. M. The mechanism of biliary secretion

of reduced glutathione: analysis of transport process in isolated rat liver canalicular membrane vesicles. Eur. J. Biochem., *134*: 467–471, 1983.

18. Inoue, M., Kinne, R., Tran, T., Biempica, L., and Arias, I. M. Rat liver canalicular membrane vesicles: isolation and topological characterization. J. Biol. Chem., *258*: 5183–5188, 1983.
19. Kamimoto, Y., Gatmaitan, Z., Hsu, J., and Arias, I. M. The function of GP170, the multidrug resistance gene product, in rat liver canalicular membrane vesicles. J. Biol. Chem., *264*: 11693–11698, 1989.
20. Donowitz, M., Emmer, E., McCullen, J., Reinlib, L., Cohen, M. E., Rood, R. P., Madara, J., Sharp, G. W., Murer, H., and Malmstrom, K. Freeze-thaw and high-voltage discharge allow macromolecule uptake into ileal brush-border vesicles. Am. J. Physiol., *252*: G723–735, 1987.
21. Shu, S., Gatmaitan, Z., and Arias, I. M. The function of GP170, the multidrug resistance gene product, in rat small intestinal brush-border membrane vesicles. (in press).
22. Mazzanti, R., Gatmaitan, Z., Croop, J. M., Shu, H., and Arias, I. M. Quantitative image analysis of Rhodamine 123 transport by adriamycin-sensitive and resistant NIH 3T3 and human hepatocellular carcinoma (Alexander) cells. J. Cell Pharmacol., *1*: 50–56, 1990.
23. Nogae, I., Kohno, K., Kikuchi, J., Kuwano, M., Akiyama, S-I., Kiue, A., and Suzuki, K-I. Analysis of structural features of dihydropyridine analogs needed to reverse multidrug resistance and to inhibit photoaffinity labeling of P-glycoprotein. Biochem. Pharmacol., *38*: 519–527, 1989.
24. Pearce, H. L., Safa, A. R., Bach, M. J., Winte, M. A., Cirtain, M. C., and Beck, W. T. Essential features of the P-glycoprotein pharmacophore as defined by a series of reserpine analogs that modulate multidrug resistance. Proc. Natl. Acad. Sci. U.S.A., *86*: 5128–5132, 1989.
25. Mazzanti, R., Kamimoto, Y., Gatmaitan, Z., and Arias, I. M. Bile acid inhibition of Gp 170, an ATP-dependent efflux pump in bile canaliculi (Abstract). Hepatology, *10*: 596, 1989.
26. Inoue, M., Kinne, R., Tran, T., and Arias, I. M. Taurocholate transport by rat liver canalicular membrane vesicles: evidence for presence of an independent transport system. J. Clin. Invest., *73*: 659–663, 1984.
27. Yang, C. P., Depinho, S. G., Greenberg, I. M., Arceci, R. J., and Horwitz, S. B. Progesterone interacts with P-glycoprotein in multidrug-resistant cells and in the endometrium of gravid uterus. J. Biol. Chem., *264*: 782–788, 1989.
28. Lin, S. H. and Guidotti, G. Cloning and expression of a cDNA coding for a rat liver plasma membrane ecto-ATPase: the primary structure of the ecto-ATPase is similar to that of the human biliary glycoprotein 1. J. Biol. Chem., *264*: 14408–14414, 1989.
29. Arias, I. M. Multidrug resistance genes, P-glycoprotein and the liver. Hepatology, *12*: 159–165, 1990.
30. Goldstein, L. J., Galski, H., Fojo, A., Willingham, M. *et al.* Expression of a multidrug resistance gene in human cancers. J. Natl. Cancer Inst., *81*: 116–124, 1989.

XENOBIOTICS AND CANCER, L. ERNSTER ET AL. (EDS.),
JAPAN SCI. SOC. PRESS ,TOKYO/TAYLOR & FRANCIS LTD., LONDON, pp. 241–251, 1991

# Multidrug Resistance:
# A Transport System of Antitumor Agents and Xenobiotics

Takashi Tsuruo

*Institute of Applied Microbiology, University of Tokyo, Tokyo 113 and Cancer Chemotherapy Center, Japanese Foundation for Cancer Research, Tokyo 170, Japan*

*Abstract:* Resistance of tumors to a variety of chemotherapeutic agents presents a major problem in cancer treatment. Resistance to such agents as doxorubicin, *Vinca* alkaloids, and actinomycin D can be acquired by tumor cells after treatment with a single drug. The gene responsible for multidrug resistance, termed *mdr*1, encodes a membrane glycoprotein (P-glycoprotein) that acts as a pump to transport various cytotoxic agents including various xenobiotics out of the cell. The amount of P-glycoprotein expression has been measured in tumor samples and was found to be elevated in intrinsically drug-resistant cancers of the colon, kidney, and adrenal as well as in some tumors that acquired drug resistance after chemotherapy. The protein was also found to be elevated in cells treated with xenobiotics.

P-glycoprotein has been shown to bind anticancer drugs and several resistance-reversing agents including calcium channel blockers, and to be an ATPase. We recently reconstituted the purified P-glycoprotein into artificial liposomes. Reconstituted P-glycoprotein showed ATPase activity, ATP-dependent drug-transport activity, and calcium channel blocker-binding activity. This model provides many advantages for studies of the biochemical functions of P-glycoprotein. In addition to these basic interests, the protein is of considerable interest as a target for cancer chemotherapy because it appears to be involved in both acquired multidrug resistance and intrinsic drug resistance in human cancer. The selective killing of tumor cells expressing P-glycoprotein could be very important in future cancer therapy.

When tumor cells acquire resistance to naturally occurring anticancer drugs such as *Vinca* alkaloids or anthracycline, they generally show cross-resistance to other antitumor agents (*1*). Reduced intracellular drug accumulation resulting from increased active drug efflux across plasma membranes is an important factor in the mechanism of this pleiotropic drug resistance (*2–5*). However, the molecular mechanisms of this active efflux pump are not fully understood.

Multidrug-resistant cells show characteristic changes in surface glycoproteins. An overexpression of a plasma membrane glycoprotein of relative molecular mass ($M_r$ 170,000–180,000) (P-glycoprotein) is consistently found in different multidrug-resistant human and animal cell lines (*6–15*). Full-length cDNAs for mouse and human P-glycoprotein genes inserted into viral expression systems and transfected into drug-sensitive cells have been shown to confer multidrug resistance (*16–18*). Sequence analysis of cDNAs showed that P-glycoprotein has homology with some bacterial transport proteins and has two binding sites for nucleoside triphosphates (*19–21*). Furthermore, it is a binding protein for chemotherapeutic agents such as vinblastine (*22–25*). These results indicate that P-glycoprotein is directly involved in drug transport mechanisms in multidrug-resistant cells (Fig. 1) (for reviews see refs. *26* and *27*). In spite of these findings, the mechanism of its molecular action has remained obscure. Biochemical analysis of the enzymatic activity associated with P-glycoprotein has not been reported, except for the ATPase activity of the protein (*28*).

This report describes the characteristics and reactions of several compounds which show an affinity for P-glycoprotein and the chemotherapeutic effects in tumor expressing this protein. Also described is the purification of P-glycoprotein using the monoclonal antibody (MRK-16). The purified P-glycoprotein was reconstituted into liposome, and the reconstituted material showed ATPase activity, ATP-dependent drug-transport activity and calcium channel blocker-binding activity. This reconstituted model offers many advantages for studies of the biochemical functions of P-glycoprotein, as well as for the discovery and characterization of the compounds, including xenobiotics, which show an affinity for it and show a chemotherapeutic effect by targeting it.

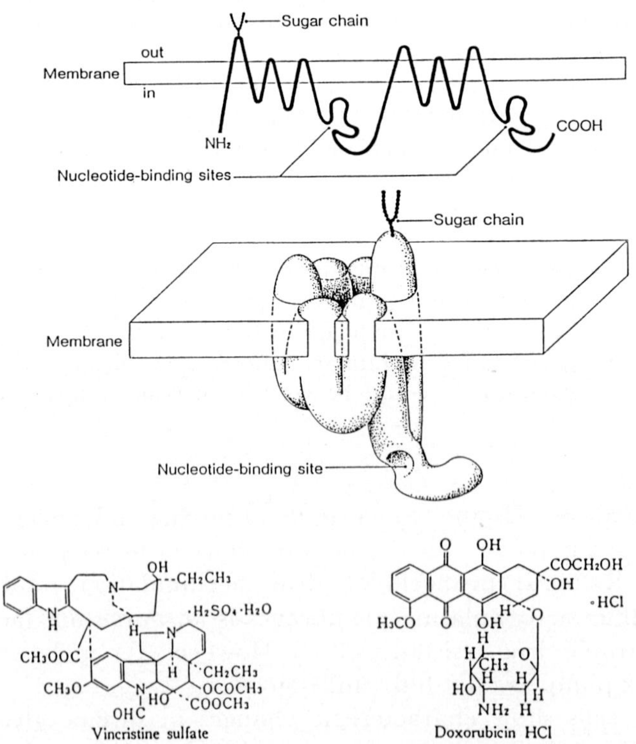


FIG. 1. Speculative model for transmembrane localization of P-glycoprotein. Vincristine and adriamycin which show no structural or functional similarities and various chemical and xenobiotics can be transported outside the cells by P-glycoprotein.

*Expression of P-glycoprotein in Cells and Organs*

P-glycoprotein has been speculated as being closely associated with the drug transport function of resistant cells. As the gene was isolated from drug-sensitive normal cells, the protein is thought to be present in normal cells (*17*). According to observations by Pastan's group, the *mdr*1 gene is expressed at high levels in human adrenal grand and kidney, and at intermediate levels in lung, liver, jejunum, colon, and rectum (*29*). Several human tumors derived from these tissues also express the *mdr*1 gene. Its increased expression in some normal organs implies that P-glycoprotein has a normal function in these organs. Recently it was reported that P-glycoprotein is also partly expressed in carcinogen-initiated hepatocytes and regenerating liver cells (*30, 31*). These findings are of considerable interest in understanding the protein's cellular function.

We have developed monoclonal antibodies against adriamycin-resistant human myelogenous leukemia K562 (K562 /ADM)(*14*). Two monoclonal antibodies designated MRK16 and MRK17 are specifically reactive against K562/ADM and a human ovarian cancer cell line resistant to adriamycin ($2780^{AD}$). Both antibodies recognized P-glycoprotein: MRK16 modulated vincristine and actinomycin D transport in the resistant cells, while MRK17 specifically inhibited the growth of these cells. These data indicate that P-glycoprotein is involved in the drug transport mechanisms and the proliferation of multidrug-resistant tumor cell lines. Since our monoclonal antibodies MRK16 and MRK17 are reactive to viable tumor cells and exhibit unique effects on the cellular function of multidrug-resistant cells, they should be useful in the study of the mechanism of multidrug resistance as well as in the diagnosis of refractory stages of malignancies.

Using monoclonal antibody MRK16, high levels of P-glycoprotein were detected in liver, colon, jejunum, kidney, pancreatic ductules, and adrenal (Table 1) (*32*). In the liver, the protein was detected on the biliary canalicular surface of the hepatocytes and on the apical surface of small biliary ductules; in the colon and jejunum, it was found on the apical surface of columnar epithelial cells; in the kidney, it was only detected on the apical surface of the epithelial cells of the proximal tubules. In addition, P-glycoprotein was found on the apical surface of small pancreatic ductules. In all these tissues, the protein was present in a highly polarized fashion, but in adrenal, the protein was not found in a polarized distribution.

These findings suggest again that P-glycoprotein has a role in the secretion of metabolites and certain other chemicals, including toxic environmental compounds,

TABLE 1. Localization of P-glycoprotein as Revealed by MRK17 (*32*)

| P-glycoprotein detected | P-glycoprotein not detected |
|---|---|
| Liver, biliary canalicular surface of hepatocytes: apical surface of small biliary ductules | Stomach<br>Lung |
| Jejunum and colon: apical surface of columnar epithelial cells | Central nervous system (cerebral cortex, cerebellum, spinal cord) |
| Kidney: brush border of proximal tubules | Ovary and uterus |
| Pancreas: apical surface of small ductules | Spleen |
| Adrenal: diffusely on the surface of cells in medulla and cortex | Skin<br>Placenta |
| | All other cells of liver, jejunum, colon, kidney, and pancreas |

xenobiotics and chemotherapeutic agents, outside the cells. Recently, we found that MRK16 also detects P-glycoprotein in the capillaries of some human brain samples (*33*). Although its precise localization in brain capillaries will require further study, it is possible that it is present in a polarized fashion on endothelial cells, and that it may serve some physiological role in clearance of toxic products or environmental poisons from the central nervous system at the blood-brain barrier. The implication of this finding holds considerable interest for the elucidation of the real nature of the blood-brain barrier.

*Substances Interacting with P-glycoprotein to Overcome Drug Resistance*

P-glycoprotein is assumed to possess a drug efflux function. If we could find inhibitors of this drug efflux function, such compounds would be of great interest in overcoming drug resistance. In 1981 and 1982, we found that calcium channel blockers and calmodulin inhibitors could inhibit the efflux of antitumor agents, thus overcoming drug resistance (*4*, *5*). Since then various compounds including quinidine, tamoxifen, cyclosporin A (CsA), and so on have also been reported to overcome drug resistance (*34–37*) (see ref. *37* for review) (Table 2). It is now believed that these

TABLE 2. Potentiation of Antitumor Agents by Various Agents

| Antitumor agent | Potentiating agent |
|---|---|
| Vincristine, vinblastine | Verapamil and its analogues |
| | Trifluoperazine |
| | Nifedipine and its analogues |
| | Diltiazem |
| | Perhexiline |
| | Quinidine |
| Adriamycin, daunomycin | Verapamil and its analogues |
| | Trifluoperazine |
| | Nifedipine and its analogues |
| | Diltiazem |
| | Perhexiline |
| | Quinidine |
| Bleomycin, peplomycin | Verapamil |
| | Pimozide |
| | Melittin |
| | Chloropromazine |
| Etoposide | Verapamil |
| | Nifedipine and its analogues |
| | Diltiazem |
| Vindesine, taxol | Verapamil |
| | Nifedipine and its analogues |
| | Diltiazem |
| Actinomycin D, mitoxantrone | Verapamil |
| Aclacinomycin A | Nifedipine and its analogues |
| Mitomycin C, menogarol | Diltiazem |
| Rhodamine | Verapamil |
| Cisplatin | w5, w7 |
| | Verapamil |
| Chloroquine | Verapamil |

agents can interact with P-glycoprotein and thus inhibit the drug efflux function of the protein. Actually, some calcium channel blockers, including verapamil, can bind to P-glycoprotein, and the binding of some antitumor agents can be inhibited competitively by calcium channel blockers and other potentiating agents. The molecular mechanisms of action of calcium channel blockers as well as that of P-glycoprotein remain to be solved.

The use of calcium channel blockers and related compounds to overcome drug resistance is a practical approach (*37*). Combination chemotherapy with calcium channel blockers is potentially useful against refractory acute lymphocytic leukemia of children, various advanced solid tumors, small cell lung cancer and brain tumors. However, the combination therapy induces side effects such as reversible hypotension and arrhythmia. It is therefore important that more effective agents (calcium channel blockers and structurally related compounds) with fewer side effects than the present calcium channel blockers be found. The calcium influx blocking action of the calcium channel blockers, which is closely related to hypotension, is not involved in the mechanism of potentiation of antitumor agents. Thus, it should be possible to find potentiating agents without calcium influx blocking action. Research along this line, as well as the search for more effective drugs with fewer side effects is now in progress worldwide.

For this purpose, newly synthesized quinoline derivatives have been investigated for their efficacy to reverse multidrug resistance. One of the most effective quinoline derivatives, MS-073 (Fig. 2), was compared with verapamil in its multidrug resistance action *in vitro* and *in vivo*. MS-073 at 0.1 $\mu$M almost completely reversed *in vitro* resistance to vincristine (VCR) in VCR-resistant P388 (P388/VCR) cells. The compound also reversed *in vitro* VCR, adriamycin (ADM), etoposide, and actinomycin D resistance in ADM-resistant human myelogenous leukemia K562 (K562/ADM) cells, ADM-resistant human ovarian carcinoma A2780 cells, and colchicine-resistant human KB cells. Administered i.p. daily for 5 days with VCR, MS-073 enhanced the chemotherapeutic effect of VCR in P388/VCR-bearing mice. Life prolongation of 19 to 50% was obtained by the combination of 100 $\mu$g/kg of VCR with 3 to 100 mg/kg of MS-073, as compared to the control (Table 3). These effects of MS-073 in reversing multidrug resistance were remarkably higher, especially at low doses, than those of verapamil both *in vivo* and *in vivo*.

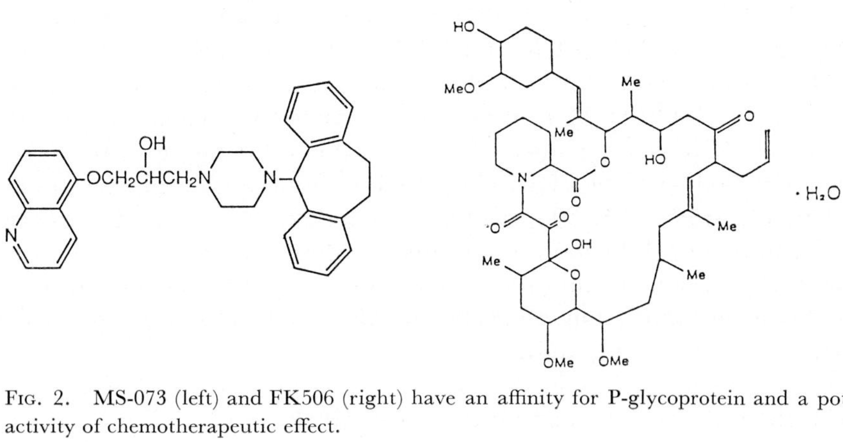


FIG. 2. MS-073 (left) and FK506 (right) have an affinity for P-glycoprotein and a potentiating activity of chemotherapeutic effect.

TABLE 3. Effect of MS-073 on Antitumor Activity of VCR in P388/VCR-bearing Mice

| Drug and dose (mg/kg) | | Mean survival time (days) | T/C (%) |
|---|---|---|---|
| Control | | 10.5 | 100 |
| MS-073 (100) | | 10.5 | 100 |
| VCR (0.1) | | 11.5 | 110 |
| +MS-073 | (3) | 12.5* | 119 |
| | (10) | 14.5* | 138 |
| | (30) | 15.5* | 148 |
| | (100) | 16.0* | 152 |

$10^6$ P388/VCR was implanted i.p. and drugs were given i.p. on days 1 to 5.
* Significant difference by Student's *t* test.

TABLE 4. Effect of FK-506 on Antitumor Activity of VCR in P388/VCR-bearing Mice

| Drug and dosage (mg/kg) | | Mean survival time (days) | T/C (%) |
|---|---|---|---|
| Control | | 11.0 | 100 |
| FK-506 | (20) | 12.5 | 114* |
| Cyclosporin A | (20) | 12.8 | 116* |
| Verapamil | (75) | 10.3 | 94* |
| VCR | (0.2) | 12.2 | 111* |
| +FK-506 | (20) | 16.6 | 151* |
| | (10) | 16.2 | 147* |
| | (5) | 15.4 | 140* |
| +Cyclosporin A | (20) | 8.0 | 73* |
| | (10) | 8.0 | 73* |
| | ( 5) | 12.2 | 111 |
| +Verapamil | (75) | 13.6 | 124* |
| | (50) | 13.4 | 122* |

$10^6$ P388/VCR was implanted i.p. and drugs were given i.p. on days 1 to 5.
* Significant difference by Student's *t* test.

MS-073 enhanced accumulation of [$^3$H]VCR in K562/ADM cells. Photolabeling of P-glycoprotein with 200 nM [$^3$H]azidopine in K562/ADM plasma membranes was completely inhibited by 10 $\mu$M MS-073.

Another interesting compound is FK-506, a novel immunosuppressive agent (Fig. 2). FK-506 at 3 $\mu$g/ml and 10 $\mu$g/ml completely reversed the resistance against vincristine *in vitro* in P388/VCR and ADM-resistant human ovarian cancer A2780 cells ($AD_{10}$), respectively. FK-506 also enhanced the cytotoxicity of VCR in highly resistant human K562/ADM *in vitro*, and enhanced the chemotherapeutic effect of VCR in P388/VCR-bearing mice (Table 4). When 20 mg/kg of the compound was combined with 200 $\mu$g/kg of VCR, 151% of T/C value was obtained. Under the protocol used in the study, FK-506 was more potent than CsA and verapamil; it also efficiently inhibited [$^3$H]azidopine binding to P-glycoprotein. The binding of VCR to K562/ADM plasma membrane was inhibited by FK-506 as effectively as CsA. Moreover, the accumulation of VCR in $AD_{10}$ cells was increased by FK-506 as efficiently as CsA and verapamil.

These results indicate that MS-073 and FK-506 directly interact with P-glycoprotein in the same way verapamil does, inhibit the active efflux of vincristine from resistant cells, increase the vincristine accumulation in resistant cells, and thus overcome multidrug resistance *in vitro* and *in vivo*. These two agents are of considerable interest for further studies for their potential clinical application.

### *Characterization of P-glycoprotein and Its Reconstitution into Liposome*

P-glycoprotein possesses an ATP-binding site, ATPase activity (*28, 38*), a binding site for vincristine and adriamycin (*23, 24, 39, 40*), a binding site for calcium channel blockers (*24, 41*), and phosphorylation sites which might be involved in regulative function (Table 5) (*42*).

We have purified the P-glycoprotein from human myelogenous leukemia K562 cells resistant to ADM by means of one-step immunoaffinity chromatography using a monoclonal antibody against P-glycoprotein. The procedure yielded an electrophoretically homogenous P-glycoprotein sample. By solubilization with 3-[3-cholamidopropyl)dimethyl-ammonio]-1-propane sulfonate, the purified P-glycoprotein was found to have ATPase activity. The ATP hydrolysis may be coupled with the active efflux of anticancer drugs across the plasma membrane of multidrug-resistant cells. GTP was also hydrolyzed by the P-glycoprotein, although less efficiently than ATP. The ATPase activity of the protein had an optimal pH range around neutrality (pH 6.5–7.4). The detergent concentration of 3-[(3-cholamidopropyl)dimethyl-ammonio]-1-propane sulfonate used for protein solubilization was essential for enzyme recovery. Maximum activity (2–10 mM) was obtained when 0.1–0.2% 3-[3(-cholamidopropyl)dimethyl-ammonio]-propane sulfonate was used, while higher concentrations markedly inhibited the activity, which was dependent on $Mg^{2+}$. Manganese and cobalt substitute for magnesium as ionic cofactors. Divalent cations such as $Ca^{2+}$, $Zn^{2+}$, $Ni^{2+}$, $Cd^{2+}$, and $Cu^{2+}$ inhibited the $Mg^{2+}$-catalyzed ATP hydrolysis. *N*-ethylmaleimide and vanadate inhibited the ATPase activity, while sodium azide or ouabain had no effect. Anticancer agents such as vincristine and ADM also did not affect the enzyme activity. In contrast, verapamil and trifluoperazine, agents which inhibit active drug efflux and restore drug sensitivity in resistant cells, caused an increase in the P-glycoprotein ATPase activity indicating that this protein is actually the target molecule of these agents.

The ATPase activity of the purified P-glycoprotein was 1.7 nmol/mg/min when 100 $\mu$M ATP was used (*38*). This specific activity was much lower than that for other membrane pumps such as Na/K-ATPase. The specific activity of the ATPase precipitated by MRK16-protein A-Sepharose was calculated, and maximum was 50 nmol/mg/min, much higher than that of the purified P-glycoprotein (1.7 nmol/mg/min). The cause of this difference is not clear; one possibility is that denaturation of the enzyme may have occurred during the purification procedure, which caused changes in the profile of ATP-dependency of the purified enzyme.

TABLE 5. Activities of P-glycoprotein

| | |
|---|---|
| 1. | ATPase activity |
| 2. | Substrate protein for C-kinase |
| 3. | VCR and ADM binding activity |
| 4. | Binding activities for various chemicals |

For precise characterization of its nature, we recently attempted to reconstitute purified P-glycoprotein into artificial liposomes. To obtain fully active P-glycoprotein, we used the peptide elution procedure in immunoaffinity chromatography with MRK16 which was shown to be reactive to the fourth external domain of the protein. In this procedure, the peptide corresponding to the fourth external domain of P-glycoprotein was used for elution, instead of acid elution which was used previously for the protein's purification (*38*). The purified P-glycoprotein retained about 80% of the estimated ATPase activity of P-glycoprotein. We reconstituted this purified P-glycoprotein into liposomes consisting of phosphatidylcholine: phosphatidylethanolamine: phosphatidylserine=7: 3: 1. The reconstituted P-glycoprotein showed ATPase activity, ATP-dependent drug-transport activity and calcium channel blocker-binding activity. Although the reconstitution experiment is still preliminary in nature, this model can provide advantages for studies of biochemical functions and the nature of compounds including xenobiotics which interact with P-glycoprotein.

*Acknowledgments*

I thank the staff of the Cancer Chemotherapy Center and the University of Tokyo for their excellent collaboration in this study. This study was supported by grants from the Ministry of Education, Science and Culture, and the Ministry of Health and Welfare, Japan. I thank Ms. T. Toyama for her expert secretarial assistance and Dr. M. Naito for his critical reading of the manuscript.

## REFERENCES

1. Riordan, J. R. and Ling, V. Genetic and biochemical characterization of multidrug resistance. Pharmacol. Ther., *28*: 51–75, 1985.
2. Skovsgaard, T. Mechanism of cross-resistance between vincristine and daunorubicin in Ehrlich ascites tumor cells. Cancer Res., *38*: 4722–4727, 1978.
3. Inaba, M., Kobayashi, H., Sakurai, Y., and Johnson, R. K. Active efflux of daunorubicin and Adriamycin in sensitive and resistant sublines of P388 leukemia. Cancer Res., *39*: 2200–2203, 1979.
4. Tsuruo, T., Iida, H., Tsukagoshi, S., and Sakurai, Y. Overcoming of vincristine resistance in P388 leukemia *in vivo* and *in vitro* through enhanced cytotoxicity of vincristine and vinblastine by verapamil. Cancer Res., *41*: 1967–1972, 1981.
5. Tsuruo, T., Iida, H., Tsukagoshi, S., and Sakurai, Y. Increased accumulation of vincristine and Adriamycin in drug resistant tumor cells following incubation with calcium antagonists and calmodulin inhibitors. Cancer Res., *42*: 4730–4733, 1982.
6. Juliano, R. L. and Ling, V. A surface glycoprotein modulating drug permeability in Chinese hamster ovary cell mutants. Biochim. Biophys. Acta, *455*: 152–162, 1976.
7. Beck, W. T., Mueller, T. J., and Tanzer, L. R. Altered surface membrane glycoproteins in *Vinca* alkaloid-resistant human leukemic lymphoblasts. Cancer Res., *39*: 2070–2076, 1979.
8. Biedler, J. L. and Peterson, R. H. F. Altered plasma membrane glycoconjugates of Chinese hamster cells with acquired resistance to actinomycin D, daunomycin, and vincristine. *In;* A. C. Sartorelli, J. S. Lazo, and J. R. Bertino (eds.), Molecular Actions and Targets for Cancer Chemotherapeutic Agents, Bristol Myers Cancer Symposia, Vol. 2, pp. 453–482, Academic Press, Inc., New York, 1981.
9. Garman, D. and Center, M. S. Alterations in cell surface membranes in Chinese hamster lung cells resistant to Adriamycin. Biochem. Biophys. Res. Commun., *105*:

157–163, 1982.

10. Debenham, P. G., Kartner, N. S., Siminovitch, L., Riordan, J. R., and Ling, V. DNA-mediated transfer of multiple drug resistance and plasma membrane glycoprotein expression. Mol. Cell. Biol., *2*: 881–889, 1982.
11. Kartner, N., Riordan, J. R., and Ling, V. Cell surface P-glycoprotein associated with multidrug resistance in mammalian cell lines. Science, *221*: 1285–1288, 1983.
12. Kartner, N., Evernden-Porelle, D., Bradley, G., and Ling, V. Detection of P-glycoprotein in multidrug-resistant cell lines by monoclonal antibodies. Nature, *316*: 820–823, 1985.
13. Tsuruo, T., Iida-Saito, H., Kawabata, H., Oh-hara, T., Hamada, H., and Utakoji, T. Characteristics of resistance to Adriamycin in human myelogenous leukemia K62 resistant to Adriamycin and the isolated clones. Jpn. J. Cancer Res., *77*: 682–692, 1986.
14. Hamada, H. and Tsuruo, T. Functional role for the 170- to 180-kDa glycoprotein specific to drug-resistant tumor cells as revealed by monoclonal antibodies. Proc. Natl. Acad. Sci. U.S.A., *83*: 7785–7789, 1986.
15. Hamada, H. and Tsuruo, T. Growth inhibition of multidrug-resistant cells by monoclonal antibodies against P-glycoprotein. *In;* I. B. Roninson (ed.), Molecular and Cellular Biology of Multidrug Resistance in Tumor Cells. Plenum Press, New York, 1991, in press.
16. Shen, D-W., Fojo, A., Roninson, I. B., Chin, J. E., Soffin, R., Pastan, I., and Gottesman, M. M. Multidurg resistance in DNA mediated transformants is linked to transfer of the human *mdr*1 gene. Mol. Cell. Biol., *6*: 4039–4045, 1986.
17. Gros, P., Neriah, Y. B. B., Croop, J. M., and Housman, D. E. Isolation and expression of a complimentary DNA (*mdr*) that confers multidrug resistance. Nature, *323*: 728–731, 1986.
18. Ueda, K., Cardarelli, C., Goteesman, M. M., and Pastan, I. Expression of a full-length cDNA for the human *mdr*1 (P-glycoprotein) gene confers multidrug resistance. Proc. Natl. Acad. Sci. U.S.A., *84*: 3004–3008, 1987.
19. Gros, P., Croop, J., and Housman, D. Mammalian multidrug resistance gene: complement cDNA sequence indicates strong homology to bacterial transport proteins. Cell, *47*: 371–380, 1986.
20. Chen, C., Chin, J. E., Ueda, K., Clark, D. P., Pastan, I., Gottesman, M. M., and Roninson, I. B. Internal duplication and homology with bacterial transport protein in the *mdr*1 (P-glycoprotein) gene from multidrug-resistant human cells. Cell, *47*: 381–389, 1986.
21. Garlach, J. H., Endicott, J. A., Juranka, P. F., Henderson, G., Sarani, F., Deuchars, K. L., and Ling, V. Homology between P-glycoprotein and a bacterial haemolysin transport protein suggests a model for multidrug resistance. Nature, *324*: 485–489, 1986.
22. Safa, A. R., Glover, C. J., Meyers, M. B., Biedler, J. L., and Felsted, R. L. Vinblastine photoaffinity labeling of a high molecular weight surface membrane glycoprotein specific for multidrug-resistant cells. J. Biol. Chem., *261*: 6137–6140, 1986.
23. Cornwell, M. M., Safa, A. R., Felsted, R. L., Gottesman, M. M., and Pastan, I. Membrane vesicles from multidrug-resistant human cancer cells contain a 150- to 170-kDa protein detected by photoaffinity labeling. Proc. Natl. Acad. Sci. U.S.A., *83*: 3847–3850, 1986.
24. Cornwell, M. M., Pastan, I., and Gottesman, M. M. Certain calcium channel blockers bind specifically to multidrug-resistant human KB carcinoma membrane vesicles and inhibit drug binding to P-glycoprotein. J. Biol. Chem., *262*: 2166–2170, 1987.

25. Willingham, M. C., Richert, N. D., Cornwell, M. M., Tsuruo, T., Hamada, H., Gottesman, M. M., and Pastan, I. Immunocytochemical localization of P170 at the plasma membrane of multidrug-resistant human cells. J. Histochem. Cytochem., *35*: 1451–1456, 1987.
26. Roninson, I. B. (ed.). Molecular and Cellular Biology of Multidrug Resistance in Tumor Cells, Plenum Press, New York, 1991.
27. Tsuruo, T. Mechanisms of multidrug resistance and implications for therapy. Jpn. J. Cancer Res., *79*: 285–296, 1988.
28. Hamada, H. and Tsuruo, T. Purification of the 170- to 180-kilodalton membrane glycoprotein associated with multidrug resistance: 170- to 180-kilodalton membrane glycoprotein is an ATPase. J. Biol. Chem., *263*: 1454–1458, 1988.
29. Fojo, A. T., Ueda, K., Salmon, D. J., Poplack, D. G., Gottesman, M. M., and Pastan, I. Expression of a multidrug-resistance gene in human tumors and tissues. Proc. Natl. Acad. Sci. U.S.A., *84*: 265–269, 1987.
30. Thorgeirsson, S. S., Huber, B. E., Sorrell, S., Fojo, A., Pastan, I., and Gottesman, M. M. Expression of the multidrug-resistant gene in hepatocarcinogenesis and regenerating rat liver. Science, *236*: 1120–1122, 1987.
31. Fairchild, G., Ivy, S. P., Rushmore, T., Lee, G., Koo, P., Goldsmith, M. E., Myers, C. E., Farber, E., and Cowan, K. H. Carcinogen-induced *mdr* overexpression is associated with xenobiotic resistance in rat preneoplastic liver nodules and hepatocellular carcinomas. Proc. Natl. Acad. Sci. U.S.A., *84*: 7701–7705, 1987.
32. Thiebaut, F., Tsuruo, T., Hamada, H., Gottesman, M., Pastan, I., and Willingham, M. C. The location of the multidrug resistance gene-product P-glycoprotein in normal tissues. Proc. Natl. Acad. Sci. U.S.A., *84*: 7735–7738, 1987.
33. Thiebaut, F., Tsuruo, T., Hamada, H., Gottesman, M., Pastan, I., and Willingham, M. C. Immunohistochemical localization in normal tissues of different epitopes in the multidrug transport protein P170: evidence for localization in brain capillaries and crossreactivity of one antibody with a muscle protein. J. Histochem. Cytochem., *37*: 159–174, 1989.
34. Tsuruo, T., Iida, H., Naganuma, K., Tsukagoshi, S., and Sakurai, Y. Promotion by verapamil of vincristine responsiveness in tumor cell lines inherently resistant to the drug. Cancer Res., *43*: 808–813, 1983.
35. Tsuruo, T., Iida, H., Tsukagoshi, S., and Sakurai, Y. Potentiation of vincristine and adriamycin effects in human hemopoietic tumor cell lines by calcium antagonists and calmodulin inhibitors. Cancer Res., *43*: 2267–2272, 1983.
36. Tsuruo, T., Iida, H., Nojiri, M., Tsukagoshi, S., and Sakurai, Y. Circumvention of vincristine and adriamycin resistance *in vitro* and *in vivo* by calcium influx blockers. Cancer Res., *43*: 2905–2910, 1983.
37. Tsuruo, T. Reversal of multidrug by calcium channel blockers and other agents. *In;* I. B. Roninson (ed.), Molecular and Cellular Biology of Multidrug Resistance in Tumor Cells, Plenum Press, New York, 1991, in press.
38. Hamada, H. and Tsuruo, T. Characterization of the activity of the Mr170,000 to 180,000 membrane glycoprotein (P-glycoprotein) associated with multidrug resistance in K562/ADM cells. Cancer Res., *48*: 4926–4932, 1988.
39. Naito, M., Hamada, H., and Tsuruo, T. ATP/$Mg^{2+}$-dependent binding of vincristine to the plasma membrane of multidrug-resistant K562 cells. J. Biol. Chem., *263*: 11887–11891, 1988.
40. Naito, M. and Tsuruo, T. Competitive inhibition by verapamil of ATP-dependent high affinity vincristine binding to the plasma membrane of multidrug-resistant K562 cells without calcium ion involvement. Cancer Res., *49*: 1452–1455, 1989.

41. Yusa, K. and Tsuruo, T. Reversal mechanism of multidrug resistance by verapamil: direct binding of verapamil to P-glycoprotein on specific sites and transport of verapamil outward across the plasma membrane of K562/ADM cells. Cancer Res., *49*: 5002–5006, 1989.

42. Hamada, H., Hagiwara, K., Nakajima, T., and Tsuruo, T. Phosphorylation of the $M_r$170,000 to 180,000 glycoprotein specific to multidrug-resistant tumor cells: effect of verapamil, trifluoperazine, and phorbol esters. Cancer Res., *47*: 2860–2865, 1987.

XENOBIOTICS AND CANCER, L. ERNSTER ET AL. (EDS.),
JAPAN SCI. SOC. PRESS, TOKYO/TAYLOR & FRANCIS LTD., LONDON, pp. 253–262, 1991

# Glutathione-linked Enzymes in Normal and Tumor Cells and Their Role in Resistance against Genotoxic Agents

Bengt MANNERVIK,*1 Kiflu BERHANE,*1 Victor M. CASTRO,*1 Birgit OLIN,*1 Marianne RIDDERSTRÖM,*1 Rita VIGNANI,*1 John W. KOZARICH,*2 and Ulrik RINGBORG*3

*Department of Biochemistry, Uppsala University, Biomedical Center, S-751 23 Uppsala, Sweden,*1 Department of Chemistry and Biochemistry, University of Maryland, College Park, Maryland 20742, U.S.A.,*2 and Department of General Oncology, Radiumhemmet, Karolinska Hospital, S-104 01 Stockholm, Sweden*3*

*Abstract:* Glutathione is the most abundant low molecular mass thiol in human cells. It is involved in the inactivation of genotoxic electrophilic compounds, and a variety of glutathione-linked enzymes catalyze such detoxication reactions. Within this group, the enzymes occurring in highest intracellular concentrations are the glutathione transferases, which catalyze the detoxication of a broad spectrum of alkylating and oxidizing compounds such as epoxides, reactive alkenes and organic hydroperoxides. Multiple forms of glutathione transferase with distinct substrate specificities exist, and their differential expression in cells contributes to differences in detoxication capacities in tissues. Glyoxalase I catalyzes the inactivation of 2-oxoaldehydes and may also be considered as part of the cellular detoxication system. Characterization of the different enzymes and their differential expression in normal and tumor cells will help to clarify their cellular functions and their significance to human cancer. Clear differences in the occurrence of the various enzyme forms in normal and tumor cells have been demonstrated and variations between different tumors appear to be linked to their degree of resistance to alkylating cytostatic drugs. Modulation of catalytic activities *in vitro* by administration of enzyme inhibitors may help to overcome this resistance.

Glutathione is the most abundant intracellular thiol found in mammalian tissues. Its reactive sulfur atom makes glutathione a good nucleophile with the capacity of reacting with electron-deficient molecules in the cell. Such reactions effect the inactivation of electrophiles, which otherwise might cause toxicity by reacting with cellular constituents such as DNA and proteins. Many chemical carcinogens are intrinsically electrophilic or give rise to electrophilic compounds by metabolic activation, and the detoxication of such compounds by glutathione-linked reactions is a mechanism for prevention of cancer. The cell has a repertoire of enzymes catalyzing glutathione-linked detoxication reactions, and it has been proposed that an original function of these enzymes was to provide protection against products of oxidative metabolism (*1, 2*). Tumor cells, like normal cells, contain glutathione-linked enzymes and certain forms of drug resistance in cancer cells have been ascribed to the activity of these enzymes. Thus, glutathione-linked enzymes appear to play important roles both in prevention of cancer and in the resistance mechanisms of tumors treated in the clinic.

*Glutathione-linked Enzymes and Detoxication of Genotoxic Agents*

A wide variety of chemical compounds with the potential of causing mutations and cancer occur in mammalian cells. Traditionally, such genotoxic compounds have been regarded as having a xenobiotic origin. However, it is obvious that many mutagenic compounds are formed by oxidative processes involving normal cell constituents and therefore have an endobiotic origin. A number of glutathione-linked enzymes are involved in reactions which lead to detoxication of such compounds (*3*). The glyoxalase system converts 2-oxoaldehydes into corresponding 2-hydroxy acids, formaldehyde dehydrogenase transforms formaldehyde into formate, and glutathione peroxidase catalyzes the reduction of hydroperoxides into corresponding alcohols and water. Glutathione transferases catalyze a broad spectrum of reactions, many of which lead to the generation of stable thioether conjugates which by further metabolism result in suitable excretion products. Finally, thioltransferase facilitates thiol-disulfide interchange and, in the presence of glutathione in reduced form, has a role in the maintenance of low molecular mass thiols and protein thiols in their reduced state. The need for regeneration of reduced glutathione from its disulfide form is accomplished by glutathione reductase at the expense of reducing equivalents from NADPH. Impairment of the enzymatic functions may compromise the cellular protection against chemical challenges. On the other hand, elevated concentrations of glutathione-linked enzymes may result in increased resistance against toxic agents.

*Glyoxalase I*

The glyoxalase system is composed of two enzymes, glyoxalase I and glyoxalase II, catalyzing the formation of S-2-hydroxyacyl-glutathione and hydrolysis of the same compound, respectively (*4*). The first reaction is the crucial one in the detoxication of 2-oxoaldehydes, since it effects elimination of the electrophilic 2-oxoaldehydic functional group. The full biological significance of the glyoxalase system remains unclear, but it is obvious that it may serve in the inactivation of genotoxic 2-oxoaldehydes which can originate from endo- as well as xenobiotics (*4*). It is known that 2-oxoaldehydes inhibit cell growth (*5*), but it is not clear if this capacity is used in the biological control of cell proliferation. Nevertheless, an effective glyoxalase system will prevent accumulation of antiproliferative concentrations of 2-oxoaldehydes. In this respect, it is noteworthy that, whereas normal cells and tissues display only a limited variation in their concentrations of glyoxalase I (*6*), tumor cell lines express widely different levels of the enzyme (*7*). Data in Table 1 span a more than 50-fold range in cytosolic specific activities of glyoxalase I.

*Glutathione Transferases*

The ensemble of glutathione transferases that exists in an organism has the potential of inactivating a wide variety of genotoxic chemical compounds. Three classes

TABLE 1. Cytosolic Specific Activities of GSH-linked Enzymes in Human Cell Lines

| Cell line | Activity (nmol/min/mg) | |
|---|---|---|
| | GSH transferase (CDNB) | Glyoxalase I (methylglyoxal) |
| Chang liver | 118 | 41 |
| Hep G2 | 14 | 40 |
| LS174T | 319 | 34 |
| Raji | 1.3 | 350 |
| Hu549Pat | 330 | 6 |
| U937 | 107 | 115 |

GSH, glutathione. Data selected from ref. *7*.

(Alpha, Mu, and Pi) of cytosolic enzymes and one membrane-associated (microsomal) enzyme are well recognized (*8*), and recent evidence suggests a fourth cytosolic class (*9, 10*). The isoenzyme distribution of the glutathione transferases varies quantitatively as well as qualitatively from tissue to tissue (*11, 12*), implying differential protection against toxic compounds that may be inactivated by enzyme-catalyzed glutathione conjugations. A measure of the total glutathione transferase activity is obtainable by use of 1-chloro-2,4-dinitrobenzene (CDNB) as substrate, and Table 1 demonstrates substantial differences in the cytosolic specific activities among various cell lines. Such quantitative differences and the variation among the glutathione transferases in their respective substrate specificity profiles may therefore provide an explanation for differences in cells of distinct origins in their resistance against electrophilic compounds.

Glutathione transferases are inducible by various compounds (*13, 14*) in a differential manner such that a given inducer causes the expression of only certain isoenzymes (*15*). In animal models, dietary constituents from plants have been shown to provide protection against chemically induced cancer as well as to effect induction of glutathione transferases (*16*). As an example of such inducers and their selective effects, cafestol palmitate has been shown to preferentially induce a class Mu glutathione transferase in the mouse (*17*).

Glutathione transferases have been shown to catalyze the inactivation of compounds that are recognized as carcinogens, or at least known to form DNA-adducts. Many of these electrophilic compounds are formed intracellularly by oxygen-dependent enzymatic reactions. For example, the simplest $\alpha$, $\beta$-unsaturated carbonyl compound, acrolein, is one of the substrates that gives rise to the highest catalytic efficiency (as measured by $k_{cat}/K_m$) of human glutathione transferase $\pi$ (*18*). Another group of substrates with the same electrophilic $\alpha$, $\beta$-unsaturated carbonyl group are the 4-hydroxyalkenals, which are excellent substrates for the class Alpha rat glutathione transferase 8–8 (*19, 20*) and which belong to the most active substrates found for any glutathione transferase (*21*). Polyunsaturated fatty acids subjected to lipid peroxidation give rise to 4-hydroxyalkenals. Organic molecules containing carbon-carbon double bonds may undergo epoxidation resulting in the reactive oxirane structure. Polycyclic aromatic hydrocarbons such as benzo(a)pyrene are known to give rise to carcinogenic arene oxides by means of cytochrome P-450 mediated monooxygenase reactions. The ultimate carcinogen (+)*anti*-7,8-dihydroxy-9,10-oxy-7,8,9,10-tetrahydrobenzo(a)pyrene in hepatocytes is metabolized predominantly by glutathione conjugation (*22*), a reaction catalyzed most efficiently by class Mu and class Pi glutathione transferases (*23, 24*). With respect to the human enzymes, it is noteworthy that glutathione transferase $\mu$ is equally active with the (—)*anti*- and the (+)*anti*-enantiomers, whereas glutathione transferase $\pi$ is stereoselective for the (+)-*anti*-enantiomer (*23*). In view of the differential expression of the various forms of glutathione transferase, it is also worth emphasizing that glutathione transferase $\mu$ displays more than 100-fold higher specific activity with certain epoxides than the known class Alpha glutathione transferases (*25*).

### *Polymorphic Expression of Glutathione Transferase $\mu$*

In the analysis of cytosol fractions from human livers it was discovered that three out of five human subjects expressed a glutathione transferase with a near-neutral isoelectric point and a substrate specificity distinct from previously known hepatic enzymes (*26*). The enzyme was named glutathione transferase $\mu$, and the significance of its distinct substrate specificity was highlighted when it was established that the enzyme was particularly active with genotoxic and mutagenic epoxides (*27, 28*). Consequently, it was proposed that individuals lacking glutathione transferase $\mu$ should be more susceptible to certain toxic compounds. Subsequent studies suggest that smokers deficient in glutathione transferase $\mu$ are subject to greater risk of developing lung cancer (*29, 30*). The polymorphic expression of glutathione transferase $\mu$ has been shown to be genetic in nature (*31, 32*) and analysis of genomic DNA indicates that the null genotype is due to a gene deletion (*33*). On the basis of cDNA sequences corresponding to glutathione transferase $\mu$ (*33, 34*) and an assumed intron/exon structure similar to genomic DNA encoding rat subunit 4 (*35*), oligodeoxynucleotide primers complementary to the 5′ end of exon 4 and the 3′ end of exon 5 of the human glutathione transferase $\mu$ gene were designed for analysis by the polymerase chain reaction, PCR (*36*). Almost identical primers for studies of the glutathione transferase $\mu$ gene have been synthesized independently (*37*). Figure 1 shows the positive results of an analysis of genomic DNA from two cell lines, Raji (a Burkitt's lymphoma) and RPMI 8322 (a malignant melanoma), which both appear to produce glutathione transferase $\mu$, as judged from immunoblots. In our studies we have found that in addition to the expected exon 4-intron 4-exon 5 fragment in glutathione transferase $\mu$ positive samples, a related 170 base pair, apparently intronless, fragment may occur. Under suitable conditions this presumed pseudogene product may serve as an internal control for proper functioning of the PCR.

Two allelic variants of the active gene have been recognized (*31, 32*). The corresponding proteins, glutathione transferases $\mu$ and $\psi$, differ in their amino acid sequences only in position 173, where the less acidic glutathione transferase $\mu$ has a lysine residue, whereas the more acidic glutathione transferase $\psi$ has an asparagine residue (*33, 34*). Both of the proteins have been expressed in *Escherichia coli* by use of recombinant DNA techniques, and the recombinant proteins are in all physicochemical and catalytic properties indistinguishable from the corresponding proteins isolated from human liver (*38*). So far, no functional differences between glutathione transferase $\mu$ and $\psi$ have been demonstrated.

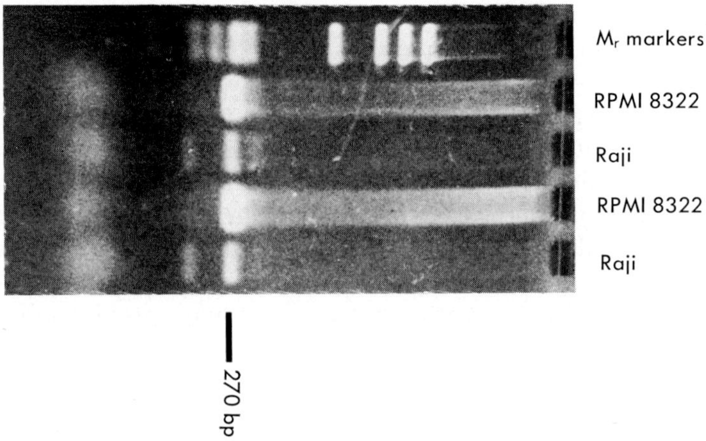


FIG. 1. Demonstration of the glutathione transferase μ gene in preparations of genomic DNA from the RPMI8322 and Raji cell lines by use of the PCR. The primers used for lanes 2 and 3 were 5′-CTG CCC TAC TTG ATT GAT GG-3′ and 5′-TGG ATT GTA GCA GAT CAT GC-3′, complementary to exons 4 and 5, respectively, in the glutathione transferase μ gene. The primers used for lanes 4 and 5 were obtained from Dr. W. D. Henner (*37*). They were almost identical to the sequences above, the difference being that the exon 4 primer contained an additional G in the 3′ end and the exon 5 primer contained an additional C in the 5′ end. The photograph shows ethidium bromide stained DNA fragments in 1.5% agarose gels after electrophoresis of aliquots from the PCR reaction mixture. The major band of approximately 270 base pair size contains the expected amplified fragment containing the major parts of exons 4 and 5 flanking an intron sequence: 5′-GTG AGT GTG GGT GGC TGC AAT GTG TAG GGG GAA GGT GGC CTC CTC CTT GGC TGG GCT GTG ATG CTG AGA TTG AGT CTG TGT TTT GTG GGT GGC AG-3′, identical in both cell lines. The latter sequence has previously been reported as part of the genomic DNA of normal somatic cells in glutathione transferase μ positive individuals (*37*). A fainter band (approximately 170 base pairs) below the main PCR product was obtained from the Raji cell samples. This fragment lacks the intron sequence and is believed to represent a pseudogene found in normal cells.

### *Glutathione-linked Enzymes and Drug Resistance*

Compelling evidence that glutathione-linked reactions contribute to resistance to certain drugs has been obtained. Of particular interest in relation to the chemotherapy of cancer are bifunctional alkylating drugs, many of which have been shown to give rise to glutathione conjugates or to metabolites resulting from the further biotransformation of these conjugates. Glutathione transferase π is the predominant form in most tumor cells investigated (see ref. *7* for a review), and this enzyme was therefore originally believed to play a major role in the resistance mechanism. However, in terms of catalytic activity, glutathione transferase π has only been shown to exhibit high specific activities with acrolein and base propenals (Table 2), electrophilic compounds that are only indirectly linked to cytostatic drugs. Acrolein is a product of the metabolic activation of cyclophosphamide, and base propenals arise from DNA by radical reactions elicited by bleomycin (*39*). Even if both acrolein and base propenals are cytotoxic DNA-reactive compounds, it is not clear to what extent they may contribute to the antitumor effects of these cytostatics.

In rodent systems clear evidence for the involvement of glutathione transferases in the resistance mechanism has been obtained. A rat glioma cell line with acquired resistance against 1,3-bis (2-chloroethyl)-1-nitrosourea (BCNU) was found to have elevated levels of class Mu glutathione transferase subunits 3 and 4 in comparison with its parental cell line (*40*). In complementary experiments, it was demonstrated that the corresponding purified class Mu glutathione transferases were the most active rat isoenzymes in the degradation of this cytostatic drug. Even if the class Pi enzyme predominates, it seems possible that cytostatic drug resistance in many cases may be linked to the less abundant glutathione transferases of classes Mu and Alpha (*7*). Increased expression of minor forms with substrate specificity profiles suitable for in-

TABLE 2. Specific Activities ($\mu$mol/min/mg) for Human GSTs Assayed with Base Propenals as Substrates

| GST | 3-Substituent of propenal | | | |
|---|---|---|---|---|
| | Adenin-9′-yl | Cytosin-1′-yl | Uracil-1′-yl | H-(acrolein) |
| $\varepsilon$ | 0.87 | 0.45 | 0.65 | 0.86 |
| $\mu$ | 14.2 | 3.0 | 7.3 | 7.1 |
| $\pi$ | 102 | 29 | 35 | 26 |

GST, glutathione transferase.

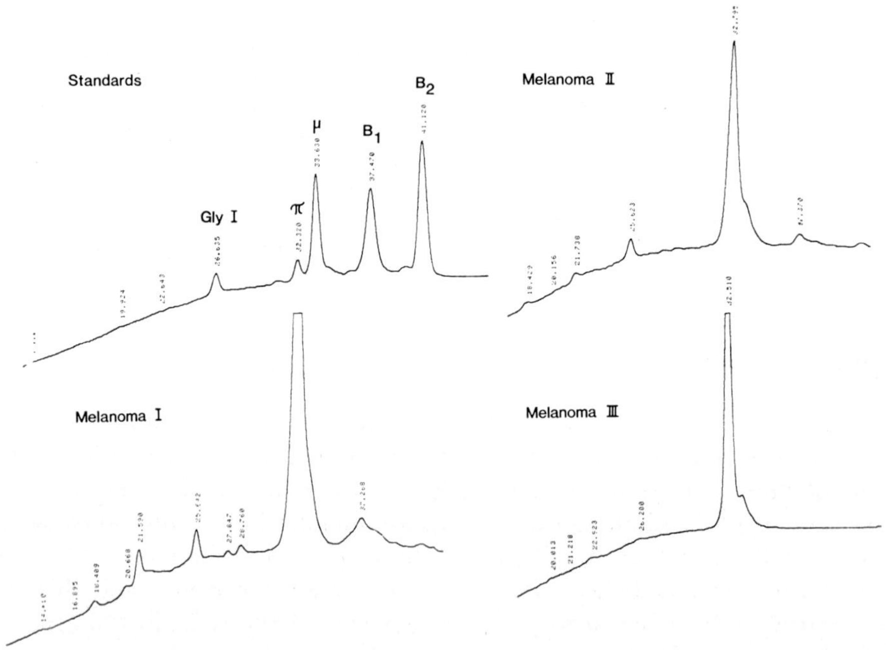


FIG. 2. Analysis by high performance liquid chromatography on a Dynamax 300A reverse phase C18 column of samples from human malignant melanoma tumors. Glutathione transferase subunits are separated by gradient elution with acetonitrile (35 to 55%, v/v) in the presence of 0.1% (v/v) trifluoroacetic acid. Elution was monitored at 214 nm. The upper left chromatogram shows the positions of reference proteins: glyoxalase I (Gly I), glutathione transferases $\pi$, $\mu$ and two class Alpha subunits, $B_1$ and $B_2$. Cytosol fractions from tumors of three malignant melanoma patients were purified by affinity chromatography on S-hexylglutathione-Sepharose before the analysis. Although each sample is dominated by glutathione transferase $\pi$, differences in the enzyme profiles in the tumor samples are clearly visible.

activation of particular drugs may be a mechanism for acquisition of enhanced drug resistance.

It has been demonstrated that the glutathione transferase pattern may vary from one malignancy to another. However, we have also found that the pattern may differ between tumors from individuals with the same disease. For example, of a total of fifteen lymphoma tumors, four expressed high levels of glutathione transferase $\mu$ and others contained high levels of class Alpha glutathione transferases (K. Berhane, U. Ringborg, B. Christensson, and B. Mannervik, unpublished results). Similar differences among tumors from different patients with malignant melanoma have also been demonstrated (Fig. 2). It is even possible that different tumors from the same individual may display differences in glutathione transferase composition. Clonal selection of cells expressing enzymes that contribute to drug resistance will give tumors a selective advantage during a regime of chemotherapy. Thus, analyses of tumor cells from cancer patients may help characterize the factors contributing to the resistance phenotype of the individual. Design and rational use of inhibitors for detoxication enzymes that contribute to drug resistance in tumors may serve as a basis for an improved patient-specific treatment of neoplastic disease.

*Acknowledgments*

The work described in this paper has been supported by grants from the Swedish Cancer Society, the Swedish Natural Science Research Council, and the Göran Gustafsson Foundation.

## REFERENCES

1. Mannervik, B. Glutathione and the evolution of enzymes for detoxication of products of oxygen metabolism. Chem. Scripta, *26B*: 281–284, 1986.
2. Mannervik, B. The roles of different classes of glutathione transferase in the detoxication of reactive products of oxidative metabolism. Chem. Scripta, *27A*: 121–123, 1987.
3. Mannervik, B., Carlberg, I., and Larson, K. Glutathione: General review of mechanism of action. *In;* D. Dolphin, R. Poulson, and O. Avramović (eds.), Coenzymes and Cofactors, Vol. 3A, pp. 475–516, John Wiley & Sons, New York, 1989.
4. Mannervik, B. Glyoxalase I. *In;* W. B. Jakoby (ed.), Enzymatic Basis of Detoxication, Vol. 2, pp. 263–273, Academic Press, New York, 1980.
5. French, F. A. and Freedlander, B. L. Carcinostatic action of polycarbonyl compounds and their derivatives. I. 3-Ethoxy-2-ketobutyraldehyde and related compounds. Cancer Res., *18*: 172–175, 1958.
6. Larsen, K., Aronsson, A.-C., Marmstål, E., and Mannervik, B. Immunological comparison of glyoxalase I from yeast and mammals and quantitative determination of the enzyme in human tissues by radioimmunoassay. Comp. Biochem. Physiol., *82B*: 625–638, 1985.
7. Castro, V. M., Söderström, M., Carlberg, I., Widersten, M., Platz, A., and Mannervik, B. Differences among human tumor cell lines in the expression of glutathione transferases and other glutathione-linked enzymes. Carcinogenesis, *11*: 1569–1576, 1990.
8. Mannervik, B., Ålin, P., Guthenberg, C., Jensson, H., Tahir, M. K. Warholm, M., and Jörnvall, H. Identification of three classes of cytosolic glutathione, transferase common to several mammalian species: correlation between structural data and enzymatic properties. Proc. Natl. Acad. Sci. U.S.A., *82*: 7202–7206, 1985.

9. Hiratsuka, A., Sebata, N., Kawashima, K., Okuda, H., Ogura, K., Watabe, T., Satoh, K., Hatayama, I., Tsuchida, S., Ishikawa, T., and Sato, K. A new class of rat glutathione *S*-transferase Yrs-Yrs inactivating reactive sulfate esters as metabolites of carcinogenic arylmethanols. J. Biol. Chem., *265*: 11973–11981, 1990.
10. Meyer, D. J., Coles, B., Pemble, S. E., Gilmore, K. S., Fraser, G. M., and Ketterer, B. Theta, a new class of glutathione transferases purified from rat and man. Biochem. J., *274*: 409–414, 1991.
11. Mannervik, B., Guthenberg, C., Jensson, H., Warholm, M., and Ålin, P. Isozymes of glutathione S-transferases in rat and human tissues. *In;* A. Larsson, S. Orrenius, A. Holmgren, and B. Mannervik (eds.), Functions of Glutathione: Biochemical, Physiological, Toxicological, and Clinical Aspects, pp. 75–88, Raven Press, New York, 1983.
12. Tu, C.-P. D., Weiss, M. J., Li, N., and Reddy, C. C. Tissue-specific expression of the rat glutathione *S*-transferases. J. Biol. Chem., *258*: 4659–4662, 1983.
13. Benson, A. M., Batzinger, R. P., Ou, S.-Y. L., Bueding, E., Cha, Y.-N., and Talalay, P. Elevation of hepatic glutathione *S*-transferase activities and protection against mutagenic metabolites of benzo(a)pyrene by dietary antioxidants. Cancer Res., *38*: 4486–4495, 1978.
14. Guthenberg, C., Morgenstern, R., DePierre, J. W., and Mannervik, B. Induction of glutathione *S*-transferases A, B and C in rat liver cytosol by *trans*-stilbene oxide. Biochim. Biophys. Acta, *631*: 1–10, 1980.
15. DiSimplicio, P., Jensson, H., and Mannervik, B. Identification of the isoenzymes of glutathione transferase induced by *trans*-stilbene oxide. Acta Chem. Scand., *B37*: 255–257, 1983.
16. Wattenberg, L. W. Inhibition of neoplasia by minor dietary constituents. Cancer Res., *43* (Suppl.): 2448s–2453s, 1983.
17. DiSimplicio, P., Jensson, H., and Mannervik, B. Effects of inducers of drug metabolism on basic hepatic forms of mouse glutathione transferase. Biochem. J., *263*: 679–685, 1989.
18. Berhane, K. and Mannervik, B. Inactivation of the genotoxic aldehyde acrolein by human glutathione transferases of classes Alpha, Mu, and Pi. Mol. Pharmacol., *37*: 251–254, 1990.
19. Ålin, P., Danielson, U. H., and Mannervik, B. 4-Hydroxyalk-2-enals are substrates for glutathione transferase. FEBS Lett., *179*: 267–270, 1985.
20. Jensson, H., Guthenberg, C., Ålin, P., and Mannervik, B. Rat glutathione transferase 8–8, an enzyme efficiently detoxifying 4-hydroxyalk-2-enals. FEBS Lett., *203*: 207–209, 1986.
21. Danielson, U. H., Esterbauer, H., and Mannervik, B. Structure-activity relationships of 4-hydroxyalkenals in the conjugation catalysed by mammalian glutathione transferases. Biochem. J., *247*: 707–713.
22. Jernström, B., Martinez, M., Svensson, S.-Å., and Dock, L. Metabolism of benzo(a)-pyrene-7,8-dihydrodiol and benzo(a)pyrene-7,8-dihydrodiol-9,10-epoxide to protein-binding products and glutathione conjugates in isolated rat hepatocytes. Carcinogenesis, *5*: 1079–1085, 1984.
23. Robertson, I. G. C., Guthenberg, C., Mannervik, B., and Jernström, B. Differences in stereoselectivity and catalytic efficiency of three human glutathione transferases in the conjugation of glutathione with 7$\beta$,8$\alpha$-dihydroxy-9$\alpha$,10$\alpha$-oxy-7,8,9,10-tetrahydrobenzo(a)pyrene. Cancer Res., *46*: 2220–2224, 1986.
24. Robertson, I. G. C., Jensson, H., Mannervik, B., and Jernström, B. Glutathione transferases in rat lung: the presence of transferase 7-7, highly efficient in the conjugation

of glutathione with the carcinogenic (+)-7$\beta$,8$\alpha$-dihydro-9$\alpha$,10$\alpha$-oxy-7,8,9,10-tetrahydrobenzo(a)pyrene. Carcinogenesis, *7*: 295–299, 1986.

25. Mannervik, B. and Danielson, U. H. Glutathione transferases—structure and catalytic activity. CRC Crit. Rev. Biochem., *23*: 283–337, 1988.
26. Warholm, M., Guthenberg, C., Mannervik, B., von Bahr, C., and Glaumann, H. Identification of a new glutathione *S*-transferase in human liver. Acta Chem. Scand., *B34*: 607–610, 1980.
27. Warholm, M., Guthenberg, C., Mannervik, B., and von Bahr, C. Purification of a new glutathione *S*-transferase (transferase $\mu$) from human liver having high activity with benzo(a)-pyrene-4,5-oxide. Biochem. Biophys. Res. Commun., *98*: 512–519, 1981.
28. Warholm, M., Guthenberg, C., and Mannervik, B. Molecular and catalytic properties of glutathione transferase $\mu$ from human liver: an enzyme efficiently conjugating epoxides. Biochemistry, *22*: 3610–3617, 1983.
29. Seidegård, J., Pero, R. W., Miller, D. G., and Beattie, E. J. A glutathione transferase in human leukocytes as a marker for the susceptibility to lung cancer. Carcinogenesis, *7*: 751–753, 1986.
30. Seidegård, J., Pero, R. W., Markowitz, M. M., Roush, G., Miller, D. G., and Beattie, E. J. Isoenzyme(s) of glutathione transferase (class Mu) as a marker for the susceptibility to lung cancer: a follow up study. Carcinogenesis, *11*: 33–36, 1990.
31. Board, P. G. Biochemical genetics of glutathione *S*-transferase in man. Am. J. Hum. Genet., *33*: 36–43, 1981.
32. Strange, R. C., Faulder, C. G., Davis, B. A., Hume, R., Brown, J. A. H., Cotton, W., and Hopkinson, D. A. The human glutathione *S*-transferases: studies on the tissue distribution and genetic variation of the GST1, GST2 and GST3 isozymes. Ann.Hum. Genet., *48*: 11–20, 1984.
33. Seidegård, J., Vorachek, W. R., Pero, R. W., and Pearson, W. R. Hereditary differences in the expression of the human glutathione transferase active on *trans*-stilbene oxide are due to a gene deletion. Proc. Natl. Acad. Sci. U.S.A., *85*: 7293–7297, 1988.
34. DeJong, J. L., Chang, C.-M., Whang-Peng, J., Knutsen, T., and Tu, C.-P. D. The human liver glutathione *S*-transferase gene superfamily: expression and chromosome mapping of an $H_b$ subunit cDNA. Nucleic Acids Res., *16*: 8541–8554, 1988.
35. Lai, H.-C. J., Qian, B., Grove, G., and Tu, C.-P. D. Gene expression of rat glutathione *S*-transferases. Evidence for gene conversion in the evolution of the $Y_b$ multigene family. J. Biol. Chem., *263*: 11389–11395, 1988.
36. Mannervik, B., Board, P. G., Berhane, K., Björnestedt, R., Castro, V. M., Danielson, U. H., Hao, X.-Y., Kolm, R., Olin, B., Principato, G. B., Ridderström, M., Stenberg, G., and Widersten, M. Classes of glutathione transferases: structural and catalytic properties of the enzymes. *In;* J. D. Hayes, C. B. Pickett, and T. J. Mantle (eds.), Glutathione *S*-Transferases and Drug Resistance, pp. 35–45, Taylor & Francis, London, 1990.
37. Comstock, K. E., Sanderson, B. J. S., Claflin, G., and Henner W. D. GST1 gene deletion determined by polymerase chain reaction. Nucleic Acids Res., *18*: 3670, 1990.
38. Widersten, M., Björnestedt, R., Holmström, E., Board, P. G., Pearson, W. R., and Mannervik, B. Structure-activity studies on mammalian glutathione transferases based on construction of point-mutated and chimeric enzymes. *In;* M. Ingelman-Sundberg, J.-Å. Gustafsson, and S. Orrenius (eds.), Drug Metabolizing Enzymes: Genetics, Regulation and Toxicology, p. 141, Karolinska Institutet, Stockholm, 1990.
39. Murugesan, N., Xu, C., Ehrenfeld, G. M., Sugiyama, H., Kilkuskie, R. E., Rodriguez, L. O., Chang, L.-H., and Hecht, S. M. Analysis of products formed during bleomycin-mediated DNA degradation. Biochemistry, *24*: 5735–5744, 1985.
40. Smith, M. T., Evans, C. G., Doane-Setzer, P., Castro, V. M., Tahir, M. K., and

Mannervik, B. Denitrosation of 1, 3-bis(2-chloroethyl)-1-nitrosourea by class Mu glutathione transferases and its role in cellular resistance in rat brain tumor cells. Cancer Res., *49*: 2621–2625, 1989.

XENOBIOTICS AND CANCER, L. ERNSTER ET AL. (EDS.),
JAPAN SCI. SOC. PRESS, TOKYO/TAYLOR & FRANCIS LTD., LONDON, pp. 263–275, 1991

# The Role of Xenobiotic Glucuronidating Enzymes in Drug Resistance of Tumour Tissues and Cells

Brian BURCHELL, Susan BAIRD, and Michael W. H. COUGHTRIE

*Department of Biochemical Medicine, Ninewells Hospital and Medical School, University of Dundee, Dundee, DD1 9SY, Scotland*

*Abstract:* Xenobiotic and endobiotic glucuronidation is regulated by many cellular features such as (a) access of substrates to a family of microsomal enzymes, the UDP-glucuronosyltransferases (UDPGTs) and (b) mechanisms of transport and excretion of glucuronides from the cell. We have isolated molecular biological probes identifying human UDPGTs to facilitate the examination of mechanisms regulating the functional expression of UDPGTs during natural development, in genetic diseases and in cancer cells. UDPGTs are encoded by a multigene family. Seven rat and four human UDPGT cDNAs have been cloned and expressed in cell culture to determine their substrate specificity and ability to glucuronidate xenobiotics. Analysis of the amino acid sequences of cloned UDPGTs has provided information about their method of synthesis and topological orientation with the lumen of the endoplasmic reticulum (ER). The location of hepatic UDPGT raises interesting questions about the role of possible transporters essential for functional glucuronidation. Measurement of the UDPGT activities and UDPGT mRNA in carcinoma tissue and in hepatic nodules from rats suggest that increases in the level of a phenol-UDPGT may contribute to drug resistance in cancer. Human UDPGTs stably expressed in cell lines have been used to study the glucuronidation of carcinogens and anticancer drugs. Human phenol UDPGT will catalyse the glucuronidation of carcinogens. The high levels of expression of human phenol UDPGT in tissue culture cells could also lead to an increased resistance to xenobiotic toxicity caused by mitoxantrone, mitomycin C, and adriamycin. This molecular cell biology approach is being used to further assess the glucuronidation and effective toxicity of anticancer drugs.

Conjugation with glucuronic acid and sulphate is central to the body's defence against toxicity from a variety of sources including drugs, environmental pollutants, carcinogens, and endogenous compounds such as bilirubin, steroids, and neurotransmitters (*1*, *2*). Glucuronides and sulphates exhibit increased polarity and water-solubility compared with the parent compound, thereby facilitating excretion in the urine or bile. The enzyme systems responsible for these reactions (the UDP-glucuronosyltransferases, UDPGTs, and sulphotransferases, STs) comprise a number of different isoenzymes, each with distinct but often overlapping substrate specificities.

The enzymes are expressed primarily in the liver, however isoenzyme-dependent extrahepatic expression is also observed, and may play a significant role in protection against cell toxicity, particularly in major ports of entry to the body such as the lungs and gastrointestinal tract (*1*).

*Hepatobiliary Transport and Metabolism of Xenobiotic Compounds*

An attempt to summarise the current state of our knowledge of this subject is illustrated by the hypothetical hepatocyte in Fig. 1. Drugs, xenobiotics, and endobiotics enter the cell by several different mechanisms after dissociation from blood carrier proteins occurs in the sinusoids. Mechanisms of uptake are: a) adsorptive endocytosis, b) passive diffusion, and c) carrier mediated uptake (*3*). A family of sinusoidal membrane proteins of 48–54 kDa has been recognised by photoaffinity labelling with

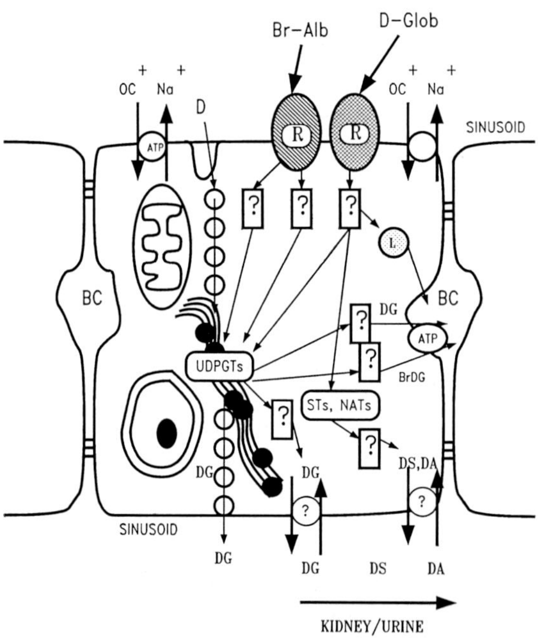


FIG. 1. Hepatocellular uptake, transport, biotransformation, and excretion of xenobiotics and drugs (D). In the model hepatocyte drugs (D), bilirubin (Br), or organic cation ($OC^+$) bound to blood globulins or albumin are dissociated in the sinusoidal space and taken into the cell *via* specific receptors (R), $Na^+$/ATP dependent transport systems or endocytosis. Following uptake, mechanisms of transcellular transport to and from most organelles remains unknown as indicated by the question marks [?]. Carrier proteins, vesicular movements, and simple diffusion have been proposed. Conjugation of drugs with sulphate, glucuronic acid, or acetate is catalysed by microsomal UDPGTs or STs and *N*-acetyltransferases (NATs). Excretion of acetylated, sulphated, or glucuronidated drugs (DA, DS, DG) is *via* the sinusoidal or bile canalicular membrane surfaces. Excretion from the cell may occur by simple diffusion, vesicular transport and microtubules or ATP dependent carriers. BrDG, bilirubin diglucuronide; BC, bile canaliculus; L, lysosome.

xenobiotics (*4*). Some of these xenobiotics were rapidly taken up into liver cells and were extensively biotransformed prior to excretion in bile. These saturable receptor mediated uptake processes were absent from hepatoma cells, where only a non-saturable undefined passive diffusion of certain xenobiotics occurred (*4*).

The transcellular transport of xenobiotic compounds to their target organelles such as endoplasmic reticulum (ER) is represented by a series of question marks on Fig. 1 indicating our lack of knowledge. Possible pathways include cytosolic diffusion, transport by soluble binding proteins and/or vectorial movement within vesicles (*5*). The current textbook view indicates binding of many xenobiotics and organic cations bind to hepatic glutathione-S-transferases (GSTs; ligandin), which apparently transport and present these molecules to microsomal enzymes. These binding proteins are believed to also decrease efflux back into plasma (see *6*).

After transport and/or biotransformation, xenobiotics and their metabolites need to be excreted from the cell. Extensive studies of canalicular excretion have been undertaken. A variety of canalicular transport systems for organic anions and cations have recently been characterised including electrogenic transporters for bile acids (*5*), anion transporters and ATP-dependent transport systems for organic anions and cytotoxic drugs (*i.e.*, MDR product, P-170, see Arias this volume) (*7*) and glutathione conjugates (*8*). Indeed, a 100 kDa protein involved in bile salt transport has been isolated, cloned, and functionally reconstituted (*9, 10*).

A more detailed characterisation of the cell specific transport systems should considerably enhance the understanding of the molecular disruption which occurs in cancer cells leading to changes in biotransformation and excretion of xenobiotics, and to drug resistance.

### *Xenobiotic UDP-glucuronosyltransferases in the Hepatic Endoplasmic Reticulum*

Xenobiotic glucuronidation in liver is catalysed by a family of enzymes, the UDPGTs. Several of the rat and human enzymes have been highly purified and partially characterised in considerable efforts to determine their substrate specificity, although problems of reconstitution of these lipid-dependent UDPGTs still causes uncertainties in interpretation of the results (*11*). Further characterisation of the UDPGTs has been achieved by cloning of cDNAs encoding these enzymes. The molecular genetic studies in combination with the protein purification work has considerably improved our understanding of these microsomal membrane bound enzymes.

Cloned rat UDPGT cDNAs have been expressed in COS cell cultures to assess substrate specificities. The newly expressed enzymes can be assayed using antibodies or by assay of UDPGT activities. To date, seven rat UDPGT cDNA clones encoding different transferases have been obtained (*11, 12*).

The cloned molecular probes for unique UDPGTs have elucidated the molecular basis of genetic defects of androsterone glucuronidation (*13*) and phenol glucuronidation in Gunn rats (14–16). Computer-based analysis and comparison of UDPGT sequences (after translation of cDNA sequence to amino acid sequence) has allowed a number of predictions concerning mechanism of synthesis, general structure and membrane topology of UDPGTs which have been verified by biochemical experimentation (*11, 17*). The majority of the transferase proteins and the catalytic function are located within the lumen of the ER. Substrate binding apparently occurs within a variable region between N-terminal amino acids 60–120 and UDPGA binding between amino acids 350–410 (*17*).

*UDP-glucuronosyltransferases and Other Conjugases in Hepatocyte Nodules and Hepatoma Cells*

Much of the work on the processes involved in neoplasia has concerned chemical carcinogenesis (*e.g.*, *18*, *19*). The multistep hypothesis which has emerged from these studies requires that the carcinogen (or its bioactivated metabolite) initiate primary lesions (*e.g.*, *via* macromolecular binding, strand breaks, *etc.*). These initiated cells proliferate and expand into focal lesions and, in the case of the liver (the most widely studied model system), into hepatocellular nodules. A crucial step in the proliferation of the primary lesions appears to involve the initiated cells acquiring resistance to the cytotoxic actions of carcinogens and hepatotoxins (*19*, *20*). This resistance is essential for the development of nodules, since it overrides the mitoinhibitory effects of the carcinogen, and allows the initiated cells to respond to mitogenic stimuli (*19*).

Measurements of drug-metabolising enzyme activities in experimentally-induced rat hepatocyte nodules suggest that a contribution towards this resistance to carcinogens results from alterations in the levels of expression of these enzymes. The activities of the cytochrome P-450-dependent monooxygenase system are severely reduced in hepatocyte nodules, down to $<10\%$ for certain activities (*21*, *22*), whereas many of the Phase 2 enzyme activities are significantly increased. For example, UDPGT activity towards 1-naphthol was increased 5-fold over control tissue (*23*, see Fig. 2). In contrast, however, other isoenzyme-specific UDPGT activities remained unchanged or only slightly elevated, such as those towards bilirubin and 4-hydroxybiphenyl (Fig. 2).

Recently, work using cDNA and oligonucleotide probes for a rat phenol UDPGT cDNA has shown that mRNA coding for this enzyme is induced by 3-methylcholanthrene and that elevated levels are permanently expressed in rat hepatocyte nodules and hepatoma cells (Table 1).

Similarly, GST, epoxide hydrolase and DT-diaphorase have all been observed to

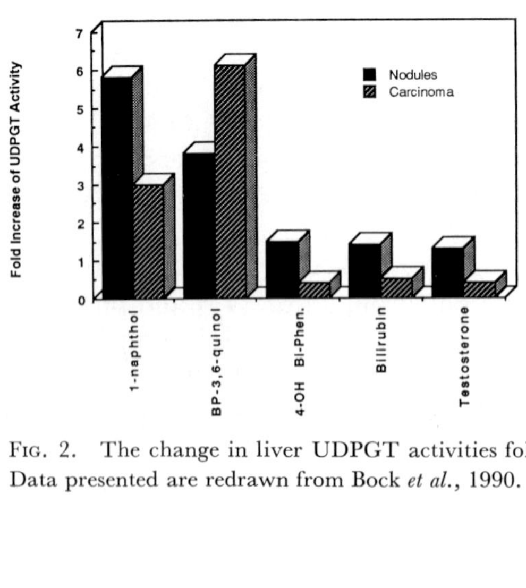


FIG. 2. The change in liver UDPGT activities following nodular and carcinoma development. Data presented are redrawn from Bock *et al.*, 1990.

TABLE 1. Elevated Phenol UDPGT mRNA in Hepatocyte Nodules and H4IIE cells

| Sample | UDPGT mRNA levels (Arb. units) |
|---|---|
| Liver | 1 |
| 3MC-liver | 10 |
| Hepatocyte nodules | 4 |
| H4IIE cells | 7 |

Data were obtained from Harding *et al.* (*14*) and Bock *et al.* (*63*).

exhibit increased activity in preneoplastic hepatocyte nodules (*24–28*). Little is known about the expression of STs in tumour tissue, although they are known to be involved in the metabolic activation of compounds such as N-hydroxy-2-acetylaminoflourene (*29*). Recently, a cDNA clone corresponding to a rat liver hydroxysteroid ST which activates carcinogenic polycyclic hydroxymethyl-arenes has been isolated and sequenced (*30*).

The mechanism (or stimuli) for these changes in enzyme activity is not well understood; however, for the GST specific increases in mRNA levels for certain of the subunits have been observed (*28*), and these authors speculated that gene amplification might be responsible, similar to the amplification of the dihydrofolate reductase gene in the acquired resistance to methotrexate (*30*).

All of these enzyme systems (with the exception of the STs) are inducible, in an isoenzyme-dependent manner, in normal hepatic (and often extrahepatic) tissue by a variety of xenobiotics including mutagens and carcinogens such as 2-acetylaminofluorene, 3-methylcholanthrene and 2,3,7,8-tetrachlorodibenzo-*p*-dioxin (TCDD), and a host of drugs, for example, phenobarbitone and the hypolipideamic agent clofibrate. This induction is usually the result of an increased rate of transcription of the particular gene or genes. Therefore the "machinery" exists for the regulation of these enzymes, but how (or if) it is involved in their regulation during carcinogenesis is not known. For induction by some of these xenobiotics, the mechanism is quite well understood—*e.g.*, TCDD exerts its effects *via* interaction with a cytosolic receptor, followed by association of the TCDD/receptor complex with the cell nucleus (*e.g.*, *32*), presumably stimulating gene expression by interaction with regulatory area(s) of responsive genes. Investigation of the expression, structure, and organisation of these genes in human tumours will yield insight into the processes involved in their regulation and functions during carcinogenesis.

### *Drug Metabolizing Enzymes and Drug Resistance*

The use of chemotherapeutic agents has been a great success in the treatment of cancer. Unfortunately, however, many tumours do not respond to chemotherapy, and others acquire resistance following an initial period of susceptibility. Consequently, the area of cytotoxic drug resistance has received considerable attention in recent years in an attempt to understand the molecular events which give rise to this phenomenon, in the hope that more effective chemotherapeutic treatments can be devised.

Tumour cells grown in culture can acquire resistance to either single drugs, or to a series of related or unrelated agents (termed multi-drug resistance). It is not surprising, therefore, that more than one factor appears to be involved in the development of drug resistance. Early work with methotrexate (MTX) resistance in cultured cells showed that the development of resistance correlated with an increase in the expression of the target enzyme, dihydrofolate reductase (DHFR), which was in turn the result of amplification of the DHRF gene (*31*). Cells which are made MTX resistant are not resistant to structurally different anti-cancer drugs. However, if mutant cells are selected which are resistant to agents such as doxorubicin, colchicine, or actinomycin D, these cell lines become resistant not only to the selecting drug but to other drugs and hydrophobic compounds (*e.g.*, *33* for reviews). It has been shown that the high level of resistance in these cell lines is usually associated with the amplification and overexpression of a small group of genes termed *mdr* (*34*, *35*). It has been suggested that at least one member of this family is a drug transport protein, responsible for increased efflux of drugs from resistant cells (see *33* for overview). However, UDPGT activity towards 1-naphthol was also increased 4-fold in daunorubicin-resistant P388 murine lymphocytic leukaemia cells (*36*).

Changes in gene expression, gene rearrangements (*37*) and gene losses (*38*, *39*) have all been shown to have important functions in tumourigenesis and susceptibility to cancer. An understanding of the molecular origins of alterations in drug metabolizing enzyme levels in cancer will allow prediction of how tumour cells are likely to respond to chemotherapy, as well as allowing assessment of the role of these enzyme systems in tumour development.

### *Conjugation of Anti-cancer Drugs*

The metabolism of chemotherapeutic agents is often complex, and in many cases poorly understood. The cytochromes P-450 and the GSTs are often the principal enzyme systems involved in the metabolism of anti-cancer drugs (see *40* for reviews). However, many compounds are subject to conjugation with glucuronic acid and/or sulphate (catalysed by UDPGTs and STs), either as the parent compound or as hydroxylated metabolites formed by the action of the cytochrome P-450-dependent monooxygenase system. Examples include the anthracyclines and their metabolites, the metabolites and derivatives of ellipticine, metabolites of anti-steroidals such as cyproterone (*40*), and the anthroquinone mitoxantrone (*41*). To the best of our knowledge, the metabolism of anti-cancer drugs by UDPGTs or STs in tumour tissue has never been investigated, and indeed *in vitro* studies on the conjugation of these compounds in any tissue are scarce. Mitoxantrone has been demonstrated to be a substrate for a 3-methylcholanthrene-inducible UDPGT in rat liver, and is likely to be a good model substrate for studying glucuronidation of anti-cancer drugs by tumour tissue. No information exists concerning its conjugation in human tissue.

### *Cloning, Expression, and Substrate Specificity of Human Liver UDPGT cDNAs*

Screening of human liver cDNA expression libraries with rat antibodies (*42*) or cDNAs (*43*) has enabled the isolation of several human liver UDPGT cDNAs. A human phenol UDPGT gene has been localised to chromosome 2 (*44*). Full length cDNAs have been transiently expressed in COS cells and their substrate specificity examined (Table 2). The four human liver UDPGT cDNAs expressed show primary

TABLE 2. Substrate Specificity of Cloned Expressed Human UDPGTs

| cDNA clone | Substrate | Reference |
|---|---|---|
| HLUG4 | 4 Nitrophenol<br>4-Methylumbelliferone<br>1-Naphthylamine<br>Estriol | *61* |
| HLUGP1 | 1-Naphthol<br>4-Methylumbelliferone<br>4-Nitrophenol<br>2-Naphthol<br>4-Ethylphenol<br>4-Methylphenol | *43* |
| ULUG25 | Hyodeoxycholic acid | *4* |
| $UDPGT_h$-2 | 4-Hydroxyestrone<br>Estriol<br>2-Hydroxyestriol<br>4-Hydroxyestradiol<br>6α-Hydroxyestriol | *62* |

specificity for xenobiotic phenols, estriol, hyodeoxycholic acid, and catechol estrogens. The expression of human phenol UDPGT (HLUGP1) allowed a crude analysis of the dimensions and electronic configurations of a series of naphthols or phenols accepted by a human phenol UDPGT. (*43*)

Similarly, the substrate specificity of a human UDPGT apparently encoding a transferase catalysing the glucuronidation of hyodeoxycholic acid was examined. Transient expression of the enzyme in COS-7 cells was poor and therefore we have obtained a transfected and cloned V-79 cell line in which the H25 UDPGT cDNA encoding hyodeoxycholate UDPGT is stably expressed. This procedure leads to more than 10-fold higher expression of the transferase protein and activity in these cell lines (*45*).

We have recently constructed a cell line which is stably transfected with cloned HLUGP1. Homogenates of modified NIH3T3 cell line show activity towards the substrate 1-naphthol which is 10 times greater than values obtained with transiently expressing cell and comparable to values observed in human liver homogenates. Such cell lines, constructed with each individual isoform, will provide a very useful tool which will allow extensive investigation of substrate specificities.

Further, stably expressed human UDPGTs can be assayed for their ability to catalyse glucuronidation of carcinogens and anti-cancer drugs. In collaboration with Bock's laboratory we have demonstrated that human phenol UDPGT will catalyse the glucuronidation of benzo(a)pyrene 3,6 quinone, paracetamol, naproxen (*46*).

### *Increased Resistance to Xenobiotic and Anti-cancer Drug-induced Toxicity in Recombinant 3T3 Cells Stably-expressing Human Phenol UDPGT*

The resistance of recombinant 3T3 cells expressing human phenol UDPGT to toxic xenobiotics was assessed using the MTT assay (*47*). In a preliminary experiment, 3T3 cells containing higher levels of human phenol UDPGT showed a 10-fold increase

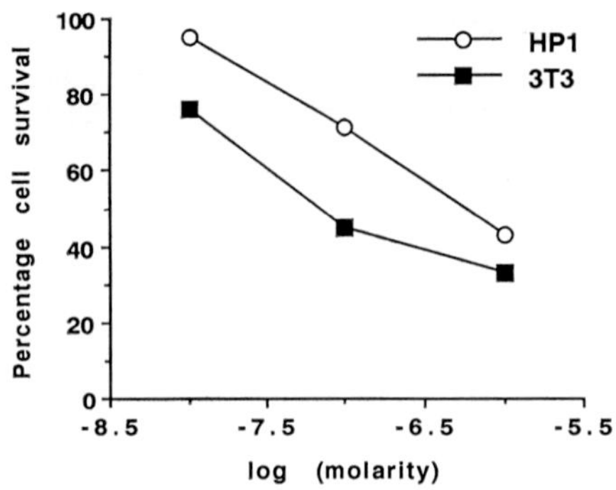


FIG. 3. Increased survival of 3T3 cells stably transfected with human phenol UDPGT after exposure to mitoxantrone. The drugs were dissolved in water and diluted in serum free Dulbecco's modified Eagles' medium. Formazan crystals were dissolved in 50 $\mu$l dimethyl sulfoxide (DMSO). The optical density (O. D.) of the wells was measured with an Eliza plate reader at 570 nm. The mean absorbance for each drug concentration was calculated from five wells. Cell survival for each drug concentration was calculated and expressed as a percentage of control wells (*i.e.*, no mitozantrone added).

in survival against 1.0 $\mu$M mitoxantrone (see Fig. 3) when compared to non-transfected 3T3 cells. Similarly, increased survival rates (5–10 fold) were observed against up to 1.5 $\mu$M mitomycin C and up to 5 fold against adriamycin (data not shown). These results indicate that increased expression of human phenol UDPGT in 3T3 cells has provided additional protection against these cytotoxic anticancer drugs, presumably by enhancing their rate of glucuronidation and excretion from the cells. Further work is underway to measure glucuronidation and further assess the protection against cytotoxic xenobiotics acquired from overexpression of human UDPGTs in tissue culture cells.

### *Transport of Xenobiotic Glucuronides from Endoplasmic Reticulum to Cell Membrane for Excretion*

Many drugs and endogenous compounds reaching the ER undergo phase I metabolism catalysed by the mono-oxygenase system prior to conjugation with glucuronic acid to form water soluble metabolites. Other compounds such as paracetamol and bilirubin are immediately glucuronidated. The transverse topologies of mono-oxygenases (*48*) and bilirubin UDPGT (*49*) in the ER have recently been investigated and the proposed orientation of the proteins is illustrated in Fig. 4. Mono-oxygenases catalyse oxidation/hydroxylation reactions on the cytoplasmic surface of the ER, whereas the products of these systems would apparently require transport into the ER for subsequent glucuronidation catalysed by the luminally located UDPGT.

How do hydroxylated metabolites or amphipathic carboxylic acids such as bilirubin reach the UDPGT? A transporter for the co-substrate UDP-glucuronic acid (UDPGA; formed in the cytoplasmic compartment) has been implicated for many years (*50*), although compelling proof of its existence is still not available.

Do additional transporters of aglycones exist in the ER? UDPGA is broken down in the ER to UMP and phosphate. The existence of an ER phosphate pyrophosphate/exporter has been demonstrated from molecular analysis of glycogen storage disease

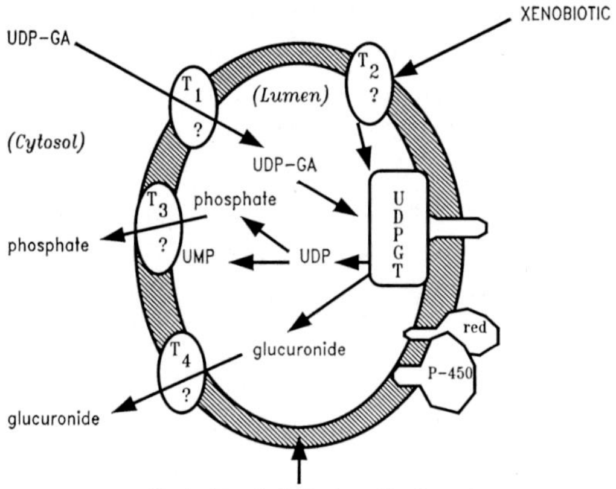


FIG. 4. Possible transporters involved in function regulation of UDPGT activitives in ER. $T_1$—UDP-glucuronic acid transporter? $T_2$—Xenobiotic transporter? $T_3$—Phosphate transporter. $T_4$—Xenobiotic glucuronide transporters?

type 1c (*51*) and is likely to be implicated in the transport of phosphate from the ER. Therefore, it is likely that various ER transporters have yet to be identified. Once formed inside the ER, how are the water soluble glucuronides released from the ER and excreted from the cell? Recent work has suggested that bilirubin glucuronide and bile salts are secreted in vesicles that are selectively transported to the bile canaliculus by microtubular transport (*52*, *53* and Fig. 4), although more extensive studies concerning the direct role of vesicles are necessary. The dynamic microtubular vesicular membrane network recently recognised in CEF cells could be involved in this function (*54*, *55*). Unfortunately, not all drugs are excreted *via* the bile; many are excreted *via* the kidneys and urine. Thus two different paths of cellular excretion of small molecules must exist, one for transport to the circulation and one *via* the bile canaliculus. How are small molecules sorted and do both pathways involve vesicular transport? Recent evidence from our laboratories studying hepatic microsomes from a hyperbilirubinaemic infant indicated that bilirubin glucuronide export from the ER was blocked, whilst export of 1-naphthol glucuronide continued, suggesting that small molecule sorting can take place in the ER by selective transport systems (unpublished work). It is possible that small molecules are excreted from the liver cell by the same exocytotic mechanisms used in excretion of newly synthesised proteins such as albumin (*56*) and IgA to the bile by transcytosis (*57*).

## *Conclusion*

It has been reported that for primary human hepatomas, *all* the drug metabolizing enzyme activities measured (cytochrome P-450, UDPGT, GST, epoxide hydrolase, ST) were decreased (*58*). Alterations in gene expression in human lung carcinoma have also been observed (*59*, *60*), where the conjugation of 1-naphthol in normal lung tissue was primarily *via* sulphation, whereas in the cancerous tissue glucuronidation was the principal pathway. Such alterations in gene expression in tumour tissue may have important consequences for the local effectiveness of chemotherapeutic agents.

The work reported here demonstrates how a molecular biological approach using cloned and expressed human conjugating enzymes will facilitate the measurement of carcinogen or anticancer drug conjugation and allow assessment of the cellular protection against toxic xenobiotics afforded by elevated levels of these enzymes.

*Acknowledgment*

We thank the Cancer Research Campaign for grants supporting this work. M.W.H.C. is a Caledonian Research Foundation Research Fellow.

REFERENCES

1. Dutton, G. J., Glucuronidation of Drugs and Other Compounds. C. R. C. Press, Boca Raton, Florida, U.S.A., 1980.
2. Mulder, G. J. and Jakoby, W. B. Sulphation. *In;* G. J. Mulder (ed.), Conjugations in Drug Metabolism, pp. 107–161, Taylor & Francis, Ltd., London, 1990.
3. Mol, W. E. M. and Meijer, D. K. F. Hepatic transport mechanisms for bivalent organic cations. Biochem. Pharmacol., *39*: 383–390, 1990.
4. Falk, E., Gerok, W., Kurg, G., Meijer, D. F. K., Muller, M., Neumann, J., and Zimmerman, H. Hepatobiliary transport of amphipathic and hydrophobic compounds. *In;* K. W. Bock, W. Gerok, and S. Matern (eds.), Hepatic Metabolism and Disposition of Endo- and Xenobiotics, Kluwer Academic Publishers, Lancaster, U. K., 1991, in press.
5. Meier, P. J. Biliary excretion of drugs. *In*; K. W. Bock, W. Gerok, and S. Matern (eds.), Hepatic Metabolism and Disposition of Endo- and Xenobiotics, Kluwer Academic Publishers, Lancaster, U. K., 1991, in press.
6. Burchell, B. and Burchell, A. Molecular pathologies of the hepatic endoplasmic reticulum. Curr. Opin. Cell Biol., *1*: 712–717, 1989.
7. Kitamura, T., Jansen, P. L. M., Hardenbrook, C., Kamimoto, Y., Gatmaitan, Z., and Arias, I. M. Defective ATP-dependent bile canalicular transport of organic anions in mutant (TR-) rats with conjugated hyperbilirubinaemia. Proc. Natl. Acad. Sci. U.S.A., *87*: 3557–3561, 1990.
8. Kobayashi, K., Sogame, Y., Hara, H., and Hayashi, K. Mechanism of glutathione-S-conjugate transport in canalicular and basolateral rat liver plasma membranes. J. Biol. Chem., *265*: 7737–7741, 1990.
9. Hong, W. and Doyle, D. cDNA cloning for a bile canaliculus domain specific membrane glycoprotein of rat hepatocytes. Proc. Natl. Acad. Sci. U.S.A., *84*: 7962–7966, 1987.
10. Ruetz, S., Hugentobler, G., and Meier, P. J. Functional reconstitution of the canalicular bile salt transport system of rat liver. Proc. Natl. Acad. Sci. U.S.A., *85*: 6147–6151, 1988.
11. Burchell, B. and Coughtrie, M. W. H. UDP-glucuronosyltransferases. Pharmacol. Ther., *43*: 261–289, 1989.
12. Sutherland, L., Wooster, R., Jackson, M. R., Harding, D., Fournel-Gigleux, S., and Burchell, B. Cloning and expression of UDP-glucuronosyltransferase cDNAs. *In;* K. W. Bock, W. Gerok, and S. Matern (eds.), Hepatic Metabolism and Disposition of Endo- and Xenobiotics. Kluwer Academic Publishers, Lancaster, U.K., 1991, in press.
13. Corser, R. B., Coughtrie, M. W. H., Jackson, M. R., and Burchell, B. The molecular basis of the inherited deficiency of androsterone UDP-glucuronosyltransferase in Wistar rats. FEBS Lett., *213*: 448–452, 1987.
14. Harding, D., Jackson, M., Corser, R., and Burchell, B. Phenol UDP-glucuronosyltransferase deficiency in Gunn rats: mRNA levels are considerably reduced. Biochem.

Pharmacol., *38*: 1013–1017, 1989.

15. Iyanagi, T., Watanabe, T., and Uchiyama, Y. The 3-methylcholanthrene-inducible UDP-glucuronosyltransferase deficiency in the hyperbilirubinaemic (Gunn) rat is caused by a -1 frameshift mutation. J. Biol. Chem., *264*: 21302–21307, 1989.
16. El Awady, M., Roy Chowdhury, J., Kesari, K., van Es, H., Jansen, P. L. M., Lederstein, M., Arias, I. M., and Roy Chowdhury, N. Mechanism of the lack of induction of UDP-glucuronosyltransferase activity in Gunn rats by 3-methylcholanthrene. Identification of a truncated protein. J. Biol. Chem., *265*: 10752–10758, 1990.
17. Tephly, T. R. and Burchell, B. UDP-glucuronosyltransferases: a family of detoxifying enzymes. Trends Pharmacol. Sci., *11*: 276–279, 1990.
18. Farber, E. and Cameron, R. The sequential analysis of cancer development. Adv. Cancer Res., *31*: 125–226, 1980.
19. Solt, D. and Farber, E. New principle for the analysis of chemical carcinogenesis. Nature, *263*: 701–703, 1986.
20. Tsuda, H., Lee, G., and Farber, E. Induction of resistant hepatocytes as a new principle for a possible short-term *in vivo* test for carcinogens. Cancer Res., *40*: 1157–1164, 1980.
21. Cameron, R., Sweeney, G. D., Jones, K., Lee, G., and Farber, E. A relative deficiency of cytochrome P-450 and aryl hydrocarbon [Benzo(a)pyrene] hydroxylase in hyperplastic nodules induced by 2-acetylaminofluorene in rat liver. Cancer Res., *36*: 3888–3893, 1976.
22. Bock, K. W., Lilienblum, W., Pfeil, H., and Eriksson, L. C. Increased uridine diphosphate-glucuronyltransferase activity in preneoplastic liver nodules and Morris hepatomas. Cancer Res., *42*: 3747–3752, 1982.
23. Eriksson, L. C., Torndal, U-B., and Andersson, G. N. Isolation and characterization of endoplasmic reticulum and Golgi apparatus from hepatocyte nodules in male Wistar rats. Cancer Res., *43*: 3335–3347, 1983.
24. Levin, W., Lu, A. Y., Thomas, P. E., Ryan, D., Kizer, D. E., and Griffin, M. J. Identification of epoxide hydrase as the preneoplastic antigen in rat liver. Proc. Natl. Acad. Sci. U.S.A., *75*: 3240–3243, 1978.
25. Astrom, A., DePierre, J. W., and Eriksson, L. Characterization of drug-metabolizing systems in hyperplastic nodules from the livers of rats receiving 2-acetylaminofluorene in their diet. Carcinogenesis, *4*: 577–581, 1983.
26. Oesch, F., Vogel-Bindel, U. V., Guenthner, T. M., Cameron, P., and Farber, E. Characterization of microsomal epoxide hydrolase in hyperplastic liver nodules of rats. Cancer Res., *43*: 313–319, 1983.
27. Pickett, C. B., Williams, J. B., Lu, A. Y., and Cameron, R. G. Regulation of glutathione transferase and DT-diaphorase mRNAs in persistent hepatocyte nodules during chemical hepatocarcinogenesis. Proc. Natl. Acad. Sci. U.S.A., *81*: 5091–5095, 1984.
28. Gutmann, H. R., Malejka-Giganti, D., Barry, E. J., and Rydell, R. E. On the correlation between the hepatocarcinogenicity of the carcinogen N-2-fluorenylacetamide, and its metabolic activation by the rat. Cancer Res., *32*: 1554–1561, 1972.
29. Ogura, K., Kajita, J., Narihata, H., Watabe, T., Ozawa, S., Nagata, K., Yamazoe, Y., and Kato, R. cDNA cloning of the hydroxysteroid sulfotransferase STa sharing a strong homology in amino acid sequence with the senescence marker protein SMP-2 in rat livers. Biochem. Biophys. Res. Commun., *166*: 1494–1500, 1990.
30. Schimke, R. T., Kaufman, R. J., Alt, F. W., and Kellems, R. T. Gene amplication and drug resistance in cultured murine cells. Science, *202*: 1051–1055, 1978.
31. Poland, A. and Knutson, J. C. 2,3,7,8-Tetrachlorodibenzo-*p*-dioxin and related halogenated aromatic hydrocarbons: examination of the mechanism of toxicity. Annu. Rev. Pharmacol. Toxicol., *22*: 517–554, 1982.

32. Pastan, I. and Gottesman, M. Multiple-drug resistance in human cancer. N. Engl. J. Med., *316*: 1388–1393, 1987.

33. Roninson, I. B., Chin, J. E., Choi, K. G., Gros, P., Housman, D. E., Fojo, A., Shen, D. W., Gottesman, M. M., and Pastan, I. Isolation of human mdr DNA sequences amplified in multidrug-resistant KB carcinoma cells. Proc. Natl. Acad. Sci. U.S.A., *83*: 4538–4542, 1986.

34. Thorgeirsson, S. S., Huber, B. E., Sorrell, S., Fojo, A., Pastan, I., and Gottesman, M. M. Expression of the multidrug-resistant gene in hepatocarcinogenesis and regenerating rat liver. Science, *236*: 1120–1122, 1987.

35. Gessner, T., Vaughan, L. A., Bechler, B. C., Bartels, C. J., and Baker, R. M. Elevated pentose cycle and glucuronosyltransferase in daunorubicin-resistant P-388 cells. Cancer Res., *50*: 3921–3927, 1990.

36. T'Ang, A., Varley, J. M., Chakraborty, S., Murphree, A. L., and Fung, Y. K. Structural rearrangement of the retinoblastoma gene in human breast carcinoma. Science, *242*: 263–266, 1988.

37. Kok, K., Osinga, J., Carritt, B., Davis, M. B., van der Hout, A. H., van der Veen, A. Y., Landsvater, R. M., de Leij, L. F., Berendsen, H. H., Postmus, P. E., Poppema, S., and Buys, C.H.C.M. Deletion of a DNA sequence at the chromosomal region 3p21 in all major types of lung cancer. Nature, *330*: 578–581, 1987.

38. Vogelstein, B., Fearon, E. R., Hamilton, S. R., Kern, S. E., Preisinger, A. C., Leppert, M., Nakamura, Y., White, R., Smits, A. M., and Bos, J. L. Genetic alterations during colorectal-tumor development. N. Engl. J. Med., *319*: 525–532, 1988.

39. Powis, G. Anthracycline metabolism and free radical formation. *In;* G. Powis and R. A. Prough (eds.), Metabolism and Action of Anti-Cancer Drugs, pp. 211–260, Taylor and Francis, London, 1987.

40. Wolf, C. R., Macpherson, J. S., and Smyth, J. F. Evidence for the metabolism of mitozantrone by microsomal glutathione transferases and 3-methylcholanthrene-inducible glucuronosyl transferases. Biochem. Pharmacol., *35*: 1577–1581, 1986.

41. Jackson, M. R., McCarthy, L. R., Harding, D., Wilson, S., Coughtrie, M. W. H., and Burchell, B. Cloning of a human liver microsomal UDP-glucuronosyltransferase cDNA. Biochem. J., *242*: 581–588, 1987.

42. Harding, D., Fournel-Gigleux, S., Jackson, M. R., and Burchell, B. Cloning and substrate specificity of a human phenol UDP-glucuronosyltransferase expressed in COS-7 cells. Proc. Natl. Acad. Sci. U.S.A., *85*: 8381–8385, 1988.

43. Harding, D., Jerimiah, S. J., Povey, S., and Burchell, B. Chromosomal mapping of a human phenol UDP-glucuronosyltransferase, *GT1*. Ann. Hum. Genet., *54*: 17–21, 1990.

44. Fournel-Gigleux, S., Waddell, L., Sabolovic, N., Burchell, B., and Siest, G. Stable expression of two human liver glucuronosyltransferases in V79 cell cultures. Mol. Pharmac., *39*: 177–183, 1991.

45. Forster, A., El Mouelhi, M., Fournel-Gigleux, S., Siest, G., Burchell, B., and Bock, K. W. Paracetamol glucuronidation in man: *in vivo* and *in vitro* studies. *In;* K. W. Bock, W. Gerok, and S. Matern (eds.), Hepatic Metabolism and Disposition of Endo- and Xenobiotics, Kluwer Academic Publishers, 1991, in press.

46. Carmichael, J., De Graff, W. G., Gazdar, A. F., Minna, J. D., and Mitchell, J. B. Evaluation of a tetrazolium-based semiautomated colorimetric assay: assessment of chemosensitivity testing. Cancer Res., *47*: 936–942, 1987.

47. De Lemos-Chiarandini, C., Frey, A. B., Sabatini, D. D., and Kreibich, G. Determination of the membrane topology of the phenobarbital-inducible rat liver cytochrome P-450 isoenzyme PB-4 using site specific antibodies. J. Cell. Biol., *104*: 209–219, 1987.

48. Shepherd, S. R. P., Baird, S. J., Hallinan, T., and Burchell, B. An investigation of the transverse topology of bilirubin UDP-glucuronosyltransferase in rat hepatic endoplasmic reticulum. Biochem. J., *259*: 617–620, 1989.
49. Burchell, B., Weatherill, P. J., and Berry, C. Evidence indicating that UDP *N*-acetylglucosamine does not appear to stimulate hepatic microsomal UDP-glucuronosyltransferase by interaction with the catalytic unit of the enzyme. Biochim. Biophys. Acta, *735*: 309–313, 1983.
50. Burchell, A. Molecular pathology of glucose-6-phosphatase. FASEB J., *4*: 2978–2988, 1990.
51. Crawford, J. M. and Gollan, J. L. Hepatocyte cotransport of taurocholate and bilirubin glucuronides: role of microtubules. Am. J. Physiol., *18*: G121–G131, 1988.
52. Lamri, Y., Roda, A., Dumont, M., Feldman, G., and Erlinger, S. Immunoperoxidase localisation of bile salts in rat liver cells—evidence for a role of the Golgi apparatus in bile salt transport. J. Clin. Invest., *82*: 1173–1182, 1988.
53. Dabora, S. L. and Sheetz, M. P. The microtubule-dependent formation of a tubulovesicular network with characteristics of the ER from cultured cell extracts. Cell, *54*: 27–35, 1988.
54. Lee, C. and Chen, L. B. Dynamic behaviour of endoplasmic reticulum in living cells. Cell, *54*: 37–46, 1988.
55. Yokota, S. and Fahimi, D. H. Intracellular transport of albumin through the secretory apparatus of rat liver parenchymal cells. An immunocytochemical study. Cell Struct. Funct., *12*: 251–264, 1987.
56. Bartles, J. R. and Hubbard, A. L. Plasma membrane protein sorting in epithelial pathways. Do secretory pathways hold the key? Trends Biochem. Sci., *13*: 181–184, 1988.
57. El Mouelhi, M., Didolkar, M. S., Elias, E. G., Guengerich, F. P., and Kauffman, F. C. Hepatic drug-metabolizing enzymes in primary and secondary tumours of human liver. Cancer Res., *47*: 460–466, 1987.
58. Cohen, G. M., Gibby, E. M., and Mehta, R. Routes of conjugation in normal and cancerous tissues from human lung. Nature, *291*: 662–664, 1981.
59. Gibby, E. M. and Cohen, G. M. Conjugation of 1-naphthol by human bronchus and bronchoscopy samples. Biochem. Pharmacol., *33*: 739–743, 1984.
60. Coffmann, B. L., Tephly, T. R., Irshaid, Y. M., Green, M. D., Smith, C., Jackson, M. R., Wooster, R., and Burchell, B. Characterisation and primary sequence of a human hepatic microsomal estriol UDP-glucuronosyltransferase. Arch. Biochem. Biophys., *281*: 170–175, 1990.
61. Ritter, J. K., Sheen, Y. Y., and Owens, I. S. Cloning and expression of human liver UDP-glucuronosyltransferase in COS-1 cells. J. Biol. Chem., *266*: 7900–7906, 1990.
62. Bock, K. W., Munzel, P. A., Rohrdanz, E., Schrenck, D., and Eriksson, L. C. Persistently increased expression of a 3-methylcholanthrene-inducible phenol UDP-glucuronosyltransferase in rat hepatocyte nodules and hepatocellular carcinomas. Cancer Res., *50*: 3569–3573, 1990.

# XENOBIOTICS AS A CAUSE OF HUMAN CANCER

XENOBIOTICS AND CANCER, L. ERNSTER ET AL. (EDS.), JAPAN SCI. SOC. PRESS, TOKYO/TAYLOR & FRANCIS LTD., LONDON, pp. 279–288, 1991

# Heterocyclic Amines Produced in Cooked Food: Unavoidable Xenobiotics

Takashi SUGIMURA, Keiji WAKABAYASHI, Hiroko OHGAKI, Shozo TAKAYAMA, Minako NAGAO, and Hiroyasu ESUMI

*National Cancer Center Research Institute, Tokyo 104, Japan*

*Abstract:* Humans are continuously exposed to naturally occurring and industrial xenobiotics in their daily lives. Heterocyclic amines, which are formed during the cooking of proteinaceous foods, have been categorized as a new class of naturally occurring xenobiotics. They are divided into 2-amino-3-methylimidazo[4,5-*f*]quinoline (IQ)- and non-IQ-types. The amounts and proportion of total mutagenicity contributed by the IQ-type heterocyclic amines in cooked food are greater than those of the non-IQ-types. Precursors of the IQ-type heterocyclic amines including IQ, 2-amino-3,8-dimethylimidazo[4,5-*f*]quinoxaline (MeIQx) and 2-amino-1-methyl-6-phenylimidazo[4,5-*b*]pyridine (PhIP) are creatinine, amino acids and sugars in meat and fish. Both types of heterocyclic amines are carcinogenic in mice and rats. All heterocyclic amines except PhIP frequently induce cancers in the liver, while PhIP induces lymphomas in mice and carcinomas of the colon and mammary gland in rats. Based on quantitative analysis of heterocyclic amines in cooked food and levels of excretion of unchanged heterocyclic amines in human urine, total heterocyclic amine intake was calculated to be around 0.4–16 $\mu$g/person per day. As in the case of other naturally occurring xenobiotics, the degree of exposure is small and is presumably insufficient alone to account for the development of human cancer. Nevertheless, a linear relationship has been demonstrated between DNA adduct levels and a wide range of doses of MeIQx in animals. In addition, combined treatment with five heterocyclic amines yielded additive or synergistic effects in the development of glutathione S-transferase placental form (GST-P) positive foci. Taking these results and current observations of multiple genetic alterations in human cancers into consideration together, heterocyclic amines are probably involved in the development of human cancer in the presence of other carcinogens, tumor promoters and factors stimulating cancer progression.

## *Historical Aspects*

There are many xenobiotics reaching the human body from the environment. Humans have been continuously exposed to naturally occurring xenobiotics contained in food, tobacco smoke, alcoholic beverages, coffee, tea, and smoke from burning wood, while modern industry has introduced many new types of industrial xenobiotics into our environment. These include food additives, pesticides, pharmaceutical preparations, and air pollutants originating in combustion engines. A great deal of attention has been devoted to xenobiotics produced by modern industry. We, however, have been emphasizing that naturally occurring mutagens/carcinogens, including mycotoxins, substances of plant origin and food-derived substances should not be overlooked and that they must also play an important role in the development of human cancer, as reported in a previous symposium in this series (*1*).

In the early 1970s, we postulated that smoke produced in the kitchen by broiling fish and meat contained mutagens, and possibly carcinogens, the same as cigarette smoke. We collected smoke particles produced by broiling fish over a gas burner on a glass-fiber filter by suction using a motor pump. The material collected was dissolved with dimethyl sulfoxide and subjected to the Salmonella mutation test after appropriate dilution (*2, 3*). Mutagenicity was demonstrated in *Salmonella typhimurium* TA98 with S9 mix but not without S9 mix. Mutagenic activity was also detected in cooked fish and meat especially in the charred part on the surface, and this mutagenic activity was recovered chiefly in the basic fraction. It was also found earlier that mutagens exhibiting activity in *S. typhimurium* TA98 with S9 mix were formed by pyrolysis of amino acids and proteins and not by pyrolysis of starch, vegetable oil or nucleic acids (*2, 4, 5*).

### *Isolation and Identification of Mutagenic Heterocyclic Amines*

By monitoring mutagenic activity in *S. typhimurium* TA98 with S9 mix during purification, a series of mutagenic heterocyclic amines were isolated from pyrolysates of amino acids and proteins and from cooked fish and meat. Two imidazopyridine compounds have been isolated from a pyrolysate of tryptophan, *i.e.*, 3-amino-1, 4-dimethyl-5*H*-pyrido[4,3-*b*]indole (Trp-P-1) and 3-amino-1-methyl-5*H*-pyrido[4,3-*b*]indole (Trp-P-2) (*6*), and two dipyridoimidazole compounds have been isolated from a pyrolysate of glutamic acid, *i.e.*, 2-amino-6-methyldipyrido[1,2-*a*: 3′,2′-*d*]imidazole (Glu-P-1) and 2-aminodipyrido[1,2-*a*: 3′,2′-*d*]imidazole (Glu-P-2) (*7*). The presence of two amino-α-carboline derivatives, 2-amino-9*H*-pyrido[2,3-*b*]indole (AαC) and 2-amino-3-methyl-9*H*-pyrido[2,3-*b*]indole (MeAαC) in soybean globulin pyrolysate has also been reported (*8*). On the other hand, mutagens have been purified directly from broiled sun-dried sardines and identified as two imidazoquinoline compounds, 2-amino-3-methylimidazo[4,5-*f*]quinoline (IQ) and 2-amino-3,4-dimethylimidazo-[4,5-*f*]quinoline (MeIQ) (*9, 10*). 2-Amino-3,8-dimethylimidazo[4,5-*f*]quinoxaline (MeIQx) was isolated as one of the major mutagens in fried beef (*11*), and much later, another major mutagen, 2-amino-1-methyl-6-phenylimidazo[4,5-*b*]pyridine (PhIP) was also isolated from fried beef by Felton's group at Lawrence Livermore National Laboratory (*12*).

These mutagens were all heterocyclic amines and have been classified into non-IQ- and IQ-types. Their structures are given in Figs. 1 and 2, and their chemical names and abbreviations are listed in Table 1. All of these are newly registered compounds, except AαC. Non-IQ-type heterocyclic amines lost their mutagenicity after treatment with 2 mM nitrite under acidic conditions, while IQ-type heterocyclic amines were not inactivated under the same conditions (*13*). The inactivation of non-IQ-type

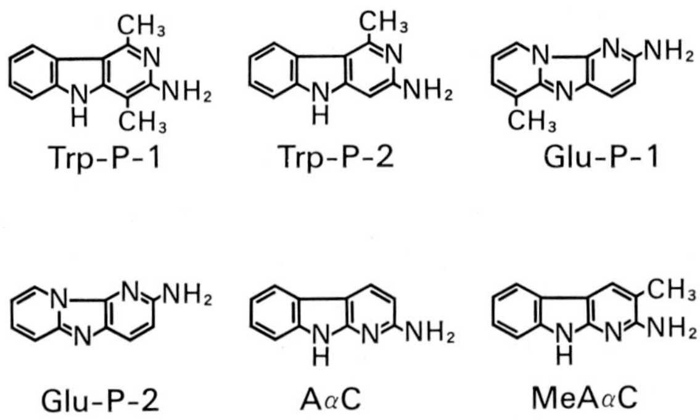


FIG. 1. Structures of non-IQ-type heterocyclic amines.

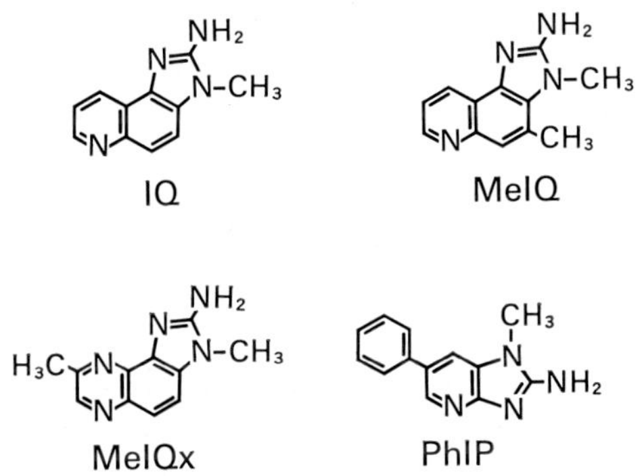


FIG. 2. Structures of IQ-type heterocyclic amines.

TABLE 1. Chemical Names and Abbreviations for Heterocyclic Amines

| Chemical name | Abbreviation |
|---|---|
| 3-Amino-1,4-dimethyl-5*H*-pyrido[4,3-*b*]indole | Trp-P-1 |
| 3-Amino-1-methyl-5*H*-pyrido[4,3-*b*]indole | Trp-P-2 |
| 2-Amino-6-methyldipyrido[1,2-*a*: 3′,2′-*d*]imidazole | Glu-P-1 |
| 2-Aminodipyrido[1,2-*a*: 3′,2′-*d*]imidazole | Glu-P-2 |
| 2-Amino-9*H*-pyrido[2,3-*b*]indole | AαC |
| 2-Amino-3-methyl-9*H*-pyrido[2,3-*b*]indole | MeAαC |
| 2-Amino-3-methylimidazo[4,5-*f*]quinoline | IQ |
| 2-Amino-3,4-dimethylimidazo[4,5-*f*]quinoline | MeIQ |
| 2-Amino-3,8-dimethylimidazo[4,5-*f*]quinoxaline | MeIQx |
| 2-Amino-1-methyl-6-phenylimidazo[4,5-*b*]pyridine | PhIP |

compounds was due to conversion of the amino group to a hydroxy group. Both IQ- and non-IQ-type heterocyclic amines were degraded by treatment with hypochlorite. Based on the differential effects of nitrite and the effect of hypochlorite on IQ- and non-IQ-type heterocyclic amines, the percentage contribution of each type of heterocyclic amine to the total mutagenicity of the basic fractions of various heated materials can be analyzed (*13*). The precursors of IQ-type heterocyclic amines were found to be creatinine, amino acids, and sugars in meat and fish (*14–16*). Creatinine could supply the aminoimidazole moiety and the remaining parts are probably formed from reaction products of amino acids and sugars or from amino acids themselves.

*Carcinogenicity of Heterocyclic Amines*

Heterocyclic amines chemically synthesized on a large scale were subjected to long-term dietary carcinogenicity testing using $CDF_1$ mice and F344 rats of both sexes. In these experiments, one or two doses ranging from 0.01 to 0.08% of the pellet diet were used. The weight gain of animals fed heterocyclic amines in these doses was only slightly suppressed or unaffected throughout the experiments.

Tumors were induced in the liver, forestomach, lung, lymphoid tissue, hematopoietic system, and blood vessels in the brown adipose tissue of mice. In the case of rats, tumors were induced in the liver, small and large intestines, Zymbal gland, clitoral gland, skin, oral cavity, and mammary gland (*17–19*). It should be noted that liver cancers were commonly produced in mice and/or rats by all heterocyclic amines except PhIP. PhIP induced lymphomas in mice of both sexes (*20*) and colon and mammary carcinomas in rats (*21*). Colon adenocarcinomas induced by PhIP are shown in Fig. 3.

It is interesting that blood vessel tumors, hemagioendothelial sarcomas, arising mainly in interscapular brown adipose tissue were found only in mice fed Glu-P-1, Glu-P-2, AαC, and MeAαC, but not in rats fed any of the heterocyclic amines. No tumors of the small and large intestines were induced in mice, but they were frequently found in rats. Squamous cell carcinomas of the Zymbal gland, clitoral gland and skin were frequently observed in rats, but the carcinomas in these tissues were not found in mice. In the case of mice, squamous cell carcinomas developed in the forestomach. It is worth noting that the squamous cell carcinomas of the forestomach of mice fed MeIQ often metastasized to the liver (*22*). Hepatocellular carcinomas induced by all heterocyclic amines in mice occurred more often in females than males, and this may be related to the fact that dietary heterocyclic amines induce higher levels of liver microsomal cytochrome P-450 in females than males (*23*). However, the mechanism of the above species difference in the carcinogenicity of heterocyclic amines remains to be fully elucidated.

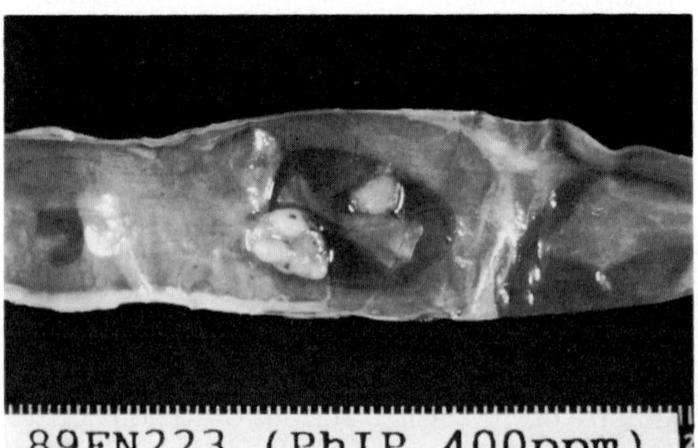


FIG. 3. Colon adenocarcinomas induced by PhIP in F344 rat.

*Level of Human Exposure to Heterocyclic Amines*

In order to estimate levels of human exposure to carcinogenic heterocyclic amines, heterocyclic amines were quantitatively analyzed in various kinds of cooked meat and fish using a method which combined blue cotton treatment and HPLC (*24–27*). Eight carcinogenic heterocyclic amines were detected by this method at levels of 0.03–69.2 ng/g cooked food. PhIP was the most abundant at 0.56–69.2 ng/g cooked food, and MeIQx was the second highest at 0.64–6.44 ng/g cooked food. Five heterocyclic amines, IQ, Trp-P-1, Trp-P-2, A$\alpha$C, and MeA$\alpha$C, were also detected in cigarette smoke condensate at levels of 0.23–10.50 ng/cigarette (*25, 28*). In addition to cooked food and cigarette smoke condensate, roasted coffee beans have been reported to contain MeIQ (*29*), and airborne particles have been found to contain Trp-P-1 and Trp-P-2 (*30*). Thus, carcinogenic heterocyclic amines are widely distributed in our environment suggesting that humans are continuously exposed to them.

To confirm the continuous exposure of humans to carcinogenic heterocyclic amines, we analyzed the levels of four heterocyclic amines, *i.e.*, MeIQx, PhIP, Trp-P-1, and Trp-P-2 in the urine of ten healthy volunteers using a method similar to the one used to quantitatively analyze heterocyclic amines in cooked food (*31*). The healthy volunteer subjects consisted of five males 33 to 80 years old and five females 13 to 67 years old who consumed ordinary diets with no dietary restrictions. All four heterocyclic amines were detected in the 24-hr urine samples of all these volunteers, and the levels were: MeIQx, 11–47 ng; PhIP, 0.12–1.97 ng; Trp-P-1, 0.04–1.43 ng; and Trp-P-2, 0.03–0.68 ng. In contrast, none of the four compounds was found in the urine samples of three inpatients receiving only parenteral alimentation. These findings indicate that humans are continuously exposed to low levels of carcinogenic heterocyclic amines derived from ordinary food (*31*).

Based on previously reported ratios (1.8–4.9%) of excretion of unchanged MeIQx in human urine to the oral dose (*32*), the daily intake of MeIQx by the above healthy volunteers was estimated to be 0.2–2.6 $\mu$g/person. The daily intake of MeIQx was also calculated to be 0.1–1.3 $\mu$g/person on the assumption that humans consume 200 g of cooked meat or fish per day. Thus, the two daily exposure levels, the one calculated from levels of excretion in the urine and the other based on amounts in cooked meat and fish, are comparable. The daily exposure to PhIP was calculated to be 0.1–13.8 $\mu$g/person, based on the same assumption about quantity of cooked food consumed as in the case of MeIQx. When we compared exposure levels to MeIQx and PhIP with their $TD_{50}$ values, the daily exposure levels were found to be far less than their $TD_{50}$ values. This suggests that the degree of human exposure to MeIQx and PhIP alone is insufficient to account for the development of human cancer.

*Possible Contribution of Heterocyclic Amines to Human Carcinogenesis*

MeIQx was administered to rats in doses of 0.4, 4, 40, and 400 ppm in the diet for 1 and 12 weeks, and DNA adduct formation in the liver was examined using the $^{32}$P-postlabeling method (*33*). A linear dose-response relationship was demonstrated between the amounts of MeIQx administered and levels of MeIQx-DNA adduct at both 1 week and 12 weeks. A linear relationship was also reported by Felton's group to exist between doses of MeIQx ranging from 500 ng/kg to 5 mg/kg body weight administered by stomach intubation and DNA adduct levels in the livers of mice (*34*). These observations suggest that even in amounts as low as daily exposure levels, heterocyclic amines are capable of forming DNA adducts in the human body.

We recently reported the effect of a combination of five heterocyclic amines on appearance of glutathione S-transferase placental form (GST-P) positive foci in a rat liver medium-term assay using diethylnitrosamine and partial hepatectomy (*35*). Rats were given each heterocyclic amine in a dose 1/5 or 1/25 the dose used in the carcinogenesis experiment. Other groups of rats were administered five heterocyclic amines in combination with a dose of 1/5 or 1/25 each. It was clearly demonstrated that combined treatment with five heterocyclic amines had an additive or synergistic effect on the development of GST-P positive foci compared to the individual chemicals at 1/5 or 1/25 the dose.

In addition to the above observations, painting the skin of the back of mice with a limited amount of Trp-P-2, which was not sufficient to produce skin tumors in the animals, produced tumors on the backs when 12-*O*-tetradecanoylphorbol-13-acetate (TPA) was subsequently painted on (*36*). Furthermore, administration of a limited amount of IQ combined with partial hepatectomy followed by phenobarbital resulted in the development of liver cancers in rats, although IQ alone in the same dose did not induce these cancers (*37*). Thus, heterocyclic amines may contribute to human cancer development when many other environmental mutagens/carcinogens, tumor promoters, and cancer progression factors are also present.

*Multi-step Carcinogenesis in Human Cancer: Its Implications in Risk Estimation for Xenobiotics Including Heterocyclic Amines*

Many reports are now available concerning the presence of multiple genetic alterations in human cancers and the multi-step nature of human carcinogenesis. Three typical examples are described below. In 1986, we observed mutation at the 12th codon of the c-Ki-*ras* gene and amplification of this mutated c-Ki-*ras* gene and c-*myc* gene in a very aggressive malignant pancreatic cancer (*38*). Recently, a point mutation in the p53 gene, a tumor suppressor gene, was also found in a cell line of this cancer (*39*). Thus, a total of four genetic alterations have been demonstrated in this pancreatic cancer. In small cell carcinoma of the lung, loss of heterozygosity (LOH) was found on chromosomes 3p, 13q, and 17p (*40, 41*). Crucial genes residing on chromosomes 13q and 17p are the genes encoding retinoblastoma and p53 proteins, respectively. The gene on chromosome 3p has not been identified yet. In the case of the LOH at the locus covering the tumor suppressor gene, one allele is missing and the other is either missing or genetically altered. This means that at least six genetic alterations are required for full malignancy of small cell lung carcinoma. Vogelstein *et al.* reported that several genetic alterations, alteration of chromosome 5, activation of the c-Ki-*ras* gene, and LOHs on chromosomes 17 and 18, occur successively in human colon carcinogenesis (*42*).

Premalignant cells acquiring several genetic alterations, still insufficient to result in fully malignant cancer, must already be present in the human body and be much more sensitive to xenobiotics, including heterocyclic amines, than normal cells. A mathematical model was proposed by Sakai *et al.* (unpublished data) on the susceptibility of premalignant cells with several genetic alterations to chemical carcinogens to produce fully malignant cancer cells. If we assume that 10 genetic alterations are necessary for complete malignancy of the cell, cells having 7, 8, and 9 preexisting genetic changes are $10^2$, $10^6$, and $10^9$ times more sensitive to carcinogenic agents than normal cells, respectively. Since numerous kinds of xenobiotics coexist with numerous kinds of autobiotics, exposure to any mutagenic and carcinogenic xenobiotics should be kept to a minimum. Fortunately, exposure to carcinogenic heterocyclic amines can be lessened by cooking meat and fish in microwave ovens and by removing the charred part of cooked meat and fish. In other words, realistic measures to minimize exposure to heterocyclic amines without inconveniencing people are available. However, complete elimination of all heterocyclic amines is impossible and a certain level of exposure to them is, regrettably, unavoidable. It should be realized that this situation with heterocyclic amines may also apply to other naturally occurring xenobiotics.

*Acknowledgments*

The studies described in this paper were supported by Grants-in-Aid for Cancer Research from the Ministry of Health and Welfare and the Ministry of Education, Science and Culture of Japan, and a Grant-in-Aid from the Ministry of Health and Welfare for a Comprehensive 10-Year Strategy for Cancer Control, Japan.

## REFERENCES

1. Sugimura, T. Naturally occurring genotoxic carcinogens. *In;* E. C. Miller, J. A. Miller, I. Hirono, T. Sugimura, and S. Takayama (eds.), Naturally Occurring Carcinogens-Mutagens and Modulators of Carcinogenesis, pp. 241–261, Japan Sci. Soc. Press, Tokyo/Univ. Park Press, Baltimore, 1979.
2. Sugimura, T., Nagao, M., Kawachi, T., Honda, M., Yahagi, T., Seino, Y., Sato, S., Matsukura, N., Matsushima, T., Shirai, A., Sawamura, M., and Matsumoto, H. Mutagen-carcinogens in food, with special reference to highly mutagenic pyrolytic products in broiled foods. *In;* H. H. Hiatt, J. D. Watson, and J. A. Winsten (eds.), Origins of Human Cancer, pp. 1561–1577, Cold Spring Harbor Laboratory, Cold Spring Harbor, NY, 1977.
3. Nagao, M., Honda, M., Seino, Y., Yahagi, T., and Sugimura, T. Mutagenicities of smoke condensates and the charred surface of fish and meat. Cancer Lett., *2*: 221–226, 1977.
4. Nagao, M., Honda, M., Seino, Y., Yahagi, T., Kawachi, T., and Sugimura, T. Mutagenicities of protein pyrolysates. Cancer Lett., *2*: 335–340, 1977.
5. Kosuge, T., Tsuji, K., Wakabayashi, K., Okamoto, T., Shudo, K., Iitaka, Y., Itai, A., Sugimura, T., Kawachi, T., Nagao, M., Yahagi, T., and Seino, Y. Isolation and structure studies of mutagenic principles in amino acid pyrolysates. Chem. Pharm. Bull., *26*: 611–619, 1978.
6. Sugimura, T., Kawachi, T., Nagao, M., Yahagi, T., Seino, Y., Okamoto, T., Shudo, K., Kosuge, T., Tsuji, K., Wakabayashi, K., Iitaka, Y., and Itai, A. Mutagenic principle(s) in tryptophan and phenylalanine pyrolysis products. Proc. Jpn. Acad., *53*: 58–61, 1977.
7. Yamamoto, T., Tsuji, K., Kosuge, T., Okamoto, T., Shudo, K., Takeda, K., Iitaka, Y., Yamaguchi, K., Seino, Y., Yahagi, T., Nagao, M., and Sugimura, T. Isolation and

structure determination of mutagenic substances in L-glutamic acid pyrolysate. Proc. Jpn. Acad., *54B*: 248–250, 1978.

8. Yoshida, D., Matsumoto, T., Yoshimura, R., and Matsuzaki, T. Mutagenicity of amino-α-carbolines in pyrolysis products of soybean globulin. Biochem. Biophys. Res. Commun., *83*: 915–920, 1978.
9. Kasai, H., Yamaizumi, Z., Wakabayashi, K., Nagao, M., Sugimura, T., Yokoyama, S., Miyazawa, T., Spingarn, N. E., Weisburger, J. H., and Nishimura, S. Potent novel mutagens produced by broiling fish under normal conditions. Proc. Jpn. Acad., *56B*: 278–283, 1980.
10. Kasai, H., Yamaizumi, Z., Wakabayashi, K., Nagao, M., Sugimura, T., Yokoyama, S., Miyazawa, T., and Nishimura, S. Structure and chemical synthesis of Me-IQ, a potent mutagen isolated from broiled fish. Chem. Lett., 1391–1394, 1980.
11. Kasai, H., Yamaizumi, Z., Shiomi, T., Yokoyama, S., Miyazawa, T., Wakabayashi, K., Nagao, M., Sugimura, T., and Nishimura, S. Structure of a potent mutagen isolated from fried beef. Chem. Lett., 485–488, 1981.
12. Felton, J. S., Knize, M. G., Shen, N. H., Lewis, P. R., Andresen, B. D., Happe, J., and Hatch, F. T. The isolation and identification of a new mutagen from fried ground beef: 2-amino-1-methyl-6-phenylimidazo[4,5-*b*]pyridine (PhIP). Carcinogenesis, *7*: 1081–1086, 1986.
13. Tsuda, M., Negishi, C., Makino, R., Sato, S., Yamaizumi, Z., Hirayama, T., and Sugimura, T. Use of nitrite and hypochlorite treatments in determination of the contributions of IQ-type and non-IQ-type heterocyclic amines to the mutagenicities in crude pyrolyzed materials. Mutat. Res., *147*: 335–341, 1985.
14. Jägerstad, M., Olsson, K., Grivas, S., Negishi, C., Wakabayashi, K., Tsuda, M., Sato, S., and Sugimura, T. Formation of 2-amino-3,8-dimethylimidazo[4,5-*f*]quinoxaline in a model system by heating creatinine, glycine and glucose. Mutat. Res., *126*: 239–244, 1984.
15. Grivas, S., Nyhammar, T., Olsson, K., and Jägerstad, M. Isolation and identification of the food mutagens IQ and MeIQx from a heated model system of creatinine, glycine and fructose. Food Chem., *20*: 127–136, 1986.
16. Shioya, M., Wakabayashi, K., Sato, S., Nagao, M., and Sugimura, T. Formation of a mutagen, 2-amino-1-methyl-6-phenylimidazo[4,5-*b*]pyridine (PhIP) in cooked beef, by heating a mixture containing creatinine, phenylalanine and glucose. Mutat. Res., *191*: 133–138, 1987.
17. Sugimura, T. Studies on environmental chemical carcinogenesis in Japan. Science, *233*: 312–318, 1986.
18. Sugimura, T. Carcinogenicity of mutagenic heterocyclic amines formed during the cooking process. Mutat. Res., *150*: 33–41, 1985.
19. Ohgaki, H., Takayama, S., and Sugimura, T. Carcinogenicities of heterocyclic amines in cooked food. Mutat. Res., *259*: 399–410, 1991.
20. Esumi, H., Ohgaki, H., Kohzen, E., Takayama, S., and Sugimura, T. Induction of lymphoma in $CDF_1$ mice by the food mutagen, 2-amino-1-methyl-6-phenylimidazo-[4,5-*b*]pyridine. Jpn. J. Cancer Res., *80*: 1176–1178, 1989.
21. Ito, N., Hasegawa, R., Sano, M., Tamano, S., Esumi, H., Takayama, S., and Sugimura, T. A new colon and mammary carcinogen in cooked food, 2-amino-1-methyl-6-phenylimidazo[4,5-*b*]pyridine (PhIP). Carcinogenesis, in press.
22. Ohgaki, H., Hasegawa, H., Suenaga, M., Kato, T., Sato, S., Takayama, S., and Sugimura, T. Induction of hepatocellular carcinoma and highly metastatic squamous cell carcinomas in the forestomach of mice by feeding 2-amino-3,4-dimethylimidazo-[4,5-*f*]quinoline. Carcinogenesis, *7*: 1889–1893, 1986.

23. Degawa, M., Kojima, M., Hishinuma, T., and Hashimoto, Y. Sex-dependent induction of hepatic enzymes for mutagenic activation of a tryptophan pyrolysate component, 3-amino-1, 4-dimethyl-5*H*-pyrido[4,3-*b*]indole, by feeding in mice. Cancer Res., *45*: 96–102, 1985.
24. Takahashi, M., Wakabayashi, K., Nagao, M., Yamamoto, M., Masui, T., Goto, T., Kinae, N., Tomita, I., and Sugimura, T. Quantification of 2-amino-3-methylimidazo-[4,5-*f*]quinoline (IQ) and 2-amino-3,8-dimethylimidazo[4, 5-*f*]quinoxaline (MeIQx) in beef extracts by liquid chromatography with electrochemical detection (LCEC). Carcinogenesis, *6*: 1195–1199, 1985.
25. Sugimura, T., Sato, S., and Wakabayashi, K. Mutagens/carcinogens in pyrolysates of amino acids and proteins and in cooked foods: heterocyclic aromatic amines. *In;* Y-T. Woo, D. Y. Lai, J. C. Arcos, and M. F. Argus (eds.), Chemical Induction of Cancer, Vol. IIIC, pp. 681–710, Academic Press, San Diego, 1988.
26. Zhang, X-M., Wakabayashi, K., Liu, Z-C., Sugimura, T., and Nagao, M. Mutagenic and carcinogenic heterocyclic amines in Chinese cooked foods. Mutat. Res., *201*: 181–188, 1988.
27. Hayatsu, H., Arimoto, S., and Wakabayashi, K. Methods for separation and detection of heterocyclic amines *In;* H. Hayatsu (ed.), Mutagens in Food: Detection and Prevention, pp. 101–112, CRC Press, Boca Raton, 1991.
28. Yamashita, M., Wakabayashi, K., Nagao, M., Sato, S., Yamaizumi, Z., Takahashi, M., Kinae, N., Tomita, I., and Sugimura, T. Detection of 2-amino-3-methylimidazo[4,5-*f*]-quinoline in cigarette smoke condensate. Jpn. J. Cancer Res. (Gann), *77*: 419–422, 1986.
29. Kikugawa, K., Kato, T., and Takahashi, S. Possible presence of 2-amino-3, 4-dimethylimidazo[4,5-*f*]quinoline and other heterocyclic amine-like mutagens in roasted coffee beans. J. Agric. Food Chem., *37*: 881–886, 1989.
30. Manabe, S., Uchino, E., and Wada, O. Carcinogenic tryptophan pyrolysis products in airborne particles and rain water. Mutat. Res., *226*: 215–221, 1989.
31. Ushiyama, H., Wakabayashi, K., Hirose, M., Itoh, H., Sugimura, T., and Nagao, M. Presence of carcinogenic heterocyclic amines in urine of healthy volunteers eating normal diet, but not of inpatients receiving parenteral alimentation. Carcinogenesis, in press.
32. Murray, S., Gooderham, N. J., Boobis, A. R., and Davies, D. S. Detection and measurement of MeIQx in human urine after ingestion of a cooked meat meal. Carcinogenesis, *10*: 763–765, 1989.
33. Yamashita, K., Adachi, M., Kato, S., Nakagama, H., Ochiai, M., Wakabayashi, K., Sato, S., Nagao, M., and Sugimura, T. DNA Adducts formed by 2-amino-3, 8-dimethylimidazo[4,5-*f*]quinoxaline in rat liver: Dose-response on chronic administration. Jpn. J. Cancer Res., *81*: 470–476, 1990.
34. Turteltaub, K. W., Felton, J. S., Gledhill, B. L., Vogel, J. S., Southon, J. R., Caffee, M. W., Finkel, R. C., Nelson, D. E., Proctor, I. D., and Davis J. C. Accelerator mass spectrometry in biomedical dosimetry: Relationship between low-level exposure and covalent binding of heterocyclic amine carcinogens to DNA. Proc. Natl. Acad. Sci. U.S.A., *87*: 5288–5292, 1990.
35. Ito, N., Hasegawa, R., Shirai, T., Fukushima, S., Hakoi, K., Takaba, K., Iwasaki, S., Wakabayashi, K., Nagao, M., and Sugimura, T. Enhancement of GST-P positive liver cell foci development by combined treatment of rats with five heterocyclic amines at low doses. Carcinogenesis, in press.
36. Takahashi, M., Furukawa, F., Miyakawa, Y., Sato, H., Hasegawa, R., and Hayashi, Y. 3-Amino-1-methyl-5*H*-pyrido[4, 3-*b*]indole initiates two-stage carcinogenesis in

mouse skin but is not a complete carcinogen. Jpn. J. Cancer Res. (Gann), *77*: 509–513, 1986.

37. Tsuda, H., Asamoto, M., Ogiso, T., Inoue, T., Ito, N., and Nagao, M. Dose-dependent induction of liver and thyroid neoplastic lesions by short-term administration of 2-amino-3-methylimidazo[4,5-*f*]quinoline combined with partial hepatectomy followed by phenobarbital or low dose 3′-methyl-4-dimethylaminoazobenzene promotion. Jpn. J. Cancer Res. (Gann), *79*: 691–697, 1988.
38. Yamada, H., Sakamoto, H., Taira, M., Nishimura, S., Shimosato, Y., Terada, M., and Sugimura, T. Amplifications of both c-Ki-*ras* with a point mutation and c-*myc* in a primary pancreatic cancer and its metastatic tumors in lymph nodes. Jpn. J. Cancer Res. (Gann), *77*: 370–375, 1986.
39. Murakami, Y., Hayashi, K., and Sekiya, T. Detection of aberrations of the p53 alleles and the gene transcript in human tumor cell lines by single-strand conformation polymorphism analysis. Cancer Res., *51*: 3356–3361, 1991.
40. Yokota, J., Wada, M., Shimosato, Y., Terada, M., and Sugimura, T. Loss of heterozygosity on chromosomes 3, 13, and 17 in small-cell carcinoma and on chromosome 3 in adenocarcinoma of the lung. Proc. Natl. Acad. Sci. U.S.A., *84*: 9252–9256, 1987.
41. Mori, N., Yokota, J., Oshimura, M., Cavenee, W. K., Mizoguchi, H., Noguchi, M., Shimosato, Y., Sugimura, T., and Terada, M. Concordant deletions of chromosome 3p and loss of heterozygosity for chromosomes 13 and 17 in small cell lung carcinoma. Cancer Res., *49*: 5130–5135, 1989.
42. Vogelstein, B., Fearon, E. R., Hamilton, S. R., Kern, S. E., Preisinger, A. C., Leppert, M., Nakamura, Y., White, R., Smits, A. M. M., and Bos, J. L. Genetic alterations during colorectal-tumor development. N. Engl. J. Med., *319*: 525–532, 1988.

XENOBIOTICS AND CANCER, L. ERNSTER ET AL. (EDS.),
JAPAN SCI. SOC. PRESS, TOKYO/TAYLOR & FRANCIS LTD., LONDON, pp. 289–301, 1991

# Metabolic Processing and Carcinogenicity of Heterocyclic Amines in Nonhuman Primates

Richard H. ADAMSON,*[1] Elizabeth G. SNYDERWINE,*[1]
Unnur P. THORGEIRSSON,*[1] Herman A. J. SCHUT,*[2] Robert J. TURESKY,*[3]
Snorri S. THORGEIRSSON,*[1] Shozu TAKAYAMA,*[4] and Takashi SUGIMURA*[4]

*National Cancer Institute, Bethesda Maryland 20892, U.S.A.,*[1] Medical College of Ohio, Toledo, Ohio 43614, U.S.A.,*[2] Nestle Research Center, Lausanne, Switzerland,*[3] and National Cancer Center Research Institute, Tokyo 104, Japan*[4]*

*Abstract:* The potential for human exposure to heterocyclic amine (HAA) mutagens derived from cooking food prompted an evaluation of the disposition and carcinogenicity of three of the HAAs in nonhuman primates, especially cynomolgus monkeys. The three HAAs currently under study are 2-amino-3-methylimidazo[4,5-*f*]quinoline (IQ), 2-amino-3,8-dimethylimidazo[4,5-*f*]quinoxaline (8-MeIQx) and 2-amino-1-methyl-6-phenylimidazo[4,5,*b*]pyridine (PhIP). These three HAAs were selected on the basis of several factors including structure, mutagenic activity *in vitro*, concentration in cooked meat, activity in rodent carcinogenicity tests and availability. Studies on the disposition of IQ demonstrated that it was extensively metabolized in monkeys and excreted in urine and feces as metabolites. These metabolites represent predominantly detoxification products of IQ. The extent of *in vivo* activation of IQ and PhIP was assessed by measuring DNA adducts in various tissues and white blood cells of monkeys following administration of the compounds. Both compounds form high levels of DNA adducts in a number of organs, particularly the liver, kidney, and heart. The carcinogenicity of IQ, 8-MeIQx and PhIP in nonhuman primates has been under study for 5 years, 24 months, and 7 months, respectively. Thus far, IQ has induced hepatocellular carcinoma in 3 of 20 monkeys at doses of 10 mg/kg daily, 5 days/week and in 10 of 20 monkeys at 20 mg/kg on the same schedule. Thus, IQ is a potent liver carcinogen in nonhuman primates and a potential carcinogen for humans.

During the past several years, 17 heterocyclic aromatic amine (HAA) mutagens have been isolated and identified from cooked fish, beef, fowl and other meat, and from beef extract (*1–8*). Several of these HAA mutagens have also been found to be carcinogenic in rodent bioassays (*6, 9–13*). These studies and the potential of human exposure to several HAAs derived from cooking as well as extensive experience in evaluating other potential human carcinogens in nonhuman primates (*14–16*) prompted us to study the disposition, DNA adduct formation and carcinogenic potential of 2-amino-3-methylimidazo[4,5-*f*]quinoline (IQ), 2-amino-3,8-dimethylimidazo-[4,5-*f*]quinoxaline (8-MeIQx), and 2-amino-1-methyl-6-phenylimidazo[4,5,*b*]-pyridine (PhIP) (Fig. 1) in nonhuman primates, a species phylogenically close to humans.

*Selection of Compounds*

We selected three compounds for study in nonhuman primates based on several factors including structure, mutagenic activity *in vitro*, concentration in cooked food, carcinogenic activity in rodent tests and availability. Thus, IQ, 8-MeIQx, and PhIP were selected for study following evaluation of the literature values of their concentra-

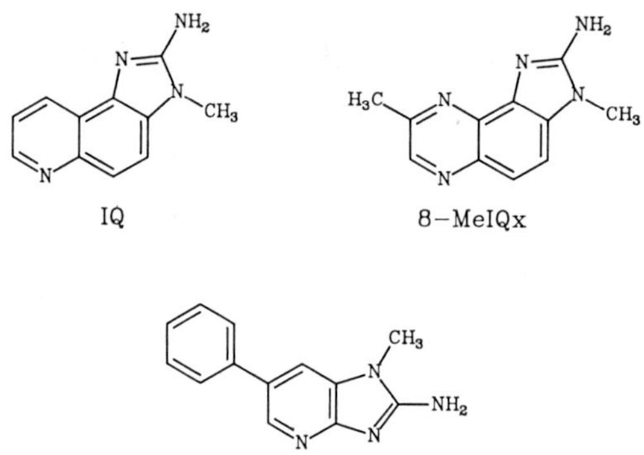


FIG. 1. The chemical structure of IQ, 8-MeIQx, and PhIP.

TABLE 1. Amount of Three HAA Mutagens in Cooked Meat and Extracts[a]

| Compound | Food | Amount (ng/g) |
|---|---|---|
| IQ | Fried ground beef | 0.02–0.6 |
| | Broiled sardine | 4.9–20 |
| | Broiled salmon | 0.3–1.8 |
| | Bact. grade beef extract | 41–142 |
| 8-MeIQx | Fried ground beef | 0.1–2.4 |
| | Smoked dried mackerel | 0.8 |
| | Food grade beef extract | 3.1–28 |
| | Bact. grade beef extract | 58.7–527 |
| PhIP | Fried ground beef | 15 |

[a] Summarized from ref. *8*.

TABLE 2. Mutagenic Contribution of Several Individual HAA Mutagens in Fried Ground Beef[a]

| Compound | Specific activity (REV/μg) | Mutational activity (REV/kg) | % mutational activity |
|---|---|---|---|
| IQ | 200,000 | 20,000 | 6.0 |
| 8-MeIQx | 70,000 | 70,000 | 21.1 |
| DiMeIQx | 130,000 | 65,000 | 19.7 |
| TMIP | 100,000 | 50,000 | 15.0 |
| PhIP | 4,000 | 60,000 | 18.1 |

[a] Summarized from ref. *7*.

TABLE 3. Carcinogenicity of Three HAA Mutagens in Rodents

| Compound | Species | Route and dose | Site tumors found | Reference |
|---|---|---|---|---|
| IQ | Mouse | Diet, 0.03% | Liver, lung, forestomach | *9* |
| | Rat | Diet, 0.03% | Intestine, liver, oral cavity, Zymbal gland | *10* |
| 8-MeIQx | Mouse | Diet, 0.06% | Liver, lung, lymphoma, leukemia | *11* |
| | Rat | Diet, 0.04% | Liver, Zymbal gland, clitoral gland, skin | *12* |
| PhIP | Mouse | Diet, 0.04% | Lymphomas | *13* |
| | Rat | Diet, 0.04% | Breast, colon | (a) |

(a) Unpublished observation.

tion, compared to other HAAs, in cooked fish and beef (Table 1), their specific activity in the TA 1538 Ames/*Salmonella* test, the percent mutational activity of various HAAs in fried ground beef (*7*) (Table 2) and the spectrum of tumors (Table 3) induced in rodent bioassays (*6, 9–13*).

Currently, IQ, 8-MeIQx, and PhIP are being evaluated in studies of their disposition, DNA adduct formation and carcinogenic potential as an initial step in evaluation of the biological effects of HAAs in nonhuman primates (*17*).

*Animal Studies*

The monkeys being used are primarily cynomolgus monkeys (*Macaca fascicularis*) which were born in a closed colony, mother-reared, and assigned to the HAA study as they became approximately one year of age. For the carcinogenic studies, IQ, 8-MeIQx, and PhIP are prepared daily as a suspension in hydroxypropyl cellulose (HPC) and administered by gavage 5 times a week at a dose of 10 or 20 mg/kg body weight. Two groups of 20 monkeys, at doses of 10 and 20 mg/kg, are being used for the IQ study and two groups of 10 monkeys, at the same doses, are being used for the 8-MeIQx study and the PhIP study. Untreated monkeys and HPC-treated monkeys are being maintained as the control group (*17*). In disposition studies, previously untreated monkeys were administered $^{14}$C-IQ (2.2 μmol—120 μCi/kg body weight) by gavage. Urinary and fecal metabolites are purified from animals being chronically administered 10 mg/kg IQ for carcinogenicity studies. Additional monkeys are used for other disposition and DNA adduct studies.

*Metabolism and Disposition of IQ in Cynomolgus Monkeys*

Pharmacokinetic studies with IQ in the cynomolgus monkey show that IQ is rapidly absorbed from the gastrointestinal tract. Peak blood levels are observed by 1 hr following oral administration of IQ and the majority of the dose is rapidly cleared from the blood by 8 hr (Fig. 2). IQ is predominantly excreted in the urine which accounts for approximately 57% of the dose by 72 hr, while the feces accounts for 9% of this dose during the same time period (Fig. 3).

Analysis of urine and feces indicates that IQ is extensively metabolized in monkeys

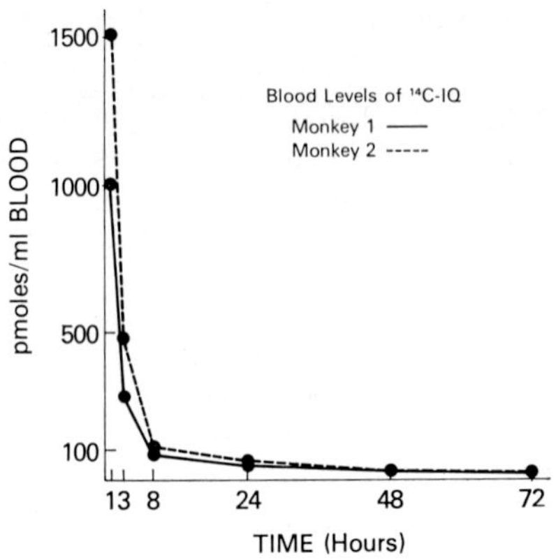


FIG. 2. Blood levels of $^{14}$C-IQ equivalents in 2 cynomolgus monkeys.

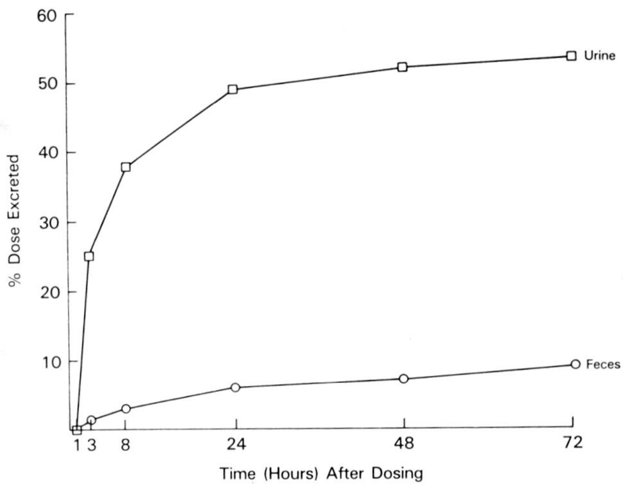


FIG. 3. Mean percent dose excreted in 2 cynomolgus monkeys at times after $^{14}$C-IQ administration.

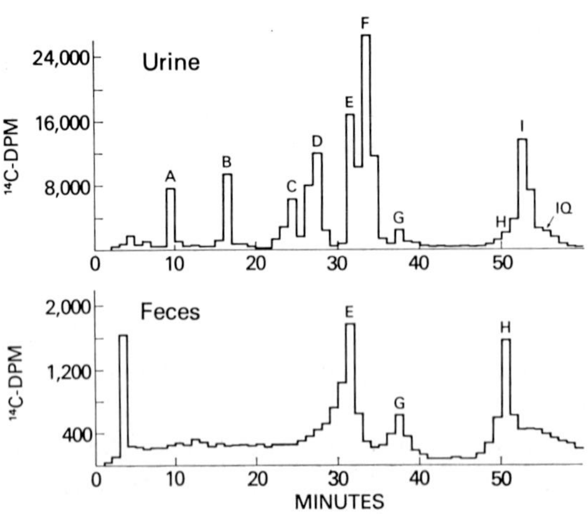


FIG. 4. HPLC analysis of urinary and fecal metabolites of IQ. Metabolites identified by NMR and MS are 3N-demethyl-2N-glucuronide-IQ (B), IQ-sulfamate (E), IQ-5-sulfate (F), and 3N-demethyl-7-OH-IQ (G).

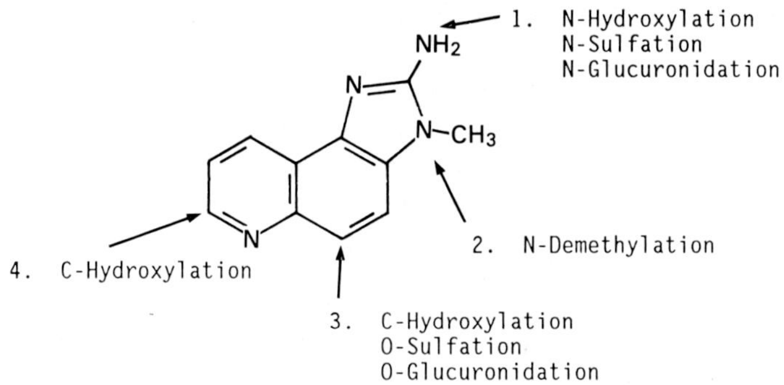


FIG. 5. Sites of metabolism of IQ in cynomolgus monkeys.

TABLE 4. Routes of IQ Metabolism in Monkeys

| Cytochrome P-450 | Conjugation | Enteric bacterium |
|---|---|---|
| C-hydroxylation | Sulfation (N- and O-[b]) | Ring oxidation[c] |
| N-hydroxylation[a] | Glucuronidation (N- and O-) | |
| N-demethylation | Acetylation (N- O-[b]) | |

[a] Route of activation. [b] Secondary step in activation of N-hydroxylamine. [c] Possible route of activation.

and excreted as conjugated and free metabolites (Fig. 4). These metabolites appear to be detoxification products of IQ metabolism because they are less mutagenic than the parent compound in the Ames/*Salmonella* mutagenicity assay. At least nine metabolites have been found in urine and at least three have been found in feces. A number of IQ metabolites in urine and feces of monkeys have been purified by HPLC and structurally characterized by nuclear magnetic resonance and mass spectrometry. The sites of IQ metabolism are shown in Fig. 5. Metabolites appear to arise from a combination of cytochrome P-450 mediated C-hydroxylation or N-demethylation followed by phase II conjugation with either sulfate or glucuronide (Table 4). Sulfate and glucuronide conjugates are the major detoxified metabolites excreted in urine. IQ-sulfamate is also a predominant detoxification product of IQ metabolism found in monkey feces. Similar studies are in progress with 8-MeIQx and PhIP.

*Formation of DNA Adducts by HAAs*

The primary route of mutagenic and possibly carcinogenic activation of HAAs is *via* microsomal cytochrome P-450 mediated N-hydroxylation to form N-hydroxylamines. Because of their reactivity with DNA, N-hydroxylamines of HAAs have been implicated as proximate/ultimate carcinogenic metabolites. Studies with IQ have shown that N-hydroxy-IQ forms adducts with DNA directly and following further metabolism by various esterifications (*18*). The DNA adduct pattern of N-hydroxy-IQ *in vitro* is identical to that found in rodents and nonhuman primates administered IQ (*19*). Thus, N-hydroxy-IQ appears to be the metabolite responsible for IQ-DNA adducts *in vivo*. In the current report, we have measured tissue levels of DNA adducts in order to estimate the extent of *in vivo* activation of IQ, MeIQx, and PhIP and to acquire information on the possible genotoxic effects of these compounds in nonhuman primates.

To maximize the sensitivity of the DNA adduct measurements we employed the $^{32}P$-postlabeling method (*20*). At present, we have obtained data for IQ and PhIP in the monkey tissues and these are summarized in Tables 5 and 6.

Although the data in Tables 5 and 6 are representative data from only 2 monkeys receiving IQ or PhIP, the results have a number of potential important implications. It is clear that both IQ and PhIP form DNA adducts in a number of tissues including,

TABLE 5. IQ-DNA Adducts in Monkey Tissues[a)]

| Organ | RAL ($\times 10^7$)[b)] | | | | |
|---|---|---|---|---|---|
| | I | II | IV | V | Total |
| Liver | 21.4167 | 2.6892 | 3.4021 | 1.0968 | 28.6048 |
| Lung | 0.4463 | 0.0069 | 0.0124 | — | 0.465 |
| Stomach | 5.0017 | 0.4598 | 0.3912 | — | 5.852 |
| Small intestine | 5.0300 | 0.5533 | 0.5878 | 0.2146 | 6.382 |
| Large intestine | 2.8667 | 0.2913 | 0.2723 | 0.1478 | 3.578 |
| Kidney | 20.6500 | 1.7734 | 1.8289 | — | 24.252 |
| Spleen | 11.4533 | 1.1404 | 0.6915 | — | 13.285 |
| Pancreas | 4.3450 | 0.6423 | 0.4491 | 0.1563 | 5.592 |
| Heart | 12.8017 | 1.1811 | 0.8817 | — | 14.864 |
| Muscle | 0.1308 | 0.0083 | 0.0217 | 0.2135 | 0.374 |
| Salivary | 3.2150 | 0.5781 | 0.4112 | 0.2061 | 4.410 |
| Brain | 2.8167 | 0.2377 | 0.1517 | — | 3.206 |
| Esophagus | 7.1933 | 0.6102 | 0.4243 | 0.1271 | 8.354 |
| Bladder | 12.6950 | 0.9590 | 0.8284 | — | 14.482 |
| Adrenal | 9.2750 | 0.7872 | 0.6231 | 0.1675 | 10.852 |

a) The tissues were obtained from monkey ♯1443DD that had been treated with IQ for 35 months at 20 mg/kg p.o. 5 days a week. The last dose of IQ was administered 6 days prior to the monkey being killed with an overdose of sodium pentobarbital. b) RAL: relative adduct labeling. The numbering of the IQ adducts (I–V) is based on the adduct pattern obtained in the rat (*20*). In the monkey tissues, adducts I, II, IV, and V were detected whereas adduct III was not. Adduct I which is the major adduct in all the tissues has been identified as the C8 guanine adduct (*18*, *19*).

TABLE 6. PhIP Adducts in Monkey Tissues[a)]

| Organ | RAL ($\times 10^7$) | | | |
|---|---|---|---|---|
| | I | II | III | Total |
| Liver | 2.6078 | 1.1928 | 1.2585 | 5.0591 |
| Stomach | 0.4995 | 0.3272 | N.D. | 0.8267 |
| Small intestine | 0.8147 | 0.5524 | 0.0828 | 1.4499 |
| Large intestine | 0.3840 | 0.3814 | N.D. | 0.7654 |
| Kidney | 1.0312 | 1.0626 | 0.3928 | 2.4866 |
| Spleen | 0.0921 | N.D. | N.D. | 0.0921 |
| Pancreas | 1.3596 | 0.8415 | 0.7872 | 2.9883 |
| Heart | 4.7992 | 4.8669 | 2.2979 | 11.9640 |
| Muscle | N.D. | N.D. | N.D. | N.D. |
| Salivary gland | 0.8231 | 0.3929 | 0.0396 | 3.1737 |
| Brain | 0.1641 | 0.2068 | 0.0396 | 0.4105 |

a) The tissues were obtained from monkey ♯1469DD following daily administration of 20 mg/kg p.o. of PhIP for a total of 9 days (Monday through Friday, then Monday through Thursday). The last dose of PhIP was administered 24 hr prior to the monkey being killed with an overdose of sodium pentobarbital.

in the case of IQ, the target organ for tumor development (*i.e.*, the liver). The levels of IQ DNA adducts are generally highest in the liver, but this was not the case for PhIP. Both compounds formed high levels of DNA adducts in a number of other organs, in particular the kidney and heart. In addition, DNA adducts for both IQ and PhIP were measured in the white blood cells (WBC) of monkeys being fed the compounds. We are presently examining the possibility of using the measurement of DNA adducts in WBC to estimate the level of metabolic activation that takes place *in vivo* which might be useful in evaluating individual differences in the extent of metabolic activation of these compounds.

The interpretation of the biological significance of these DNA adducts is at present uncertain, since apart from hepatocellular carcinoma, no tumors have thus far been observed in the IQ-treated monkeys (see below). It seems, however, reasonable to entertain the possibility that tumors may occur in other organs in which high levels of adducts are formed, and also that diseases other than cancer may be associated with the formation of these adducts. This may particularly apply to degenerative diseases of the cardiovascular system. Further research endeavors in this area are clearly indicated.

### *Carcinogenicity Studies in Nonhuman Primates*

Three HAAs, IQ, 8-MeIQx, and PhIP are being evaluated for carcinogenic effects in nonhuman primates, primarily cynomolgus monkeys. As of October 1, 1990, the longest period of time monkeys have been on study with 8-MeIQx is 24 months and for PhIP, 7 months. The highest total dose of MeIQx and PhIP received by a cynomolgus monkey was 11.5 grams and 4.9 grams, respectively. The time period is probably too short for tumor development in this species by chemical carcinogens administered orally. In contrast, IQ has been on study in cynomolgus monkeys for 5 years (*17*) and tumors have developed at both doses being administered, *i.e.*, 10 or 20 mg/kg daily, 5 times/week. Table 7 summarizes the data on tumors induced at both doses. Thus far, 3 monkeys, or 15 percent, have developed tumors at the low dose (10 mg/kg), while 10 monkeys, or 50 percent, have developed tumors at the 20 mg/kg dose. All the tumors that developed are primary hepatocellular carcinomas. Hepatocellular carcinoma has not been found in any of the breeders or control monkeys (more than 300) in this colony over the past 25 years, nor in the HPC control monkeys.

The first monkey was diagnosed with massive tumor involvement replacing up to 80% of the liver after two and a half years of dosing with IQ (10 mg/kg). The tumor had broken through the capsule of the liver and invaded the stomach and diaphragm. There was also evidence of intrahepatic vascular invasion and metastases to the lungs and hilar lymph nodes. Another monkey which received 10 mg/kg of IQ presented

TABLE 7. Tumors Induced by IQ in Cynomolgus Monkeys

| Dose | No. treated | No. with tumors | % with tumors | Average total dose | Average latent period |
|---|---|---|---|---|---|
| 10 mg/kg | 20 (14M, 6F)[a)] | 3 (3M) | 15 | 30 g | 45 months |
| 20 mg/kg | 20 (8M, 12F) | 10 (6M, 4F) | 50 | 35 g | 37 months |

a) Numbers in parenthesis are sex of monkeys on study.

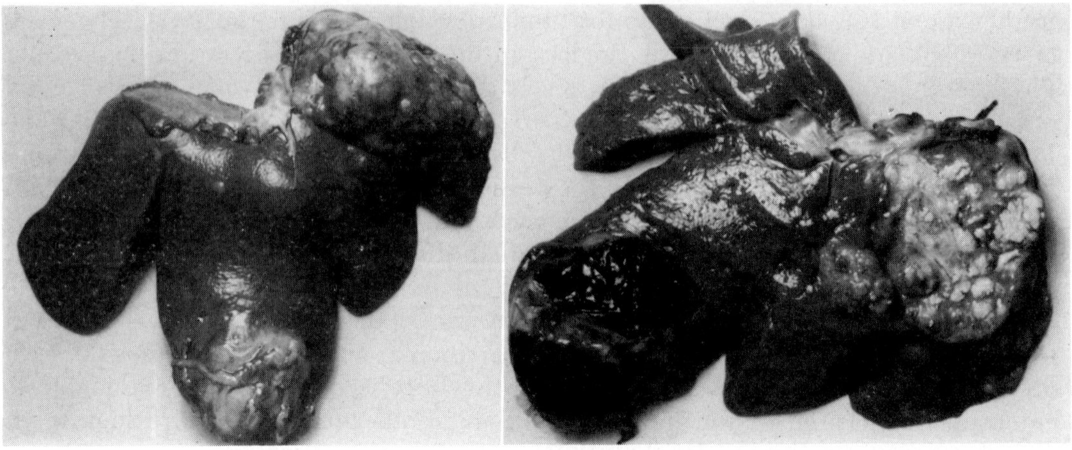

FIG. 6. Case No. 1409BB. Anterior surface (left) and cross section (right) of the liver showing two tumor masses measuring 7 and 5.5 cm in largest diameter. This monkey died as a result of peritoneal bleeding from a hemorrhagic liver mass seen at the inferior edge of the liver.

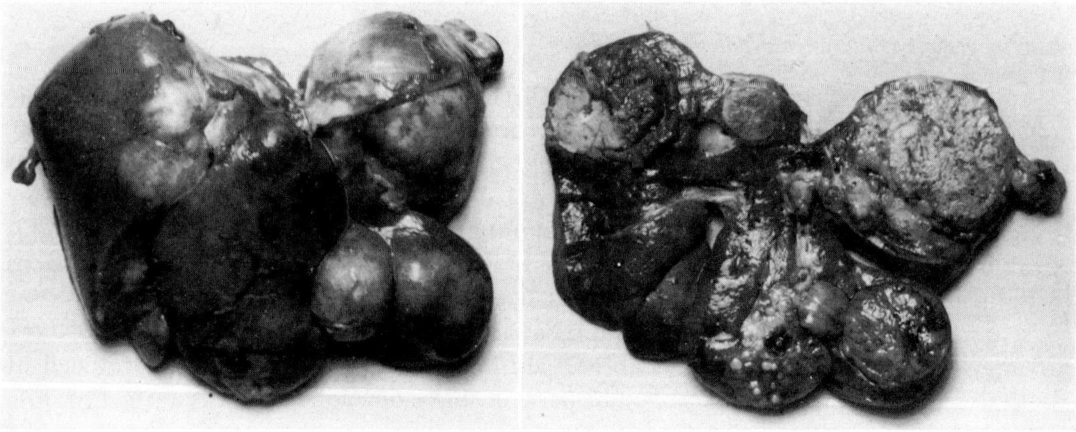

FIG. 7. Case No. 1434CC. Anterior surface (left) and cross section (right) of the liver showing five nodules of hepatocellular carcinoma ranging in diameter from 2–7 cm. The largest nodules show extensive necrosis.

with similar findings, except for a lack of tumor invasion into neighboring organs. Most of the hepatocellular carcinoma cases could be classified as nodular, *i.e.*, there were multiple discrete nodules throughout the liver (Figs. 6 and 7), although in some instances nodular conglomerates had formed occupying a large proportion of the liver. The tumors were soft, frequently with large areas of necrosis, except for a few scirrhous nodules of very firm consistency.

Microscopically, all of the IQ-induced tumors were confirmed to be hepatocellular carcinoma. A trabecular pattern was most frequent (Fig. 8), sometimes with pseudoglandular formation. In some cases, a solid pattern of well- to moderately well-differentiated hepatocellular carcinoma was identified. There was a lack of supporting connective tissue within the tumors exhibiting trabecular and solid histological

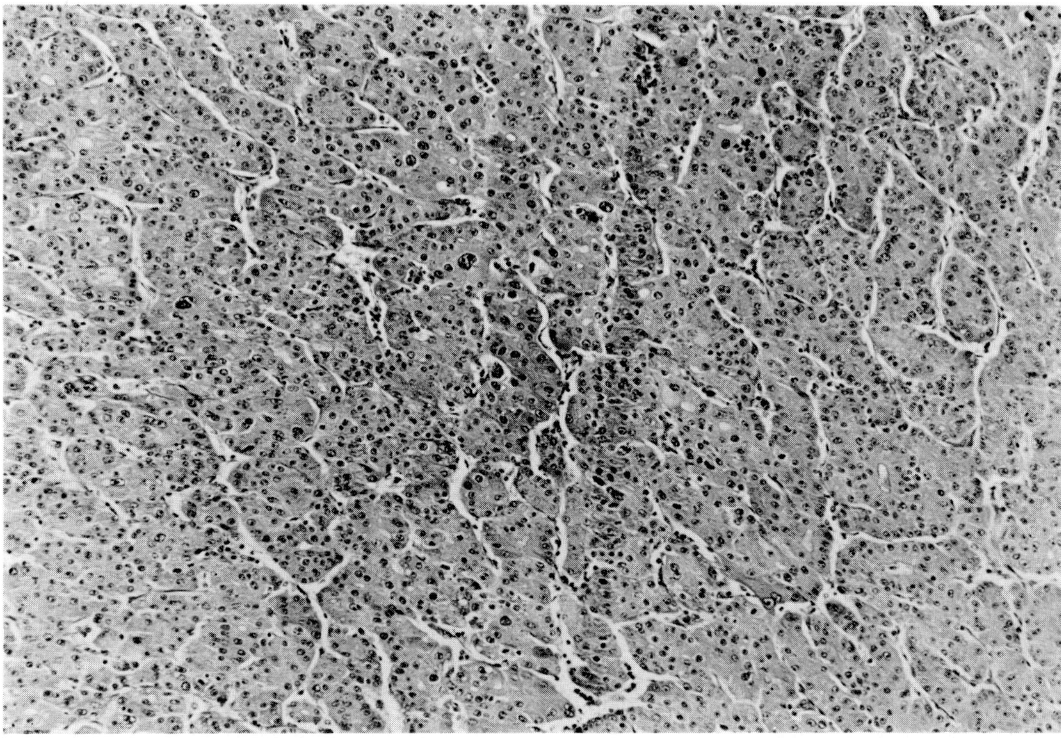

FIG. 8. Case No. 1429CC. Trabecular pattern of a well-differentiated hepatocellular carcinoma. (H & E, ×100)

growth patterns. However, some of the tumor nodules were partially surrounded with a fibrous capsule. Due to tumor expansion pressure atrophy of the adjacent liver parenchyma was commonly seen. The scirrhous nodules contained abundant fibrous tissue surrounding a mixed tumor cell population of spindle shape and hepatocellular differentiation. Generally, the tumor nodules exhibited a well- to moderately well-differentiated hepatocellular carcinoma, except in one case where severe atypia and giant tumor cells were observed. In this case, all of the tumor nodules were heavily infiltrated with lymphocytes. Pulmonary metastases were detected in several of the necropsied monkeys (Fig. 9). Intravascular tumor thrombi were also noted in cases where there was no evidence of gross metastases.

The liver parenchyma that was not involved with neoplastic changes was relatively normal, except for clear cell foci that were commonly seen (Fig. 10). The foci varied in size from a few cells to well-defined nodules measuring up to 1 or 2 millimeters in diameter. They were composed of cells with abundant clear cytoplasm and eccentric nuclei, often slightly smaller and darker than normal. PAS staining of the clear cell foci with and without diastase revealed the presence of cytoplasmic glycogen. Hyperplastic nodules of the liver were rarely seen in the tumor-bearing animals, although they were commonly visualized at laparoscopy prior to gross tumor development.

At necropsy, lymph nodes of the colonic submucosa and mesentery were found to be enlarged (Fig. 11). On cut section, the lymph nodes were of normal color and con-

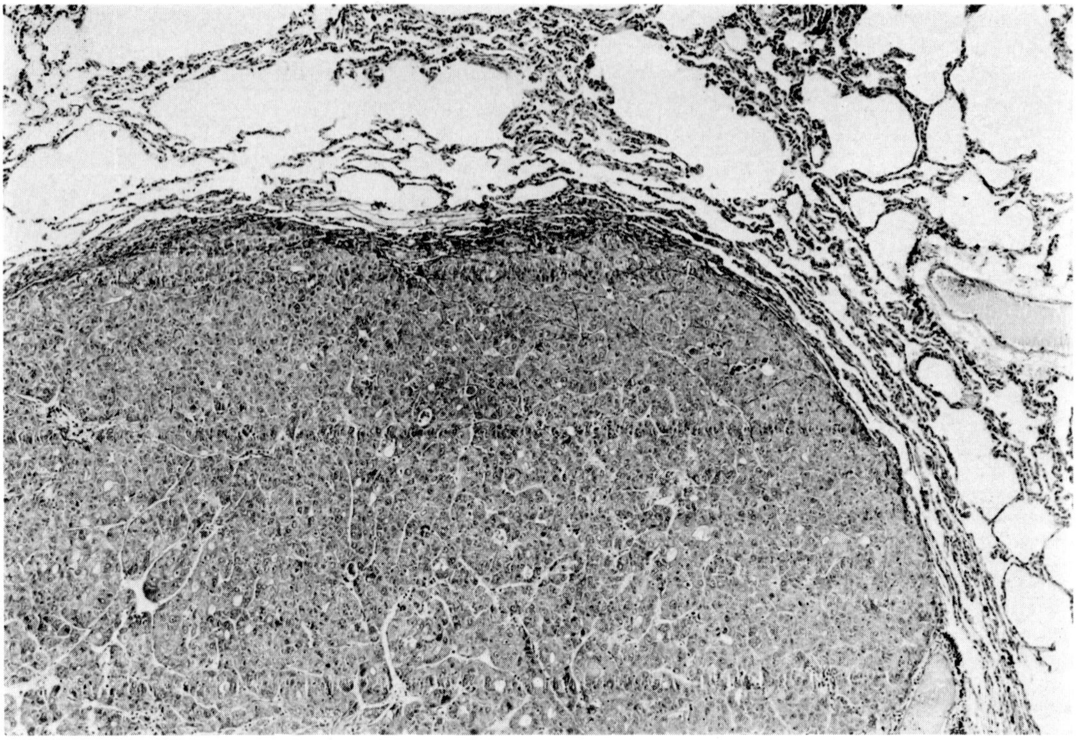

FIG. 9. Case No. 1394BB. Lung metastasis showing trabecular and diffuse patterns of hepatocellular carcinoma. (H & E, ×50)

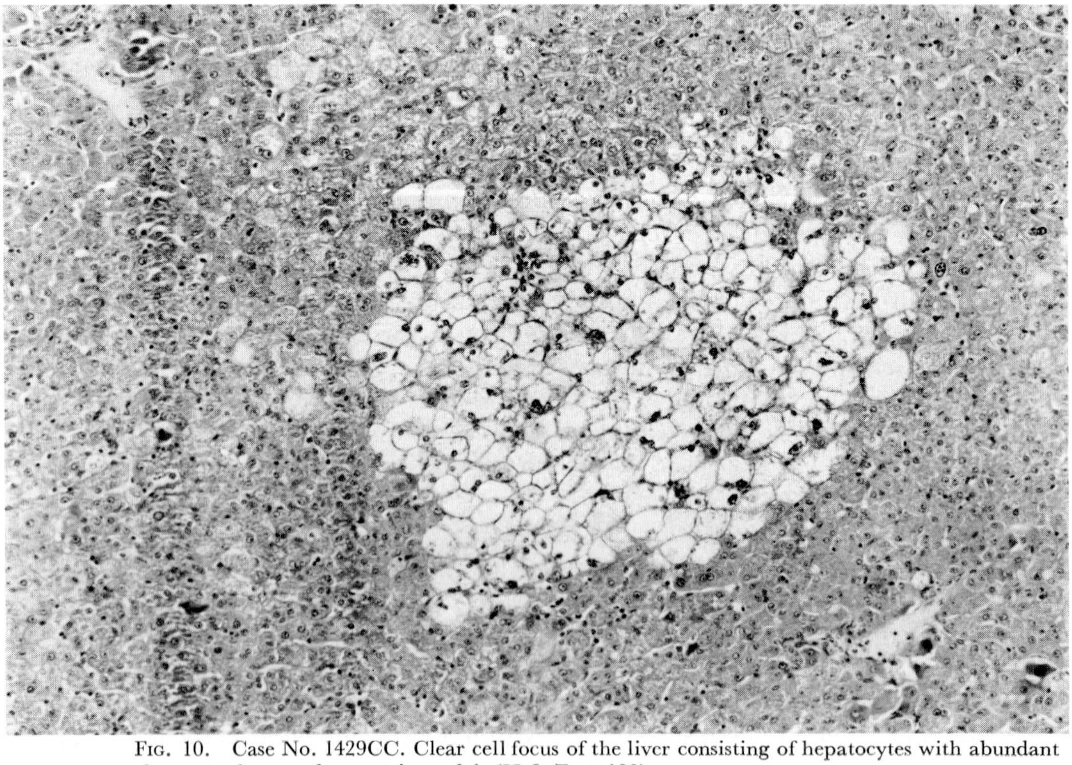

FIG. 10. Case No. 1429CC. Clear cell focus of the liver consisting of hepatocytes with abundant clear cytoplasm and eccentric nuclei. (H & E, ×100)

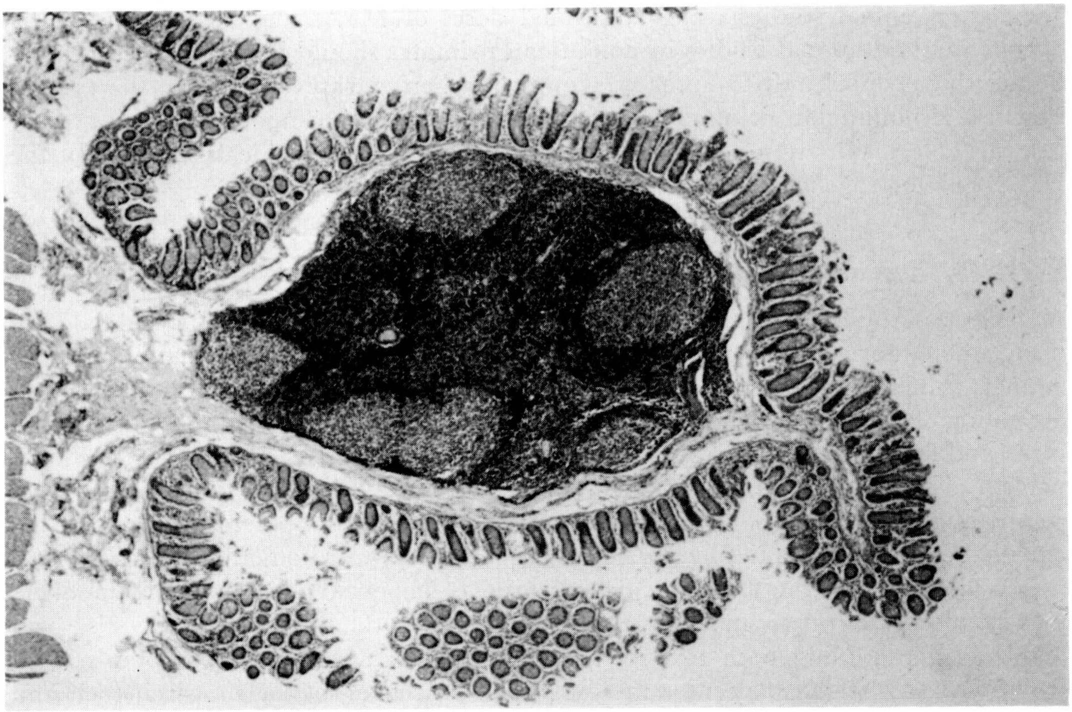

FIG. 11. Case No. 1425CC. Submucosal lymph node of colon showing reactive hyperplasia and follicular enlargement. (H & E ×8)

TABLE 8. Methods to Minimize Intake of HAAs

| |
|---|
| Vary method of cooking meat. |
| Microwave fish and poultry more often. If barbecuing chicken or pork, microwave prior to barbecuing. Stew, boil and poach meat more often. |
| Do not allow drippings from meat to become dry before making gravy. |
| Eat beef medium instead of well done. |

sistency. Microscopically, they exhibited reactive hyperplasia and large lymphoid follicles. No other gross or light microscopic abnormalities have been detected thus far in the IQ-treated groups. The remaining monkeys continue to be monitored by laparoscopy every 3 months for detection of tumor development.

*Significance of HAAs in the Human Diet*

The amounts and types of HAAs in foods prepared by industry and individuals still is inexact. Nevertheless, both industry and individuals may take various measures to lower the amounts of HAAs in their food. A summary of actions that individuals can take to minimize their intake of HAAs is given in Table 8. Eating beef medium instead of well done and use of the microwave for cooking fish and poultry, especially prior to barbecuing, are steps that are easy and will significantly reduce the amount of HAAs formed.

Better animal studies using additional doses of HAAs and completion of the ongoing and additional studies in nonhuman primates should help in risk extrapolation of these compounds to humans. However, when extrapolating from the present rodent and nonhuman primate data, it is clear that these compounds post a greater risk for cancer causation in humans than the majority of chemicals banned by the U.S. regulatory agencies.

### *Conclusion*

Three of the HAA mutagens (IQ, 8-MeIQx, and PhIP) found in cooked food are being studied for carcinogenic effects in nonhuman primates. The formation of DNA adducts in tissues of monkeys following administration of IQ or PhIP indicates that activation of these compounds occurs *in vivo*. Analysis of metabolites of IQ in monkey urine and feces also indicates that extensive metabolism occurs and that a significant portion of the compound is detoxified. Studies of the carcinogenic potential of these compounds in cynomolgus monkeys demonstrated that IQ is a potent liver carcinogen equalled only in our studies by the hepatocarcinogen N-nitrosodiethylamine (*14–16*).

While data on the carcinogenic potential of chemical compounds in monkeys may be most relevant to humans, additional factors in the human diet may also play a role in determining both toxicity and carcinogenicity of these compounds. This includes agents which may alter the metabolic processing of the procarcinogen and thereby modulate the binding of the reactive metabolite(s) at critical macromolecular sites. Studies concerning the risk of HAAs to human health should consider these factors as well.

### *Acknowledgments*

This work was supported in part by National Cancer Institute Contract No. NO1-CP-51013 to Hazleton Laboratories America, Inc., Vienna, Virginia; by a Grant-in-Aid from the Ministry of Health and Welfare for a Comprehensive 10-Year Strategy for Cancer Control, Japan; and by the Foundation for Promotion of Cancer Research, Japan.

## REFERENCES

1. Sugimura, T., Nagao, M., Kawachi, T., Honda, M., Yahagi, T., Seino, Y., Sato, S., Matsukura, N., Matsushima, T., Shirai, A., Sawamura, M., and Matsumoto, H. Mutagen-carcinogens in foods with special reference to highly mutagenic pyrolytic products in broiled foods. *In;* H. H. Hiatt *et al.* (eds.), Origins of Human Cancer, pp. 1561–1577, Cold Spring Harbor, New York, 1977.
2. Sugimura, T., Kawachi, T., Nagao, M., Yahagi, T., Okamoto, T., Shudo, K., Kosuge, T., Tsuki, K., Wakabayashi, K., Litaka, Y., and Itai, A. Mutagenic principles in tryptophan and phenylamine pyrolysis products. Proc. Jpn. Acad., *53*: 58–61, 1977.
3. Commoner, B., Vithayathil, A. J., Dolara, P., Nair, S., Madyastha, P., and Cuca, G. C. Formation of mutagens in beef and beef extract during cooking. Science, *201*: 913–916, 1978.
4. Kasai, H., Nishimura, S., Wakabayashi, K., Nagao, M., and Sugimura, T. Chemical synthesis of 1-amino-3-methylimidazo[4,5-*f*]quinoline (IQ), a potent mutagen isolated from broiled fish. Proc. Jpn. Acad., *58*: 382–384, 1980.
5. Bjeldanes, L. F., Morris, M. M., Felton, J. S., Healy, S. K., Stuermer, D. H., Berry, P., Timourian, H., and Hatch, F. T. Mutagens from the cooking of food. II. Survey by

Ames/*Salmonella* test of mutagen formation in the major protein-rich foods of the American diet. Food Chem. Toxicol., *20*: 357–363, 1982.

6. Sugimura, T., Sato, S., and Wakabayashi, K. Mutagens/carcinogens in pyrolysates of amino acids and proteins and cooked foods: heterocyclic aromatic amines. *In;* Y. T. Woo *et al.* (eds.), Chemical Induction of Cancer, Structural Bases, and Biological Mechanisms, pp. 681–710, Academic Press, San Diego, 1988.
7. Felton, J. S., Knize, M. G., Shen, N. H., Andresen, B. D., Bjeldanes, L. F., and Hatch, F. T. Identification of the mutagens in cooked beef. Environ. Health Perspect., *67*: 17–24, 1986.
8. Felton, J. S. and Knize, M. G. Heterocyclic amine mutagens/carcinogens in foods. *In;* C. S. Cooper and P. L. Grover (eds.), Handbook of Experimental Pharmacology, Vol. 94/I, pp. 471–502, Springer Verlag, Berlin/Heidelberg, 1990.
9. Ohgaki, H., Kusama, K., Matsukura, N., Morino, K., Hasegawa, H., Sato, S., Takayama, S., and Sugimura, T. Carcinogenicity in mice of a mutagenic compound, 2-amino-3-methylimidazo[4, 5-*f*]quinoline, from broiled sardine, cooked beef and beef extract. Carcinogenesis, *5*: 921–924, 1984.
10. Takayama, S., Nakatsuru, Y., Masuda, M., Ohgaki, H., Sato, S., and Sugimura, T., Demonstration of carcinogenicity in F344 rats of 2-amino-3-methylimidazo[4,5-*f*]-quinoline, from broiled sardine, fried beef and beef extract. Gann, *75*: 467–470, 1984.
11. Ohgaki, H., Hasegawa, H., Suenaga, M., Sato, S., Takayama, S., and Sugimura, T. Carcinogenicity in mice of a mutagenic compound, 2-amino-3,8-dimethylimidazo[4, 5-*f*]quinoxaline (MeIQx) from cooked foods. Carcinogenesis, *8*: 665–688, 1987.
12. Kato, T., Ohgaki, H., Hasegawa, H., Sato, S., Takayama, S., and Sugimura, T. Carcinogenicity in rats of a mutagenic compound, 2-amino-3,8-dimethylimidazo[4, 5-*f*]quinoxaline. Carcinogenesis, *9*: 71–73, 1988.
13. Esumi, H., Ohgaki, H., Kohzen, E., Takayama, S., and Sugimura, T. Induction of lymphoma in $CDF_1$ mice by the food mutagen, 2-amino-1-methyl-6-phenylimidazo[4, 5-*b*]pyridine. Jpn. J. Cancer Res., *80*: 1176–1178, 1989.
14. Adamson, R. H. and Sieber, S. M. The use of nonhuman primates for chemical carcinogenesis studies. *In;* F. Coulston (ed.), Regulatory Aspects of Carcinogenesis and Food Additives, pp. 275–296, Academic Press, New York, 1979.
15. Adamson, R. H. and Sieber, S. M. Chemical carcinogenesis studies in nonhuman primates. *In;* R. Langenbach *et al.* (eds.), Organ and Species Specificity in Chemical Carcinogenesis, pp. 129–156, Plenum Publishing Corp., New York, 1983.
16. Adamson, R. H. Induction of hepatocellular carcinoma in nonhuman primates by chemical carcinogens. Cancer Detect. Prev., *14*: 215–219, 1989.
17. Adamson, R. H., Thorgeirsson, U. P., Snyderwine, E. G., Thorgeirsson, S. S., Reeves, J., Dalgard, D. W., Takayama, S., and Sugimura, T. Carcinogenicity of 2-amino-3-methylimidazo[4,5-*f*]quinoline in nonhuman primates: induction of tumors in three macaques. Jpn. J. Cancer Res., *81*: 10–14, 1990.
18. Snyderwine, E. G., Roller, P. P., Adamson, R. H., Sato, S., and Thorgeirsson, S. S. Reaction of N-hydroxylamine and N-acetoxy derivatives of 2-amino-3-methylimidazo[4, 5-*f*]quinoline with DNA. Synthesis and identification of N-(deoxyguanosine-8-yl)-IQ. Carcinogenesis, *9*: 1061–1065, 1988.
19. Schut, H. A. J., Snyderwine, E. G., Zu, H.-X., and Thorgeirsson, S. S. Similar patterns of DNA adduct formation of 2-amino-3-methylimidazo[4, 5-*f*]quinoline in the Fischer-344 rat, $CDF_1$ mouse and cynomolgus monkey, and *Salmonella typhimurium*. Carcinogenesis, in press.
20. Schut, H. A. J., Putman, K. L., and Randerath, J. DNA adduct formation of the carcinogen 2-amino-3-methylimidazo[4, 5-*f*]quinoline in target tissues of the F344 rat. Cancer Lett., *41*: 345–352, 1988.

XENOBIOTICS AND CANCER, L. ERNSTER ET AL. (EDS.),
JAPAN SCI. SOC. PRESS, TOKYO/TAYLOR & FRANCIS LTD., LONDON, pp. 303–314, 1991

# Natural Chemicals, Synthetic Chemicals, Risk Assessment, and Cancer

Bruce N. AMES and Lois Swirsky GOLD

*Division of Biochemistry and Molecular Biology, University of California, Berkeley, California 94720 and Lawrence Berkeley Laboratory, Berkeley, California 94720, U.S.A.*

*Abstract:* The administration of chemicals at the maximum tolerated dose (MTD) in standard animal cancer tests is postulated to increase cell division (mitogenesis), which in turn increases rates of mutagenesis and thus carcinogenesis. The animal data are consistent with this mechanism, because a high proportion—about half—of all chemicals tested (whether natural or synthetic) are indeed rodent carcinogens. We conclude that at the low doses of most human exposures, where cell killing does not occur, the hazards to humans of rodent carcinogens may be much lower than is commonly assumed.

The toxicological significance of exposures to synthetic chemicals is examined in the context of exposures to naturally occurring chemicals. We calculate that 99.99% (by weight) of the pesticides in the American diet are chemicals that plants produce to defend themselves. Only 52 natural pesticides have been tested in high-dose animal cancer tests, and about half (27) are rodent carcinogens; these 27 are shown to be present in many common foods. We conclude that natural and synthetic chemicals are equally likely to be positive in animal cancer tests.

The toxicology of synthetic chemicals is compared to that of natural chemicals, which represent the vast bulk of the chemicals to which humans are exposed. It is argued that animals have a broad array of inducible general defenses to combat the changing array of toxic chemicals in plant food (nature's pesticides) and that these defenses are effective against both natural and synthetic toxins. Synthetic toxins such as dioxin are compared to natural chemicals, such as indole carbinol (in broccoli) and ethanol. The finding that in high-dose tests, a high proportion of both natural and synthetic chemicals are carcinogens, mutagens, teratogens, and clastogens (30–50% for each group) undermines current regulatory effects based on these tests to protect public health from low doses of synthetic chemicals.

Testing chemicals for carcinogenicity at near-toxic doses in rodents does not provide enough information to predict the excess numbers of human cancers that might occur at low-dose exposures (*1*, *2*). The attempt to prevent cancer by eliminating low levels of synthetic chemicals by "risk assessment", using worst-case, 1 in a million risk scenarios based on rodent tests is not scientifically justified. In addition, this cancer prevention strategy is enormously costly, is counterproductive because it diverts resources from much more important risks, and, in the case of synthetic pesticides makes fruits and vegetables more expensive, thus serving to decrease consumption of foods that help to prevent cancer.

The great concern about traces of synthetic chemicals does not take into account: 1) that the natural world of chemicals makes up the vast bulk of chemicals humans are exposed to (*3*); 2) that the toxicology of synthetic and natural toxins is not fundamentally different (*4*); 3) that about half of the *natural* chemicals tested chronically in rats and mice at the maximum tolerated dose (MTD) are carcinogens (*1, 3*); 4) that testing at the MTD can frequently cause chronic cell killing and consequent cell replacement (a risk factor for cancer that is limited to the high dose) and that ignoring this greatly exaggerates risks (*1*); 5) that an extrapolation from high to low doses should be based on an understanding of the mechanisms of carcinogenesis (*1*).

*Carcinogenesis*

*Mitogenesis increases mutagenesis:* Many "promoters" of carcinogenesis have been described and have been thought to increase mitogenesis and/or selective growth of preneoplastic cells, or both. The concept of promotion, however, has been fuzzy compared to the clearer understanding of the role of mutagenesis in carcinogenesis. The idea that mitogenesis increases mutagenesis helps to explain promotion and other aspects of carcinogenesis (*1, 2*).

A dividing cell is much more at risk of mutating than a quiescent cell (*1*). Mutagens are often thought to be only exogenous agents, but endogenous mutagens cause massive DNA damage (by formation of oxidative and other adducts) that can be converted to stable mutations during cell division (*5, 6*). We estimate that the number of DNA hits per cell per day from endogenous oxidants is normally $\sim 10^5$ in the rat and $\sim 10^4$ in the human (*5, 6*). This promutagenic damage is effectively but not perfectly repaired; the normal steady-state level of 8-hydroxydeoxyguanosine (1 out of about 20 known oxidative DNA adducts) in rat DNA has been measured as 1 per 130,000 bases or about 90,000 per cell (*6*). We have argued that this oxidative DNA damage is a major contributor to aging and the degenerative diseases associated with aging such as cancer (*5*). Thus, any agent causing chronic mitogenesis can be indirectly mutagenic (and consequently carcinogenic) because it increases the probability of converting endogenous DNA damage into mutations (Fig. 1). Nongenotoxic agents (for example, saccharin) can be carcinogens at high doses just by causing cell killing with chronic mitogenesis and inflammation, and the dose response would be expected to show a threshold (*1, 7, 8*). Genotoxic chemicals, because they hit DNA, are even more effective than nongenotoxic chemicals at causing cell killing and cell replacement at high doses. Since genotoxic chemicals also act as mutagens, they can produce a multiplicative interaction not found at low doses, leading to an upward curving dose response for carcinogenicity (*1, 8*). Furthermore, endogenous rates of DNA damage are so high that it may be difficult for exogenous mutagens to increase DNA damage rates significantly at low doses that do not increase mitogenesis. Therefore, mitogenesis, which can be increased by high doses of chemicals, is indirectly mutagenic, and seems to explain much of carcinogenesis (*1, 7, 9*). Nevertheless, potent

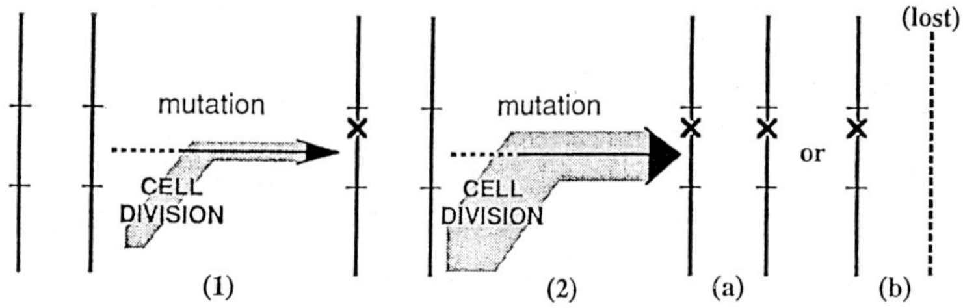


FIG. 1. Mitogenesis (induced cell division) is a major multiplier of endogenous (or exogenous) DNA damage leading to mutation. The pathway to inactivating (X) both copies of a recessive tumor-suppressor gene is shown (two vertical lines represent the pair of chromosomes carrying the genes). Cell division increases mutagenesis due to the following: DNA adducts converted to mutations before they are repaired (1 and 2a); mutations due to DNA replication (1 and 2a); vulnerability of replicating DNA to damage (1 and 2a). Mitotic recombination (2a), gene conversion (2a), and nondisjunction (2b) are more frequent, and the first two give rise to the same mutation on both chromosomes. This diagram does not attempt to deal with the complex mutational pathway to tumors.

mutagens induce tumors at moderate doses in the presence of only background rates of mitogenesis (*8*). Mutation through mitogenesis is not of interest in those cells that are discarded (*e.g.*, epithelial tissues) or killed through apoptosis (*e.g.*, liver). Detailed studies of mechanism are critically important.

*Causes of human cancer:* Henderson and co-workers (*10, 11*) and others (*1*) have discussed the importance of chronic mitogenesis for many, if not most, of the known causes of human cancer, *e.g.*, hormones in breast cancer; hepatitis B (*12*) or C viruses or alcohol in liver cancer; high salt or *Helicobacter* (*Campylobacter*) infection in stomach cancer; papilloma virus in cervical cancer; asbestos or tobacco smoke in lung cancer; and excess animal fat and low calcium in colon cancer. For chemical carcinogens associated with occupational cancer, worker exposure has been primarily at high, near-toxic, doses that might be expected to induce mitogenesis.

Epidemiologists are frequently discovering clues about the causes of human cancer, and the resulting hypotheses are then refined by animal and metabolic studies. During the next decade, it appears likely that this approach will lead to an understanding of the causes of the major human cancers. Current epidemiologic data point to several risk factors for human cancer: cigarette smoking (which is responsible for 30% of cancer deaths), dietary imbalances, infections, hormones, and occupation. "The age adjusted mortality rate for all cancers combined except lung cancer has been declining since 1950 for all individual age groups except 85 and above" (*13*). Although incidence rates for some cancers have been rising, trends in recorded incidence rates may be biased by improved registration and diagnosis. Even though mortality rates for cancers at particular sites can be shown to be increasing (for example, non-Hodgkins lymphoma, melanoma) or decreasing (for example, stomach, cervical, rectal), establishing causes remains difficult because of the many changing aspects of our lifestyle. Life expectancy continues to increase every year.

Cancer clusters in small areas are expected to be common by chance alone, and epidemiology lacks the power to establish causality in these cases (*14*). It is important to show that a pollution exposure that purportedly causes a cancer cluster is significantly greater than the background of exposures to naturally occurring rodent carcinogens.

*Causes of cancer in animal tests:* Animal cancer tests are conducted at near-toxic doses (MTD) of the test chemical for long periods of time, which can cause chronic mitogenesis (*1, 7, 9*). Chronic dosing at the MTD can be thought of as chronic wounding, which is known to be both a promoter of carcinogenesis in animals and a risk factor for cancer in humans. Thus, a high percentage of all chemicals might be expected to be carcinogenic at chronic, near-toxic doses and this is exactly what is found. About half of all chemicals tested chronically at the MTD are carcinogens (*1, 3*).

Synthetic chemicals account for 82% (350/427) of the chemicals adequately tested in both rats and mice (*1*). Despite the fact that humans eat vastly more natural than synthetic chemicals, the world of natural chemicals has never been tested systematically (*3*). Of the natural chemicals tested, approximately half are carcinogens, which is approximately the same as has been found for synthetic chemicals (*1, 3*). It is unlikely that the high proportion of carcinogens in rodent studies is due simply to selection of suspicious chemical structures: most chemicals were selected because of their use as industrial compounds, pesticides, drugs, or food additives. Moreover, historically our knowledge to predict carcinogenicity has been inadequate.

## *Nature's Pesticides*

"Plants are not just food for animals. . . . The world is not green. It is colored lectin, tannin, cyanide, caffeine, aflatoxin, and canavanine" (*15*).

### *1. Dietary pesticides are 99.99% all natural*

Nature's pesticides are one important subset of natural chemicals (*3*). Plants produce toxins to protect themselves against fungi, insects, and animal predators. Tens of thousands of these natural pesticides have been discovered, and every species of plant analyzed contains its own set of perhaps a few dozen toxins. When plants are stressed or damaged, such as during a pest attack, they may greatly increase their natural pesticide levels, occasionally to levels that can be acutely toxic to humans. We estimate that Americans eat about 1.5 g of natural pesticides per person per day, which is about 10,000 times more than they eat of synthetic pesticide residues.

Concentrations of natural pesticides in plants are usually measured in parts per thousand or million rather than parts per billion, the usual concentration of synthetic pesticide residues or of water pollutants (*1*). We estimate that humans ingest roughly 5,000 to 10,000 different natural pesticides and their breakdown products (*1*). For example, 49 natural pesticides (and metabolites) are ingested when cabbage is eaten: only 2 have been tested for carcinogenicity (*1*). Lima beans contain a completely different array of 23 natural toxins that, in stressed plants, range in concentration from 0.2 to 33 parts per thousand fresh weight; none appears to have been tested yet for carcinogenicity or teratogenicity (*16*). Many Leguminosae contain canavanine, a toxic arginine analog that, after being eaten by animals, is incorporated into protein in place of arginine. Feeding alfalfa sprouts (1.5% canavanine dry weight) or canavanine to monkeys causes a lupus erythematosus-like syndrome (*17*). Lupus in humans is characterized by a defect in the immune system that is associated with autoimmunity, antinuclear antibodies, chromosome breaks and various types of pathology. The toxicity of nonfood plants is well known: plants are among the most commonly ingested poisonous substances for children under 5 years.

Surprisingly few plant toxins have been tested for carcinogenicity (*3*). Among 1,052 chemicals tested in at least one species in chronic cancer tests, only 52 are naturally occurring plant pesticides (*3*). Among these, about half (27/52) are carcinogenic. Even though only a tiny proportion of the plant toxins in our diet has been tested so far, the 27 natural pesticides that are rodent carcinogens are present in the following foods: (those at levels greater than 10 ppm are in *italics*): *anise*, *apple*, apricot, banana, *basil*, broccoli, *Brussels sprouts*, *cabbage*, cantaloupe, *caraway*, *carrot*, *cauliflower*, *celery*, *cherries*, cinnamon, cloves, cocoa, *coffee* (brewed), collard greens, *comfrey herb tea*, currants, *dill*, *eggplant*, *endive*, *fennel*, *grapefruit juice*, *grapes*, guava, *honey*, honeydew melon, *horseradish*, kale, lentils, *lettuce*, *mango*, *mushrooms*, *mustard* (brown), *nutmeg*, *orange juice*, *parsley*, *parsnip*, peach, *pear*, peas, *pepper* (black), pineapple, *plum*, *potato*, radish, raspberries, *rosemary*, *sage*, *sesame seeds* (heated), *tarragon*, tea, *thyme*, tomato, and turnip. Thus, it is probable that almost every fruit and vegetable in the market contains natural plant pesticides that are rodent carcinogens. The levels of these 27 rodent carcinogens in the above plants are commonly thousands of times higher than the levels of synthetic pesticides.

Caution is necessary in interpreting the implications of ingesting natural pesticides that are rodent carcinogens. It is not argued here that these dietary exposures are necessarily of much relevance to human cancer. What is important in our analysis is that exposures to natural rodent carcinogens may cast doubt on the relevance of far lower levels of exposures to synthetic rodent carcinogens. Particular natural pesticides that are carcinogenic in rodents can be bred out of crops if studies of mechanism indicate that they may be significant hazards to humans.

2. *Residues of synthetic pesticides*

The U.S. Food and Drug Administration (FDA) has assayed food for 200 chemicals, including the synthetic pesticide residues thought to be of greatest importance and the residues of some industrial chemicals such as polychlorinated biphenyls (PCBs) (*18*). The FDA found residues for 105 of these chemicals: the U.S. intake of the sum of these 105 chemicals averages about 0.09 mg per person per day, which we compare to 1.5 g of natural pesticides (*i.e.*, 99.99% natural). Other analyses of synthetic pesticide residues are similar (*19*). About half (0.04 mg) of this daily intake of synthetic pesticides is composed of 4 chemicals (*18*) that were not carcinogenic in rodent tests: ethylhexyl diphenyl phosphate, chlorpropham, malathion, and dicloran. Thus, the intake of known or potential rodent carcinogens from synthetic residues is only about 0.05 mg a day (averaging about 0.06 ppm in plant food).

Synthetic pesticides have markedly lowered the cost of plant food, thus increasing consumption. Eating more fruits and vegetables and less fat appears to be the best way to lower risks of cancer and heart disease, other than giving up smoking.

*Cooking food:* The cooking of food is also a major dietary source of potential rodent carcinogens. Cooking produces about 2 g (per person per day) of mostly untested burnt material that contains many rodent carcinogens—*e.g.*, polycyclic hydrocarbons, heterocyclic amines (*20, 21*), furfural, nitrosamines and nitroaromatics—as well as a plethora of mutagens (*20, 22*). Thus, the number and amounts of carcinogenic (or total) synthetic pesticide residues appear to be minimal compared to the background of naturally-occurring chemicals in the diet. Roasted coffee, for example, is known to contain 826 volatile chemicals; 21 have been tested chronically and 16 are rodent carcinogens; caffeic acid, a non-volatile rodent carcinogen, is also present (*3*). A typical cup of coffee contains at least 10 mg (40 ppm) of rodent carcinogens (mostly caffeic acid, catechol, furfural, hydroquinone, and hydrogen peroxide) (*3*). Thus, the 10 mg of known natural rodent carcinogens in a cup of coffee (only a few percent of the chemicals have been tested) would be equivalent in amount ingested to about a year's worth of synthetic pesticide residue carcinogens (assuming half of the potentially carcinogenic synthetic residues will be).

The evidence on coffee and human health has been recently reviewed, and the evidence to date is insufficient to show that coffee is a risk factor for cancer in humans. The same caution discussed above about the implications for humans of natural rodent carcinogens in the diet apply to coffee and the products of cooked food.

*The case of dioxin:* Cabbage and broccoli contain a chemical whose breakdown products bind to the body's Ah receptor, induce the defense enzymes under the control of the receptors, and possibly cause mitogenesis—just as does dioxin (2,3,7,8-tetrachlorodibenzo-*p*-dioxin, TCDD), one of the most feared industrial contaminants. TCDD is of great public concern because it is carcinogenic and teratogenic in rodents at extremely low doses. The doses humans ingest are, however, far lower than the lowest doses that have been shown to cause cancer and reproductive damage in rodents.

TCDD exerts many or all of its harmful effects in mammalian cells through binding to the Ah receptor (*23*). A wide variety of natural substances also bind to the Ah receptor, (*e.g.*, tryptophan oxidation products (*24*)), and insofar as they have been examined, they have similar properties to TCDD. A cooked steak, for example, contains polycyclic hydrocarbons that bind to the Ah receptor and mimic TCDD. In addition, a variety of flavones and other plant substances in the diet, such as indole carbinol (IC), also bind to the Ah receptor. IC is the main breakdown compound of glucobrassicin, a glucosinolate that is present in large amounts in vegetables of the *Brassica* genus, including broccoli (about 25 mg per 100 g portion), Brussels sprouts (125 mg per 100 g), and cabbage (25 mg per 100 g) (*25, 26*). When tissues of these vegetables are lacerated, as occurs during chewing, they release an enzyme that breaks down the glucobrassicin. The enzyme is quite heat stable, and cooked vegetables yield most of the indole compounds that raw vegetables do (*27*). Therefore, we assume for the following calculation that 20% of glucobrassicin is converted to IC on eating. At the pH of the stomach, IC makes dimers and trimers that induce the same set of detoxifying enzymes as TCDD (*27–29*). IC, like TCDD, protects against carcinogenesis when given *before* aflatoxin or other carcinogens (*29–31*). However, when given *after* aflatoxin or other carcinogens, IC, like TCDD, stimulates carcinogenesis (*28*). This stimulation of carcinogenesis has also been shown for cabbage itself.

These IC dimers and trimers appear to be much more of a potential hazard than TCDD, assuming that binding to the Ah receptor is critical for, toxic effect. The Environmental Protection Agency's human "reference dose" (formerly "acceptable dose limit") of TCDD is 6 fg per kg per day. This should be compared with 5 mg of IC per 100 g of broccoli or cabbage (*3*). Although the affinity of one major indole dimer in binding to Ah receptors is less than that of TCDD by a factor of about 8,000 (Bjeldanes and Bradfield, personal communication), the effective dose to the Ah receptor from a helping of broccoli would be about 1,500 times higher than that of TCDD, taking into account an extra factor of 1,000 for the very long lifetime of TCDD in the body (several years) and assuming that the lifetime of the hydrophobic indole dimers is as short as 1 day. Another IC dimer has recently been shown to bind to the Ah receptor with about the same affinity as TCDD (Bjeldanes, personal communication). However, it is not clear whether at the low doses of human exposure either IC or TCDD is hazardous; they may even be protective. It seems likely that many more of these natural "dioxin simulators" will be discovered in the future.

If TCDD is compared with ethanol it seems of minor interest as a teratogen or carcinogen. Alcoholic beverages are the most important known human chemical teratogen (*32*). In contrast, there is no persuasive evidence that TCDD is either carcinogenic or teratogenic in humans, although it is both at near-toxic doses in rodents. If one compares the teratogenic potential of TCDD to that of alcohol (after adjusting for their respective teratogenic potency as determined in rodent tests), then a daily consumption of the Environmental Protection Agency's reference dose of TCDD (6 fg per kg) would be equivalent in teratogenic potential to a daily consumption of alcohol from 1/3,000,000th of a beer. That is equivalent to drinking a single beer (15 g ethyl alcohol) over a period of 8,000 years.

Alcoholic beverages in humans are a risk factor for cancer as well as for birth defects. A comparison of the carcinogenic potential for rodents of TCDD with that of alcohol (adjusting for the potency in rodents) (*4*) shows that ingesting the TCDD reference dose of 6 fg per kg per day is equivalent to ingesting 1 beer every 345 years. Since the average consumption of alcohol in the United States is equivalent to more than 1 beer per person per day, and since 5 drinks a day are a carcinogenic risk in humans, the experimental evidence does not of itself seem to justify the great concern over TCDD at levels in the range of the reference dose.

### *The Toxicology of Synthetic and Natural Toxins Is Similar*

It is often assumed that, because plants are part of human evolutionary history whereas synthetic chemicals are recent, the mechanisms that animals have evolved to cope with the toxicity of natural chemicals will fail to protect us against synthetic chemicals. "For the first time in the history of the world, every human being is now subjected to contact with dangerous chemicals, from the moment of conception until death" (*33*). We find this assumption flawed for several reasons.

*Defenses that animals have evolved are mostly of a general type*, as might be expected, since the number of natural chemicals that might have toxic effects is so large (*4*). General defenses offer protection not only against natural but also against synthetic chemicals, making humans well buffered against toxins (*4*). These defenses include the following: (a) the continuous shedding of cells exposed to toxins: the surface layers of the mouth, esophagus, stomach, intestine, colon, skin, and lungs are discarded every few days. (b) The induction of a wide variety of general detoxifying mechanisms, such as antioxidant defenses or the Phase II electrophile-detoxifying systems, *e.g.*, glutathione transferases. Cells that are exposed to small doses of an oxidant, such as radiation or hydrogen peroxide, induce antioxidant defenses and become more resistant to higher doses, whether the oxidant in synthetic or natural. Natural or synthetic electrophiles induce Phase II detoxifying enzymes that are effective against both. (c) The active excretion of planar hydrophobic molecules (natural or synthetic) out of liver and intestinal cells. (d) DNA repair: this is effective against DNA adducts formed from both synthetic and natural chemicals, and is inducible in response to DNA damage.

Anticarcinogenic chemicals in the diet, *e.g.*, antioxidants, help to protect humans against carcinogens, but do not distinguish between synthetic and natural carcinogens. It has been argued that synergism between synthetic carcinogens could multiply hazards, but this is equally true of natural carcinogens.

The fact that defenses are usually general, rather than specific for each chemical, makes good evolutionary sense. The reason that predators of plants evolved general defenses against toxins is presumably to be prepared to counter a diverse and ever-changing array of plant toxins in an evolving world; if a herbivore had defenses against only a set of specific toxins it would be at a great disadvantage in obtaining new foods when favored foods became scarce or evolved new toxins.

Various natural toxins, some of which have been present throughout vertebrate evolutionary history, nevertheless cause cancer in vertebrates. Mold aflatoxins, for example, have been shown to cause cancer in trout, rats, mice, monkeys, and possibly in humans. Eleven mold toxins out of 16 tested have been reported to be carcinogenic (*3*). Many of the common elements are carcinogenic (*e.g.*, salts of lead, cadmium, beryllium, nickel, chromium, selenium, and arsenic), or clastogenic at high doses, despite their presence throughout evolution (*3, 4*). Selenium and chromium are essential trace elements in animal nutrition.

Humans have not had time to evolve into a "toxic harmony" with all of the plants in their diet. Indeed, very few of the plants that humans eat would have been present in an African hunter-gatherer's diet. The human diet has changed drastically in the last few thousand years, and most humans are eating many recently introduced plants that their ancestors did not—*e.g.*, coffee, cocoa, tea, potatoes, tomatoes, corn, avocados, mangoes, olives, and kiwi fruit. In addition, cruciferous vegetables such as cabbage, broccoli, kale, cauliflower, and mustard were used in ancient times "primarily for medicinal purposes" and were spread as foods across Europe only in the Middle Ages (*3, 4*). Natural selection works far too slowly for humans to have evolved specific resistance to the food toxins in these newly introduced plants.

DDT bioconcentrates in the food chain due to its unusual lipophilicity; however, natural toxins can also bioconcentrate. DDT is often viewed as the typically dangerous synthetic pesticide because it persists for years; it is representative of a class of chlorinated pesticides. Natural pesticides, however, also bioconcentrate if lipophilic: for example, the teratogens from potato, solanine (and its aglycone solanidine), and chaconine are found in the tissues of potato eaters (*34–36*). Although DDT was unusual with respect to bioconcentration, it was remarkably non-toxic to mammals, saved millions of lives, and has not been shown to cause harm to humans (*37*). To a large extent DDT, the first major synthetic insecticide, replaced lead arsenate, a major pesticide used before the modern era; lead arsenate is even more persistent than DDT, and although natural, both lead and arsenic are carcinogenic. When the undesirable bioconcentration and persistence of DDT and its lethal effects on some birds were recognized, it was prudently phased out, and less persistent chemicals were developed to replace it. Examples are the synthetic pyrethroids that disrupt the same sodium channel in insects as DDT, are degraded rapidly in the environment, and can often be used at a concentration as low as a few grams per acre.

Positive results are remarkably common in high-dose screening tests for carcinogens, clastogens (agents that break chromosomes), teratogens, and mutagens. About half of the chemicals tested, whether natural or synthetic, are carcinogens in chronic, high-dose rodent tests (*1*, *3*) and about half are clastogens in tissue culture tests (*38*). A high proportion of positives is also reported for rodent teratogenicity tests: 38% of the 2,800 chemicals tested in laboratory animals "have been teratogenic" in the standard, high-dose protocol (*39*). It is therefore reasonable to assume that a sizeable percentage of both synthetic and natural chemicals will be reproductive toxins at high doses. Mutagens may also be common: of 340 chemicals tested for carcinogenicity in both rats and mice and for mutagenicity in *Salmonella*, 46% were mutagens, and mutagens were nearly twice as likely to be carcinogenic than were non-mutagens (*40*; Gold, unpublished). Of these 340 chemicals, 70% were either mutagens or carcinogens or both. How much this high frequency of positive results is due to bias in selecting chemicals is not known. Even if selection bias doubled the percentage of positives, which we think is unlikely, the high proportion of positives would still mean that almost everything natural we eat contains carcinogens, mutagens, teratogens, and clastogens. Thus, testing a random group of natural pesticides and pyrolysis products from cooking should be a high priority for these various tests so an adequate comparison can be made to synthetic toxins.

These arguments undermine many assumptions of current regulatory policy and necessitate a rethinking of policy designed to reduce human cancer. Minimizing pollution is a separate issue and is clearly desirable for reasons other than effects on public health. There is a sizeable literature on why focussing on worst-case, 1 in a million risks, rather than major risks "impedes intelligent risk reduction" (*41*).

It is by no means clear that many significant risk factors for human cancer will be discovered by screening assays. Dietary imbalances, such as antioxidant (*32*, *42*, *43*) and folate (*44*) deficiencies, are likely to be major contributors to human cancer, and understanding these should be, but is not, a major priority of research. Understanding why caloric restriction dramatically lowers mitogenesis rates and cancer rates and extends life-span in experimental animals (*45–47*) should also be a major research priority. More studies on mechanisms of carcinogenesis should also be of high priority.

*Acknowledgment*

This paper was adapted in part from references *1–4* which present the arguments in more detail.

## REFERENCES

1. Ames, B. N. and Gold, L. S. Chemical carcinogenesis: too many rodent carcinogens. Proc. Natl. Acad. Sci. U.S.A., *87*: 7772–7776, 1990.
2. Ames, B. N. and Gold, L. S. Too many rodent carcinogens: mitogenesis increases mutagenesis. Science, *249*: 970–971, 1990.

3. Ames, B. N., Profet, M., and Gold, L. S. Dietary pesticides (99.99% all natural). Proc. Natl. Acad. Sci. U.S.A., *87*: 7777–7781, 1990.
4. Ames, B. N., Profet, M., and Gold, L. S. Nature's chemicals and synthetic chemicals: comparative toxicology. Proc. Natl. Acad. Sci. U.S.A., *87*: 7782–7786, 1990.
5. Ames, B. N. Endogenous oxidative DNA damage, aging, and cancer. Free Rad. Res. Commun., *7*: 121–128, 1989.
6. Fraga, C. G., Shigenaga, M. K., Park, J.-W., Degan, P., and Ames, B. N. Oxidative damage to DNA during aging: 8-hydroxy-2′-deoxyguanosine in rat organ DNA and urine. Proc. Natl. Acad. Sci. U.S.A., *87*: 4533–4537, 1990.
7. Butterworth, B. E. and Slaga, T. (eds.). Chemically Induced Cell Proliferation: Implications for Risk Assessment, Alan R. Liss, New York, 1990.
8. Cohen, S. M. and Ellwein, L. B. Cell proliferation in carcinogenesis, Science, *249*: 1007–1011, 1990.
9. Bernstein, L., Gold, L. S., Ames, B. N., Pike, M. C., and Hoel, D. G. Some tautologous aspects of the comparison of carcinogenic potency in rats and mice. Fund. Appl. Toxicol., *5*: 79–86, 1985.
10. Henderson, B. E., Ross, R., and Bernstein, L. Estrogens as a cause of human cancer: The Richard and Hinda Rosenthal Foundation Award Lecture. Cancer Res., *48*: 246–253, 1988.
11. Preston-Martin, S., Pike, M. C., Ross, R. K., Jones, P. A., and Henderson, B. E. Increased cell division as a cause of human cancer. Cancer Res., *50*: 7415–7421, 1990.
12. Dunsford, H. A., Sell, S., and Chisari, F. V. Hepatocarcinogenesis due to chronic liver cell injury in hepatitis B virus transgenic mice. Cancer Res., *50*: 3400–3407, 1990.
13. National Cancer Institute, 1987 Annual Cancer Statistics Review Including Cancer Trends: 1950–1985, NIH Pub. No. 88–2789, National Institutes of Health, Bethesda, Maryland, 1988.
14. Higginson, J. Changing concepts in cancer prevention: limitations and implications for future research in environmental carcinogenesis. Cancer Res., *48*: 1381–1389, 1988.
15. Janzen, D. H. Promising directions of study in tropical animal plant interactions. Ann. Missouri Bot. Gard., *64*: 706–736, 1977.
16. Green, M. B. and Hedin, P. A. (eds.). Natural Resistance of Plants to Pests: Roles of Allelochemicals, ACS Symposium 296, American Chemical Society, Washington, D. C., 1986.
17. Malinow, M. R., Bardana, E. J., Jr., Pirofsky, B., Craig, S., and McLaughlin, P. Systemic lupus erythematosus-like syndrome in monkeys fed alfalfa sprouts: role of a nonprotein amino acid. Science, *216*: 415–417, 1982.
18. Gunderson, E. L. FDA total diet study, April 1982–April 1984, Dietary intakes of pesticides, selected elements, and other chemicals. J. Assoc. Off. Anal. Chem., *71*: 1200–1209, 1988.
19. Nigg, H. N., Beier, R. C., Carter, O., Chaisson, C., Franklin, C., Lavy, T., Lewis, R. G., Lombardo, P., McCarthy, J. F., Maddy, K. T., Moses, M., Norris, D., Peck, C., Skinner, K., and Tardiff, R. G. *In*: S. R. Baker and C. F. Wilkinson (eds.). The Effects of Pesticides on Human Health, Vol. XVIII, pp. 35–130, Princeton Scientific Publishing Co. Inc., Princeton, New Jersey, 1990.
20. Sugimura, T. Successful use of short-term tests for academic purposes: their use in identification of new environmental carcinogens with possible risk for humans. Mutat. Res., *205*: 33–39, 1988.
21. Takayama, S., Nakatsuru, Y., and Sato, S. Carcinogenic effect of the simultaneous administration of five heterocyclic amines to F344 rats. Jpn. J. Cancer Res. (Gann), *78*: 1068–1072, 1987.

22. Environ. Health Perspect. Dietary Mutagens (special issue), *67*: 1986.
23. Knutson, J. C. and Poland, A. Response of murine epidermis to 2,3,7,8-tetrachlorodibenzo-*p*-dioxin: Interaction of the *Ah* and *hr* loci. Cell, *30*: 225–234, 1982.
24. Rannug, A., Rannug, U., Rosenkranz, H. S., Winqvist, L., Westerholm, R., Agurell, E., and Grafstrom, A.-K. Certain photooxidized derivatives of tryphtophan bind with very high affinity to the Ah receptor and are likely to be endogenous signal substances. J. Biol. Chem., *262*: 15422–15427, 1987.
25. Carlson, D. G., Daxinbichler, M. E., Van Etten, C. H., Kwolek, W. F., and Williams, P. H. Glucosinolates in crucifer vegetables: Broccoli, Brussels sprouts, cauliflower, collards, kale, mustard greens, and kohlrabi. J. Am. Soc. Hort. Sci., *112*: 173–178, 1987.
26. McDanell, R., McLean, A. E. M., Hanley, A. B., Heaney, R. K., and Fenwick, G. R. Chemical and biological properties of indole glucosinolates (glucobrassicins): A review. Food Chem. Toxicol., *26*: 59–70, 1988.
27. Bradfield, C. A. and Bjeldanes, L. F. High-performance liquid chromatographic analysis of anticarcinogenic indoles in *Brassica olereacea*. J. Agric. Food Chem., *35*: 46–49, 1987.
28. Bradfield, C. A. and Bjeldanes, L. F. Structure-activity relationships of dietary indoles: a proposed mechanism of action as modifiers of xenobiotic metabolism. J. Toxicol. Environ. Health, *21*: 311–323, 1987.
29. Michnovicz, J. J. and Bradlow, H. L. Induction of estradiol metabolism by dietary indole-3-carbinol in humans. J. Natl. Cancer Inst., *82*: 947–949, 1990.
30. Dashwood, R. H., Arbogast, D. N., Fong, A. T., Hendricks, J. D., and Bailey, G. S. Mechanisms of anti-carcinogenesis by indole-3-carbinol: Detailed *in vivo* DNA binding dose-response studies after dietary administration with aflatoxin B1. Carcinogenesis, *9*: 427–432, 1988.
31. Bailey, G. S., Hendricks, J. D., Shelton, D. W., Nixon, J. E., and Pawlowski, N. E. Enhancement of carcinogenesis by the natural anticarcinogen indole-3-carbinol. J. Natl. Cancer Inst., *78*: 931–934, 1987.
32. National Research Council. Diet and Health, Implications for Reducing Chronic Disease Risk, National Academy Press, Washington, D. C., 1989.
33. Carson, R. Silent Spring, pp. 15, Houghton Mifflin, Boston, Massachusetts 1962.
34. Matthew, J. A., Morgan, M. R. A., McNerney, R., Chan, H. W.-S., and Coxon, D. T. Determination of solandine in human plasma by radioimmunoassay. Food Chem. Toxicol., *21*: 637–640, 1983.
35. Harvey, M. H., Morris, B. A., McMillan, M., and Marks, V. Measurement of potato steroidal alkaloids in human serum and saliva by radioimmunoassay. Human Toxicol., *4*: 503–512, 1985.
36. Claringbold, W. D. B., Few, J. D., and Renwick, J. H. Kinetics and retention of solanidine in man. Xenobiotica, *12*: 293–302, 1982.
37. Jukes, T. H. Insecticides in health, agriculture and the environment. Naturwissenschaften, *61*: 6–16, 1974.
38. Ishidate, M. Jr. Harnois, M. C., and Sofuni, T. A comparative analysis of data on the clastogenicity of 951 chemical substances tested in mammalian cell cultures. Mutat. Res., *195*: 151–213, 1988.
39. Schardein, J. L. Chemically Induced Birth Defects. Marcel Dekker, New York, 1985.
40. Gold, L. S., Bernstein, L., Magaw, R. and Slone, T. H. Interspecies extrapolation in carcinogenesis: prediction between rats and mice. Env. Health Perspect., *81*: 211–219, 1989.
41. Zeckhauser, R. J. and Viscusi, W. K., Risk within reason. Science, *248*: 559–564, 1990.

42. National Research Council. Diet, Nutrition, and Cancer. National Academy Press, Washington, D. C., 1982.
43. Reddy, B. S. and Cohen, L. A. (eds.). Diet, Nutrition, and Cancer: A Critical Evaluation, Vols. I and II, CRC Press, Boca Raton, Florida, 1986.
44. MacGregor, J. T., Schlegel, R., Wehr, C. M., Alperin, P., and Ames, B. N. Cytogenetic damage induced by folate deficiency in mice is enhanced by caffeine. Proc. Natl. Acad. Sci. U.S.A., *87*: 9962–9965, 1990.
45. Roe, F. J. C. Non-genotoxic carcinogenesis: implications for testing and extrapolation to man. Mutagenesis, *4*: 407–411, 1989.
46. Lok, E., Scott, F. W., Mongeau, R., Nera, E. A., Malcolm, S., and Clayson, D. G. Calorie restriction and cellular proliferation in various tissues of the female Swiss Webster mouse. Cancer Lett., *51*: 67–73, 1990.
47. Heller, T. D., Holt, P. R., and Richardson, A. Food restriction retards age-related histological changes in rat small intestine. Gastroenterology, *98*: 387–391, 1990.

# BIOMONITORING

XENOBIOTICS AND CANCER, L. ERNSTER ET AL. (EDS.),
JAPAN SCI. SOC. PRESS, TOKYO/TAYLOR & FRANCIS LTD., LONDON, pp. 317–328, 1991

# Monitoring Carcinogen Actions on DNA by $^{32}$P-postlabeling

Kurt Randerath and Erika Randerath

*Division of Toxicology, Department of Pharmacology, Baylor College of Medicine, Houston, Texas 77030, U.S.A.*

*Abstract:* Among several recently developed analytical methods, $^{32}$P-postlabeling analysis is a highly sensitive method for the detection and measurement of covalent carcinogen-DNA adducts and other DNA modifications. Since the method does not require radioactive carcinogens, it is suitable for DNA of humans exposed to environmental or occupational genotoxicants. The basic procedure entails the enzymatic incorporation of $^{32}$P-label into monomeric or dimeric hydrolysis products of DNA, followed by chromatographic mapping and autoradiography of the $^{32}$P-labeled digestion products and quantitation by scintillation spectrometry. Microgram amounts of DNA are analyzed; thus the assay is well suited for limited amounts of cells or tissue. Various versions of the assay afford different sensitivities of adduct detection. Under optimal conditions, one aromatic or bulky/hydrophobic adduct in $10^8$–$10^{10}$ nucleotides can be detected and measured (corresponding to 0.3–30 amol adduct/microgram DNA or 0.1–10 nmol adduct/mol DNA-P). The assay has been successfully applied to a variety of mutagenic (genotoxic) as well as non-mutagenic carcinogens. In humans, the $^{32}$P-postlabeling assay has been applied to DNA specimens from cigarette smokers, iron foundry workers, and coke oven workers. Estimation of total aromatic adduct levels in exposed individuals gave values of 1 adduct in $10^6$–$10^8$ DNA nucleotides. These values are similar to the total levels of persistent adducts in tissues of animals after exposure to initiating or carcinogenic doses of authentic aromatic genotoxicants. Among the non-mutagenic carcinogens investigated are estrogens, 2,3,7,8-tetrachlorodibenzo-*p*-dioxin (TCDD), choline-devoid diet, carbon tetrachloride, and peroxisome proliferators. In addition, age-dependent DNA modifications (I-compounds) are being detected by $^{32}$P-postlabeling in animals that have not been knowingly exposed to mutagens/carcinogens. I-compound profiles and levels are dependent on species, tissue, sex, and diet. Reduced levels of I-compounds have been consistently noted in the target organ of carcinogen-exposed animals and in resulting neoplasms, suggesting that I-compound loss may play a role in carcinogenesis.

Numerous lines of evidence indicate that naturally occurring and man-made chemicals play a significant role in the etiology of human cancer (*1*). In experimental animals and cultured human cells, most chemical carcinogens are activated chemically or metabolically to electrophiles which react with DNA, RNA and proteins, resulting in the formation of covalent adducts, and ample experimental evidence suggests that formation of premutagenic DNA adducts is a critical event in the initiation of multistage chemical carcinogenesis (*2*, *3*).

While several excellent short-term *in vitro* assays employing bacteria, lower eukaryotes or mammalian cells in culture are available for the detection of genotoxic activity of chemicals (*4–6*), they do not accurately mimic the *in vivo* situation, which entails complex biological interactions such as absorption, distribution, bioactivation, detoxication, DNA repair, and loss of genetically damaged cells by attrition. In addition, these parameters are strongly dependent on species, age, sex, nutritional status, cell type, and tissue as well as on chronobiological effects. Radioactive carcinogens or antibodies specific to known adducts or classes of adducts have been utilized for detection of carcinogen-induced DNA damage *in vivo* (*7*, *8*); however, since these techniques cannot be readily applied to the large number of chemicals in the human environment, alternative techniques are needed.

$^{32}$P-postlabeling represents a general and sensitive approach for the measurement of DNA lesions formed with nonradioactive mutagens/carcinogens (*9–11*), entailing $^{32}$P-labeling of normal and modified (adducted) nucleotides, chromatographic separation, and quantitation by scintillation spectrometry. The $^{32}$P-assay has been applied to DNA preparations modified by over 100 test chemicals, comprising arylamines, arylamides, nitroaromatics, nitrosamines, azocompounds, dyestuffs, polycyclic aromatic hydrocarbons, heterocyclic polycyclic aromatics, epoxides, and methylating agents, as well as mycotoxins, alkenylbenzenes, antibiotics, estrogens, peroxisome proliferators, carbon tetrachloride, and polychlorinated dibenzo-*p*-dioxins. DNA alterations associated with exposures to complex mixtures and unidentified sources have also been detected by $^{32}$P-postlabeling. In addition, endogenous DNA modifications (I-compounds) have been detected in untreated animals (*12*) and the modulation of these compounds by non-mutagenic carcinogens has been studied (*13–17*). This review presents the basic principles of the assay, followed by an overview of various applications. Examples are mainly from the authors' laboratory.

### *General Method*

The basic method (Fig. 1) (*9–11*, *18*, *19*) entails the nucleolytic digestion of DNA to 3′-mononucleotides, subsequent conversion of these digestion products to 5′-$^{32}$P-labeled 3′, 5′-bisphosphate derivatives with [$\gamma$-$^{32}$P]ATP as the donor of label and T4 polynucleotide kinase as the catalyst, separation of the labeled nucleotides by polyethyleneimine (PEI)-cellulose thin layer chromatography (TLC), autoradiography to detect adducts and normal nucleotides, and scintillation spectrometry for quantitation. Separation of aromatic or bulky/hydrophobic adducts from the usually large excess of normal DNA nucleotides is accomplished by PEI-cellulose TLC employing non-denaturing solvents as the mobile phase. The various versions of the assay are illustrated in Fig. 2. In procedures 1 and 2, adducts are labeled in the presence of the normal DNA nucleotides, while in procedures 3, 4, and 5, normal nucleotides are removed before $^{32}$P-labeling. Physical (procedure 3) (*20*) and enzymatic (procedures 4 and 5) (*19*, *21*) techniques have been described. The latter

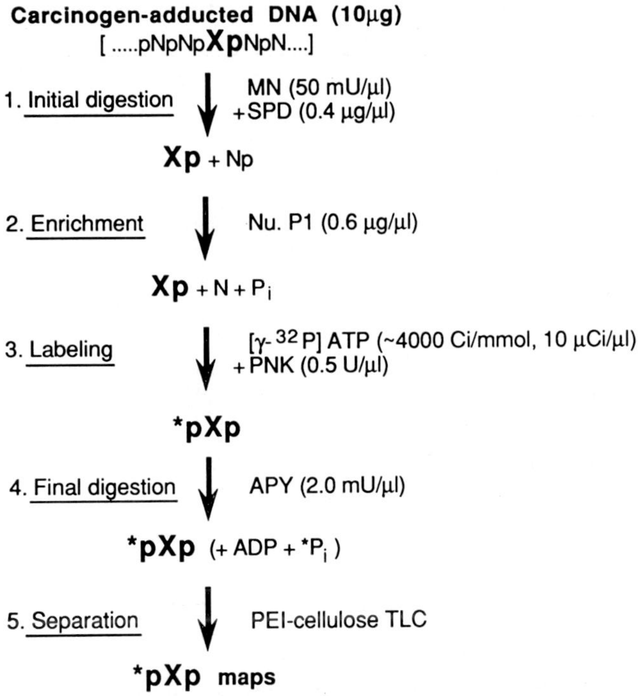


FIG. 1. The various steps of the $^{32}$P-postlabeling assay for DNA adducts: DNA hydrolysis, adduct enrichment (obligatory for low levels of adducts), $^{32}$P-labeling, final digestion to destroy excess ATP, and TLC mapping. For further details, see text and Fig. 2. Asterisks denote $^{32}$P-labeled groups.

three procedures afford the greatest sensitivity of adduct detection (1 adduct in $10^9$–$10^{10}$ DNA nucleotides, requiring 5–10 $\mu$g DNA per individual assay). Recoveries of certain adducts depend on adduct structure. The procedure is selected on the basis of amounts and types of adducts present in the DNA. For example, individual enrichment procedures utilize different principles and thus, some differences in their performance are observed. Nucleotides containing carcinogen moieties attached at exocyclic nitrogen or oxygen atoms are recovered to similar extents by procedures 3–5, while procedures 3 and 5 afford a better recovery of guanine-C8 substituted aromatic amine adducts.

The choice of chromatographic procedure is key to optimal adduct resolution. TLC on PEI-cellulose has been used most extensively for this purpose. Concentrated electrolyte solutions containing 7–8.5 M urea (*11, 18, 22*) appear best suited as solvents in the separation of non-polar adducts containing polycyclic aromatic moieties, while more polar adducts are resolved with solvents containing lower concentrations of electrolytes and urea (*23*). Derivatives of widely divergent polarities in a DNA sample may require several mapping systems (*23*). High performance liquid chromatography has been used to separate small alkylated (*24*) as well as polycyclic aromatic (*25*) adducts in combination with $^{32}$P-postlabeling.

Adduct levels are calculated as relative adduct labeling (RAL) values, which represent the ratio of count rates of adducted nucleotides to count rates of total

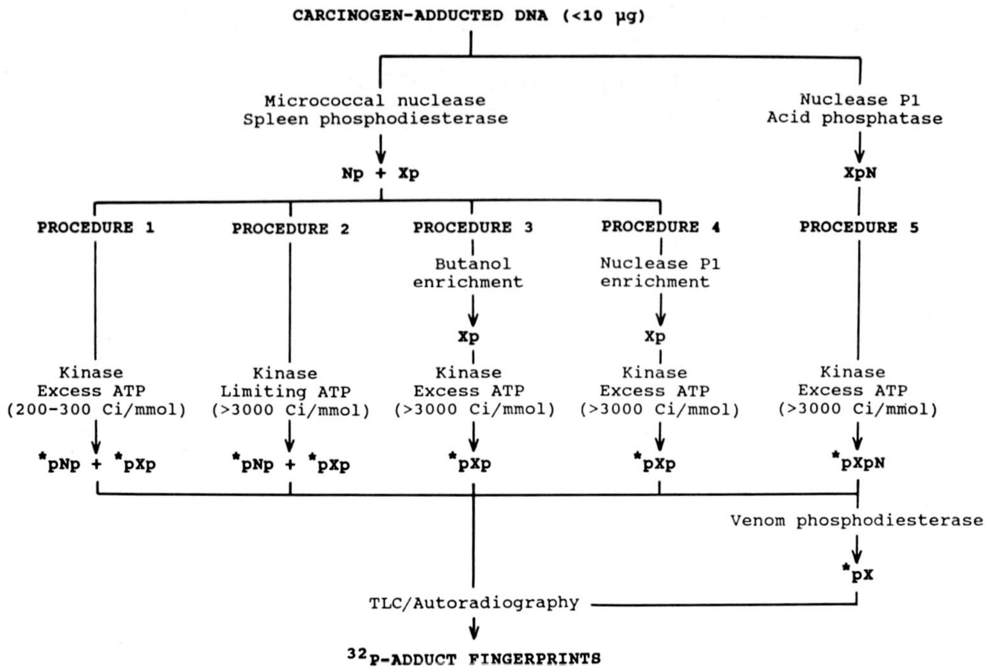


FIG. 2. Scheme of various versions of the $^{32}$P-postlabeling assay outlined in this article. Procedures 1–4 yield $^{32}$P-labeled deoxyribonucleoside 3′, 5′-bisphosphates (pNp and pXp), while procedure 5 yields adducted dinucleotides (pXpN) and adducted deoxyribonucleoside 5′-monophosphates (pX). N, normal DNA constituent; X, adduct moiety. Asterisks denote $^{32}$P-labeled groups.

(adducted plus normal) nucleotides (*11, 19*). The radioactivity of normal nucleotides is evaluated by analyzing an aliquot of the labeled DNA digest (*11, 19*). In procedures 4 and 5, the specific activity of [$\gamma$-$^{32}$P]ATP is utilized for RAL calculations. The RAL $\times$ $10^n$ value is equal to the number of adducts in $10^n$ DNA nucleotides, provided adducts are labeled and recovered quantitatively; otherwise, a correction factor is applied (*19*).

*Authentic Mutagenic (Genotoxic) Carcinogens*

Carcinogens whose DNA binding has been examined by $^{32}$P-postlabeling have been listed in a review (*22*). For example, a number of $^{32}$P-labeled adducts was detected in digests of DNA from mouse skin tissues at several time points after topical treatment with polycyclic aromatic hydrocarbons, such as benzo[a]pyrene, 7, 12-dimethylbenz[a]anthracene, and 3-methylcholanthrene, and some of these adducts were highly persistent in target tissue DNA (*26, 27*). Rapid partial removal of adducts from skin or epidermal DNA occurred during the first 2 weeks after carcinogen application, while adducts remaining thereafter underwent little change. Some polycyclic aromatic hydrocarbon-DNA adducts persisted in mouse epidermis and dermis for at least 1 year after brief dermal carcinogen exposure (*27*). Such results imply that persistent adducts occupy genomic sites in quiescent cells such that they are inaccessible to DNA repair processes. Persistence of adducts, however, is not consistently associated with tumorigenicity (*28*). Strong associations have been observed by $^{32}$P-postlabeling between the extent of initial binding to target organ DNA and hepatocarcinogenicity of dibenzo[c, g]carbazole (*29*) and safrole (*30, 31*). Thus it may frequently be a combination of high initial DNA binding affinity of the carcinogen and persistence of resulting adducts that significantly contributes to the development of neoplasia.

### *Cigarette Smoke-induced DNA Lesions*

The $^{32}$P-postlabeling assay is applicable to adducts induced by exposure to complex mixtures of DNA-damaging chemicals. Cigarette smoke-induced DNA adducts were initially detected in both experimental animals (*32*) and humans (*32–34*) by procedure 2 (Fig. 2). The more sensitive nuclease P1/bisphosphate version of the $^{32}$P-postlabeling assay (procedure 4) subsequently allowed the detection of much lower levels of smoking-related DNA adducts (*35, 36*). Adduct maps obtained by this procedure from human and mouse tissues (Fig. 3) show two extensive diagonal radioactive zones (DRZ 1 and DRZ 2) of cigarette smoke-related $^{32}$P-labeled material, consistent with the presence of numerous, only partially resolved aromatic DNA adducts of varying polarities. Similar patterns of DNA lesions in human and mouse tissues suggest common characteristics of tobacco-associated carcinogen activation and adduct formation in different mammalian species (*35, 36*).

The smoking-associated DNA adducts were found to occur in a dose- and time-dependent manner in surgical specimens of lung, bronchus, and larynx from smokers

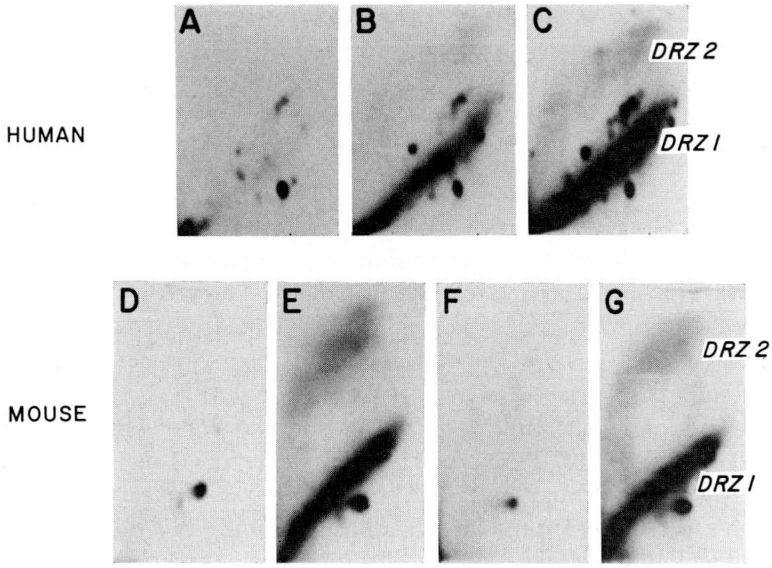


FIG. 3. Autoradiograms of $^{32}$P-labeled DNA adducts from lung of smokers and lung and heart of mice treated dermally with cigarette smoke condensate ("tar"). Adducts were purified by nuclease P1 treatment (*19*) and mapped as previously described (*35*). A: nonsmoker; B: smoker (50 pack years); C: smoker (75 pack years); D: mouse lung control; E: lung after exposure to 6 daily doses of cigarette "tar" corresponding to 0.75 cigarette each; F: heart control; G: heart after treatment as in E. DRZ: diagonal radioactive zone (see text).

with cancer of these organs (*36*). The highest levels of aromatic adducts observed were about 1.2 adducts in $10^7$ DNA nucleotides. The extent of DNA damage in lung and larynx paralleled cancer risk and mortality, which are known to increase with the number of cigarettes smoked and the duration of smoking (*37, 38*). Similarly, the long-time persistence of smoking-associated DNA adducts of up to 14 years (*36*) was in accord with the slow decline of lung and larynx cancer risk and mortality after cessation of smoking (*37, 38*). These data confirmed that smoking-associated DNA adducts in major target organs of human carcinogenesis, as assayed by $^{32}$P-postlabeling, provide a valid dosimeter for human initiator/carcinogen exposure.

The tissue distribution of smoking-associated DNA adducts in autopsy samples from heavy smokers was found to parallel that seen in mice treated dermally with cigarette smoke condensate (CSC) (*35, 36*), *i.e.*, adduct levels in lung and heart DNA of both species were significantly higher than in other human and mouse tissues, such as kidney, liver, and spleen. Thus the mouse appears to provide a suitable model system for studying DNA damage and mechanisms of smoking-associated human carcinogenesis.

### *DNA Alterations in White Blood Cells of Iron Foundry and Coke Oven Workers*

White blood cells (WBC) provide an easily accessible source of DNA for biomonitoring of human exposure to environmental or occupational genotoxicants *via* a minimally invasive technique. WBC DNA of workers in a Finnish foundry (*39, 40*) and a Polish cokery (*41*) as well as corresponding controls was assayed by the nuclease P1/bisphosphate version of the $^{32}$P-postlabeling assay (procedure 4). Foundry workers were categorized into high, medium, or low exposure groups, based on exposure levels to airborne benzo[a]pyrene (BP) levels. Highly significant correlations were observed between exposure and WBC adduct levels, and the data when analyzed by job category showed correlations between the estimated exposure in a particular job and adduct levels (*39, 40*). The highest adduct levels measured in exposed individuals were about 1 adduct in $10^6$ DNA nucleotides. While adducts derived from BP were identified in the $^{32}$P-adduct profile, most of the adducts formed a complex pattern of unidentified spots. The results were in agreement with epidemiological studies showing that foundry workers are at an elevated risk of cancer. The cokery study involved the comparison of three populations, cokery workers, exposed occupationally to high levels of polycyclic aromatic hydrocarbons, residents of towns near the cokery (local controls), and residents from a rural area (countryside controls) (*41*). Local controls exhibited WBC adduct levels similar to the cokery workers, with maximum levels reaching about 1 adduct in $10^7$ DNA nucleotides, while levels in countryside controls were 2–3 times lower. As adduct patterns were similar in cokery workers and local controls, environmental pollution by the cokery significantly contributed to DNA adduct levels in local controls. The results obtained with WBC DNA of both foundry and cokery workers show that the $^{32}$P-postlabeling assay constitutes a powerful tool to assess human occupational exposure to genotoxic agents (mutagens and carcinogens) at the molecular target (DNA).

*Estrogen-induced DNA Alterations*

Kidney DNA from estrogen-treated male Syrian hamsters provides an example for the detection of chemically unidentified adducts by the $^{32}$P-postlabeling assay (*42*). These animals develop renal carcinoma with high incidence after 6–8 months of exposure to natural or synthetic estrogens. $^{32}$P-postlabeling showed that stilbene and steroid estrogens, in spite of their divergent structures, all led to the formation of a set of chromatographically identical DNA adducts, and this was confirmed by re-chromatography of the individual estrogen-induced adducts in various systems (*42*). Thus, the adducts did not contain bound estrogen moieties but rather were derivatives of an estrogen-induced unknown electrophilic metabolite (or metabolites). This appeared to involve the activation of such a metabolite(s) by cytochrome P-450 but not prostaglandin endoperoxide synthase (*43*). Since these adducts were only observed in the target organ, they were postulated to be involved in the initiation of renal tumors. Whether a similar mechanism of DNA damage also pertains to estrogen-induced tumorigenesis in other systems has not as yet been elucidated.

*I-compounds*

Tissue DNA of untreated animals contains covalent modifications, termed I-compounds (*12*), that were detected by $^{32}$P-postlabeling. These DNA modifications, being absent or only marginally detectable in newborn animals, accumulate in an age-dependent manner and their amounts and patterns depend on species, strain, tissue, and sex (Fig. 4) (*12, 15, 44–46*). Furthermore, diet composition has recently been found to be a major determinant of profiles and levels of certain I-compounds (*46*). These findings strongly support our original interpretation (*12*) that I-compounds are formed from endogenous electrophiles resulting from metabolism of nutrients and other natural dietary components. In addition, various lines of experimental evidence have excluded exogenous carcinogens as the source of these DNA modifications (*15, 44, 46*). I-Compounds exhibit a wide range of polarities, indicating structural diversity (*15, 23*). Precise structural definition of I-compounds has not yet been possible because the amounts isolated from tissues have been too low for analysis by current methods such as mass spectrometry.

Because of their dual character, resembling carcinogen-DNA adducts on the one hand and normal DNA modifications on the other, I-compounds could conceivably play different functional roles *in vivo* (*15*). As adduct analogues, they may be involved in natural aging and "spontaneous" tumor formation (*12*). The estrogen-induced DNA adducts of endogenous origin in male hamster kidney (*42*) were recently found to be chromatographically identical to I-compounds in kidney of untreated female hamsters which do not develop renal tumors, where they increased with age (*44*). Thus, while being associated with hormonal carcinogenesis in the male kidney, no harmful effects could be attributed to their presence in the female kidney. As progesterone prevents tumor development in the male hamster model (*47*), this finding may conceivably be explained in part by the natural presence of this hormone in female animals.

There are also various lines of experimental evidence which suggest a functional

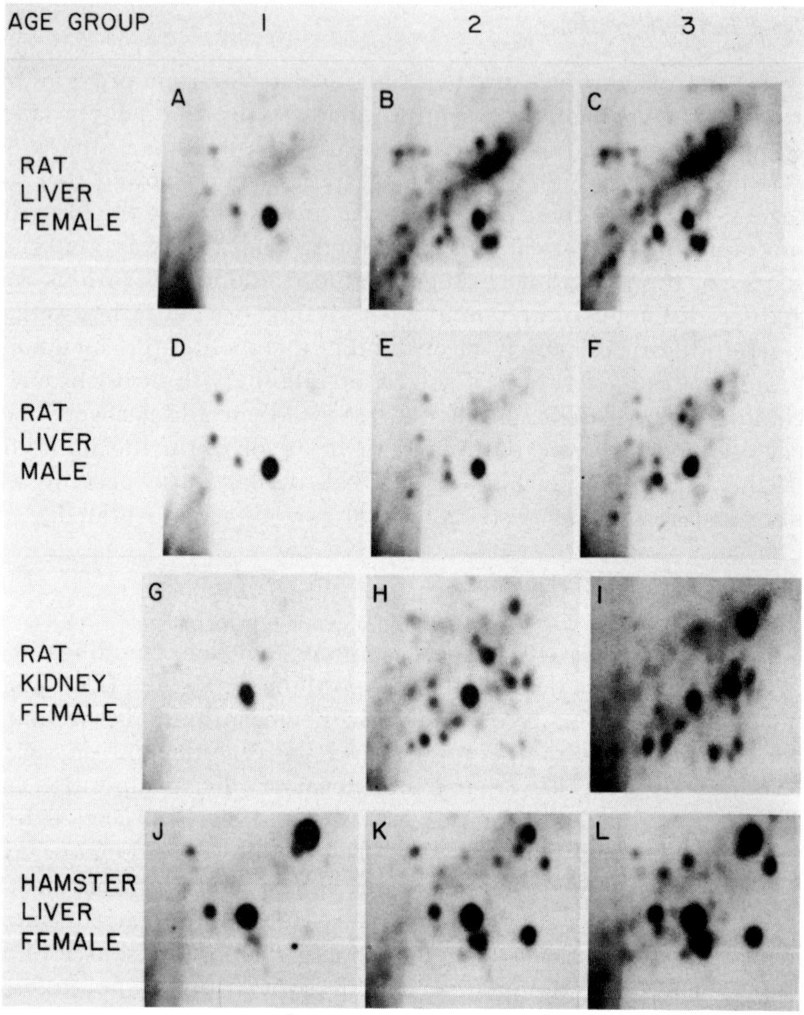


FIG. 4. Age-, sex-, tissue-, and species-dependent autoradiographic profiles of I-compounds in DNA of untreated Sprague-Dawley rats (panels A–I) and Syrian hamsters (panels J–L). Ages (months) of the animals were: 1=1; 2=4 (rats) or 2.5 (hamsters); 3=10 (rats) or 9.5 (hamsters). DNA was analyzed by the procedure depicted in Fig. 1 (procedure 4, see Fig. 2). The $^{32}$P-labeled compounds shown represent the low polarity fraction of I-compounds (*13, 23*).

or beneficial role of I-compounds: (i) rat liver mitochondrial DNA exhibits, in addition to two mitochondria-specific spots which also increase with animal age, similar profiles and levels of I-compounds as does nuclear DNA (*48*), suggesting cellular control mechanisms which regulate I-compound levels for the benefit of the cell; (ii) I-compounds may exert protective effects against carcinogenesis, as inferred from the presence of comparatively low levels of I-compounds in organs of certain strains of mice with a high incidence of "spontaneous" neoplasms (*49*); (iii) dietary restriction, which prolongs life and reduces tumor incidence in many species, enhances levels of I-compounds in rat liver and kidney DNA (*50*); (iv) I-compound levels are reduced by non-mutagenic carcinogens (see next section); and (v) hepatomas contain very low levels of I-compounds (see next section).

### *Modulation of I-compound Profiles by Non-mutagenic Carcinogens*

Potent non-mutagenic carcinogens such as 2,3,7,8-tetrachlorodibenzo-*p*-dioxin (TCDD) (*13, 51*), choline-devoid diet (*14, 16*), carbon tetrachloride ($CCl_4$) (*17*), and peroxisome proliferators (*52*) were all found to reduce I-compound levels substantially in rodent liver, the target organ of carcinogenesis. Reduction of I-compound levels by TCDD correlated with carcinogenicity not only in an organ- but also sex-specific manner in rats (*13, 51*). While a carcinogenic dose fed for 6 months to rats reduced the levels of individual I-compound fractions by 37–77% in female liver (target organ), kidney or male liver (non-targets) were unaffected. Similarly, feeding a choline-devoid diet, which is hepatocarcinogenic in male but not female rats, reduced I-compound levels drastically in male but not female liver. Since neither TCDD nor choline-devoid diet led to carcinogen adduct formation in the target organ, loss of I-compounds may represent a novel biomarker for carcinogenesis by non-mutagenic mechanisms. Reduction of I-compound levels by these agents did not appear to be solely due to cell proliferation but also to effects on I-compound biosynthesis because: (i) levels of individual I-compounds were not affected to the same extent (*13, 17*). (ii) I-Compound levels did not recover for many months after switching rats from choline-devoid to choline-supplemented diet (*16*). (iii) Persistently low hepatic I-compound levels were also observed at 22 weeks after treatment of ICR mice with another non-mutagenic hepatocarcinogen, $CCl_4$, long after DNA synthesis had returned to normal (*17*).

The interpretation that the capacity of synthesizing I-compounds is at least partially lost in the above systems is supported by the low levels or lack of I-compounds in choline-devoid diet- (*16*) and peroxisome proliferator-induced (*52*) liver tumors, as well as Morris hepatomas exhibiting a wide spectrum of growth rates (*53*). The consistent loss of I-compounds in the above carcinogenesis models and their lack in tumors support an anticarcinogenic role of these DNA modifications (*15*).

### *Acknowledgments*

The authors' work cited in this review has been supported by USPHS grants CA 32157 and CA 43263 awarded by the National Cancer Institute, AG 07750 awarded by the National Institute on Aging, and ES 04917 awarded by the National Institute of Environmental Health Sciences.

## REFERENCES

1. Doll, R. and Peto, R. The Causes of Cancer. Oxford University Press, Oxford, 1981.
2. Miller, E. C. and Miller, J. A. Searches for ultimate chemical carcinogens and their reactions with cellular macromolecules. Cancer, *47*: 2327–2345, 1981.
3. Hemminki, K. Nucleic acid adducts of chemical carcinogens and mutagens. Arch. Toxicol., *52*: 249–285, 1983.
4. Ames, B. N. Identifying environmental chemicals causing mutations and cancer. Science, *204*: 587–593, 1979.

5. De Serres, F. J. and Ashby, J. Evaluation of Short-Term Tests for Carcinogens: Report of the International Collaborative Program. Elsevier, New York, 1981.
6. Stich, H. F. and San, R. H. C. Short-Term Tests for Chemical Carcinogens. Springer-Verlag, New York, 1981.
7. Baird, W. M. The use of radioactive carcinogens to detect DNA modifications by chemical carcinogens. *In;* P. L. Grover (ed.), Chemical Carcinogens and DNA, Vol. 1, pp. 59–83, CRC Press, Boca Raton, Florida, 1979.
8. Poirier, M. C. Antibodies to carcinogen-DNA adducts. J. Natl. Cancer Inst., *67*: 515–519, 1981.
9. Randerath, K., Reddy, M. V., and Gupta, R. C. $^{32}P$-labeling test for DNA damage. Proc. Natl. Acad. Sci. U.S.A., *78*: 6126–6129, 1981.
10. Reddy, M. V., Gupta, R. C., and Randerath, K. $^{32}P$-base analysis of DNA. Anal. Biochem., *117*: 271–279, 1981.
11. Gupta, R. C., Reddy, M. V., and Randerath, K. $^{32}P$-postlabeling analysis of nonradioactive aromatic carcinogen-DNA adducts. Carcinogenesis, *3*: 1081–1092, 1982.
12. Randerath, K., Reddy, M. V., and Disher, R. M. Age- and tissue-related DNA modifications in untreated rats: detection by $^{32}P$-postlabeling assay and possible significance for spontaneous tumor induction and aging. Carcinogenesis, *7*: 1615–1617, 1986.
13. Randerath, K., Putman, K. L., Randerath, E., Mason, G., Kelley, M., and Safe, S. Organ-specific effects of long term feeding of 2,3,7,8-tetrachlorodibenzo-*p*-dioxin and 1,2,3,7,8-pentachlorodibenzo-*p*-dioxin on I-compounds in hepatic and renal DNA of female Sprague-Dawley rats. Carcinogenesis, *9*: 2285–2289, 1988.
14. Li, D., Chandar, N., Lombardi, B., and Randerath, K. Reduced accumulation of I-compounds in liver DNA of rats fed a choline-devoid diet. Carcinogenesis, *10*: 605–607, 1989.
15. Randerath, K., Li, D., and Randerath, E. Age-related DNA modifications (I-compounds): Modulation by physiological and pathological processes. Mutat. Res., *238*: 245–253, 1990.
16. Li, D., Xu, D., Chandar, N., Lombardi, B., and Randerath, K. Persistent reduction of indigenous DNA modification (I-compound) levels in liver DNA from male Fischer rats fed choline-devoid diet and in DNA of resulting neoplasms. Cancer Res., *50*: 7577–7580, 1990.
17. Nath, R. G., Li, D., and Randerath, K. Acute and long-term effects of carbon tetrachloride on DNA modifications (I-compounds) in male mouse liver. Chem.-Biol. Interactions, *76*: 343–357, 1990.
18. Reddy, M. V., Gupta, R. C., Randerath, E., and Randerath, K. $^{32}P$-postlabeling test for covalent DNA binding of chemicals *in vivo*: application to a variety of aromatic carcinogens and methylating agents. Carcinogenesis, *5*: 231–243, 1984.
19. Reddy, M. V. and Randerath, K. Nuclease $P_1$-mediated enhancement of sensitivity of $^{32}P$-postlabeling test for structurally diverse DNA adducts. Carcinogenesis, *7*: 1543–1551, 1986.
20. Gupta, R. C. Enhanced sensitivity of $^{32}P$-postlabeling analysis of aromatic carcinogen-DNA adducts. Cancer Res., *45*: 5656–5662, 1985.
21. Randerath, K., Randerath, E., Danna, T. F., van Golen, K. L., and Putman, K. L. A new sensitive $^{32}P$-postlabeling assay based on the specific enzymatic conversion of bulky DNA lesions to radiolabeled dinucleotides and nucleoside 5′-monophosphates. Carcinogenesis, *10*: 1231–1239, 1989.
22. Gupta, R. C. and Randerath, K. Analysis of DNA adducts by $^{32}P$-labeling and thin-layer chromatography. *In;* E. C. Friedberg and P. C. Hanawalt (eds.), DNA Repair, A Laboratory Manual of Research Procedures, Vol. 3, pp. 399–418, Marcel Dekker,

Inc., New York, 1988.

23. Randerath, K., Lu, L.-J. W., and Li, D. A comparison between different types of covalent DNA modifications (I-compounds, persistent carcinogen adducts and 5-methylcytosine) in regenerating rat liver. Carcinogenesis, *9*: 1843–1848, 1988.
24. Wilson, V. L., Basu, A. K., Essigmann, J. M., Smith, R. A., and Harris, C. C. $O^6$-alkyldeoxyguanosine detection by $^{32}$P-postlabeling and nucleotide chromatographic analysis. Cancer Res., *48*: 2156–2161, 1988.
25. Dunn, B. P. and San, R. H. C. HPLC enrichment of hydrophobic DNA-carcinogen adducts for enhanced sensitivity of $^{32}$P-postlabeling analysis. Carcinogenesis, *9*: 1055–1060, 1988.
26. Randerath, E., Agrawal, H. P., Reddy, M. V., and Randerath, K. Highly persistent polycyclic aromatic hydrocarbon-DNA adducts in mouse skin: detection by $^{32}$P-postlabeling analysis. Cancer Lett., *20*: 109–114, 1983.
27. Randerath, E., Agrawal, H. P., Weaver, J. A., Bordelon, C. B., and Randerath, K. $^{32}$P-postlabeling analysis of DNA adducts persisting for up to 42 weeks in the skin, epidermis and dermis of mice treated topically with 7, 12-dimethylbenz(a)anthracene. Carcinogenesis, *6*: 1117–1126, 1985.
28. Wogan, G. N. and Gorelick, N. J. Chemical and biochemical dosimetry of exposure to genotoxic chemicals. Environ. Health Perspect., *62*: 5–18, 1985.
29. Schurdak, M. E. and Randerath, K. Tissue-specific DNA adduct formation in mice treated with the environmental carcinogen, 7H-dibenzo(c, g)carbazole. Carcinogenesis, *6*: 1271–1274, 1985.
30. Randerath, K., Haglund, R. E., Phillips, D. H., and Reddy, M. V. $^{32}$P-postlabelling analysis of DNA adducts formed in the livers of animals treated with safrole, estragole and other naturally-occurring alkenylbenzenes. I. Adult female CD-1 mice. Carcinogenesis, *5*: 1613–1622, 1984.
31. Phillips, D. H., Reddy, M. V., and Randerath, K. $^{32}$P-postlabelling analysis of DNA adducts formed in the livers of animals treated with safrole, estragole and other naturally-occurring alkenylbenzenes. II. Newborn male B6C3F$_1$ mice. Carcinogenesis, *5*: 1623–1628, 1984.
32. Randerath, E., Avitts, T. A., Reddy, M. V., Miller, R. H., Everson, R. B., and Randerath, K. Comparative $^{32}$P-analysis of cigarette smoke induced DNA damage in human tissues and mouse skin. Cancer Res., *46*: 5869–5877, 1986.
33. Everson, R. B., Randerath, E., Santella, R. M., Cefalo, R. C., Avitts, T. A., and Randerath, K. Detection of smoking related covalent DNA adducts in human placenta. Science, *231*: 54–57, 1986.
34. Everson, R. B., Randerath, E., Santella, R. M., Avitts, T. A., Weinstein, I. B., and Randerath, K. Quantitative associations between DNA damage in human placenta and maternal smoking and birth weight. J. Natl. Cancer Inst., *80*: 567–576, 1988.
35. Randerath, E., Mittal, D., and Randerath, K. Tissue distribution of covalent DNA damage in mice treated dermally with cigarette "tar": preference for lung and heart DNA. Carcinogenesis, *9*: 75–80, 1988.
36. Randerath, E., Miller, R. H., Mittal, D., Avitts, T. A., Dunsford, H. A., and Randerath, K. Covalent DNA damage in tissues of cigarette smokers as determined by $^{32}$P-postlabeling assay. J. Natl. Cancer Inst., *81*: 341–347, 1989.
37. United States Department of Health and Human Services. The Health Consequences of Smoking: Cancer. A Report of the Surgeon General, Office on Smoking and Health, Rockville, Maryland, 1982.
38. IARC Monographs on the Evaluation of the Carcinogenic Risk of Chemicals to Humans. Tobacco Smoking, Vol. 38. International Agency for Research on Cancer,

Lyon, France, 1985.

39. Savela, K., Hemminki, K., Hewer, A., Phillips, D. H., Putman, K. L., and Randerath, K. Interlaboratory comparison of the $^{32}$P-postlabeling assay for aromatic DNA adducts in white blood cells of iron foundry workers. Mutat. Res., *224*: 485–492, 1989.
40. Hemminki, K., Randerath, K., Reddy, M. V., Putman, K. L., Santella, R. M., Perera, F. P., Young, T.-L., Phillips, D. H., Hewer, A., and Savela, K. Postlabeling and immunoassay analysis of polycyclic aromatic hydrocarbons—adducts of deoxyribonucleic acid in white blood cells of foundry workers. Scand. J. Work Environ. Health, *16*: 158–162, 1990.
41. Hemminki, K., Grzybowska, E., Chorazy, M., Twardowska-Saucha, K., Sroczynski, J. W., Putman, K. L., Randerath, K., Phillips, D. H., Hewer, A., Santella, R. M., Young, T. L., and Perera, F. P. DNA adducts in humans environmentally exposed to aromatic compounds in an industrial area of Poland. Carcinogenesis, *11*: 1229–1231, 1990.
42. Liehr, J. G., Avitts, T. A., Randerath, E., and Randerath, K. Estrogen-induced endogenous DNA adduction: possible mechanism of hormonal cancer. Proc. Natl. Acad. Sci. U.S.A., *83*: 5301–5305, 1986.
43. Liehr, J. G., Hall, E. R., Avitts, T. A., Randerath, E., and Randerath, K. Localization of estrogen-induced DNA adducts and cytochrome P-450 activity at the site of renal carcinogenesis in the hamster kidney. Cancer Res., *47*: 2156–2159, 1987.
44. Randerath, K., Liehr, J. G., Gladek, A., and Randerath, E. Age-dependent covalent DNA alterations (I-compounds) in rodent tissues: species, tissue and sex specificities. Mutat. Res., *219*: 121–133, 1989.
45. Li, D., Xu, D., and Randerath, K. Species and tissue specificities of I-compounds as contrasted with carcinogen adducts in liver, kidney and skin DNA of Sprague-Dawley rats, ICR mice and Syrian hamsters. Carcinogenesis, *11*: 2227–2232, 1990.
46. Li, D. and Randerath, K. Association between diet and age-related DNA modifications (I-compounds) in rat liver and kidney. Cancer Res., *50*: 3991–3996, 1990.
47. Kirkman, H., Growth characteristics in the Syrian hamster. *In;* Estrogen-Induced Tumors of the Kidney in the Syrian Hamster, Natl. Cancer Inst. Monogr., No 1, pp. 1–57, 1959.
48. Gupta, K. P., van Golen, K. L., Randerath, E., and Randerath, K. Age-dependent covalent DNA alterations (I-compounds) in rat liver mitochondrial DNA. Mutat. Res., *237*: 17–27, 1990.
49. Li, D. and Randerath, K. Strain differences of I-compounds in relation to organ sites of spontaneous tumorigenesis and non-neoplastic disease in mice. Carcinogenesis, *11*: 251–255, 1990.
50. Randerath, E., Hart, R. W., Turturro, A., Danna, T. F., Reddy, R., and Randerath, K. Effects of aging and caloric restriction on I-compounds in liver, kidney, and white blood cell DNA of male Brown-Norway rats. Mech. Ageing Devel., 1991, in press.
51. Randerath, K., Putman, K. L., Randerath, E., Zacharewski, T., Harris, M., and Safe, S. Effects of 2,3,7,8-tetrachlorodibenzo-*p*-dioxin on I-compounds in hepatic DNA of Sprague-Dawley rats: sex-specific effects and structure-activity relationships. Toxicol. Appl. Pharmacol., *103*: 271–280, 1990.
52. Randerath, E., Randerath, K., Reddy, R., Danna, T. F., Rao, M. S., and Reddy, J. K. Induction of rat liver DNA alterations by chronic administration of peroxisome proliferators as detected by $^{32}$P-postlabeling. Mutat. Res., *247*: 65–76, 1991.
53. Randerath, K., Randerath, E., and Danna, T. F. Lack of I-compounds in DNA from a spectrum of Morris hepatomas. Carcinogenesis, *11*: 1041–1044, 1990.

XENOBIOTICS AND CANCER, L. ERNSTER ET AL. (EDS.),
JAPAN SCI. SOC. PRESS, TOKYO/TAYLOR & FRANCIS LTD., LONDON, pp. 329–338, 1991

# Carcinogenic Aromatic Amine Metabolism and DNA Adduct Detection in Humans

Fred F. KADLUBAR

*National Center for Toxicological Research (HFT-100), Jefferson, Arkansas 72079, U.S.A.*

*Abstract:* Human exposure to carcinogenic aromatic amines can occur from a variety of sources, including cigarette smoke and cooked foods. Initial metabolism occurs primarily in the liver and involves *N*-hydroxylation by cytochrome P-450IA2 and *N*-acetylation by acetyltransferase, which serve as competing activation and detoxification reactions, respectively. Both enzymes are polymorphic in humans and individual phenotype can be readily assessed using caffeine ingested in coffee followed by urinary metabolite analysis. *N*-hydroxy arylamines can then be transported through the blood where they can form protein adducts with hemoglobin or undergo renal filtration into the urinary bladder lumen where, at acidic pH, they can react covalently with urothelial DNA. Carcinogen-DNA adduct levels in human bladder are smoking-related and the C8-deoxyguanosine derivative of 4-aminobiphenyl (ABP) is a major product.

Alternatively, *N*-hydroxy arylamines can be conjugated in the liver by glucuronyl transferases which provides a mechanism for biliary transport to the colon lumen where $\beta$-glucuronidases can regenerate the aglycone. In the colon mucosa, acetyltransferases can further activate the *N*-hydroxy metabolite by *O*-acetylation; and persons with the rapid acetylation phenotype are known to be at higher risk for colorectal cancer. Detection of specific arylamine-DNA adducts in human colon should provide direct evidence for the role of these carcinogens in the etiology of this disease.

## *Aromatic Amines as Risk Factors for Human Urinary Bladder and Colorectal Cancers*

Urinary bladder cancer and colorectal cancer are significant health problems worldwide and represent the sixth and second leading cause of cancer deaths, respectively, in the United States (*1*). Occupational exposure to aromatic amines and nitroaromatic hydrocarbons has long been recognized as a causative factor for urinary bladder cancer; and several specific chemicals, such as 4-aminobiphenyl (ABP) and 2-naphthylamine, have been clearly implicated as human bladder carcinogens (*2*). While industrial production of these particular chemicals has been essentially eliminated, potential human exposure to this class of carcinogens continues today from a variety of sources (*3*). These include: a) potential occupational exposure to 4,4′-methylene*bis*(2-chloroaniline), 4,4′-methylenedianiline, and benzidine-based azo dyes, which have extensive industrial usage; b) mainstream and sidestream cigarette smoke, which contains known carcinogens such as *o*-toluidine, ABP, 2-naphthylamine, and several heterocyclic amines; c) coal and shale oil, which contain ABP, 2-naphthylamine, and 2-aminofluorene; d) cooked foods containing heterocyclic amines such as PhIP, MeIQx, IQ, and Glu-P-1; e) agricultural chemicals that include *p*-chloro-*o*-toluidine, a carcinogenic breakdown product of the insecticide Chlordimeform, and several herbicides of the nitrobiphenyl ether, dinitroaniline, and triazine classes; and f) diesel exhaust, airborne particulates, coal fly ash, soil, and wastewater contaminated with polycyclic nitroaromatic hydrocarbons, of which the mono- and di-nitropyrenes, 6-nitrochrysene, and 2- and 3-nitrofluoranthenes are known to possess appreciable carcinogenic activity.

Of these, tobacco usage is regarded as major risk factor for urinary bladder cancer, with 40% to 85% of all cancer cases being attributable to smoking cigarettes. Moreover, smokers have a 2 to 10-fold increased risk over non-smokers for developing bladder tumors (*4*). Metabolic factors have also been associated with increased risk. The drug acetylation polymorphism, which is known to predispose individuals to several aromatic amine drug toxicities (*e.g.*, procainamide-induced lupus, isoniazide-induced polyneuritis, and hepatitis), is distributed disproportionately among bladder cancer cases and controls. A significantly higher proportion of slow acetylator phenotypes is generally found among patients with a history of bladder cancer, especially when exposure to aromatic amines has been documented (*5*).

For cancer of the colon and rectum, the lack of dietary fiber, cruciferous vegetables, and physical exercise, as well as high dietary fat and caloric intake have all been shown to serve as major risk factors. In addition, genetic determinants, involving activation of the K-*ras* oncogene and/or inactivation of the *p*53 tumor suppressor gene, have been strongly implicated in predisposing individuals toward development of colorectal cancer (*6*, *7*). Aromatic amines and nitroaromatic hydrocarbons have likewise been suggested as causative agents. Carcinogenic heterocyclic amines are known to be formed as pyrolysis products during the cooking of foods; and consumption of fried, smoked, cured, and barbecued beef and pork have been associated with increased cancer risk for colorectal tumors (*8*). In addition, agricultural occupations are over-represented in cancer patients vs. controls; and exposure to nitroaromatic herbicides has been cited as a potential risk factor (*8*, *9*). Moreover, the aromatic amine acetylator polymorphism is also distributed disproportionately among cancer cases and controls, with the rapid acetylator phenotype being much more prevalent in patients with a history of colorectal cancer (*5*).

### *Metabolic Activation of Aromatic Amines and Nitroaromatic Hydrocarbons in Relation to Human Urinary Bladder and Colorectal Carcinogenesis*

The predominant pathway for the metabolic activation of most carcinogenic aromatic amines in humans is thought to involve a hepatic microsomal cytochrome P-450IA2-catalyzed *N*-oxidation to form the *N*-hydroxy arylamine (*10*, *11*). Human cytochrome P-450IA2, originally characterized as the phenacetin *O*-deethylase, has

TABLE 1. Rates of *N*-Oxidation of Carcinogenic Aromatic and Heterocyclic Amines by Human Hepatic Microsomal Cytochrome P-450IA2[a)]

| Substrate | Rate of *N*-oxidation (nmol/min/mg protein) |
|---|---|
| PhIP | 5.34±0.64 |
| 4-Aminobiphenyl | 5.00±0.32 |
| MeIQx | 2.98±0.49 |
| 2-Naphthylamine | 2.49±0.28 |
| Glu-P-1 | 2.42±0.14 |
| IQ | 2.30±0.21 |
| Trp-P-2 | 0.28±0.14 |

[a)] Rates of *N*-oxidation were determined with hepatic microsomes from the same individual ($n$=3 or 4; ±SD). Data taken from refs. *12* and *21*.

also been suggested to be polymorphic in humans. It exhibits wide interindividual variation, is inducible by cigarette smoking, and is completely absent in about 5% of the Caucasian population (*12*). PhIP and ABP have recently been shown to be excellent substrates for this monooxygenase and have the highest turnover numbers, followed by MeIQx, 2-naphthylamine, Glu-P-1, IQ, and Trp-P-2 (Table 1).

Aromatic amines and their *N*-hydroxy derivatives are also formed from carcinogenic nitroaromatic hydrocarbons. However, this process involves metabolic reduction, which can be carried out by a variety of different microsomal and cytosolic nitroreductases in several tissues and also by intestinal microflora (*13*). Re-oxidation of the amine by cytochrome P-450 may then occur and has been suggested as a rate-limiting step in the formation of the *N*-hydroxy arylamine (*14*).

The *N*-hydroxy metabolites are regarded as proximate carcinogens and mutagens (*15*) and can bind directly to DNA, in an acid-catalyzed reaction, to form covalent adducts (Fig. 1). In the liver cytosol, *N*-acetylation of the primary aromatic amine by the polymorphic acetyltransferase can also occur; and, while the *N*-acetylated amine can likewise undergo *N*-oxidation, the rates of formation of these *N*-hydroxy arylamides are generally much lower than that of the parent arylamine. Thus, hepatic *N*-acetylation represents a direct competing pathway for arylamine *N*-oxidation and for the formation of the reactive *N*-hydroxy arylamine.

For aromatic amines that serve as urinary bladder carcinogens (Fig. 2), the *N*-hydroxy metabolite appears to be poorly conjugated by hepatic glucuronyl transferases and readily enters the circulation. Here, it is apparently absorbed quickly into the erythrocyte and oxidized to the nitroso derivative, which undergoes a facile addition reaction with hemoglobin. This results in formation of an arylamine-cysteinyl adduct that can account for 2–10% of the carcinogen dose (*16*). The remaining *N*-hydroxy metabolite is transported to the kidney where it can be filtered into the urinary bladder lumen. Once in the bladder, the *N*-hydroxy arylamine appears to react directly with urothelial DNA and forms adducts in direct proportion to the voiding interval (*17*). Further metabolic activation in the bladder could occur by *O*-esterification of the *N*-hydroxy metabolite or by peroxidation of the arylamine; however, experimental evidence indicates that these are minor pathways *in vivo*.

For arylamines that serve as colorectal carcinogens (Fig. 3), the *N*-hydroxy metabolite appears to be efficiently conjugated by hepatic glucuronyl transferases and

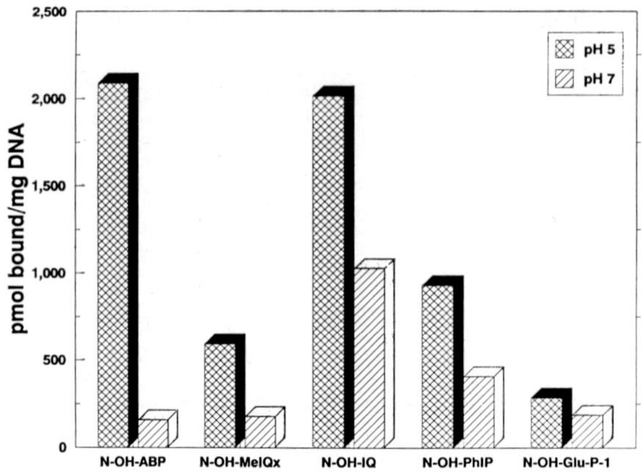


FIG. 1. Covalent binding of *N*-hydroxy aromatic and heterocyclic amines to calf thymus DNA *in vitro* at pH 5 and pH 7. Data from ref. *21*.

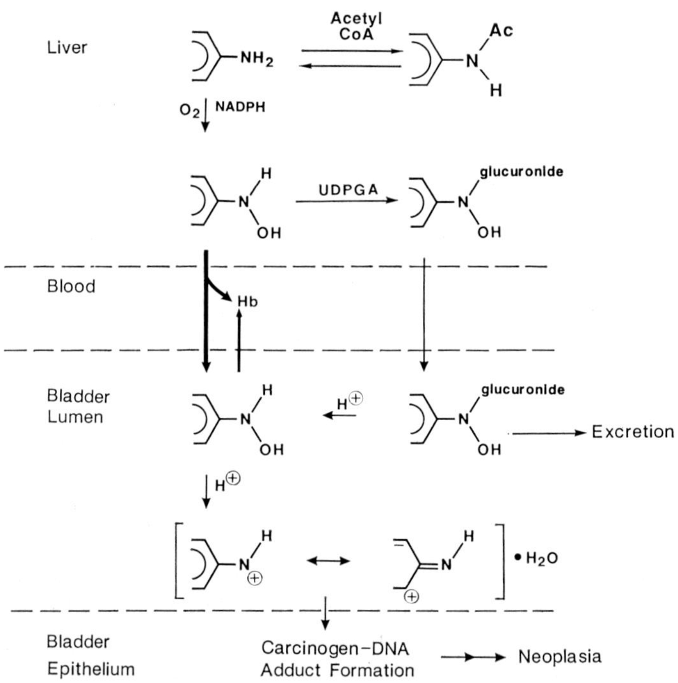


FIG. 2. Proposed metabolic activation pathways for aromatic amine-induced urinary bladder carcinogenesis.

the *N*-hydroxy *N*-glucuronide enters the intestinal lumen as a major biliary metabolite. Here, bacterial $\beta$-glucuronidases can hydrolyze this conjugate and regenerate the *N*-hydroxy arylamine, which would be expected to be rapidly reabsorbed into the colon mucosa. Several lines of evidence have indicated that *O*-acetylation of *N*-hydroxy arylamines in the colon by acetyl CoA-dependent *O*-acetyltransferase results in the formation of highly reactive *N*-acetoxy arylamines that form colon DNA adducts (*18*, *19*). This *O*-acetyltransferase is also present in human liver where it appears to

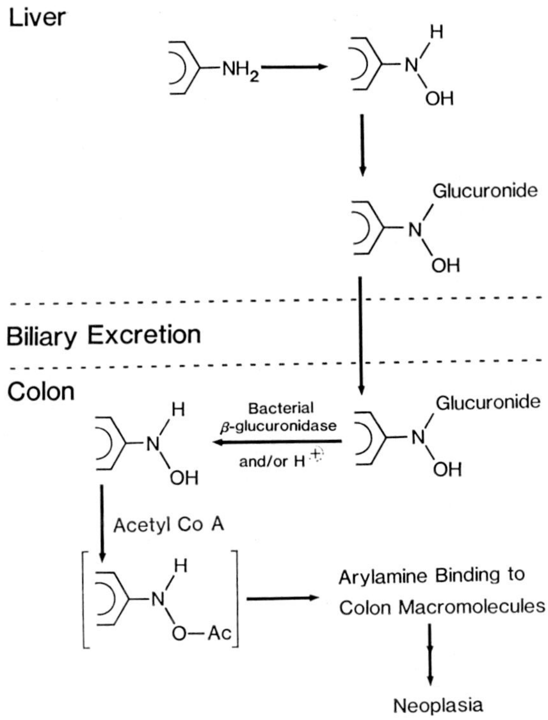


FIG. 3. Proposed metabolic activation pathways for aromatic amine-induced colorectal carcinogenesis.

TABLE 2. Human Colon Mucosa *O*-acetyltransferase Activity[a)]

| Substrate | Acetyl CoA-dependent DNA binding (pmol/mg DNA) |
|---|---|
| *N*-hydroxy-4-aminobiphenyl | 24±9 |
| *N*-hydroxy-PhIP | 20±7 |
| *N*-hydroxy-MeIQx | 14±6 |
| *N*-hydroxy-IQ | 14±5 |
| *N*-hydroxy-Glu-P-1 | 10±3 |

[a)] Activities were determined with cytosol preparations from 7 different human colon samples. Data taken from ref. *20*.

be identical with the polymorphic *N*-acetyltransferase (*20*). Accordingly, rapid *N*-acetylation in the liver might be expected to decrease the amount of *N*-hydroxy metabolite available for conjugation and transport to the colon lumen. However, aromatic amine colon carcinogens appear to be relatively poor substrates for *N*-acetylation; and the biliary *N*-hydroxy arylamines are good substrates for *O*-acetylation by human colon cytosol. This tissue contains high levels of both the polymorphic and monomorphic acetyltransferases (*21*, *22*) and readily activates several of the *N*-hydroxy heterocyclic amines (Table 2). Thus, the prevalence of rapid acetylator phenotypes among patients with a history of colorectal cancer is consistent with this activation pathway and suggests that aromatic amines may play an important role in the etiology of this disease.

*Metabolic Phenotyping of Acetyltransferase and Cytochrome P-450IA2 as Biomarkers of Susceptibility to Carcinogenesis*

Since both acetyltransferase and cytochrome P-450IA2 play an important role in metabolic activation and detoxification of carcinogenic aromatic amines, there has been considerable interest in developing and improving methods for determination of metabolic phenotypes as biomarkers of individual susceptibility. Recently, caffeine has become the preferred drug for determining acetylator status (*5*, *23*). The method involves administration of caffeine in coffee, collection of urine, and HPLC analysis to determine the ratio of an acetylated metabolite, 5-acetylamino-6-formylamino-3-methyluracil (AFMU), to 1-methyxathine (1X). The method affords excellent reproducibility and the AFMU/1X ratio provides a clear discrimination of slow and rapid acetylation phenotypes. There appear to be three different genotypes associated with this polymorphism (*24*, *25*). Individuals who are homozygous in gene 1 (true rapid acetylators) or heterozygous in genes 1 and 2 and 1 and 3 (intermediate acetylators) all classify phenotypically as rapid acetylators, while heterozygotes for genes 2 and 3 or homozygotes for gene 3 are phenotypically slow acetylators. The acetylation status varies appreciably with different ethnic groups and ranges from 20% rapid acetylator phenotype in a Scandinavian population to 90% in a Japanese population (*5*).

Metabolic phenotyping for cytochrome P-450IA2 is now also feasible through the use of caffeine. We have recently shown (*12*) that liver cytochrome P-450IA2 is primarily responsible for the rate-limiting step in caffeine biotransformation in humans, which involves the hepatic 3-dimethylation of caffeine (137X) to paraxanthine (17X). Thus, the proficiency of caffeine 3-demethylation in different individuals can be used to describe their *N*-oxidation phenotype. Using a modification of the published method for determining acetylation status, it has been possible to quantify the urinary ratio of both AFMU/1X and 17X/137X in the same HPLC analysis (*26*). The ratio of 17C/137X in urine collected at 4–5 hr after caffeine dosing is regarded as a close approximation of initial metabolism in the liver, since this represents a time when 137X and 17X are predominant in the plasma and at quasi-steady state levels (*26*, *27*). A frequency distribution and probit analysis in Italian ($n=95$), Canadian ($n=75$), and Chinese populations ($n=78$) each shows a bimodal distribution which can be readily classified into slow (80–90%) and rapid (10–20%) *N*-oxidation phenotypes. Moreover, in 13 individuals given caffeine over 5 consecutive days or weekly for 5 weeks, the ratio of urinary 17X/137X was highly reproducible and permitted the correct classification of rapid metabolizers on any given day.

Thus, the determination of metabolic phenotype for both acetyltransferase and cytochrome P-450IA2 in case-control studies should provide a useful biomarker of individual susceptibility to arylamine-induced cancers. From the metabolic activation pathways described above, it is hypothesized that patients with urinary bladder cancer will have a higher frequency of rapid *N*-oxidation and slow acetylation phenotypes when compared to control patients. For patients with colorectal cancer, a higher proportion of both rapid *N*-oxidation and acetylation phenotypes is expected when compared to the control group.

*Detection of Aromatic Amine-DNA Adducts in Human Tissues*

A preferred approach in human risk assessment and cancer etiology is the detection and characterization of carcinogen-DNA adducts in human carcinogen-target tissues. In pilot studies, we have examined the presence of aromatic amine-DNA adducts in surgical biopsy samples of human urothelium and in exfoliated bladder cells isolated from urine (*3*, *28*, *29*). Both immunochemical and $^{32}$P-postlabelling methods have been utilized. With the latter method, enhancement procedures involving *n*-butanol extraction and nuclease-$P_1$ treatment (*30*, *31*) permitted detection of distinct populations of carcinogen-DNA adducts.

Nuclease-$P_1$ treatment preferentially degrades the major C8-guanine-substituted adducts of aromatic amines but greatly enhances detection of $N^2$ -guanine adducts, as found predominantly with polycyclic aromatic hydrocarbons. Accordingly, up to 6 distinct adducts were consistently observed in our nuclease $P_1$-treated, $^{32}$P-postlabelled human bladder DNA samples. Four of these were significantly elevated in active smokers as compared to ex-smokers and never-smokers (Fig. 4) and were chromatographically similar to putative hydrocarbon adducts reported earlier for placenta and lung DNA samples from cigarette smokers (*32*, *33*).

In contrast, *n*-butanol extraction and $^{32}$P-postlabelling, which preferentially enhance the detection of arylamine-C8-guanine adducts, allowed the observation of up to 9 putative adducts, none of which were found in the nuclease $P_1$-treated samples (and *vice versa*). Four of these were significantly elevated in active smokers as compared with ex-smokers and never-smokers (Fig. 5). Furthermore, adducts B3, B4, and B9 were chromatographically identical in several thin-layer systems with the major DNA adducts found after reaction with the *N*-hydroxy metabolites of 2-naphthylamine, ABP, and PhIP, each of which is known to be present in ng-quantities in cigarette smoke (*34*, *35*). In order to characterize adduct B4 further, the $^{32}$P-postlabelled component was eluted from the thin-layer chromatograms of several individuals, mixed with a synthetic [$^3$H]*N*-(deoxyguanosin-8-yl)-4-aminobiphenyl-3′, 5′-*bis*phosphate, and injected onto an HPLC. All of the radioactivity ($^{32}$P and $^3$H)

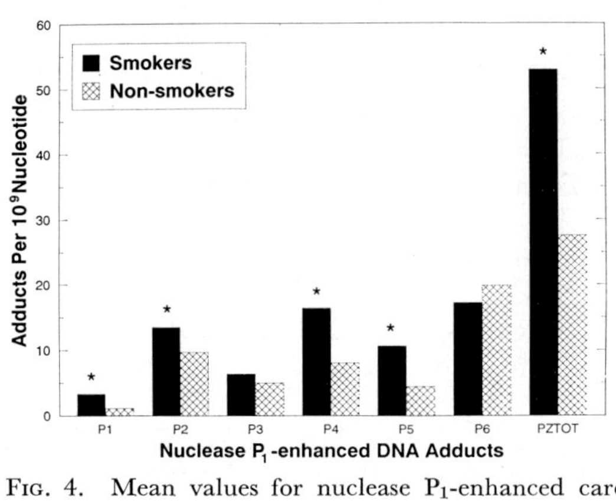


FIG. 4. Mean values for nuclease $P_1$-enhanced carcinogen-DNA adducts, comparing current smokers ($n=13$) to never-smokers ($n=9$). An asterisk indicates those adducts where there was a statistically significant difference (Mann-Whitney test) between smokers and never-smokers at the $p \leq 0.05$ level.

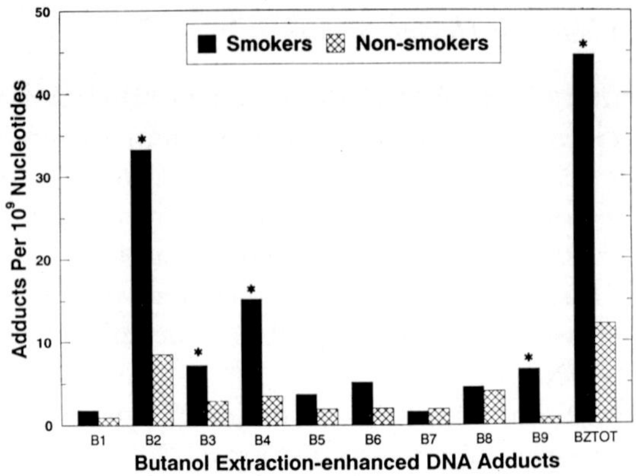


FIG. 5. Mean values for *n*-butanol-enhanced carcinogen-DNA adducts, comparing current smokers ($n=13$) to never-smokers ($n=9$). An asterisk indicates those adducts where there was a statistically significant difference (Mann-Whitney test) between smokers and never-smokers at the $p \leq 0.05$ level.

co-migrated with the ultraviolet-absorbing synthetic marker. These results provide strong evidence that ABP, a known human bladder carcinogen, is major DNA-damaging agent in the urothelium of cigarette smokers; and it suggests a molecular basis for the urinary bladder carcinogenicity of cigarette smoke.

A similar approach for the detection of arylamine-DNA adducts in human liver and colon should provide useful information on the role of heterocyclic amines and nitroaromatic herbicides in the etiology of this disease.

## REFERENCES

1. Cancer Facts and Figures, 1989. American Cancer Society, Atlanta, Georgia, 1990.
2. Garner, R. C., Martin, C. N., and Clayson, D. B. Carcinogenic aromatic amines and related compounds. *In;* C. E. Searle (ed.), Chemical Carcinogens, 2nd Edition, American Chemical Society Monograph 182, pp. 175–276, Washington D. C., 1984.
3. Kadlubar, F. F., Talaska, G., Lang, N. P., Benson, R. W., and Roberts, D. W. Assessment of exposure and susceptibility to aromatic amine carcinogens. *In;* H. Bartsch, K. Hemminki, and I. K. O'Neill (eds.), Methods for Detecting DNA Damaging Agents in Humans: Applications in Cancer Epidemiology and Prevention, IARC Scientific Publications No. 89, pp. 166–174, Lyon, 1988.
4. Mommsen, S. and Aagaard, J. Tobacco as a risk factor in carcinogenesis. Carcinogenesis, *4*: 335–338, 1983.
5. Hein, D. W. Acetylator genotype and arylamine-induced carcinogenesis. Biochim. Biophys. Acta, *948*: 37–66, 1988.
6. Meyeres, F. J., Gumerlock, P. H., Kokoris, S. P., White, R. P. D., and McCormick, F. Human bladder and colon carcinomas contain activated *ras p*21. Cancer, *63*: 2177–2181, 1989.
7. Baker, S. J., Markowitz, S., Fearon, E. R., Willson, J. K. V., and Vogelstein, B. Suppression of human colorectal carcinoma cell growth by wild-type p53. Science, *249*: 912–915, 1990.
8. Wohlleb, J. C., Hunter, C. F., Blass, B., Kadlubar, F. F., Chu, D. Z. J., and Lang, N. P. Aromatic amine acetyltransferase as a marker for colorectal cancer: Environ-

mental and demographic associations. Int. J. Cancer, *46*: 22–30, 1990.
9. Caldwell, G. G., Cannon, S. B., Pratt, C. B., and Arthur, R. D. Serum pesticide levels in patients with childhood colorectal carcinoma. Cancer, *48*: 774–778, 1981.
10. Kadlubar, F. F. and Hammons, G. J. The role of cytochrome P-450 in the metabolism of chemical carcinogens. *In;* F. P. Guengerich (ed.), Mammalian Cytochromes P-450, Vol. 2, pp. 81–130, CRC Press, Boca Raton, Florida, 1987.
11. Yamazoe, Y., Abu-Zeid, M., Yamauchi, K., and Kato, R. Metabolic activation of pyrolysate arylamines by human liver microsomes: possible involvement of a P-448-H type cytochrome P-450. Jpn. J. Cancer Res.; *79*: 1159–1167, 1988.
12. Butler, M. A., Iwasaki, M., Guengerich, F. P., and Kadlubar, F. F. Human cytochrome P-450$_{PA}$(P-450IA2), the phenacetin *O*-deethylase, is primarily responsible for the hepatic 3-demethylation of caffeine and *N*-oxidation of carcinogenic arylamines. Proc. Natl. Acad. Sci. U.S.A., *86*: 7696–7700, 1990.
13. Fu, P. P. Metabolism of nitro-polycyclic aromatic hydrocarbons. Drug Metab. Disp., *22*: 209–268, 1990.
14. Kadlubar, F. F., Fu, P. P., Jung, H., Shaikh, A. U., and Beland, F. A. The metabolic *N*-oxidation of carcinogenic arylamines in relation to nitrogen charge density and oxidation potential. Environ. Health Persp., *87*: 233–236, 1990.
15. Miller, E. C. and Miller, J. A. Searching for the ultimate chemical carcinogens and their reactions with cellular macromolecules. Cancer, *47*: 2327–2345, 1981.
16. Bryant, M. S., Vineis, P., Skipper, P. L., and Tannenbaum, S. R. Hemoglobin adducts of aromatic amines: associations with smoking. Proc. Natl. Acad. Sci., U.S.A., *85*: 9788–9791, 1988.
17. Kadlubar, F. F., Dooley, K. L., Teitel, C. H., Roberts, D. W., Benson, R. W., Butler, M. A., Bailey, J. R., Young, J. F., Skipper, P. W., and Tannenbaum, S. R. Effects of voiding interval on metabolism, pharmacokinetics, blood hemoglobin adduct formation, and liver and urinary bladder DNA adduct levels in beagle dogs administered the carcinogen, 4-aminobiphenyl. Cancer Res., in press.
18. Flammang, T. J. and Kadlubar, F. F. Acetyl coenzyme A-dependent metabolic activation of *N*-hydroxy-3,2′-dimethyl-4-aminobiphenyl and several carcinogenic *N*-hydroxy arylamines in relation to tissue and species differences, other acyl donors, and arylhydroxamic acid-dependent acyltransferases. Carcinogenesis, *7*: 919–926, 1986.
19. Shinohara, A., Saito, K., Yamazoe, Y., Kamataki, T., and Kato, R. Acetyl coenzyme A dependent activation of *N*-hydroxy derivatives of carcinogenic arylamines: mechanism of activation, species difference, tissue distribution, and acetyl donor specificity. Cancer Res., *46*: 4362–4367, 1986.
20. Flammang, T. J., Yamazoe, Y., Guengerich, F. P., and Kadlubar, F. F. The S-acetyl coenzyme A-dependent metabolic activation of the carcinogen *N*-hydroxy-2-aminofluorene by human liver cytosol and its relationship to the aromatic amine *N*-acetyltransferase phenotype. Carcinogenesis, *8*: 1967–1970, 1987.
21. Turesky, R. J., Butler, M. A., Teitel, C. H., and Kadlubar, F. F. Metabolic activation of carcinogenic heterocyclic amines in human liver and colon. Carcinogenesis, in press.
22. Pacifici, G. M., Franchi, M., Gervasi, P. G., Longo, V., diSimplicio, P., Temellini, A., and Guiliani, L. Profile of drug-metabolizing enzymes in human ileum and colon. Pharmacology, *38*: 137–145, 1989.
23. Grant, D. M., Tang, B. K., and Kalow, W. A single test for acetylator phenotype using caffeine. Br. J. Clin. Pharm., *17*: 459–464, 1984.
24. Deguchi, T., Mashima, M., and Suzuki, T. Correction between acetylater phenotypes and genotypes of polymorphic arylamine *N*-acetyltransferase in human liver. J. Biol. Chem., *265*: 127757–127760, 1990.

25. Blum, M., Grant, D. M., McBride, W., Heim, M., and Meyer, U. A. Human arylamine *N*-acetyltransferase genes: isolation, chromosomal localization, and functional expression. DNA and Cell Biology, *9*: 193–203, 1990.
26. Butler, M. A., Caporaso, N., Vineis, P., Lang, N. P., and Kadlubar, F. F. Characterization of the carcinogenic arylamine *N*-oxidation phenotype in humans by urinalysis of caffeine metabolites. Unpublished.
27. Bonati, M., Latini, R., Galletti, F., Young, J. F., Tognoni, G., and Garattini, S. Caffeine disposition after oral doses. Clin. Pharm. Therap., *32*: 98–106, 1982.
28. Talaska, G., Al-Juburi, A. Z. S. S., and Kadlubar, F. F. Smoking related carcinogen-DNA adducts in biopsy samples of human urinary bladder: identification of N-(deoxyguanosin-8-yl)-4-aminobiphenyl as a major adduct. Proc. Natl. Acad. Sci. U.S.A., in press.
29. Talaska, G. and Schamer, M. Detection of carcinogen-DNA adducts in exfoliated urothelial cells of cigarette smokers: correlation with smoking, hemoglobin adducts, metabolic status and urinary mutagenicity. Unpublished.
30. Reddy, M. V. and Randerath, K. Nuclease $P_1$-mediated enhancement of sensitivity of $^{32}P$-postlabeling test for structurally diverse DNA adducts. Carcinogenesis, *7*: 1543–1551, 1986.
31. Gupta, R. C. and Earley, K. $^{32}P$-adduct assay: comparative recoveries of structurally diverse DNA adducts in the various enrichment procedures. Carcinogenesis, *9*: 1687–1693, 1988.
32. Everson, R. B., Randerath, E., Santella, R. M., Cefalo, R. C., Avitts, T., and Randerath, K. Detection of smoking-related covalent DNA adducts in human placenta. Science, *231*: 54–57, 1986.
33. Phillips, D. H., Hewer, A., Martin, C. N., Garner, R. C., and King, M. M. Correlation of DNA adduct levels in human lung with cigarette smoking. Nature, *336*: 790–792, 1988.
34. Patrianakos, C. and Hoffmann, D. Chemical studies on tobacco smoke LXIV. On the analysis of aromatic amines in cigarette smoke. J. Anal. Toxicol., *3*: 150–154, 1979.
35. Peluso, M., Castegnaro, M., Malaveille, C., Friesen, M., Garren, L., Hautefeuille, A., Vineis, P., Kadlubar, F. F., and Bartsch, H. $^{32}P$-postlabelling analysis of urinary mutagens from smokers of black tobacco implicate 2-amino-1-methyl-6-phenylimidazo [4,5-*b*]pyridine (PhIP) as a major DNA-damaging agent. Carcinogenesis, *12*: 713–717, 1991.

XENOBIOTICS AND CANCER, L. ERNSTER ET AL. (EDS.),
JAPAN SCI. SOC. PRESS, TOKYO/TAYLOR & FRANCIS LTD., LONDON, pp. 339–350, 1991

# The Role of Molecular Epidemiology in Cancer Prevention

Frederica P. PERERA, Regina M. SANTELLA, Paul BRANDT-RAUF, Scott KAHN, Wei JIANG, Deliang TANG, and Jack MAYER

*Columbia University School of Public Health, New York, New York 10032, U.S.A.*

*Abstract:* Risk of cancer is determined by the complex interaction between "environmental" exposures and genetic and nutritional factors that modulate response to carcinogenic insults. Here, the term "environmental" encompasses lifestyle, occupation, and the ambient environment. As a promising approach in cancer prevention, a number of biologic markers are currently being evaluated in terms of their ability to identify harmful exposures and populations at risk in time to effectively intervene. These biomarkers are reflective of the molecular dose or early effect of carcinogens (such as DNA or protein adducts, gene or chromosomal alterations and oncogene activation) or they provide information on potential susceptibility (such as the genetically or nutritionally determined handling of carcinogens). Techniques as diverse as immunoassays, $^{32}$P-postlabelling and gas chromatography-mass spectroscopy (GC/MS) are being deployed to measure DNA and protein adducts in cells and tissues from persons with occupational, community or lifestyle-related exposure to chemical carcinogens. Signal changes in target oncogenes and tumor suppressor genes are also being investigated in heavily exposed, "healthy" populations and in lung cancer cases and controls using current molecular biologic techniques. Inherited predisposition to lung cancer is being evaluated through such assays as aryl hydrocarbon hydroxylase (AHH), glutathione activity and restriction fragment length polymorphism. A review of recent studies using a panoply of biomarkers provides a departure point for recommendations for future, integrated molecular epidemiologic studies of cancer.

## *The Challenge of Cancer Prevention*

Cancer prevention is one of the greatest challenges facing the research and public health communities today. For example, in the U.S. alone 500,000 persons die each year from cancer (*1*). This burden is growing. While *mortality* from cancer declined between 1950 and 1985 in the U.S., there has been a 37% overall increase in cancer *incidence* for whites and a 23% increase when lung cancer is excluded (*2*). Incidence rates have been rising more for blacks than for whites (*2*). In addition, between 1968 and 1983, mortality from brain cancer, multiple myeloma and a number of other cancers rose in persons aged 55 and older (U.S. white males and females) (*3*).

Only a small percentage of cancer is attributable to genetic factors alone; thus, most cancers can be prevented by controlling environmental exposures to carcinogens. These environmental exposures are both voluntary (lifestyle-related, such as cigarette smoking and diet) and involuntary (such as workplace or ambient exposure to industrial pollutants). Alone, or in combination with other environmental agents, cigarette smoking is the major identified cause of cancer, accounting for an estimated 30% of the total cancer burden (*4*). The remaining 70% is not well accounted for; and exercises to apportion blame to specific sources have been stymied by lack of adequate data on exposure, and by other uncertainties (*5, 6*). There has, for example, been much discussion of the role of diet in cancer. Thus far, however, the role of specific dietary constituents such as fat and fiber, vitamins and micronutrients in various human cancers has proved elusive, with epidemiologic studies frequently showing weak or inconsistent associations (*6*). The association between dietary fat and breast cancer, although limited, appears strongest, followed by that between fat intake and colon cancer (*7*).

By contrast, involuntary exposure to industrial chemicals, products of fossil fuel combustion, metals, fibers, and radiation has been definitively linked to human cancer (*8*). Indeed, of the 50 agents known to be human carcinogens, 30 are chemicals or industrial processes (*8*) which were established to be carcinogenic by occupational epidemiology. Risk from these substances is not confined to the workplace. For example, community exposure to arsenic and industrial or urban air pollution has been associated with increased risk of lung cancer (*5, 9–11*). Interactions between voluntary and involuntary exposures to carcinogens (such as smoking and uranium, asbestos and arsenic, respectively) have been established and are likely to occur commonly in the human setting (*5*). Thus, the challenge in cancer prevention lies in the early identification of environmental hazards—voluntary and involuntary—that increase an individual's risk of cancer. New approaches are needed to supplement conventional laboratory testing and epidemiology.

### *The Need for Biological Markers*

Conventional epidemiological methods are limited in their ability to identify causal factors in common cancers such as that of the lung. The long latency of cancer generally precludes reliable estimation of exposure, necessary to establish dose-response relationships and quantitative estimates of risk. Moreover, epidemiologic studies afford limited opportunity to evaluate mechanisms by which carcinogens (interacting with other environmental and host factors) exert their effect. Most importantly, conventional epidemiology precludes prevention, as it relies on tumor incidence or mortality as the dependent variable. By documenting molecular or biochemical alterations directly in human tissues, molecular epidemiology has significant potential in cancer prevention (*12–15*). Because they directly reflect factors and mechanisms involved in the human carcinogenic process, biomarkers can be useful in providing early warning of elevated cancer risk as well as in assessing the magnitude of cancer risk from specific environmental agents. In addition, biomarkers have the potential to identify individuals or subpopulations who are most biologically susceptible to environmental carcinogens—essential information when one is designing effective prevention and intervention programs. In the case of voluntary exposures such as cigarette smoking, this information allows targeting of programs aimed at behavior modification and education, while for involuntary exposures to industrial or man-made carcinogens, appropriately stringent standards can be set to protect sensitive subpopulations.

Available biologic markers of greatest relevance to cancer include carcinogen-DNA and carcinogen-protein adducts as molecular dosimeters of environmental carcinogens. Chromosomal alterations and activated oncogenes can also be feasibly monitored in humans and are sensitive to environmental exposures to mutagens/carcinogens (*16*). These lesions can be useful as markers of early preclinical effect of carcinogens, although in some cases genetic alterations in lung cancer may reflect inherent susceptibility to carcinogenic exposures. An intriguing observation has been the wide interindividual variation in these biomarkers in humans after controlling for differences in exposure (*17*). Presumably this variation stems from observed differences in the complex "handling" of xenobiotics—including metabolic activation, detoxification, DNA damage and repair, cell proliferation and immune surveillance (*18*, *19*). As will be discussed, many of these processes are under genetic control (in some cases modulated by environmental factors) and are also influenced by health status including level of nutrition. Thus biologic markers that can reflect genetic/metabolic activity or nutritional status can also be useful in establishing "ecogenetic" interactions at the molecular or biochemical level. This information may help us to identify those subgroups or individuals at greatest risk. The following discussion emphasizes studies relevant to respiratory carcinogenesis, since most of the research has involved the inhalation route. However, the molecular epidemiologic approach is applicable to all types of cancer.

### *Carcinogen-DNA and Protein Adducts*

Since most carcinogens are metabolically activated to electrophilic species capable of covalently binding to cellular macromolecules (DNA, RNA, and protein), it is not surprising that in laboratory animals the carcinogenic potency of a series of genotoxic carcinogens is generally correlated with their ability to form covalent adducts with DNA (*20–22*). DNA and protein adducts can be regarded as "black box" measurements summing up the complex "ecogenetic" process of handling xenobiotics and identifying "high responders". Carcinogen-DNA adducts (and protein adducts as a surrogate) have been widely studied in human populations with known exposure to environmental carcinogens. Since 1982, numerous studies of so-called "model populations" (cigarette smokers, workers, persons living in a heavily polluted environment, and cancer patients) have detected a broad array of adducts on DNA and protein. These chemical fingerprints include adducts formed by a number of inhaled pollutants including: polycyclic aromatic hydrocarbons (PAHs), nitrosamines, 4-aminobiphenyl, ethylene oxide, and styrene. For example, studies begun in the 1970s (*23*) have shown ethylene oxide-hemoglobin adducts to be sensitive to low level exposure to this systemically distributed carcinogen. Recently, hospital sterilization workers exposed generally to less than one part per million of ethylene oxide (8 hr time weighted average) had elevated levels of hemoglobin binding compared to controls (*24*). Sister chromatic exchanges (SCEs) and decreased DNA repair capacity were also significantly affected by exposure and the former were highly correlated with the protein adducts. As another example, a recent study of nonsmokers and smokers found an association between 4-aminobiphenyl-hemoglobin adducts and relative risk of bladder cancer (*25*). This molecular epidemiologic study thus provided evidence of the biochemical basis for the causal relationship between cigarette smoking and bladder cancer.

Although many studies have reported a significant increase in adduct levels resulting from exposure, all have observed significant interindividual variation among exposed individuals. For example, in a study of 35 foundry workers, a general "dose-response" relationship was seen between estimated workplace exposure to PAHs and PAH-DNA adducts. However, there was a 90-fold variation in PAH-DNA binding among all workers and a 30-fold variation among the low exposed workers (*17, 26*).

There have been a number of investigations of adducts in white blood cells (WBC) or lung tissue of lung cancer cases and controls. In a study of 81 cases and 67 controls, PAH-DNA adducts in WBC measured by immunoassay were not correlated to smoking status. However, among current cigarette smokers (whose P-450 metabolizing enzyme systems are likely to be similarly induced), lung cancer patients had a significantly higher mean level of adducts than controls (*27*). Another study using an immunoassay has reported increased levels of PAH-DNA adducts in lung tissue from cases *vs.* controls (*28*). These findings suggest that the ability to activate and bind this class of carcinogens may be a risk factor in disease and are consistent with evidence from *in vitro* studies of a genetic component in PAH-DNA binding that is associated with increased risk of lung cancer (*29–31*).

Studies using the $^{32}P$-postlabelling technique (which measures a broad spectrum of adducts on DNA) have shown that the DNA from lung tissue and lymphocytes of both smokers and nonsmokers contains multiple adducts, with the level and pattern varying greatly between individuals (*32–34*). In contrast to lymphocytes, adducts in lung tissue measured by the postlabelling method have shown a general association with history of cigarette smoking (*32, 34*).

With few exceptions, studies of DNA or protein adducts have involved worker populations, cigarette smokers, or cancer patients. However, residents in a heavily polluted industrial area of Poland (Upper Silesia) had PAH-DNA adduct levels in peripheral blood (13.5 adducts per $10^8$ nucleotides) that were significantly higher than in rural unexposed controls ($4.8/10^8$) and quite close to those seen in coke oven workers in the same region ($15.2/10^8$) (*35*). This is the first report of a significant effect of ambient environmental pollution on carcinogen-DNA binding in humans.

### *Signal Genetic Alterations*

In many cases, it is not possible to distinguish completely between genetic alterations that constitute a biologic effect of exposure to environmental carcinogens from those that reflect inborn genetic predisposition. As with adducts, genetic alterations such as chromosomal aberrations, SCEs and alterations in oncogenes and tumor suppressor genes are likely to reflect both factors. Chromosomal aberrations, SCEs, and even certain oncogene changes have been increased in smokers and in workers having defined exposure to diverse carcinogens (*16*). There are also numerous reports of elevated frequencies of SCEs as well as genetic abnormalities in lung cancer cases compared to controls (*36*, *37*). These can be classified as chromosomal deletions of putative antioncogenes, activation of protooncogenes by amplification, overexpression and mutation, and growth factor expression. Unfortunately, given that these observations have been made on malignant cells, it is unclear whether the genetic alterations precede cancer development or simply reflect the genetic instability arising from the malignancy itself (*38*). Prospective studies or "nested case-control" studies are required to resolve this question.

A major focus in clinical research on cancer has been the elaboration of molecular genetics in order to understand the biology of the disease and to design more effective therapies. However, the same database can theoretically be applied to prevention by identifying risk factors with greater precision than hitherto possible. For example, the study of the molecular genetics of lung cancer has uncovered a possible interaction of inherited susceptibility and environmental carcinogens. Deletions of putative tumor suppressor genes including 3P (14–23), 13q14 (Rb), and 17p (p53) occur commonly in lung cancer. It has been hypothesized that these cases reflect the combination of an inherited predisposition to lung cancer with an environmentally triggered mutation. Individuals who are heterozygous for the specific allele in their germ line (with one normal, functional allele and one nonfunctional recessive allele) may be at heightened risk of lung cancer from exposure to environmental carcinogens such as cigarette smoke which can induce a chromosomal deletion uncovering the inherited recessive mutation. This deletion effectively inactivates a putative tumor suppressor gene, resulting in altered regulation of cell growth or differentiation (*36*). Thus, altered tumor suppressor genes appear to arise from a combination of environmental insults and inherited genetic susceptibility.

Alterations in another target gene have been associated with environmental exposure. Several studies have linked a mutagenic component in tobacco smoke to *ras* mutation in adenocarcinoma of the lung (*39–41*). In a series of studies of adenocarcinoma patients, mutation in codon 12 of K-*ras* was observed in 13/32 (41%) of smokers, compared to 1/4 former smokers and 0/6 never smokers (*39*, *40*).

In preliminary studies, we have also observed an association between cigarette smoking and mutational activation of K-*ras*. A novel polymerase chain reaction (PCR)-mediated restriction fragment length polymorphism (RFLP) assay (*42*) was able to detect mutated K-*ras* alleles in the tumor tissue but not the normal lung tissue from 5/12 patients with adenocarcinoma for whom smoking status was known. No K-*ras* mutations were seen in tumor or normal lung tissue from 6 patients with squamous cell carcinomas of the lung. Lung tissue samples from 5 controls (patients without lung cancer) were uniformly negative. There was an association between cigarette smoking history and presence of K-*ras* alleles mutant at codon 12. The median pack years (PY) of smoking for the PCR-positive adenocarcinoma patients was higher than that for the PCR-negative adenocarcinoma cases (62 PY *vs*. 23 PY).

These results are consistent with experimental observations that *ras* gene mutations, creating *ras* (p21) proteins with transforming potential, have resulted from exposure to a range of carcinogenic chemicals and agents. These include 3-methylcholanthrene, benzo(a)pyrene, dimethylbenz(a)anthracene, ionizing radiation, nitrosamines, tetranitromethane, and aflatoxin $B_1$ (*43–49*).

It may ultimately be possible to identify a series of chemical-specific mutational spectra in these target genes, thus allowing oncogenes to serve as markers of tumor etiology (*50*). For example, the majority of mutations in the K-*ras* gene in adenocarcinoma are G-T transversions, whereas in colon tumors the majority of mutations are G-A transitions (*51*). This variation may indicate involvement of different mutagens in the induction of lung tumors *vs*. colon tumors.

The observation that different oncogene changes occur at various stages of lung cancer not only endows them with prognostic value but may provide clues as to involvement of early or late-stage carcinogens in malignant transformation. For example, by contrast to *ras*, which has been implicated in the intiation of lung cancer, it appears that *myc* amplification and rearrangement occur not at the time of malignant transformation but during tumor progression (*52–54*).

A number of these oncogene changes have been identified in premalignant lesions of the lung (*55*). This has led to the search for feasible screening methods for early changes in target genes. While it is not possible to obtain lung tissue from healthy workers or smokers, one can screen sputum or urine cytology specimens as well as serum for the presence of oncogene protein products. In the case of serum, oncogene protein products such as *ras* P21 may be released into the extracellular environment by secretion, leakage from altered membranes or through cell turnover and necrosis. These oncoproteins may then be detected by modified Western blotting techniques using monoclonal antibodies to the normal or mutated protein (*56, 57*). Thus, in preliminary studies, foundry workers with PAH exposure resulting in dose-related PAH-DNA adducts were evaluated for the presence of oncogene proteins in sera. Three of 17 individuals belonging to the medium and high exposure groups showed overexpression of *ras* or *fes* compared to none of the 18 workers having low exposure and none of 10 unexposed controls (*58*). The same method was used to screen sera from lung cancer cases and controls, revealing that sera of 18 of 22 lung cancer patients (all non small cell lung carcinomas) were positive for overexpression of at least one oncogene protein (predominantly *ras* and *fes*) compared to 2 or 20 healthy controls (both smokers) ($p<0.001$) (*56, 58*).

### *Markers of Genetic Susceptibility*

As discussed above, chromosomal deletions (*e.g.*, 3p, 13q, 17p) possibly triggered by environmental mutagens and carcinogens may unmask an inherited genetic defect. Thus, these signal deletions apparently constitute markers of both genetic susceptibility and biologic effect arising from environmental exposure.

There has been considerable interest in certain metabolic or detoxification phenotypes such as aryl hydrocarbon hydroxylase (AHH) activity, debrisoquine hydroxylation and glutathione-*S*-transferase activity as possible markers of genetic susceptibility to lung cancer. The rationale for studying AHH activity is that this function is performed by one subfamily of the cytochrome P-450 microsomal enzyme system, which converts PAH to carcinogenic intermediates (*59*). The control of AHH activity in humans is polygenic and is influenced by certain environmental exposures such as smoking. Case-control studies have yielded contradictory results conterning the association between AHH activity in lymphocytes and lung cancer risk (*38*).

Another candidate marker also reflecting phase I monooxygenation (but by a different P-450 enzyme than AHH) is the hydroxylation of the anti-hypertensive drug, debrisoquine. This marker has been demonstrated to be under genetic control and to be dominated by a single gene. Case-control studies have consistently observed a higher risk of lung cancer in extensive metabolizers, with the strongest association in squamous cell and small cell cancer (*60*).

Phase II conjugation of inactive intermediates with endogenous compounds such as glucuronic acid and glutathione renders them water soluble, hence readily excretable and unable to bind covalently with DNA. Thus, in contrast to phase I monooxygenation which would be expected to correlate with cancer risk, low phase II conjugating enzyme activity is likely to enhance risk. Mu glutathione transferase ($\mu$-GT) activity appears to be dominated by a single autosomal gene (*61*). An association between low $\mu$-GT activity in peripheral blood monocytes and lung cancer risk has been reported. In a recent case-control study, 58% of smokers without lung cancer ($n=192$) has the high $\mu$-GT activity phenotype compared to only 36% of lung cancer patients ($n=191$) ($p<0.0001$) (*62*). This relationship was most pronounced in patients with adenocarcinoma. Although this result requires confirmation, it is biologically plausible since $\mu$-GT detoxifies benzo(a)pyrene, ethylene oxide, and styrene oxide —all carcinogenic constituents of cigarette smoke.

All of these metabolic studies have identified phenotype rather than genotype and are subject to bias since metabolic effects could be produced by drugs, illness-related changes in diet or smoking, or the biologic effects of cancer itself (*38*). Therefore, complementary DNA and protein sequences for P-450s (*63, 64*) are valuable because they make it possible to use probes to identify metabolic genotypes that may predispose to lung cancer.

Finally, a potential marker of susceptibility is DNA repair capacity, which is known to vary significantly among individuals (*65*). In addition to assays that measure DNA repair in lymphocytes exposed *in vitro* to a mutagen/carcinogen, it is becoming possible to probe for the expression of a human DNA repair gene directly in human tissues. As with other such markers, these may reflect both inherent predisposition and environmental challenges.

The appropriate motivation for seeking evidence for genetic predisposition to cancer is to shed light on the biology of this disease and the nature of variability in risk, rather than to "screen out" susceptible individuals or to allow continued exposure of "resistant" individuals. It is important to note that the studies to date suggest that a fairly large proportion of the population may have increased risk due to genetic factors. For example, the study of $\mu$-GT activity described above suggests that roughly half of the population has a 1.5–3 fold increased risk of lung cancer as a result of this factor (*38*).

### *Nutritional Markers*

A second "host factor" that appears to play a role in susceptibility to lung carcinogens is nutritional status. For example, molecular epidemiologic studies have provided convincing evidence of a protective effect of beta-carotene for lung cancer (*66–68*). Experimentally, vitamin A compounds (including retinol, retinoic acids, and retinyl esters) inhibit mutagenesis and/or DNA binding by PAHs (*69–72*). Vitamin E (alpha-tocopherol) is a potent antioxidant. Although human data on cancer chemoprevention by vitamin E are sparse, experimental inhibition of PAH-DNA binding by alpha-tocopherol has been demonstrated (*73*).

Therefore, it is of interest to evaluate a possible inverse relationship between levels of these vitamins and carcinogen-DNA adducts, chromosomal alterations, and mutated or overexpressed oncogenes. This effect has also not previously been explored in a properly designed longitudinal or nested case-control molecular epidemiologic study.

### *Conclusion*

It is clear that a number of biologic markers are potentially applicable to in-depth molecular epidemiologic studies of cancer causation and risk. These markers cover the spectrum from molecular dosimetry (*e.g.*, carcinogen-DNA and carcinogen-protein adducts) to irreversible biologic effects of environmental carcinogens (*e.g.*, chromosomal alterations, mutational activation of oncogenes), genetic and/or acquired susceptibility (*e.g.*, metabolic phenotype or genotype, plasma levels of vitamins) and a combination of genetic predisposition and biologic effects of exposure (*e.g.*, deletions of tumor suppressor genes). The current challenge is to link these markers directly to cancer risk. This will require a shift from the present design approaches that are largely cross-sectional surveys of "healthy" exposed and unexposed populations and case-control studies. While these studies provide valuable clues as to the etiology of lung cancer, they cannot provide the definitive link between potential risk factors and cancer. For this, it is necessary to move to longitudinal or prospective studies in which biological samples are collected at the outset of a cohort study (and ideally at subsequent serial timepoints) and long-term follow-up allows the identification of cases and controls. In this way, it is possible to ascertain the predictive relationship between biologic markers and the subsequent health outsome. Since follow-up would need to be on the order of decades, a more practical approach would be the nested case-control design in which stored samples from a prospective study undertaken years or even decades earlier are assayed retrospectively once disease outcome is known. In that instance, cancer cases could be matched to controls by age and smoking history. In conclusion, to those of us interested in cancer prevention, the possibility of molecular epidemiologic studies linking the beginning and end of the disease pathway is an exciting one.

### *Acknowledgments*

The authors are grateful to Dr. P. Brandt-Rauf, Dr. K. Hemminki, Dr. A. Jeffrey, Dr. T. Raudall, Dr. S. Smith, Dr. W. Y. Tsai, Dr. L. Wazneh, Dr. I. B. Weinstein, and Dr. T. L. Young for their valuable contributions to this research.

Support for this research was provided by NIH grants CA39174, CU5026401, CA47351, CA43013, POI ESO5294, CA13696, CA51196, ACS grants SIG/13 PDT3J3 and the Lucille P. Markey Charitable Trust.

## REFERENCES


1. American Cancer Society. Annual Report. 1988 Cancer Facts and Figures. American Cancer Society, New York, 1989.
2. National Cancer Institute: New Cancer Statistics Released. JNCI, *8*: 8, 1988.
3. Davis, D. L. and Schwartz, J. Trends in cancer mortality: U.S. white males and females, 1968–83. Lancet, *1*: 633–636, 1988.
4. Tomatis, L. The contribution of epidemiological and experimental data to the control of environmental carcinogens. Cancer Lett., *25*: 5, 1985.
5. Perera, F. P., Boffetta, P., and Nisbet, I. What are the major carcinogens in the etiology of human cancer? *In;* V. DeVita, S. Hellman, and S. A. Rosenberg (eds.), Important Advances in Oncology, pp. 249–265, J. B. Lippincott Co., Philadelphia, 1989.
6. National Research Council. Diet, Nutrition and Cancer. National Academy Press, Washington, D. C., 1982.
7. Jedrychowski, W., Becher, H., Wahrendorf, J., and Basa-Cierpialek, Z. Case-control study of lung cancer with special reference to the effect of air pollution in Poland. J. Epid. Commun. Health, *44*: 114–120, 1990.
8. International Agency for Research on Cancer. Overall evaluations of carcinogenicity: an updating of IARC monographs. Vols. 1–42, Suppl. 7, IARC, Lyon, France, 1987.
9. Brown, L. M., Pottern, L. M., and Blot, W. J. Lung cancer in relation to environmental pollutants emitted from industrial sources. Environ. Res., *34*: 250–261, 1984.
10. Cohen, L. Diet and Cancer. Sci. Am., *257*: 42–48, 1987.
11. Nisbet, I. C. T., Schneiderman, M. A., Karch, N. J., and Siegel, D. M. Review and evaluation of evidence for cancer associated with air pollution. EPA 450/5-83-006R. Research Triangle Park, NC, EPA, Office of Air Quality Planning and Standards, 1984.
12. Perera, F. P. and Weinstein, I. B. Molecular epidemiology and carcinogen-DNA adduct detection: new approaches to studies of human cancer causation. J. Chron. Dis., *35*: 581–600, 1982.
13. Harris, C. C. Biochemical and Molecular Epidemiology of Cancer. Alan R. Liss, New York, 1986.
14. Perera, F. P. Molecular cancer epidemiology: a new tool in cancer prevention. J. Natl. Cancer Inst., *78*: 887–898, 1987.
15. National Academy of Sciences, National Research Council, Committee on Biologic Markers. Biological markers in environmental health. Environ. Health Perspect., *64*: 3–9, 1987.
16. International Agency for Research on Cancer. H. Bartsch, K. Hemminki, and I. K. O'Neill. (eds.). Methods for Detecting DNA Damaging Agents in Humans: Applications in Cancer Epidemiology and Prevention, IARC Sci. Publ. No. 89, Lyon, France, 1988.
17. Perera, F. P., Mayer, J., Santella, R. M., Brenner, D., Jeffrey, A., Latriano, L., Smith, S., Warburton, D., Young, T. L., Tsai, W. Y., and Hemminki, K. Biologic markers in risk assessment for environmental carcinogens. Environ. Health Perspect., in press.
18. Harris, C. C., Weston, A., Willey, J., Trivers, G., and Mann, D. Biochemical and molecular epidemiology of human cancer: Indicators of carcinogen exposure, DNA damage, and genetic predisposition. Environ. Health Perspect., *75*: 109–119, 1987.
19. Vahakangas, K. and Pelkonen, O. Host variations in carcinogen metabolism and DNA repair. *In;* H. T. Lynch and T. Hirayama (eds.), Genetic Epidemiology of Cancer, pp. 35–54, CRC Press, Inc., Boca Raton, 1989.

20. Bartsch, H., Terracini, B., and Malaveille, C. Quantitative comparisons of carcinogenicity, mutagenicity and electrophilicity of 10 direct-acting alkylating agents and the initial 0: 7-alkylguanine ration in DNA with carcinogenic potency in rodents. Mutation Res., *110*: 181–219, 1983.
21. Lutz, W. K. *In vivo* covalent binding organic chemicals to DNA as a quantitative indicator in the process of chemical carcinogenesis. Mutation Res., *65*: 289–356, 1979.
22. Pelkonen, O., Vahakangas, K. N., and Nebert, D. W. Binding of polycyclic aromatic hydrocarbons to DNA: comparison with mutagenesis and tumorigenesis. J. Toxicol. Environ. Health, *6*: 1009–1020, 1980.
23. Ehrenberg, L. and Osterman-Golkar, S. Alkylation of molecules for detecting mutagenic agents. Teratog. Carcinog. Mutag., *1*: 105–127, 1980.
24. Mayer, J., Warburton, D., Jeffrey, A., Pero, R., Andrews, L., Walles, S., Toor, M., Latriano, L., Tang, D., Tsai, W. Y., Kuroda, M., and Perera, F. Biologic markers in ethylene oxide-exposed workers and controls. Mutat. Res., in press.
25. Bryant, M. S., Vineis, P., Skipper, P. L., and Tannenbaum, S. R. Hemoglobin adducts of aromatic amines: associations with smoking status and type of tobacco. Proc. Natl. Acad. Sci. U.S.A., *85*: 9788–9791, 1988.
26. Perera, F. P., Hemminki, K., Young, T. L., Brenner, D., Kelly, G., and Santella, R. M. Detection of polycyclic aromatic hydrocarbon-DNA adducts in white blood cells of foundry workers. Cancer Res., *48*: 2288–2291, 1988.
27. Perera, F. P., Mayer, J., Jartezki, A., Hearne, S., Brenner, D., Young, T. L., Fischmann, H. K., Grimes, M., Grantham, S., Tang, M. X., Tsai, W. Y., and Santella, R. M. Comparison of DNA adducts and sister chromatid exchange in lung cancer cases and controls. Cancer Res., *49*: 4446–4451.
28. Sinopoli, N. T., Trivers, G. E., Ficorella, C., Tomao, S., Martelli, M., Cagnazzo, P., Sama, N., Harris, C. C., and Frati, L. Immunoassay detection of carcinogen-DNA adducts in tumor and noninvolved lung tissue from lung cancer patients. Proc. Am. Assoc. Cancer Res., *31*: 97, 1990.
29. Rudiger, H. W., Nowak, D., Harmann, K., and Cerutti, P. Enhanced formation of benzo(a)pyrene-DNA adducts in monocytes of patients with a presumed predisposition to lung cancer. Cancer Res., *45*: 5890–5894, 1985.
30. Hawke, L. J. and Farrell, G. C. Increased binding of benzo(a)pyrene metabolites to lymphocytes from patients with lung cancer. Cancer Lett., *30*: 289–297, 1986.
31. Nowak, D., Schmidt-Preuss, U., and Jorres, R. Formation of DNA adducts and water-soluble metabolites of benzo(a)pyrene in human monocytes is genetically controlled. Int. J. Cancer, *41*: 169–173, 1988.
32. Randerath, E., Miller, R. H., Mittal, D., Avitts, T. A., Dunsford, H. A., and Randerath, K. Covalent (DNA) damage in tissues of cigarette smokers as determined by $^{32}$P-postlabelling assay. J. Natl. Cancer Inst., *81*: 341–347, 1989.
33. Phillips, D. H., Hewer, A., and Glover, L. Aromatic DNA adducts in human bone marrow and peripheral blood leukocytes. Carcinogenesis, *7*: 2071–2075, 1986.
34. Phillips, D. H., Hewer, A., Martin, C. N., Garner, R. C., and King, M. M. Correlation of DNA adduct levels in human lung with cigarette smoking. Nature, *336*: 790–792, 1989.
35. Hemminki, K., Twardowska-Saucha, K., Sroczyski, J. W., Grzybowka, E., Chorazy, M., Putnam, K. L., Randerath, K., Phillips, D. H., Hewer, A., Santella, R. M., Young, T. L., and Perera, F. P. DNA adducts in humans environmentally exposed to aromatic compounds in an industrial area of Poland. Carcinogenesis, *11*: 1229–1231, 1990.
36. Birrer, M. J. and Minna, J. D. Molecular genetics of lung cancer. Seminars in Oncology, *15*: 226–235, 1988.

37. Viallet, J. and Minna, J. D. Dominant oncogenes and tumor suppressor genes in the pathogenesis of lung cancer. Am. J. Respir. Cell Mol. Biol., *2*: 225–232, 1990.
38. Law, M. R. Genetic predisposition to lung cancer. Br. J. Cancer, *61*: 195–206, 1990.
39. Rodenhuis, S., Slebos, R. J. C., Boot, A. J. M., Evers, S. G., Mooi, W. J., Wagenaar, S. S., van Bodegom, P. C., and Bos, J. L. K-*ras* oncogene activation in adenocarcinoma of the lung: incidence and possible clinical significance. Cancer Res., *48*: 5738–5741, 1988.
40. Bos, J. L. *ras* oncogenes in human cancer: a review. Cancer Res., *49*: 4682–4689, 1989.
41. Perera, F. P., Santella, R. M., Brandt-Rauf, P., Kahn, S., Jiang, S., Tang, D., and Mayer, J. Molecular epidemiology of lung cancer. *In*; J. Brugge, T. Curran, E. Harlow, and F. McCormick (eds.), Origins of Human Cancer 1990, Cold Spring Harbor Laboratory, Cold Spring Harbor, New York, 1991, in press.
42. Jiang, W., Kahn, S., Guillem, J., Lu, S., and Weinstein, I. B. Rapid detection of *ras* oncogenes in human tumors: application to colon, esophageal and gastric cancer. Oncogene, *4*: 923–928, 1989.
43. Barbacid, M. *ras* genes. Annu. Rev. Biochem., *56*: 779–827, 1982.
44. Eva, A. and Trimmer, R. W. High frequency of c-K-*ras* activation in 3-methylcholanthrene-induced mouse thymomas. Carcinogenesis (London), *7*: 1931–1933, 1986.
45. Marshall, C. J., Voosden, K. H., and Phillips, D. H. Activation of c-Ha-*ras*-1 proto-oncogene by *in vitro* modification with a chemical carcinogen, benzo(a)pyrene diol epoxide. Nature, *310*: 586–589, 1984.
46. Balmain, A. and Pragnell, I. B. Mouse skin carcinomas induced *in vivo* by chemical carcinogens have a transforming Harvey-*ras* oncogene. Nature, *303*: 72–74, 1983.
47. Stowers, S. J., Glover, P. L., Reynolds, S. H., Boone, L. R., Maronpot, R. R., and Anderson, M. W. Activation of the K-*ras* protooncogene in lung tumors from rats and mice chronically exposed to tetranitromethane. Cancer Res., *47*: 3212–3219, 1987.
48. McMahon, G., Hanson, L., Lee, J. J., and Wogan, G. N. Identification of an activated c-Ki-*ras* oncogene in rat liver tumors induced by aflatoxin B1. Proc. Natl. Acad. Sci., U.S.A., *83*: 9418–9422, 1986.
49. Guerrero, L. and Pellicer, A. Mutational activation of oncogenes in animal model systems of carcinogenesis. Mutat. Res., *185*: 293–308, 1987.
50. Taylor, T. A. Oncogenes and their applications in epidemiologic studies. Am. J. Epidemiol., *130*: 6–13, 1989.
51. Bos, J. L., Fearon, E. R., Hamilton, S. R., Verlaan-de Vries, M., van Boom, J. H., van der Eb, A. J., and Vogelstein, B. J. L. Prevalence of *ras* gene mutations in human colorectal cancers. Nature (London), *327*: 293, 1987.
52. Yokota, J., Wada, M., Yoshida, T., Noguchi, M., Teresaki, T., Shimosato, Y., Sugimura, T., and Terada, M. Heterogeneity of lung cancer cells with respect to the amplification and rearrangement of *myc* family oncogenes. Oncogene, *2*: 607–611., 1988.
53. Little, C. D., Nau, M. M., Carney, D. N., Gazdar, A. F., and Minna, J. D. Amplification and expression of the c-*myc* oncogene in human lung cancer cell lines. Nature, *306*: 194–196, 1983.
54. Wong, A. J., Ruppert, J. M., Eggleston, J., Hamilton, S. R., Baylin, S. B., and Vogelstein, B. Gene amplification of c-*myc* and n-*myc* in small cell carcinoma of the lung. Science, *233*: 461–464, 1986.
55. Slamon, D. J., de Kernian, J. B., Verma, I. M., and Cline, M. J. Expression of cellular oncogenes in human malignancies. Science, *224*: 256–262, 1984.
56. Brandt-Rauf, P., Smith, S., and Perera, F. P. Molecular epidemiology and the environmental carcinogenesis of the lung. *In;* T. J. Witek and E. N. Schacter (eds.), Current

Issues in Respiratory Public Health, pp. 44–61, J. B. Lippincott, New York, 1989.

57. Brandt-Rauf, P., Smith, S., Perera, F. P., Niman, H. L., Yohannen, W., Hemminki, K., and Santella, R. M. Serum oncogene proteins in foundry workers. J. Soc. Occ. Med., *40*: 11–14, 1990.

58. Perera, F. P., Hemminki, K., Brenner, D., Young, T. L., and Weinstein, I. B. Application of biological markers to the study of lung cancer causation and prevention. IARC Sci. Publ., *89*: 451–459, 1988.

59. Gonzalez, F. J., Jaiswal, A. K., and Nebert, D. W. P450 genes: evolution, regulation, and relationship to human cancer and pharmacogenetics. Cold Spring Harbor Symp. Quant. Biol., *51*: 879–890, 1986.

60. Caporaso, N., Hayes, R. B., Dosemeci, M., Hoover, R., Ayesh, R., Hetzel, M., and Idle, J. Lung cancer risk, occupational exposure, and the debrisoquine metabolic phenotype. Cancer Res., *49*: 3675, 1989.

61. Seidegärd, J. and Pero, R. W. The hereditary transmission of high glutathione transferase activity towards trans-stilbene oxide in human mononuclear leukocytes. Hum. Genet., *69*: 66–68, 1985.

62. Seidegärd, J., Pero, R. W., Markowitz, M. M., Roush, G., Miller, D. G., and Beattie, E. J. Isoenzyme(s) of glutathione transferase (class mu) as a marker for the susceptibility to lung cancer: a follow-up study. Carcinogenesis, *11*: 33–36, 1990.

63. Nebert, D. W. and Gonzalez, F. J. P-450 genes: structure, evolution, and regulation. Annu. Rev. Biochem., *56*: 945–993, 1987.

64. Jaiswal, A. K., Nebert, D. W., McBride, O. W., and Gonzalez, F. J. Human P3-450: cDNA and complete protein sequence, repetitive sequences in the 3′ nontranslated region, and localization of gene to chromosome 15. J. Exp. Pathol., *3*: 1–17, 1987.

65. Setlow, R. B. Variations in DNA repair among humans. *In;* C. C. Harris and H. Autrup (eds.), Human Carcinogenesis, pp. 231–254, Academic Press, New York, 1983.

66. Kvale, G., Bjelke, E., and Gart, J. J. Dietary habits and lung cancer risk. Int. J. Cancer, *31*: 397–405, 1983.

67. Hinds, M. W., Kolonel, L. N., Hankin, J. E., and Lee, J. Dietary vitamin A, carotene, vitamin C and risk of lung cancer in Hawaii. Am. J. Epidemiol., *119*: 227–237, 1984.

68. Ziegler, R. G., Mason, T. J., Stemhagen, A., Hoover, R., Schoenberg, J. B., Gridly, G., Virgo, P. W., Altman, R., and Fraumeni, J. F., Jr. Dietary carotene and vitamin A and risk of lung cancer among white men in New Jersey. J. Natl. Cancer Inst., *73*: 1429–1435, 1984.

69. Rocchi, P., Arfellini, G., Capucci, A., Grilli, M. P., and Prodi, G. Effect of vitamin A palmitate on mutagenesis induced by polycyclic aromatic hydrocarbons in human cells. Carcinogenesis, *4*: 245–247, 1983.

70. Pezzuto, J. M., Chou, J. S., Jia-Xiong, J., Kudo, S., and Swanson, S. W. Effect of beta-retinyl acetate on BaP metabolism and binding to nuclear macromolecules with cultured bronchus. Cancer Res., *27*: 84, 1986.

71. Nomi, S., Matsura, T., Veyama, H., and Ueda, K. Effect of vitamin A compounds on the covalent binding of BaP to nuclear macromolecules. J. Nutr. Sci. Vitaminol., *27*: 33–41, 1981.

72. Genta, V. M., Kaufman, D. G., Harris, C. C., Smith, J. M., Sporn, M. B., and Saffioti, U. Vitamin A deficiency enhances binding of benzo(a)pyrene to tracheal epithelial DNA. Nature, *247*: 48–49, 1974.

73. Matsura, T., Uegama, H., Nomi, S., and Ueda, K. Effect of alpha-tocopherol on the binding of BaP to nuclear macromolecules. J. Nutr. Sci. Vitaminol., *25*: 495–504, 1979.

XENOBIOTICS AND CANCER, L. ERNSTER ET AL. (EDS.),
JAPAN SCI. SOC. PRESS, TOKYO/TAYLOR & FRANCIS LTD., LONDON, pp. 351–360, 1991

# Hemoglobin-carcinogen Adducts as Molecular Biomarkers in Epidemiology

Steven R. TANNENBAUM

*Department of Chemistry, Division of Toxicology, Massachusetts Institute of Technology, Cambridge, Massachusetts 02139, U.S.A.*

*Abstract:* The goal of our work is to determine the exposure of people to the ultimate form of both environmental and endogenous mutagens and carcinogens. The scientific approach is to develop methods of analysis of chemically-defined adducts of protein and DNA. Our research to date has encompassed a wide variety of compounds known or suspected to cause cancer in people: aromatic amines, heterocyclic amines, polycyclic aromatic hydrocarbons (PAH), aflatoxins, *N*-nitroso compounds, and urethane. The most advanced of those problems is that of aromatic amines in which several different types of studies on human populations have already been completed using hemoglobin (Hb) adducts of 4-aminobiophenyl (ABP) as the biomarker. These studies have revealed a correlation between the level of amine adduct and risk of bladder cancer, and most important, the role of a metabolic polymorphism, the acetylator phenotype, as an important determinant of adduct level. In the case of PAH we have developed a useful human dosimeter based upon release of bay region tetrols from Hb esters. This method is now being applied to analyze the internal dose of benzo[a]pyrene (BaP) diolepoxide and to determine the range of PAH structures subject to conversion to ultimate carcinogenic forms. Together, these studies open the door to a new era in which we will be able to examine the overall influence of metabolic polymorphisms on the internal dose of many carcinogens in individuals.

The association of environmental factors with the etiology of human cancers has been known for over 200 years, and the experimental demonstration of cancer in laboratory animals by Yamagiwa and Ichikawa is now 75 years old. Yet the question of whether environmental chemicals which have been demonstrated to be potent animal carcinogens actually contribute in a significant way to cause human cancers is still debated. With the exception of cigarette smoking and lung cancer, few sources of environmental chemicals are generally accepted as a significant, not hypothetical, disease factor. Are the favorite chemicals of experimental carcinogenesis, including polycyclic aromatic hydrocarbons (PAHs), aromatic amines, heterocyclic amines, mold toxins, nitrosamines, *etc.* merely tools for exploring the cancer paradigm or do these chemicals, at the concentrations they exist in our environment, cause sufficient genetic change to contribute to increased risk of cancer in human populations?

It is axiomatic in toxicology that the dose makes the poison. Therefore, to answer some of the questions raised above we need to know at least two things:

1. What is the dose delivered to an individual, or what is the distribution of doses in a population?
2. What is the minimum dose of a chemical required to produce a biological effect in a human?

In general we have relied on anecdotal information of the type resulting from unfortunate accidental exposures to estimate the second factor, and/or we rely on the admittedly imprecise and inaccurate approach of extrapolating from animal experiments. For the first requirement we tend to rely on the equally inaccurate and imprecise approach of measuring average concentrations of chemicals in air, water, and food.

This paper will deal with issues concerning the question of dose, and, more important, the matter of internal dose of the ultimate form of the carcinogen. Many of the papers in this Symposium deal with metabolism of carcinogens, and it is the combination of external dose and metabolism that leads to the internal dose, which in turn yields the biologically effective dose, *etc.*, as illustrated in Fig. 1.

A key issue for any biomarker is the nature of the biological sample with regard to ease of obtaining the sample, storage, size of the population which can be sampled, size of the sample, and concentration of the carcinogen product within that sample.

The approach we have used, suggested originally by Lars Ehrenberg, is to use proteins as surrogates of the dose to DNA. This concept is illustrated diagrammatically in Fig. 2. An extensive discussion of the background and theory of this approach is given in a recent review of our research in this area (*1*); however, it would be useful to concisely review here some salient points using hemoglobin (Hb) as an example.

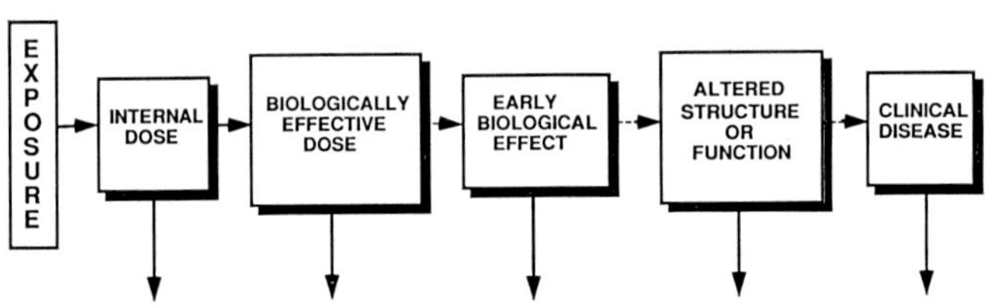


FIG. 1. Biomarkers for health effects of environmental chemicals. (NAS/NRC Env. Health Persp., *74*: 3–9, 1987)

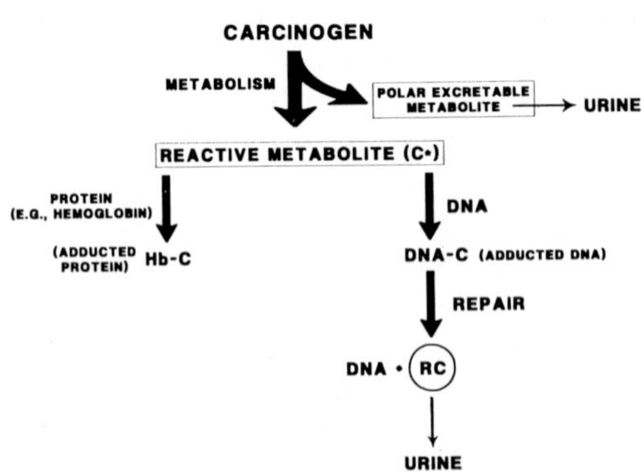


FIG. 2. Metabolism of genotoxic carcinogens leading to protein and DNA adducts.

Hb has the unique biological property of having a lifespan equivalent to the lifespan of the erythrocyte, which in humans is approximately 120 days. The age distribution of the protein is uniform; thus, if a carcinogen forms an adduct that is chemically stable, and if exposure to the carcinogen is chronic, then the amount of adduct will be proportional to Hb age; Hb molecules 120 days old will have 120 times as much adduct as Hb molecules that are only one day old. The average level of adduct will be halfway between or approximately 60 times the amount formed by the daily dose. Even if the daily dose is not constant, or if exposure is intermittent, the average level of adduct will still be 60 times the average dose over the past 120 days. The Hb dosimeter therefore reflects a 4 month record of the average exposure. Concomitantly, when exposure ceases the adduct level drops rapidly, since the initial class of erythrocytes that is lost is the oldest and thus has the highest level of adduct.

A critical issue for the validity of the dosimeter is that it should represent exactly the same chemical adduct that damages DNA. Thus the measurement of the protein adduct will be an index of damage to DNA within that tissue compartment. A major limitation to the use of Hb is that it represents only the dose to the blood compartment. Whether this will be predictive of the dose to the bladder or lungs or colon, *etc.* must be determined empirically. Alternative protein targets that we have investigated include serum albumin, which is a useful index of adduct formation in the liver, and collagen, which is present at some concentration in all tissues. This latter case is an example of a template that might be a good index of the target organ dose but which is not readily available in general populations.

For several of the carcinogens we have studied proteins have been excellent surrogates for DNA. In this paper I will discuss our research on aromatic amine exposure and risk for bladder cancer and on our progress in PAH.

### *Aromatic Amines*

The first group of carcinogens we investigated were the aromatic amines, and particularly the human bladder carcinogen, 4-aminobiphenyl (ABP). The metabolism of this compound has been studied extensively over the years by many investigators and recently the cytochrome P-450 isoform responsible for *N*-oxidation in human microsomes has been identified (*2, 3*). Figure 3 gives the Phase I and Phase II enzymes related to major routes of metabolic disposition. The pathway to DNA adduct formation occurs *via* the arylhydroxylamine (ArNHOH). The pathway to Hb adduct formation requires oxidation of the hydroxylamine in the erythrocyte to the arylnitroso compound which then reacts with a sulfhydryl group in Hb (cysteine beta-93) to yield the biologically stable cysteine sulfinamide adduct. This adduct has been fully characterized for structure (*4*), dose-response (*5*), and stability in animals (*5*) and humans (*6*). For analysis of Hb adducts of arylamines a small blood sample is withdrawn, erythrocytes collected, Hb isolated, and the aromatic amines released by acid or basic hydrolysis. The released amines are derivatized for gas chromatography-mass spectroscopy (GC-MS) and analyzed (*7*). Using this approach we have demonstrated the presence of more than 10 different aromatic amines in human blood samples and shown that monocyclic and bicyclic compounds exist as 2 separate classes with regard to exposure and/or metabolism (*8*) (Table 1).

A major purpose of our research in this area has been to test the hypothesis that

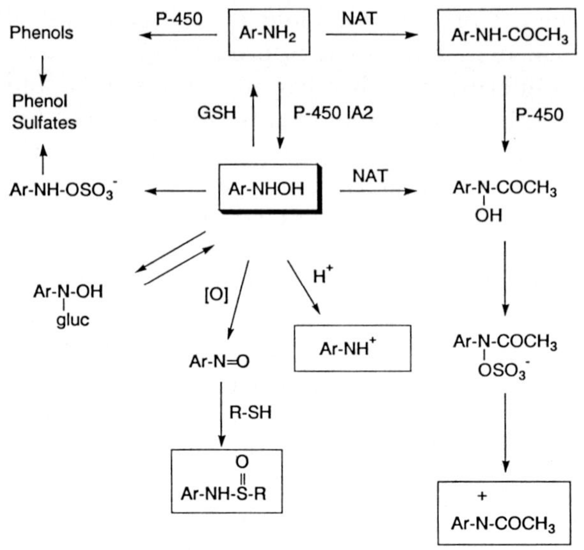


FIG. 3. Scheme for metabolism of aromatic amines. Ar, aryl; P-450, cytochrome P-450; NAT, *N*-acetyltransferase; GSH, glutathione.

TABLE 1. Pearson Correlation Coefficients between Aromatic Amines

| Amine | Correlation coefficient | |
|---|---|---|
| | 4-ABP | *o*-Toluidine |
| 4-Aminobiphenyl | 1 | 0.18 |
| 3-Aminobiphenyl | 0.45* | 0.14 |
| 2-Napthylamine | 0.29* | 0.20 |
| *p*-Toluidine | 0.05 | 0.34* |
| 3-Ethylaniline | 0.03 | 0.43* |
| 2,4-Dimethylaniline | −0.06 | 0.72* |

* statistically significant, data summarized from ref. *8*.

aromatic amines in cigarette smoke, and especially ABP, are related to risk of bladder cancer. Combining the results of several studies, the observed relationship between self-reported number of cigarettes smoked per day (CPD) and ABP adduct level is shown in Fig. 4 (*9, 10*). When all of the data are combined a striking pattern emerges. A sharp increase in adduct levels occurs in individuals smoking 1–10 CPD relative to nonsmokers. Another considerable increase is observed among those smoking 11–19 CPD. Beyond that level of cigarette consumption there is no further significant increase in adduct levels. This pattern is in contrast to that observed for ethylene/ethylene oxide, and is open to various interpretations.

The simplest explanation is that smoking patterns change as the number of cigarettes consumed increases so that actual intake of ABP remains relatively constant beyond a certain point. This is not unreasonable, but it is not supported by measurements of plasma cotinine, which appears to increase steadily with increasing cigarette consumption. It is also not supported by measurements of ethylene oxide adducts.

An alternative explanation is that changes in metabolic profiles occur as the result

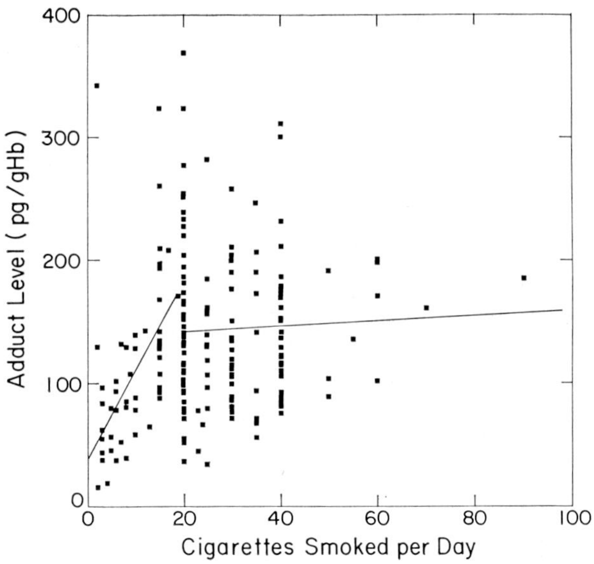


FIG. 4. ABP-Hb adducts in smokers. The data were grouped into two sets (1–19 CPD and 20–90 CPD) for linear regression analysis.

TABLE 2. Hemoglobin-4-aminobiphenyl Levels by Type of Tobacco and Acetylator Phenotype

| Smoking status | Acetylator phenotype | | Ratio S/F |
|---|---|---|---|
| | Slow | Fast | |
| Non-smoking | 32 | 20 | 1.6 |
| Blond tobacco | 112 | 86 | 1.3 |
| Black tobacco | 175 | 118 | 1.5 |

(From ref. *13*)

of heavy cigarette consumption. That such changes do occur is quite clear (*11*), but how these would influence the overall disposition of ABP is not yet known. What would be required would be a reduction in the relative yield of *N*-hydroxylamine available for reaction with Hb. There are many ways to achieve this outcome, and at present it is only possible to speculate as to which are likely. Some possible candidates for experimental investigation are diagrammed in Fig. 3. Up to this point I have considered only *N*-oxidation and ignored all of the pathways that would compete with Hb adduct formation. I would now like to examine some other metabolic routes that might be induced or otherwise differentially expressed in the general population.

An important enzymatic reaction is that of *N*-acetyltransferase, which has been dealt with earlier in this Symposium. Acetylation of the ABP would reduce hydroxylamine formation and potentially lead to other types of protein and DNA adducts (*12*). We have examined the influence of acetylator phenotype on adduct level and the results are shown in Table 2 (*13*). As predicted, there is a clear increase in Hb adducts in the slow phenotype relative to the fast phenotype, and this difference even shows up in nonsmokers. Although this difference is significant with regard to the overall population it does not, however, account for much of the variance in Fig. 3.

TABLE 3. Hemoglobin Adducts of 4-Aminobiphenyl and Relative Risk for Bladder Cancer

| | Relative adduct level | R. R. |
|---|---|---|
| Nonsmokers | 1.0 | 1.0 |
| Blond tobacco | 3.8 | 1.7 |
| Black tobacco | 5.5 | 7.1 |

Other competing reactions in Fig. 3 include the *N*-oxidative phenotype, levels of reduced glutathione in hepatocytes and erythrocytes, enzymatic glucuronidation, and sulfotransferases. Each of these is known to vary in the population as a result of genetic background and/or lifestyle factors. We cannot predict the net effect of all these variables but we are currently continuing to explore the effect of these metabolic phenotypes on Hb ABP adduct levels.

In time we hope to have a better understanding of the overall effect of metabolism on risk of bladder cancer, but we already have demonstrated that Hb ABP adducts are proportional to the risk of bladder cancer (*10*). Table 3 shows the results of a population-based study of 3 groups at different levels of risk in Torino, Italy. The implication of these results when taken with those in Fig. 4 is that the internal dose of hydroxylamine to the erythrocyte is in fact a predictor of the biologically effective dose. Preliminary evidence in fact suggests that in smokers, bladder ABP DNA adducts are correlated with Hb ABP adducts (F. Kadlubar, personal communication). Thus, although we may not currently understand all of the variables determining the internal dose, for this compound the internal dose is a predictor of risk.

### *PAH*

This group of compounds is perhaps the oldest in terms of recognition as human carcinogens (soots, tars) and in terms of experimental carcinogenesis. Their metabolism has been studied for many years and is reasonably well understood for the alternate class of PAH (*14*). Information on human metabolism is, however, quite limited, and this in turn limits our ability to determine the internal dose of a variety of PAH components. The molecular epidemiology for this group is further complicated by the fact that people are exposed to different sources with varying composition, but selected compounds appear in almost all sources. That is, compounds like benzo[a]-pyrene (BaP), chrysene (Ch), fluoranthene, benz[a]anthracene, *etc.* appear in almost all sources, ranging from diesel exhaust to charcoal-broiled steaks. In addition, the pharmacokinetics are complicated by the fact that the route of entry may be on particulate matter (soot) into the lungs or dissolved in fat (broiled food) into the gastrointestinal (GI) tract. Therefore, the internal dose to the blood compartment may not be equally representative for external doses of the same compound taken up *via* different routes of entry.

The major routes of metabolism to the most genotoxic metabolic forms occur through cytochrome P-450 enzyme working in concert with epoxide hydrolases (EHs). The most potent ultimate carcinogenic and mutagenic species are bay region dihydrodiol epoxides, however, other electrophilic reactants exist and may be important. A highly oversimplified diagram of some competing reactions for BaP is shown in Fig. 5.

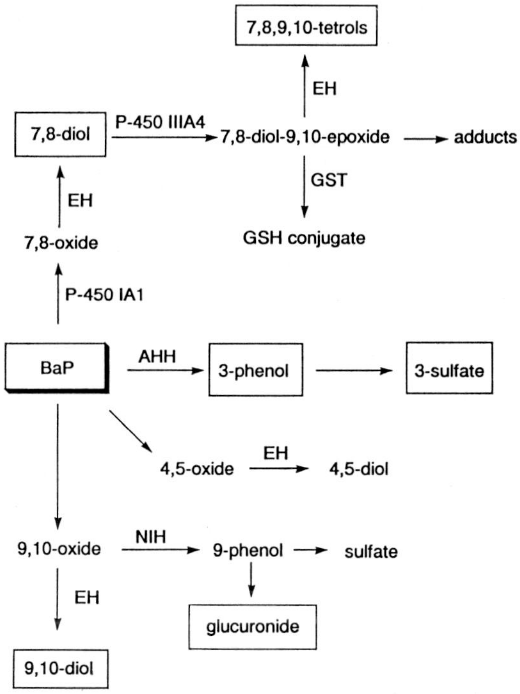


FIG. 5. Scheme for metabolism of BaP. EH, epoxide hydrolase; GST, glutathione-S-transferase; AHH, aryl hydrocarbon hydroxylase; NIH, NIH shift.

We have concentrated on the 7, 8-diol-9,10-epoxide (BPDE) as the ultimate carcinogen and determined the nature of its reactions and covalent adduct formation in human hemoglobin. These studies disclosed that the predominant biologically stable adduct is an ester at the C-10 position of BPDE linked to the aspartate alpha-47 carboxylate (*15*). Further studies disclosed that a wide array of epoxides and diolepoxides would form esters at this site. Therefore, the selective release of these esters would yield diols and tetrols which originated from the parent PAH and were metabolized *via* the P-450-EH pathway. Competing reactions (Fig. 5) such as oxidation at non-bay positions, conjugation with glutathione, *etc.* would represent potential metabolic polymorphisms that could alter the relationship between external dose and internal dose.

A method to analyze the tetrols released from labile esters of hemoglobin has been developed and applied to human samples. This method is outlined in Fig. 6 and is based on the following principles: the ester formed between the epoxide and the aspartate side-chain is a benzylic ester and is labile under neutral aqueous conditions. This is in contrast to most esters which require either acid- or base-catalyzed hydrolysis. We have demonstrated the lability of the PAH epoxide esters and their incorporation of $^{18}O$ from $H_2{}^{18}O$ during hydrolysis (*16, 17*). Therefore, we surmise that the hydrocarbon and its ester bond are buried in a hydrophobic region of the protein which stabilizes the structure. Anything which tends to destabilize the structure, such as enzymatic digestion of the protein leads to release of the tetrol. Therefore, we have chosen proteolytic digestion as the first step because it releases only benzylic alcohols.

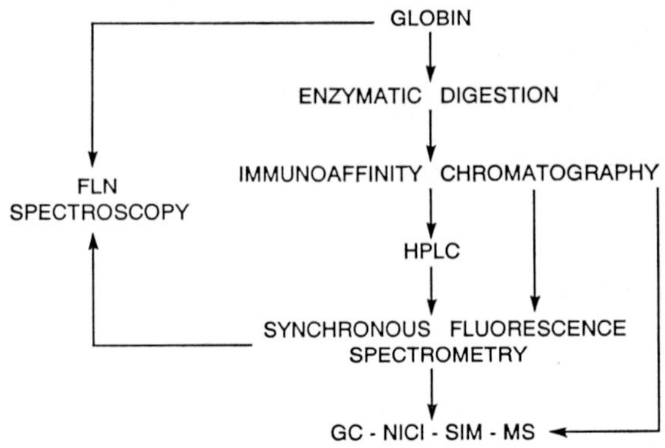


FIG. 6. Scheme for analysis of PAH tetrols from Hb. See text for explanation of terms.

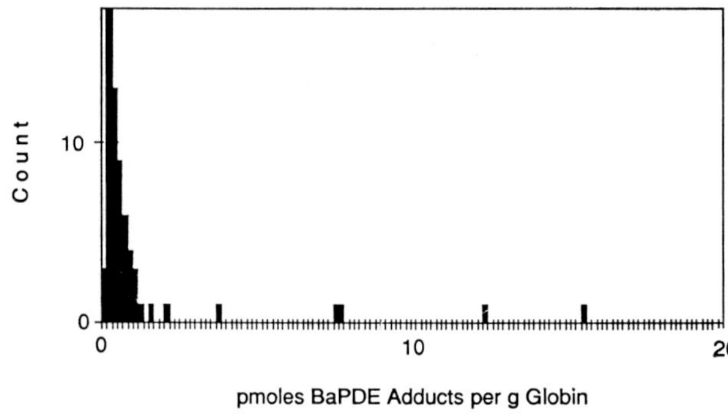


FIG. 7. Distribution of BaP tetrol released from ester adducts and analyzed by GC-MS from the blood of 63 adult donors.

Although ester release is fairly selective it results in a dilute solution of a very complex mixture of compounds including amino acids, peptides, and assorted adducts. The concentration of BaP tetrol is on the order of $10^{-12}$ moles/g globin so an extensive amount of concentration and purification is essential prior to analysis. A major step in this direction is effected through immunoaffinity chromatography (IAC) using monoclonal antibodies designed to recognize specific PAH tetrol epitopes. One such antibody was available to us from R. Santella at Columbia University and others have been constructed in our own laboratory. Immobilization of the antibody on Sepharose gives material for minicolumns which effect a one-step method for purification prior to GC-MS (*17*). For GC-MS we have successfully employed the tetra-trimethylsilyl esters for detection at the femtomole ($10^{-15}$) level (*18*).

An alternative and complementary method has been conventional and laser-induced fluorescence. The specific power of fluorescence has been its ability to identify the aromatic ring structure of the intact adduct or of the tetrol. Fluorescence has been used following IAC or following fractions collected by HPLC as a means of estimating BaP tetrol levels (*17*). A most powerful technique has been Fluorescence Line Narrowing (FLN) Spectroscopy which is capable of distinguishing even the nature of the heteroatom bound at the C-10 position of BaP triol (*19*). The explanation and application of this new approach is beyond the scope of this paper (please see ref. *19*).

Using these approaches we have begun epidemiological studies. The results on a combined group of smokers and nonsmokers is shown in Fig. 7. Although we cannot yet interpret these results we find the presence of outliers extremely interesting and suggestive of the possible importance of metabolic polymorphisms in determining internal dose.

In addition, we have also begun to systematically examine our IAC fraction for tetrols other than from BaP. We have already discovered significant amounts of Ch (*20*), 5-methylchrysene and 6-methylchrysene. On the other hand, we have failed to find any evidence of tetrols from benz[a]anthracene even though this would be expected based on external exposure measurements. Experiments with human liver microsomes (from F. Guengerich) suggest that benz[a]anthracene does not yield tetrols even after extensive metabolism, so this might be the explanation.

*Conclusion*

I have summarized here our work on 2 classes of protein adducts. We are also working on several other types of compounds, including heterocyclic amines and urethane, and we are collaborating with laboratories working on ethylene/ethylene oxide and tobacco specific nitrosamines. I hope that from these studies there will emerge a more definitive answer to my question 1: what is the delivered dose or, better, the internal dose of environmentally important compounds to various individuals in the general population?

*Acknowledgment*

S. R. Tannenbaum's research is supported by grants from the USPHS/NIH.

REFERENCES

1. Skipper, P. L. and Tannenbaum, S. R. Protein adducts in the molecular dosimetry of chemical carcinogens. Carcinogenesis, *11*: 507–518, 1990.
2. Butler, M. A., Guengerich, F. P., and Kadlubar, F. F. Metabolic oxidation of the carcinogens 4-aminobiphenyl and 4,4′-methylene-*bis*-(2-chloroaniline) by human hepatic microsomes and by purified rat hepatic cytochrome P-450 monooxygenases. Cancer Res., *49*: 25–31, 1989.
3. Butler, M. A., Iwasaki, M., Guengerich, F. P., and Kadlubar, F. F. Human cytochrome P-$450_{PA}$ (P-450IA2), the phenacetin *O*-deethylase, is primarily responsible for the hepatic 3-demethylation of caffeine and *N*-oxidation of carcinogenic arylamines. Proc. Natl. Acad. Sci., U.S.A., *86*: 7696–7700, 1989.
4. Ringe, D., Turesky, R. J., Skipper, P. L., and Tannenbaum, S. R. Structure of the single stable hemoglobin adduct formed by 4-aminobiphenyl *in vivo*. Chem. Res. Toxicol., *1*: 22–24, 1988.
5. Green, L. C., Skipper, P. L., Turesky, R. J., Bryant, M. S., and Tannenbaum, S. R. *In vivo* dosimetry of 4-aminobiphenyl in rats *via* a cysteine adduct in hemoglobin. Cancer Res., *44*: 4254–4259, 1984.
6. Maclure, K. M., Bryant, M. S., Skipper, P. L., and Tannenbaum, S. R. Decline of the hemoglobin adduct of 4-aminobiphenyl during withdrawal from smoking. Cancer Res., *50*: 181–184, 1990.
7. Stillwell, W. G., Bryant, M. S., and Wishnok, J. S. GC/MS analysis of biologically

important aromatic amines. Biomed. Environ. Mass Spectrom., *14*: 221–227, 1987.

8. Ronco, G., Vineis, P., Bryant, M. S., Skipper, P. L., and Tannenbaum, S. R. Haemoglobin adducts formed by aromatic amines in smokers: sources of inter-individual variability. Br. J. Cancer, *61*: 534–537, 1990.
9. Bryant, M. S., Skipper, P. L., Tannenbaum, S. R., and Maclure, M. Hemoglobin adducts of 4-aminobiphenyl in smokers and non-smokers. Cancer Res., *47*: 602–608, 1987.
10. Bryant, M. S., Vineis, P., Skipper, P. L., and Tannenbaum, P. L. Hemoglobin adducts of aromatic amines: associations with smoking status and type of tobacco. Proc. Natl. Acad. Sci. U.S.A., *85*: 9788–9791, 1988.
11. Conney, A. H. Induction of microsomal enzymes by foreign chemicals and carcinogenesis by polycyclic aromatic hydrocarbons: G. H. A. Clowes Memorial Lecture. Cancer Res., *42*: 4875–4917, 1982.
12. Skipper, P. L., Obiedzinski, M. W., Tannenbaum, S. R., Miller, D. W., Mitchum, R. K., and Kadlubar, F. F. Identification of the major serum albumin adduct formed by 4-aminobiphenyl *in vivo* in rats. Cancer Res., *45*: 5122–5127, 1985.
13. Vineis, P., Caporaso, N., Tannenbaum, S. R., Skipper, P., Glogowski, J., Bartsch, H., Coda, M., Talasaka, G., and Kadlubar, F. The acetylation phenotype, carcinogen-hemoglobin adducts, and cigarette smoking. Cancer Res., *50*: 3002–3004, 1990.
14. Dipple, A., Moschel, R. C., and Bigger, A. H. Polycyclic aromatic carcinogens. *In;* C. E. Searle (ed.), Chemical Carcinogens, ACS Monograph 182, pp. 41–126, American Chemical Society, Washington, D. C., 1984.
15. Skipper, P. L., Naylor, S., Gan, L-S., Day, B. W., Pastorelli, R., and Tannenbaum, S. R. Origin of the tetrahydrotetrols derived from human hemoglobin adducts of benzo[a]pyrene. Chem. Res. Toxicol., *2*: 280–281, 1989.
16. Naylor, S., Gan, L-S., Day, B. W., Pastorelli, R., Skipper, P. L., and Tannenbaum, S. R. Benzo[a]pyrene diol epoxide adduct formation in the mouse and human-hemoglobin: physicochemical basis for dosimetry. Chem. Res., Toxicol., *3*: 111–117, 1990.
17. Day, B. W., Naylor, S., Gan, L.-S., Sahali, Y., Nguyen, T. T., Skipper, P. L., Wishnok, J. S., and Tannenbaum, S. R. Molecular dosimetry of polycyclic aromatic hydrocarbon epoxides and diol epoxides *via* hemoglobin adducts. Cancer Res., *50*: 4611–4618, 1990.
18. Day, B. W., Naylor, S., Gan, L.-S., Sahali, Y., Nguyen, T. T., Skipper, P. L., Wishnok, J. S., and Tannenbaum, S. R. GC/MS analysis of diols and tetrols from reactions of polycyclic aromatic hydrocarbon epoxides with hemoglobin. J. Chromatogr. Biomed. Appl., *562*: 563–571, 1990.
19. Jankowiak, R., Day, B. W., Lu, P.-Q., Doxtader, M. M., Skipper, P. L., Tannenbaum, S. R., and Small, G. J. Fluorescence line-narrowing spectral analysis of *in vitro* human hemoglobin-benzo(a)pyrene adducts: comparison to synthetic analogues. J. Am. Chem. Soc., *112*: 5866–5869, 1990.
20. Day, B. W., Skipper, P. L., Wishnok, J. S., Coghlin, J., Hammond, S. K., Gann, P., and Tannenbaum, S. R. Identification of an *in vivo* chrysene diol epoxide adduct in human hemoglobin. Chem. Res. Toxicol., *3*: 340–343, 1990.

# Author Index

# Subject Index